Handbook of
Experimental Pharmacology

Continuation of Handbuch der experimentellen Pharmakologie

Vol. 51

Uric Acid

Contributors

W.J. Arnold · M.A. Becker · J.M. Brogard · F.L. Coe
W.H. Dantzler · H.S. Diamond · G.B. Elion
B.T. Emmerson · N.H. Ertel · I.H. Fox · J.F. Henderson
G.H. Hitchings · E.W. Holmes · W.A. Katz · G. Peters
F. Roch-Ramel · H.R. Schumacher · P.A. Simkin
L.B. Sorensen · J. Spilberg · A. Stahl · J. Stahl · T.H. Steele
J.H. Talbott · M. Tatibana · S.C. Wallace · Ts'Ai-Fan Yü

Editors

William N. Kelley
Irwin M. Weiner

With 114 Figures

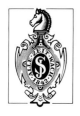

Springer-Verlag Berlin Heidelberg New York 1978

WILLIAM N. KELLEY, MD, Professor and Chairman
Department of Internal Medicine,
University of Michigan, Medical School, Ann Arbor, MI 48109, USA

IRWIN M. WEINER, MD, Professor and Chairman
Department of Pathology, Upstate Medical Center, Syracuse, NY 13210, USA

ISBN 3-540-08611-0 Springer-Verlag Berlin Heidelberg New York
ISBN 0-387-08611-0 Springer-Verlag New York Heidelberg Berlin

Library of Congress Cataloging in Publication Data. Main entry under title: Uric acid. (Handbook of Experimental Pharmacology; v. 51) Includes bibliographies and indexes. 1. Gout. 2. Uric acid metabolism. I. Arnold, William James, 1928—. II. Kelley, William N. III. Weiner, Irwin M., 1930—. QP905.H3 vol. 51 [RC629] 615'.1'08s [616'.6] 77-28641

Typesetting, printing, and bookbinding: Brühlsche Universitätsdruckerei, Lahn-Gießen.

2122/3130-543210

Preface

Uric acid has attracted the attention of scientists from a broad spectrum of disciplines, and in recent years dramatic progress has occurred within many of these disciplines. This volume is designed to fill void in the field. Major works in the past five years have provided comprehensive reviews of disorders of uric acid metabolism for the clinical (1–3) as well as short reports of recent progress for the interested scholar (4, 5). In *Uric Acid* the reader will find extensive reviews of relevant topics selected largely by virtue of recent progress in the field and written by those who, to a considerable extent, are responsible for that progress.

Seven chapters are dedicated to a description of uric acid synthesis, its control, diseases resulting from aberrations in the pathway, and effects of intermediates and end products of this pathway on other metabolic processes. The next five chapters describe our current understanding of the mechanisms by which uric acid is eliminated by the organism. Then seven chapters review the factors responsible for the human "disease" produced by uric acid in the joints and kidneys. The final four chapters provide a summary of therapeutic approaches to control gout, the most important disease caused *per se* by uric acid.

This book is not designed to be totally comprehensive. Potentially relevant areas which are not covered extensively include epidemiology, genetics, hypouricemia, and management of asymptomatic hyperuricemia. On the other hand, some repetition has been allowed where this was important for emphasis or continuity. This style should enhance the overall value of the volume.

WILLIAM N. KELLEY
I. M. WEINER

Table of Contents

Biochemistry and Physiology of Uric Acid: Production

CHAPTER 1

Uric Acid: Chemistry and Synthesis. G. H. HITCHINGS. With 10 Figures

CHAPTER 2

Regulation of Biosynthesis De Novo. E. W. HOLMES, JR. With 7 Figures

CHAPTER 3

Purine Salvage Enzymes. W. J. Arnold

CHAPTER 4

Purine Nucleotide Interconversions. J. F. Henderson. With 1 Figure

CHAPTER 5

Degradation of Purine Nucleotides. I. H. Fox. With 7 Figures

CHAPTER 6

Interrelationship of Purine and Pyrimidine Metabolism. M. Tatibana. With 3 Figures

CHAPTER 7

Abnormalities of PRPP Metabolism Leading to an Overproduction of Uric Acid.
M. A. BECKER. With 3 Figures

Biochemistry and Physiology of Uric Acid: Renal Disposal

CHAPTER 8

Urate Excretion in Nonmammalian Vertebrates. W. H. DANTZLER. With 2 Figures

CHAPTER 9

Urinary Excretion of Uric Acid in Nonhuman Mammalian Species.
F. ROCH-RAMEL and G. PETERS

CHAPTER 10

Urate Excretion in Man, Normal and Gouty. T. H. STEELE. With 12 Figures

CHAPTER 11

Abnormal Urate Excretion Associated with Renal and Systematic Disorders, Drugs, and Toxins. B. T. EMMERSON

Biochemistry and Physiology of Uric Acid: Extrarenal Disposal

CHAPTER 12

Extrarenal Disposal of Uric Acid. L. B. SORENSEN. With 1 Figure

Pathology of Uric Acid: Acute Gouty Arthritis

CHAPTER 13

Initial Events in the Development of an Acute Attack of Gouty Arthritis.
H. R. SCHUMACHER. With 5 Figures

CHAPTER 14

Role of Proteoglycans in the Development of Gouty Arthritis. W. A. KATZ.
With 7 Figures

CHAPTER 15

Role of the Leukocyte and Chemical Mediators of the Acute Gouty Attack.
I. SPILBERG. With 1 Figure

CHAPTER 16

Role of Local Factors in the Precipitation of Urate Crystals. P. A. SIMKIN.
With 10 Figures

Pathology of Uric Acid: Nephrolithiasis and Urate Nephropathy

CHAPTER 17

Uric Acid Nephrolithiasis. T.-F. YÜ. With 6 Figures

CHAPTER 18

Association of Calcium Nephrolithiasis with Disorders of Uric Acid Metabolism.
F. L. COE. With 11 Figures

CHAPTER 19

Pathology of Urate Nephropathy. J. H. TALBOTT. With 8 Figures

Pharmacology of Uric Acid

CHAPTER 20

Uricosuric Drugs. H. S. DIAMOND. With 6 Figures

CHAPTER 21

Allopurinol and Other Inhibitors of Urate Synthesis. G. B. ELION. With 3 Figures

CHAPTER 22

Enzymatic Uricolysis and Its Use in Therapy. J. M. Brogard, A. Stahl and J. Stahl.
With 5 Figures

CHAPTER 23

Pharmacology of Drugs Used in Treatment of Acute Gout. S. L. WALLACE and
N. H. ERTEL. With 6 Figures

List of Contributors

W. J. ARNOLD, MD, Director, Section of Rheumatology, Lutheran General Hospital, 1775 W. Dempster, Park Ridge, IL 60068, USA

M. A. BECKER, MD, Associate Professor of Medicine, Veterans Administration Hospital, 3350 La Jolla Village Drive, San Diego, CA 92161, USA

J. M. BROGARD, Professeur Agr., Département de Médicine Interne de la Clinique Médicale B 10—20, 1, Place de l'Hôpital, F-67005 Strasbourg Cedex

F. L. COE, MD, Director, Renal Division, Michael Reese Hospital, 29th Street and Ellis Avenue, Chicago, IL 60616, USA

W. H. DANTZLER, MD, PhD., Professor of Physiology, Department of Physiology, College of Medicine, Arizona Health Sciences Center, University of Arizona, Tucson, AZ 85724, USA

H. DIAMOND, MD, State University of New York, Downstate Medical Center, 450 Clarkson Avenue, Brooklyn, NY 11203, USA

G. B. ELION, DSc, The Wellcome Research Laboratories, Burroughs Wellcome Co., 3030 Cornwallis Road, Research Triangle Park, NC 27709, USA

B. T. EMMERSON, MD, Professor of Medicine, University of Queensland, Department of Medicine, Princess Alexandra Hospital, Ipswich Road, Woolloongabba Q 4102, Australia

N. H. ERTEL, MD, Professor of Medicine, Chief, Medical Service, Veteran's, Administration Hospital, East Orange, NJ 07103, USA

I. H. FOX, MD, Clinical Research Center, University of Michigan Hospital, W-4642 Main Hospital, Ann Arbor, MI 48109, USA

J. F. HENDERSON, PhD., Professor, The University of Alberta, Cancer Research Unit, McEachern Laboratory, Edmonton, Alberta, Canada T6G 2H7

G. H. HITCHINGS, MD, The Wellcome Research Laboratories, Burroughs Wellcome Co., 3030 Cornwallis Road, Research Triangle Park, NC 27709, USA

E. W. HOLMES, Jr., MD, Associate Professor of Medicine, Assistant Professor of Biochemistry, Division of Rheumatic and Genetic Diseases, Duke University Medical Center, Durham, NC 27710, USA

W. A. KATZ, MD, Chief, Division of Rheumatology, Department of Medicine, Medical College of Pennsylvania, 3300 Henry Avenue, Philadelphia, PA 19129, USA

G. PETERS, MD, Professor and Chairman, Institut de Pharmacologie d l'Université de Lausanne, Rue du Bugnon 21, CH-1011 Lausanne

F. ROCH-RAMEL, PhD, Associate Professor, Institut de Pharmacologie de l'Université de Lausanne, Rue du Bugnon 21, CH-1011 Lausanne

H. R. SCHUMACHER, MD, Veterans Administration Hospital, University & Woodland Avenues, Philadelphia, PA 19104

P. A. SIMKIN, MD, Associate Professor of Medicine, University of Washington, Department of Medicine, RG-20, Seattle, WA 98195, USA

L. B. SORENSEN, MD, PhD., Professor and Associate Chairman, Department of Medicine, Box 143, University of Chicago, 950 East 59th St., Chicago, IL 60637, USA

I. SPILBERG, MD, Washington University, School of Medicine, Box 8045, 660 So. Euclid Avenue, St. Louis, MO 63110, USA

A. STAHL, MD, Département de Médecine Interne de la Clinique Médicale B 10—20, 1, Place de l'Hôpital, F-67005 Strasbourg Cedex

J. STAHL, MD, Département de Médecine Interne de la Clinique Médicale B 10—20, 1, Place de l'Hôpital, F-67005 Strasbourg Cedex

T. H. STEELE, MD, The University of Wisconsin, Department of Medicine, 1300 University Avenue, Madison, WI 53706, USA

J. H. TALBOTT, AB, MD, DSc (Hon.), Professor of Medicine, University of Miami, School of Medicine Arthritis Division, P.O. Box 520875, Miami, FL 33152, USA

M. TATIBANA, MD, PhD, Professor and Chairman, IInd Department of Biochemistry, Chiba University School of Medicine, Inohana, Chiba 280, Japan

S. L. WALLACE, MD, Professor of Medicine. The Jewish Hospital and Medical Center of Brooklyn, 555 Prospect Place, Brooklyn, NY 11238, USA

T. F. YÜ, MD, Research Professor of Medicine, Mount Sinai School of Medicine Fifth Avenue and 100th St., New York N.Y. 10029, USA

CHAPTER 1

Uric Acid: Chemistry and Synthesis

G. H. HITCHINGS

A. Introduction

The year 1976 marked the bicentennial of an event of major importance, the isolation in pure form and characterization of uric acid (SCHEELE, 1776). It was this event that later was commemorated (FISCHER, 1899) in the generic name, "purine" (from *purum uricum*) for the heterocyclic system, which under modern systematic nomenclature would be called 7(9)-H-imidazo(4,5-*d*)pyrimidine. Other members of the system were sporadically recognized, xanthine in 1838 (WÖHLER and LIEBIG), guanine in 1846 (UNGER), and hypoxanthine in 1850 (SCHERER). It is a reflection of the ubiquitous distribution of deaminases that adenine was found only after relatively fresh tissue had been subjected to acid hydrolysis (KOSSEL, 1886, 1888).

The discovery of xanthine is of particular interest. It was announced in a note (WÖHLER and LIEBIG, 1838b) which followed a major paper (WÖHLER and LIEBIG, 1838b) on degradation products of uric acid—work which laid the basis for the subsequent elucidation of the structure of uric acid. By a round-about way WÖHLER and LIEBIG obtained the "larger half" of urinary concretion that had been removed by MARCET (1817). They carefully compared the substance with uric acid and concluded that it was a close relative with one less oxygen atom. They further speculated that their substance was a normal minor constituent of urine that had under some unusual circumstance given rise to the calculus. Thus was recognition of xanthinuria foreshadowed!

Uric acid for many years was considered by many to be a key metabolite, an intermediate product of protein metabolism. The relationship between xanthine and uric acid had been perceived by WÖHLER and LIEBIG, but as other members of the series accumulated, their interrelationships were speculative. It remained for two major contributions to bring order to the field. The first was the isolation of nucleic acid by MIESCHER (1874). In particular, *lachsmilch*, the spermatic fluid of Rhine salmon, gave him a starting material from which he isolated a "nuclein" which was separable into protamine and protein-free nucleic acid. Two milestones! MIESCHER himself, on the basis of a color reaction with nitric acid, suspected the presence of purine bases. PICCARD (1874), to whom he transferred this problem, made some sound observations, but his interpretations were confused. KOSSEL brought clarity to the problem 5 years later. From nucleic acid he isolated guanine (1883–1884) and adenine (1886) and cleared up the confusion between hypoxanthine and adenine which had prevailed because of similarities in chemical properties. His work strongly suggested a connection between his "alloxuric bases" and uric acid. It also established the presence of phosphoric acid as a constituent of nucleic acids and clarified the distinction (stoutly resisted by some) between nucleic acids and phosphoprotein complexes.

The early literature on the origins of uric acid is a mélange of reasonably good observations and questionable techniques combined with faulty hypotheses and interpretations. For example, HORBACZEWSKI (1889) is usually credited with the demonstration that uric acid arises from nucleic acid. His source of nucleic acid was calf spleen pulp, and the technique involved putrefaction, aeration, and the addition of arterial blood. He did show that uric acid resulted and that the omission of the aeration resulted in xanthine and hypoxanthine instead. He also left a bequest of wrangles about hydrolytic and oxidative enzymes that are still not fully resolved. He showed also that the ingestion of nucleic acid leads to increased uric acid excretion but attributed it to an alimentary leukocytosis (HORBACZEWSKI, 1891). This interpretation was prompted by his previous true observation that patients with leukemia excrete excessive amounts of uric acid, i.e., leukocytes are the sole source. One should not disparge HORBACZEWSKI; his numerous contributions were the starting point for many others.

One more historical note may be permissible. Inosinic acid (a mistranslation of inosinsäure which correctly would be called "inosic acid") was isolated from meat extract in 1847 by LIEBIG (1847). LIEBIG, however, missed the phosphate in his analysis, and it remained for later workers to find it and to identify hypoxanthine as a component.

B. Structure

The exhaustive work of WÖHLER and LIEBIG (1838a) on the oxidation products of uric acid set the stage for subsequent structural studies. Perhaps the most important fragments identified were uramil (I), alloxan (II), and urea. The fragments were fit together in two different ways by FITTIG (III) and MEDICUS (IV) (Fig. 1), neither of whom had solid support for his speculation. Definitive proof was not supplied either

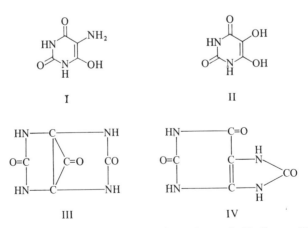

Fig. 1. Formulas for uric acid and degradation products. *I*, uramil; *II*, alloxan; *III*, Fittig formula for uric acid; *IV*, Medicus formula for uric acid

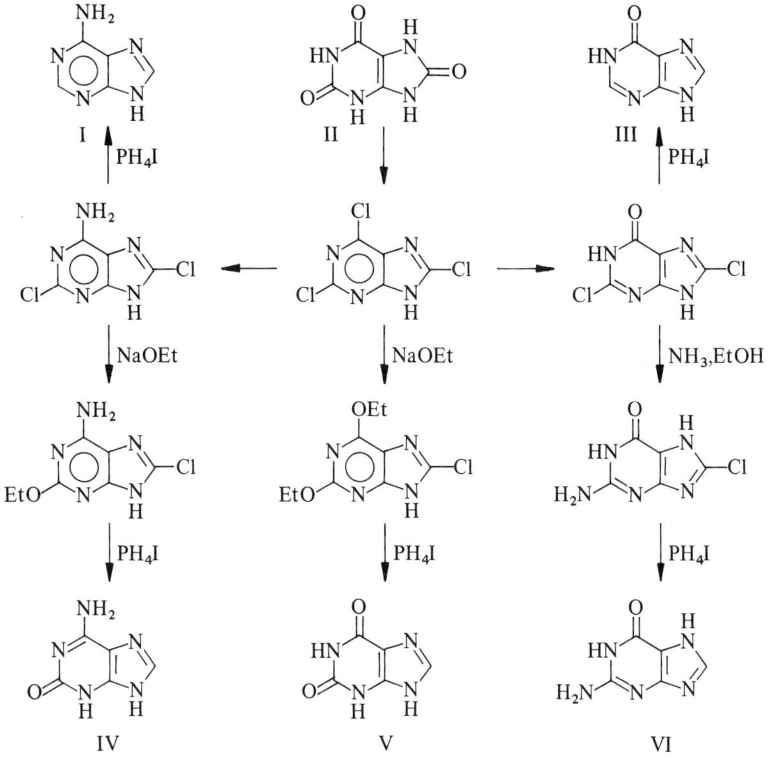

Fig. 2. Fischer's interconversions of purines. *I*, adenine; *II*, uric acid; *III*, hypoxanthine; *IV*, isoguanine; *V*, xanthine; *VI*, guanine

by two independent syntheses (HORBACZEWSKI, 1887; BEHREND and ROOSEN, 1889) of the substance. It remained for the genius of EMIL FISCHER and his school to provide not only a definitive synthesis (1895) but to wrap up the whole package of the purine derivatives then known and to add new members by means of transformation reactions, clearly demonstrating the interrelationships (Fig. 2). It is interesting that FISCHER named and used the correct structural formula (FISCHER, 1884) and added his numbering system (FISCHER, 1897) before he explained how he had arrived at the name (FISCHER, 1899) some 15 years after he had first used it.

One need add very few words to supplement the transformation scheme as set forth by FISCHER. One might add that in the course of the work the Fittig formula was laid to rest with finality by the synthesis of all of the 14 N-methyl derivatives permitted by the Medicus formula, whereas the Fittig formula, because of an element of symmetry, permitted only five.

C. Properties

Uric acid crystallizes in a variety of microscopic forms: plates, tablets, and rhombic pyramids. When heated it decomposes at about 400° C without melting. Combustion yields 0.46 cal/mole. In water at 37° C a saturated solution is 0.38 mM, corresponding to 6.45 mg/100 ml. Characteristically tenacious supersaturation occurs when impurities are present. Both the ammonium salt and the monosodium salt are somewhat more soluble in water than the free acid, but significant solubility only occurs at pH values which are entering the range of the second ionization constant ($pk_{a1} = 5.75$; $pk_{a2} = 10.3$). An early observation that the lithium salt was readily soluble gave rise to a chemically naive attempt to dissolve urate concretions by feeding lithium salts.

Among the chemical properties of uric acid two are of sufficient historic interest to be mentioned. One is the "murexide" test, which is applicable to all purines capable of oxidation to an alloxan derivative. The oxidative reagents, usually HNO_3, carry the oxidation further to purpuric acids. A yellow color is produced, which turns purple on the addition of ammonia.

One should also be aware that the yellow products obtained by GOWLAND HOPKINS when he autoclaved aqueous uric acid are, at least in part, pteridines. His observations provided a stimulus to pteridine chemistry, even though it took years to clarify the nature of the products and the reaction mechanisms (PFLEIDERER, 1959).

The chemical properties of the purine system are consistent with its formulation as a condensed imidazopyrimidine. The pyrimidine ring is π-electron deficient because of the electron-localizing effect of the two nitrogen atoms. The imidazole ring is π-electron excessive. Both properties are minimized through fusion of the two-ring systems, but the balance can be disturbed by the insertion of strong electron-donating or -withdrawing groups into either ring. For example, the 8-carbon atom in adenine and hypoxanthine can only be brominated; in xanthine it can be chlorinated, brominated, or nitrated.

Amino, oxo, and thiopurines can exist in tautomeric modifications, which unfortunately require separate nomenclature. One author (RINGERTZ, 1972) has estimated the double-bond character of 6-substituted purines as 35% for NH_2, 70% for O, and 95% for S. Strictly speaking, 6-mercaptopurine should be called "1,6-dihydro-6-thiopurine," and uric acid would become "1,2,3,6,7,8-hexahydro-2,6,8-trioxopurine." The questionable implication of the systematic nomenclature (besides the added work for the typesetter) is that hydro derivatives would ordinarily be nonaromatic. In fact, the substituted derivatives retain substantial aromatic character, not only because of tautomerism but also because multiple resonance forms exist. For practical reasons this review will attempt to use the simplest unambiguious name (often a trivial name), while disclaiming any implications towards fine details of structure.

D. Synthesis

A brief description of the chemical struggles with uric acid and related substances will provide a background to the biochemical developments which came later. Much of the early chemistry, since it was focused primarily on the synthesis of purines from pyrimidines, is irrelevant to the biosynthetic pathway revealed by the work of BUCHANAN, GREENBERG, and many others (v.i. Biosynthesis of Purines). Nevertheless the flowering of purine chemistry around the turn of the 20th century provided a wealth of new purines and an understanding of their chemical properties. The renaissance

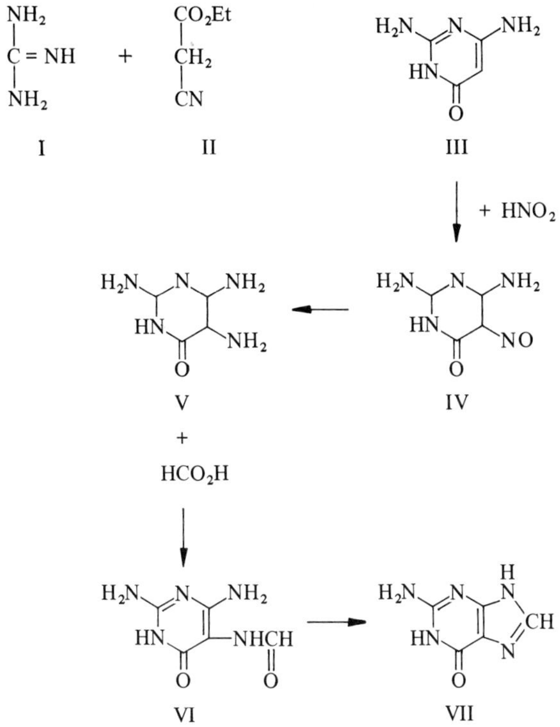

Fig. 3. Synthesis of purines from pyrimidines (Traube methods) illustrated by the synthesis of guanine. *I*, guanidine; *II*, ethylcyanoacetate; *III*, 2,4-diamino-6-oxopyrimidine; *IV*, 2,4-diamino-5-nitroso-6-oxopyrimidine; *V*, 6-oxo-2,4,5-triaminopyrimidine; *VI*, 2,4-diamino-5-formamido-pyrimidine; *VII*, guanine

that accompanied an intensifying interest in the nucleic acids drew heavily upon this background.

Perhaps it is sufficient simply to trace the history of the earliest truly definitive synthesis of uric acid and then to mention briefly the major approaches to purine synthesis that have been used.

WöHLER and LIEBIG (1838) recognized that two of the fragments they obtained from uric acid degradation, uramil (Fig. 1), and urea, needed only to be condensed, with subsequent abstraction of a molecule of water, to form uric acid. Their attempts to synthesize a ureidopyrimidine failed, and it was 25 years before BAEYER (1863) found that uramil gave a ureido derivative on reaction with KCNO in aqueous medium. BAEYER was unable to cyclize the derivatives, and another 36 years passed before this was accomplished by FISCHER and ACH (1895). By that time, the synthesis became only one of a number of mutually supporting lines of evidence that removed all lingering doubts about structure.

Although FISCHER had succeeded in the synthesis of uric acid from a pyrimidine derivative, the main attention of his school had been directed toward the transformation reactions, and his synthesis was neither very productive nor versatile. It re-

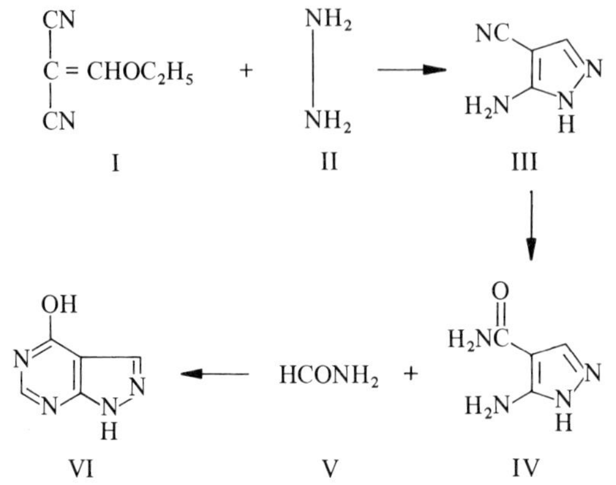

Fig. 4. Synthesis of allopurinol. *I*, ethoxymethylene malononitrile; *II*, hydrazine; *III*, 5-amino-4-cyanopyrazole; *IV*, 5-aminopyrazole-4-carboxamide; *V*, formamide; *VI*, 4-hydroxypyrazolo-[3,4-d]pyrimidine

mained then for TRAUBE to introduce his methods which met both of these objectives. Conceptually they all began with the formation of a pyrimidine ring bearing the desired functional groups or their precursors, and then forming the imidazole moiety. An example of these procedures is presented in Figure 3. They are capable of many modifications and elaborations and have been used in the synthesis of the majority of the purines that have been made (LISTER, 1971).

I. Synthesis from Imidazoles

Since the purine ring is an imidazopyrimidine, it was inevitable that the synthesis of purine from imidazoles as well as from pyrimidines would be undertaken. This subject has been reviewed by LISTER (1963). Synthetic routes from imidazoles were slow to develop. It is apparent that the limiting factor is and was the rate of development of imidazole chemistry. This becomes clear when one surveys the synthesis of purine analogs. Many of these are condensed pyrimidine systems where the precursors are the appropriate heterocycles upon which the pyrimidine ring is completed (e.g., TAYLER and McKILLOP, 1970). In fact, it is this type of reaction sequence which is followed in a synthesis of allopurinol (Fig. 4) (ROBINS, 1956).

A suitable imidazole intermediate, 4-amino-5-imidazolecarboxomide, was first synthesized in 1923 by WINDAUS and LANGENBECK, who noted that it probably could be converted to a purine. The following year the 1-methyl derivative was converted to 7-methylxanthine in poor yield (SARASIN and WEGMANN, 1924). Productive and versatile synthesis from imidazoles have not appeared, but SHAW (1950) succeeded in synthesizing adenine, hypoxanthine, and xanthine this way. Interest in this route was enhanced as it became apparent that the biosynthetic route involves the formation of imidazoles prior to the closure of the pyrimidine ring in the last step. It should be noted that substitution of the imidazole ring by ribose phosphate substantially alters its chemistry.

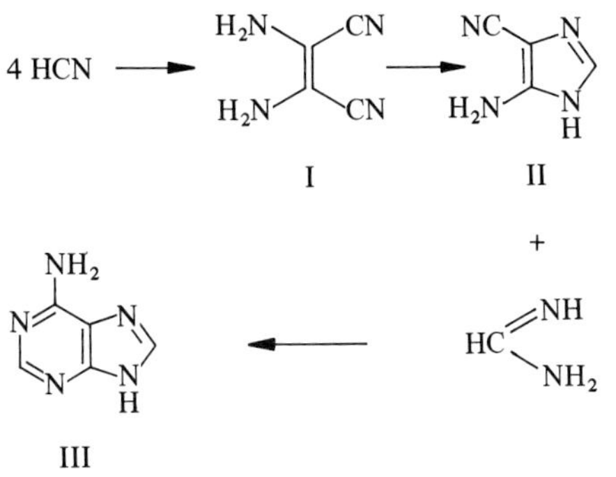

Fig. 5. Photochemical synthesis of adenine from hydrogen cyanide. *I*, diaminomaleonitrile; *II*, 4-amino-5-cyanoimidazole; *III*, adenine

II. One-Pot Synthesis

Several one-step syntheses of purines have been reported. Many of these had in mind natural conditions that could have produced purines in an abiotic or prebiotic world or were fishing for some lead as to the mechanisms of biosynthesis. HORBACZEWSKI (1882, 1885, 1887) seems to have had both in mind. By heating glycine he obtained a small yield of uric acid. Somewhat later he produced it by heating urea with trichlorolactamide. This correlated with the observations of MINKOWSKI (1886) that hepatectomized birds excreted ammonium lactate to replace much, but significantly not all, of the uric acid excreted by normal birds. This was perceived at the time as indicating that uric acid arises from two different sources in birds.

Purines have been found among the reaction products of formamide and other formate derivatives in a variety of reaction conditions. More sophisticated methods prepared putative intermediates first. Thus, hypoxanthine in good yield is formed in one step from aminomalonamideamidine and ethyl orthoformate (RICHTER and TAYLOR, 1955) or formamidomalonamideamidine and formamide (ALBERT, 1960).

Possibly of greater significance for prebiotic purine synthesis was the finding of adenine among the products formed when hydrogen cyanide reacts with ammonia (ORO and KIMBALL, 1962). This reaction has been studied intensively by ORGEL and co-workers (FERRIS and ORGEL, 1966a, 1966b), and a very plausible sequence of reactions has been worked out (Fig. 5). Adding to the plausibility is the observation that in the mass-spectrograph adenine gives all the ions corresponding to HCN and its polymers corresponding to 2,3, and 4 molecules as well as the pentamer, adenine (SHANNON and LETHAM, 1966).

As one surveys the myriad of condensations of simple molecules that has given rise to purines, he finds increasing credibility for prebiologic organic chemical evolution. A primitive atmosphere consisting of CH_4, NH_3, CO_2, HCN, H_2O, and H_2 in contact with pools of warm (not necessarily hot) water would surely have given rise to preformed purines as well as pyrimidines, proteins, lipids, etc.—building blocks of biologic systems.

One finds plausible, too, the concept that in the interim between prebiotic evolution and truly organized life, that biosynthetic sequences were developed in the direction product→precursor. Protobiosis would begin with end-products (e.g., adenine), and mechanisms for their utilization and trapping would evolve. The environment would then become depleted of these substances, and any advance toward the utilization of the precursor still available in the milieu would convey an enormous advantage. And so, stage by stage, the mechanisms for synthesis and eventual protorpy would evolve (HOROWITZ, 1945).

E. Biosynthesis of Purines

Until the advent of isotopic tracers, the only guides to biosynthetic pathways were analogies with organic chemical reactions. For purine biosynthesis, such analogies were far off the mark. An early plausible and widely accepted guess was that uric acid was formed by condensation of dialuric acid and urea (WIENER, 1902).

The first hint that other and simpler precursors were involved had come from KREBS and coworkers in the 1930's (EDSON et al., 1936; ÖRSTRÖM et al., 1939). They had shown that uric acid synthesis in fowls involved glutamine and a source of carbon (oxalacetate stimulated synthesis), and that hypoxanthine was formed in the pigeon by liver slices and converted to uric acid in the kidney by xanthine oxidase.

Isotopic nitrogen in the form of ammonium salts provided a tool that eliminated the putative roles of urea, arginine, and histidine in purine biosynthesis but suggested that purines and pyrimidines might be involved in the same metabolic processes (BARNES and SCHOENHEIMER, 1943). Again, ^{15}N provided a means to demonstrate that preformed adenine could be incorporated into nucleic acids, and that it could be transformed into polynucleotide guanine with retention of an intact purine ring (BROWN, 1954).

The mid-1940's witnessed the rapid unraveling of the main features of purine biosynthesis. By then, ^{14}C as well as ^{15}N had become available. Two independent but interacting approaches contributed. BUCHANAN and his coworkers set about to dissect the uric acid molecule in such a way that the individual atoms could be identified. Their origins could then be traced by feeding pigeons with isotopically labeled precursors. By 1946, the precursors had been identified except for those of the 1,3, and 9-N atoms (Fig. 6) (SONNE et al., 1946; BUCHANAN and SONNE, 1946; SONNE et al., 1948; SHEMIN and RITTENBERG, 1947). The findings encompassed a couple of surprises. It was unexpected that the carboxyl group of glycine would turn up fully aromatized in the 4-carbon atom. Moreover, a role for formate as an active metabolite had not been forecast.

Meanwhile, a cell-free system capable of carrying out hypoxanthine synthesis was developed from pigeon liver by GREENBERG (1948). In this system, with ^{14}C-labeled formate or CO_2, he found not only hypoxanthine but also detected another intermediate with even higher specific activity (GREENBERG, 1951). This was identified as the phosphoribosyl derivative of hypoxanthine, inosinic acid. By studying the time course of incorporation of the tracers, GREENBERG concluded that inosinic acid was the first purine derivative formed and that both inosine and hypoxanthine resulted from its catabolism. The work strongly suggested that purines were formed from nonpurine phosphoribosyl derivatives. Discovery of these and the elucidation of the sequence still presented major challenges, but the method of attack had been established.

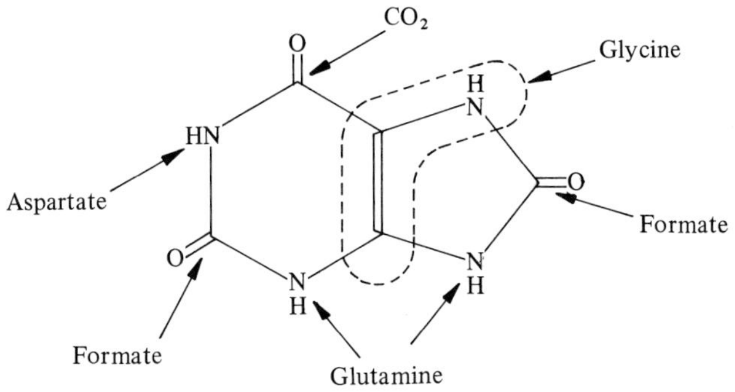

Fig. 6. The precursors of the ring atoms of uric acid

The completion of assignment of the ring of atoms of the purine skeleton became possible when a soluble enzyme preparation had been developed (SCHULMAN and BUCHANAN, 1951; GREENBERG, 1951). The lability of the nitrogen atoms of putative precursors had frustrated attempts to trace their origins in the whole pigeon. SONNE et al. (1953, 1956), using extracts, demonstrated that the amide nitrogen of glutamine contributed two of the ring N-atoms, and the other was derived from the α-amino group of asparate.

By this time the GREENBERG group (GOLDTHWAIT et al., 1954) had demonstrated the first and second steps in purine biosynthesis de novo. The synthesis of glycine-amide ribonucleotide, catalyzed by an extract of pigeon liver acetone powder, required glycine, glutamine, ribose-5-phosphate, and ATP. This was shown to be a precursor of a formylated derivative. Thus, at once the activation of ribose-5-phosphate and formate were demonstrated, and clues from other directions allowed GOLDTHWAIT et al. to find tetrahydrofolate involved in the activation of formate. The active form of ribose-5-phosphate was identified in a rather oblique manner. KORNBERG and his co-workers had detected an activated form of ribose-5-phosphate in studies of the mechanism by which orotate is converted to orotidylate. They proceeded rapidly with the purification of the enzyme that catalyzes the reaction: ribose-5-phosphate + ATP→AMP + PRPP and characterized the products definitively (KORNBERG et al., 1955a). Moreover, they lost no time in characterizing both pyrimidine and purine pyrophosphorylases (phosphoribosyltransferases) and elegantly demonstrated that adenine phosphoribosyltransferase was separable from hypoxanthine—guanine phosphoribosyltransferase (KRONBERG et al., 1955b). Almost simultaneously, REMY et al. (1955) succeeded in showing that "activated" ribose-5-phosphate was identical with the KORNBERG substance and that it could, with a second enzyme, form inosinate from hypoxanthine.

The pointers that led GOLDTHWAIT et al. (1954) to identify tetrahydrofolate as an activator of formate were many. The first was the gradual clarification of the actions of sulfonamides, and the integration of this knowledge with what had been learned about folic acid. It will be recalled that within a few years after the discovery of sulfanilamide, it had become clear that its actions were competitively reversed by p-aminobenzoic acid (pAB) and noncompetitively by purines, methionine, and thymine. This was interpreted correctly as suggesting that pAB was involved in a

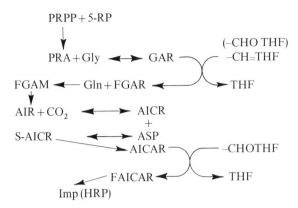

Fig. 7. Purine biosynthesis de novo. Abbreviations used are: 5-RP, ribose-5-phosphate; PRPP, 5-phosphoribosyl-1-pyrophosphate; PRA, 5-phosphoribosyl-1-amine; Gly, glycine; GAR, glycin-amideribonucleotide; THF, tetrahydrofolate; FGAR, formylglycinamideribonucleotide; Gln, glutamine; FGAM, formylglycinamidineribonucleotide; AIR, 5-aminoimidazole-1-ribonucleo-tide; AICR, 5-amino-4-imidazolecarboxylic acid-1-ribonucleotide; Asp, aspartate; S-AICR, 5-amino-4-imidazole-N-succinocarboxamide-1-ribonucleotide; AICAR, 5-amino-4-imidazolecar-boxamide-1-ribonucleotide; FAICAR, 5-formamido-4-imidazolecarboxamide-1-ribonucleotide; Imp, inosinic acid

catalytic function, and that the other substances were products of this catalysis (e.g., Winkler and De Haan, 1948; Woods, 1950). There was also little doubt that some form of folate was this catalyst. This was supported by the observation that puri-nes + thymine could supplant folic acid as a growth factor for many microorganisms (Stokstad, 1941) and was enhanced when pAB was found to be a constituent of the folic acid molecule. Still another intertwining line was built upon the observations of Stetten and Fox (1945) that *E. coli* in sulfonamide stasis excreted 5-amino-4-imida-zolecarboxamide. The eventual working out of this observation led not only to the identification of the immediate precursor of inosinate, the phosphoriboside of the imidazole derivative, but also a clear demonstration that tetrahydrofolate (leucovo-rin) was active as a carrier of formate (Buchanan and Schulman, 1953).

There remained to be determined the steps between formylglycineamide-ribonucleotide and aminoimidazoleribonucleotide and the characterization of the cofactor forms of tetrahydrofolate as well as identification of the enzymes in-volved. By 1957, the general pathway of purine biosynthesis had been established by Levenberg et al. (q.v.). The main outlines and the cofactors and reactants involved are shown in Figure 7, which scheme is now generally accepted.

A collateral development necessary to a more complete understanding of the pathways were the isolations and characterizations of the enzymes and the cofactors involved at each step. The reactions were summarized by Friedkin (1963) and Hitchings and Burchall (1965) and are shown in the skeleton form in Figure 8.

Some refinements may be necessary. Most of the studies have been carried out with pteroylmonoglutamate, whereas it is known that tetrahydropteroyl-tetraglutamate predominates in bacteria (Baugh et al., 1974). More testing of tetrah-ydropteroylpolyglutamates as substrates for specific enzymes is needed in view of the

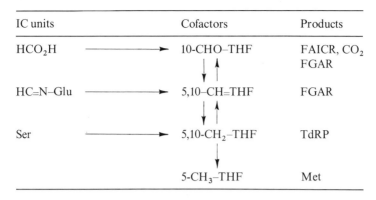

IC units	Cofactors	Products
HCO₂H ⟶	10-CHO–THF	FAICR, CO₂
		FGAR
	↓ ↑	
HC≡N–Glu ⟶	5,10–CH=THF	FGAR
	↓ ↑	
Ser ⟶	5,10-CH₂–THF	TdRP
	↓	
	5-CH₃–THF	Met

Fig. 8. Cofactors involving tetrahydrofolate derivatives. Abbreviations used are: HC=N-Glu, formiminoglutamate; Ser, serine; THF, FAICR, FGAR, see legend Figure 7; TdRP, thymidylate; Met, methionine

finding of HIMES and RABINOWITZ (1962) that the triglutamate was bound more tightly than monoglutamate to formyltetrahydrofolate synthetase. However, recent evidence suggests that polyglutamate synthesis may serve primarily to trap tetrahydrofolate intracellularly.

Recently, DEV and HARVEY (1977) scrutinized the evidence for the participation of 5, 10-methenyl THF in the GAR transformylase and concluded that at least in *E. coli* the actual substrate is 10-formyl THF.

KREBS and HEMS (1975) found that methionine controls formyltetrahydrofolate dehydrogenase and is necessary for the evolution of CO_2 from the one-carbon unit of formiminoglutamate. He views this mechanism as a control both of one-carbon units and methionine.

F. Uricotelism

To state that "uric acid is the end product of purine metabolism" is an anthropomorphic view. In most mammals, allantoin or allantoic acid is the end product (Fig. 9). Sporadically, allantoicase carries the degradation to glyoxalate and urea. In some species of animals uric acid is the end-product not only of nucleic acid metabolism but the major end-product of all nitrogen metabolism. Birds, saurian reptiles, insects, and terrestrial gastropods are uricotelic, while mammals, chelonian reptiles, and amphibia excrete mainly urea and ammonia; aquatic invertebrates down to protozoa excrete almost entirely ammonia. A few odd-ball creatures excrete other end-products such as guanine (spiders) and trimethylamine oxide (some fish). It is possible, but apparently undocumented, that the guanine of Peruvian guano represents unabsorbed guanine that is abundantly present in fish scales.

Uricotelism is an adaptation to terrestrial life; uric acid is the prime nitrogenous waste product that can be excreted in solid form, sparing water and tonicity and possibly toxicity. Its adoption by terrestrial animals correlates strictly with oviparity (NEEDHAM, 1942); indeed adult terrestrial animals with access to water would have

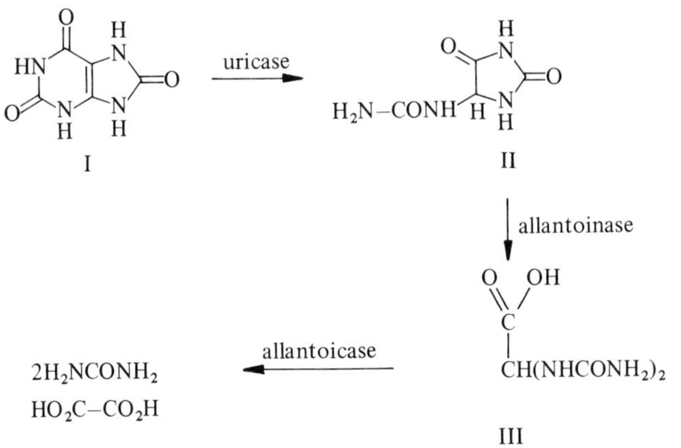

Fig. 9. Enzymatic degradation of uric acid. *I*, uric acid; *II*, allantoin; *III*, allantoic acid

no apparent need for it. The cost in energy expenditure is high, far greater than for the concentration of aqueous urea (Heinz and Pitlak, 1960). Buchanan (1958/59) estimates 56 cal/mole of inosinic acid, and although the heat of combustion of urate is only 0.46 cal/mole, it is difficult to find any step in the degradation of inosinate where the potential energy could usefully be recycled. It is plausible, then, to interpret the need to conserve water (or prevent hypertonicity) in the closed system of the hard-shelled egg as so great that uricotelism is the lesser evil. It would follow that the adult uricotelic animal has less stress but is unable to regenerate uricase once lost or to invent control mechanisms to turn the process off. Among zoo birds and reptiles, urate tophi are not uncommon.

G. Uricolysis

Uricolysis was well established in invertebrates. In the primitive hepatopancreas three enzymes were present, uricase, allantoinase, and allantoicase (Fig. 9). Deletions began sporadically among fish (e.g., salmon lacks allantoicase) and at the level of mammalia only uricase proper is retained. The retention of uricase and the evolution of the mammalian kidney must be viewed as linked. Extensive reabsorption of urate with clearances of the order of 10 in mammals contrasts sharply with clearances of roughly 50 in chickens (e.g., Martindale, 1976) accomplished mainly by tubular secretion. The obvious advantage of reabsorption is to ensure passage over hepatic uricase sufficient to split the bulk of purine end-product to readily soluble, readily cleared allantoin.

H. Measurement of Uric Acid Synthesis in Man

Serum urate concentration represents a balance between synthesis de novo plus contributions of dietary purines and excretion. Early attempts to measure the uric acid pool by injecting ^{15}N-urate (Benedict et al., 1952) quickly revealed the mobility of tophaceous deposits. The miscible urate pool thus comprises urate in solution, and that readily dissolved, and may inadequately measure total urate, since old deposits may be difficulty soluble (STETTEN, 1950). Nevertheless, deposits are resolved when serum urate levels are maintained below the solubility point of urate (RUNDLES et al., 1966).

When isotopically labeled precursors became available, quantification of urate biosynthesis in man became possible. Many of the intermediates identified earlier in works with pigeons, bacteria, and other species have given rise to urate in man and thus served the secondary purpose of confirming biochemical unity with respect to the pathway of Figure 7. Two salient points emerged from tracer experiments. Calculations of purine neogenesis are higher by 30–40% than the labeled uric acid excreted (SEEGMILLER et al., 1961). Moreover, ^{15}N-labeled uric acid is, in part, converted to urinary urea (WYNGAARDEN and STETTEN, 1953). These observations led to recognition of the hepatic circulation of uric acid with intestinal destruction, which plays a role that may become major when impaired renal function is present. The second point concerns the differences in patterns of incorporation of glycine and glutamine-N that are observed when gouty subjects are compared with normal. These encompass a more rapid appearance of the ^{15}N of ^{15}N-glycine in the urinary urate of the gouty (BENEDICT et al., 1952), an observation that at that time gave rise to the concept of a "uric acid shunt." Moreover, more of the ^{15}N of glycine appeared in N-atoms 9 and 3 in the gouty than in the normal (GUTMAN et al., 1962). This was accompanied by a diminished excretion of ^{15}NH$_4$+. Rather too much has been made of this type of observation. What the experiments are saying is not much beyond what was already known, i.e., that in many gouty subjects the synthesis of inosinate is greatly in excess of the amount that can give rise to coenzymes and nucleic acids. To account for all the apparent abnormalities would require detailed knowledge of a multitude of pool sizes and turnovers. It is probable that even in the normal the turnover of inosinate is sufficient to provide a surplus. Forces that drive, pull, or decontrol the mechanisms can only result in a disproportionate increase in spillage.

J. Uric Acid Formation from Purines

Salvage pathways, nucleotide interconversions, and control mechanisms of purine biosynthesis are discussed in detail in other chapters of this paper by HOLMES, ARNOLD, HENDERSON, FOX, TATIBANA, and BECKER. However, some general outlines are necessary to this discussion, and a skeleton scheme is presented (Fig. 10). A review of intermediary metabolism in relation to gout is also available (WYNGAARDEN and KELLEY, 1972).

The ultimate formation of urate in man depends on the action of xanthine oxidase on hypoxanthine and xanthine. This is amply established by the findings in xanthinuria (ENGLEMAN et al., 1964) and by the consequences of inhibition of this enzyme by allopurinol (ELION, this volume). This drug-induced biochemical lesion assisted in unraveling the consequences of other lesions and led to a deeper understanding of details of purine metabolism and particularly of control mechanisms.

An early finding with allopurinol-treated patients was that many, particularly over-producers, replaced uric acid with less than the stoichiometric equivalent quantities of oxypurines. This, coupled with the observation that allopurinol treat-

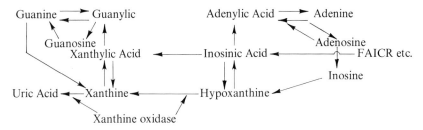

Fig. 10. Interrelationships of oxypurines and nucleotides. Abbrevations used: FAICR, see legend
Figure 7

ment enhanced the utilization of exogenous hypoxanthine and xanthine, was interpreted as reutilization of these precursors and ultimate feed-back control of purine
biosynthesis de novo (HITCHINGS, 1966; RUNDLES et al., 1969).

The substrate activities of hypoxanthine and xanthine for xanthine oxidase are
comparable, with xanthine somewhat the better (KRENITSKY et al., 1972). The concentrations of the free bases in serum are similar, 10^{-5}M (NELSON, 1976), and
possibly somewhat higher than their K_m values for milk xanthine oxidase (KRENIT-
SKY et al., 1972). However, there is a very large difference in their substrate activities
for human hypoxanthine guanine phosphoribosyltransferase (HGPRT). Xanthine is
less well bound to the enzyme by a factor of 100, and the reaction is slower, so that
the overall rate at comparable concentrations is some 1700 times as fast with hypoxanthine as with xanthine (KRENITSKY et al., 1969). With hypoxanthine, conversion
to the ribonucleotide is favored; with xanthine, oxidation to urate would be expected
to predominate.

BALIS (1968) measured pool sizes, turnover, and excretions of the two oxypurines
in a xanthinuric patient. The pool sizes were comparable (hypoxanthine, 118 mg;
xanthine, 73 mg). These would give concentrations in the range 1–2 times 10^{-5}M in
total body water. Turnover rates were quite different for the two; hypoxanthine
almost a gram/day and xanthine about a quarter of that. The daily excretion of
xanthine was comparable to the turnover; only 5% of the daily turnover of hypoxanthine was represented in the urine. The chief route from hypoxanthine to xanthine in
the xanthinuric is necessarily via inosinate dehydrogenase, and in view of the considerations in the paragraph above, it is also probably the chief route in the normal.

At present it is not possible to pinpoint the origins of the free bases other than to
say that they arise mainly from the ribonucleotides. The suggestion that the adeno-
sine-inosine loop (Fig. 10) might be an important source of hypoxanthine (BALIS,
1968) seems to have been put to rest on the basis of kinetics and inhibitor studies
(BROX and HENDERSON, 1976) and on the absence of effect on purine turnover of
deletion of adenosine kinase and adenine phosphoribosyltransferase in lymphoblastic cell lines (HIRSHFIELD et al., 1976).

Xanthine oxidase (xanthine: oxygen oxidoreductase EC 1.2.3.2) is accompanied
in many tissues and species by a similar enzyme, "aldehyde oxidase" (aldehyde:
oxygen oxidoreductase, EC 1.2.3.1). Both enzymes have molecular weights approximately 300,000 and contain iron, flavin adenine dinucleotide, and molybdenum in
the ratios 4:1:1 (DE RENZO, 1956). A closely related enzyme, xanthine dehydroge-

nase (EC 1.2.1.37), is present in avian kidney tissue. It has an iron, FAD, molybdenum ratio of 8:1:1 and requires NAD as hydrogen acceptor, but can use hydroxylamine, which is inhibitory to the oxidase, and cannot use ferricyanide, which functions well with the oxidases (LANDON and CARTER, 1960).

The literature on xanthine oxidase is voluminous, and a good deal is known about its mechanism of action. Rather major contributions to this knowledge have been made by studies involving allopurinol and particularly oxipurinol (MASSEY et al., 1970; SPECTOR and JOHNS, 1970). The literature on aldehyde oxidase is skimpy, and the possible participation of this enzyme in metabolic events is often overlooked. The substrate specificities of the two enzymes overlap but may differ for specific molecules, and the points of attack may differ (KRENITSKY et al., 1972). Both enzymes oxidize hypoxanthine to xanthine and allopurinol to oxipurinol. Two examples of the metabolic importance of aldehyde oxidase will suffice. It seems clear that the inactivity of azathioprine as an immunosuppressive agent in the rabbit is due to its oxidation by aldehyde oxidase, which is abundant in that species. Somewhat more speculative is the suggestion of SPECTOR (1977) that the formation of oxipurinol from allopurinol in a xanthinuric patient was due to the retention of aldehyde oxidase in the face of deletion of xanthine oxidase. It is clear that the product could not have been formed as had been suggested (CHALMERS et al., 1969) via the action of inosinate dehydrogenase on allopurinol ribonucleotide (HITCHINGS, 1975; MILLER and ADAMCZYK, 1976). There is a clear need for more information on aldehyde oxidase, and this should be easily obtainable through the use of appropriate substrates; for example, xanthine is oxidized by xanthine oxidase and not by aldehyde oxidase, while 3-methylhypoxanthine is an excellent substrate for aldehyde oxidase and very poorly oxidized by xanthine oxidase (KRENITSKY et al., 1972).

Two major questions regarding the role of xanthine oxidase in human metabolism have not been answered definitively. These are: Is xanthine oxidase an inducible enzyme? Can it play an important role in the regulation of purine turnover?

In uricotelic creatures, xanthine dehydrogenase is clearly dependent on diet. Thus, this enzyme increased 13-fold (units/g. chick liver) when the casein content of the feed was increased from 5% to 75% (ITOH and TSUSHIMA, 1974). The enzyme is inducible by substrates, but in starved chicks STIRPE and DELLA CORTE (1965) found only inosine and not free purines to be active. Uric acid formation can be augmented by the administration of precursors such as glutamine, asparagine, and ammonium acetate (KARASAWA et al., 1973).

Mammalian organisms also contain xanthine dehydrogenase in addition to xanthine oxidase (DELLA CORTE and STIRPE, 1972; KRENITSKY et al., 1974). Some confusion has arisen because the dehydrogenase is spontaneously (on incubation) converted to an oxidase. It has only recently been recognized that the dehydrogenase-derived oxidase differs from the oxidase present in fresh extracts (TUTTLE and KRENITSKY, 1977).

Some uncertainties regarding previous observations on changes in xanthine oxidase activities result from the current knowledge that dehydrogenase is converted to oxidase. It is clear, however, that xanthine oxidase activity in animals depends on dietary protein and molybdenum (WESTERFELD and RICHERT, 1951). The enzyme is also adaptive to some degree, since several authors have reported its level to increase with administration of purines (FEIGELSON et al., 1954; DIETRICH, 1954).

Carcassi and co-workers (1969) reported elevated hepatic xanthine oxidase levels in seven of eight subjects with primary gout and hyperuricosuria. In one of the subjects with a 12-fold increase in activity, this was associated with a defective HGPRT (Carcassi, 1976). This was interpreted as induction of xanthine oxidase consequent to elevated levels of hypoxanthine, but supporting measurements have not been presented.

The possibility was considered that treatment with allopurinol might result in elevated xanthine oxidase activities. This seems not to have occurred, since the dosage of allopurinol to control hyperuricemia in a given subject has remained stable or even diminished (Rundles et al., 1969). This provides very little evidence one way or the other, since administration of the inhibitor is followed by minimal changes in serum oxypurines. The factors that limit a rise in oxypurines are two: the high renal clearances of these substances and the extensive reutilization that occurs when xanthine oxidase is inhibited (Hitchings, 1966).

Hypoxanthine and xanthine levels in serum reflect dynamic equilibria involving binding constants of the substrates to and activities of xanthine oxidase and dehydrogenase and HGPRT. Less directly, they reflect the pool sizes of inosinate and xanthylate, which are responsive to the binding constants of these to and the activities of a substantial number of additional enzymes. Moreover, exogenous purines and renal clearances must be taken into account.

The impression one has is that xanthine oxidase is inducible in man within limits, but factors other than purines (e.g., protein) may play a role. It is not inconceivable that it plays a regulatory role in purine turnover through a pull mechanism (increased xanthine oxidase would favor its competition for substrates with respect to the anabolic enzymes). This may be a chick-egg sort of proposal. In any case, it is clear that only through the coordinated measurement of multiple parameters would one be able to do more than speculate on these control mechanisms.

References

Albert, A.: Purine-8-carboxylic acid. J. Chem. Soc. 4705 (1960)

Allison, A. C.: Purine and pyrimidine metabolism. Nature (Lond.) 262, 7—8 (1976)

Baeyer, A.: Untersuchungen über die Harnsäuregruppe. Justus Liebigs Ann. Chem. 127, 1—27 (1863)

Balis, M. E.: Aspects of purine metabolism. Fed. Proc. 27, 1067—1074 (1968)

Barnes, F. W., Jr., Schoenheimer, R.: On the biological synthesis of purines and pyrimidines. J. biol. Chem. 151, 123—139 (1943)

Baugh, C. M., Braverman, E., Nair, M. G.: The identification of poly-α-glutamyl chain lengths in bacterial folates. Biochemistry 13, 4952—4957 (1974)

Behrend, R., Roosen, O.: Synthese der Harnsäure. Justus Liebigs Ann. Chem. 251, 235—256 (1889)

Benedict, J. D., Roche, M., Yü, T. F., Bien, E. J., Gutman, A. B., Stetten, D., Jr.: Incorporation of glycine nitrogen into uric acid in normal and gouty man. Metabolism 1, 3—12 (1952)

Bergmann, F., Dikstein, S.: Studies on uric acid and related compounds. III. Observations on the specificity of mammalian xanthine oxidases. J. biol. Chem. 223, 765—780 (1956)

Bills, C. W., Gebura, S. E., Meek, J. S., Sweeting, O. J.: New synthesis of uric acid and 1, 7-dimethyl-uric acid. J. org. Chem. 27, 4633—4635 (1962)

Bishop, C., Talbot, J. H.: Uric acid: its role in biological processes and the influence upon it of physiological, pathological, and pharmacological agents. Pharmacol. Rev. 5, 231—273 (1953)

Block, K.: The metabolism of l(+)-arginine and synthesis of creatine in the pigeon. J. biol. Chem. **165**, 477—484 (1946)

Brown, G. B.: The biosynthesis of nucleic acids as a basis for an approach to chemotherapy. Ann. N.Y. Acad. Sci. **60**, 185—194 (1954)

Brox, L. W., Henderson, J. F.: The "adenosine cycle" is not a significant route of purine metabolism in mammalian cells. Canad. J. Biochem. **54**, 200—202 (1976)

Buchanan, J. M.: The enzymatic synthesis of the purine nucleotides. Harvey Lect. **54**, 104—130 (1958/59)

Buchanan, J. M.: The amidotransferases. Advanc. Enzymol. **39**, 91—183 (1973)

Buchanan, J. M., Sonne, J. C.: The utilization of formate in uric acid synthesis. J. biol. Chem. **166**, 781 (1946)

Buchanan, J. M., Schulman, M. P.: Biosynthesis of the purines. III. Reactions of formate and inosinic acid and an effect of the citrovorum factor. J. biol. Chem. **202**, 241—252 (1953)

Carcassi, A.: Xanthine-oxidase activity in a gouty patient with partial deficiency of HGPRT. Z. klin. Chem. Klin. Biochem. **14**, 283 (1976)

Carcassi, A., Marcolongo, R., Marinello, E., Riario-Sforza, G., Boggiano, C.: Liver xanthine oxidase in gouty patients. Arthr. and Rheum. **12**, 17—20 (1969)

Chalmers, R. A., Parker, R., Simmonds, H. A., Snedden, W., Watts, R. W. E.: The convertion of 4-hydroxypyrazolo[3,4-d]pyrimidine (allopurinol) into 4,6 dehydroxypyrazolo[3,4-d]pyrimidine (oxipurinol) in vivo in the absence of xanthine-oxygen oxidoreductase. Biochem. J. **112**, 527—532 (1969)

Della Corte, E., Stirpe, F.: The regulation of rat liver xanthine oxidase. Biochem. J. **126**, 739—745 (1972)

Dev, I. K., Harvey, R. J.: N^{10}-formyltetrahydrofolate as substrate for GAR-transformyl as in *E. coli*. (in press) (1977)

Dietrich, L. S.: Factors affecting the induction of xanthine oxidase of mouse liver. J. biol. Chem. **211**, 79—85 (1954)

Edson, N. L., Krebs, H. A., Model, A.: CXCVI. The synthesis of uric acid in the avian organism: hypoxanthine as an intermediary metabolite. Biochem. J. **30**, 1380—1385 (1936)

Engleman, K., Watts, R. W. E., Kleinenberg, J. R., Sjoerdsma, A., Seegmiller, J. E.: Clinical, physiological and biochemical studies of a patient with xanthinuria and pheochromocytoma. Amer. J. Med. **37**, 839—861 (1964)

Feigelson, P., Feigelson, M., Wood, T. R.: Apparent simultaneous adaptive enzyme formation in C57 mice. Science **120**, 502—503 (1954)

Ferris, J. P., Orgel, L. E.: An unusual photochemical rearrangement in the synthesis of adenine from hydrogen cyanide. J. Amer. chem. Soc. **88**, 1074 (1966a)

Ferris, J. P., Orgel, L. E.: Studies in prebiotic synthesis. I. aminomalononitrile and 4-amino-5-cyanoimidazole. J. Amer. chem. Soc. **88**, 3829—3831 (1966b)

Fischer, E.: Über die Harnsäure I. Ber. dtsch. chem. Ges. **17**, 328—338 (1884)

Fischer, E.: Über die Constitution des Caffeins, Xanthins, Hypoxanthins und verwandter Basen. Ber. dtsch. chem. Ges. **30**, 523—549 (1897)

Fischer, E.: Synthese in der Puringruppe. Ber. dtsch. chem. Ges. **32**, 435—504 (1899)

Fischer, E., Ach, L.: Neue Synthese der Harnsäure u. ihrer Methylderivate. Ber. dtsch. chem. Ges. **28**, 2473—2480 (1895)

Friedkin, M.: Enzymic aspects of folic acid. Ann. Rev. Biochem. **32**, 185—214 (1963)

Goldthwait, D. A., Peabody, R. A., Greenberg, G. R.: Glycine ribotide intermediates in the de novo synthesis of inosinic acid. J. Amer. chem. Soc. **76**, 5258—5259 (1954)

Greenberg, G. R.: Incorporation of carbon-labeled formic acid and carbon dioxide into hypoxanthine in pigeon liver homogenates. Arch. Biochem. Biophys. **19**, 337—339 (1948)

Greenberg, G. R.: Synthesis of purine in dialyzed liver extracts. Fed. Proc. **10**, 192 (1951)

Greenberg, G. R.: De novo synthesis of hypoxanthine via inosine-5-phosphate and inosine. J. biol. Chem. **190**, 611—631 (1951)

Gutman, A. B., Yü, T. F., Adler, M., Javitt, N. B.: Intramolecular distribution of uric acid-U^{15} after administration of glycine-N^{15} and ammonium-N^{15} chloride to gouty and non-gouty subjects. J. clin. Invest. **41**, 623—636 (1962)

Harvey, A. M., Christensen, H. N.: Uric acid transport system: apparent absence in erythrocytes of the Dalmatian coach hound. Science **145**, 826—827 (1964)

Heinz,E., Pitlak,C.S.: Energy expenditure in active transport mechanisms. Biochim. biophys. Acta (Amst.) **44**, 324—334 (1960)

Himes,R.H., Rabinowitz,J.C.: Formylteterhydrofolate synthetase. II. Characteristics of the enzyme and the enzymic reation. J. biol. Chem. **237**, 2903—2914 (1962)

Hirshfield,M., Spector,E., Seegmiller,J.E.: Purine synthesis and excretion in human lymphoblasts. Mutants deficient in adenosine kinase (AK) and adenine phosphoribosyl transferase (APRT). J. Clin. Chem. Clin. Biochem. **14**, 297 (1976)

Hitchings,G.H.: Effects of allopurinol in relation to purine biosynthesis. Ann. rheum. Dis. **25**, 601—607 (1966)

Hitchings,G.H.: Pharmacology of allopurinol. Arthr. and Rheum. **18**, 863—870 (1975)

Hitchings,G.H., Burchall,J.J.: Inhibition of folate biosynthesis and function as a basis for chemotherapy. Advanc. Enzymol. **27**, 417—468 (1965)

Horbaczewski,J.: Synthese der Harnsäure. Ber. dtsch. chem. Ges. **15**, 2678 (1882)

Horbaczewski,J.: Über künstliche Harnsäure und Methylharnsäure. Mh. Chem. **6**, 356—362 (1885)

Horbaczewski,J.: Über eine neue Synthese und über die Konstitution der Harnsäure. Wien. Monatsh. **8**, 201—207 (1887)

Horbaczewski,J.: Untersuchungen über die Entstehung der Harnsäure im Säugetierorganismus. Mh. Chem. **10**, 624—641 (1889)

Horbaczewski,J.: Bildung der Harnsäure und Xanthinbasen sowie die Entstehung der Leucocytosen in Säugetierorganismus. Mh. Chem. **12**, 221—275 (1891)

Horowitz,N.H.: The evolution of biochemical synthesis. Proc. nat. Acad. Sci. (Wash.) **31**, 153—157 (1945)

Itoh,R., Tsushima,K.: Comparisons of adaptations to diet of enzymes involved in uric acid production from IMP in chickens and rats. J. Biochem. (Tokyo) **75**, 715—721 (1974)

Jezewska,M.M.: Xanthine accumulation during hypoxanthine oxidation by milk xanthine oxidase. Europ. J. Biochem. **36**, 385—390 (1973)

Karasawa,Y., Tasaki,I., Yokota,H.-O., Shibata,F.: Comparative effect of intravenously administered nitrogenous compounds on uric acid synthesis in chickens fed a 20% protein diet. J. Nutr. **103**, 1208—1211 (1973)

Kornberg,A., Lieberman,I., Simms,E.S.: Enzymatic synthesis and properties of 5-phosphoribosylpyrophosphate. J. biol. Chem. **215**, 389—402 (1955a)

Kornberg,A., Lieberman,I., Simms,E.S.: Enzymatic synthesis and purine nucleotides. J. biol. Chem. **215**, 417—427 (1955b)

Kossel,A.: Über Guanin. Hoppe-Seylers Z. physiol. Chem. **8**, 404—410 (1884)

Kossel,A.: Weitere Beiträge zur Chemie des Zellkernes. II. Über das Adenine. Hoppe-Seylers Z. physiol. Chem. **10**, 248—264 (1886)

Krebs,H.A., Hems,R.: The regulation of the degradation of methionine and of the one-carbon units derived from histidine, serine, and glycine. Advanc. Enzyme Regul. **14**, 493—513 (1975)

Krenitsky,T.A., Neil,S.M., Elion,G.B., Hitchings,G.H.: A comparison of the specificities of xanthine oxidase and aldehyde oxidase. Arch. Biochem. Biophys. **150**, 585—599 (1972)

Krenitsky,T.A., Papionannou,R., Elion,G.B.: Human hypoxanthine phosphoribosyltransferase. I. purification, properties and specificity. J. biol. Chem. **244**, 1263—1270 (1969)

Krenitsky,T.A., Tuttle,J.V., Cattau,E.L.,Jr., Wang,P.: A comparison of the distribution and electron acceptor specificities of xanthine oxidase and aldehyde oxidase. Comp. Biochem. Physiol. [B] **49**, 687—703 (1974)

Landon,E.J., Carter,C.E.: The preparation, properties, and inhibition of hypoxanthine dehydrogenase of avian kidney. J. biol. Chem. **235**, 819—824 (1960)

Levenberg,B., Hartman,S.C., Buchanan,J.M.: Biosynthesis of the purines. X. Further studies in vitro on the metabolic origin of nitrogen atoms 1 and 3 of the purine ring. J. biol. Chem. **220**, 379—390 (1956)

Liebig,J.: Inosinsäure. Justus Liebigs Ann. Chem. **62**, 317—323 (1847)

Lister,J.H.: Synthesis of purines from pyrimidines. Rev. pure appl. Chem. **11**, 178—195 (1961)

Lister,J.H.: Synthesis of purines from imidazoles. Rev. pure appl. Chem. **13**, 30—47 (1963)

Lister,J.H.: Fused pyrimidines. II. Purines. New York: Wiley-Interscience 1971

McBurney,M.W., Whitmore,G.F.: Isolation and biochemical characterization of folate deficient mutants of Chinese hamster cells. Cell **2**, 173—182 (1974)

Marcet, A.: An Essay on the Chemical History and Medical Treatment of Calculus Disorders, pp. 95—101. London: Longham, Hurst, Rees, Orme and Brown 1817

Martindale, L.: Renal urate synthesis in the fowl *(Gallus domesticus)*. Comp. Biochem. Physiol. [A] **53**, 389—391 (1976)

Massey, V., Komai, H., Palmer, G., Elion, G. B.: On the mechanism of inactivation of xanthine oxidase by allopurinol and other pyrazolo[3,4-d]pyrimidines. J. biol. Chem. **245**, 2837—2844 (1970)

Medicus, L.: Zur Constitution der Harnsäuregruppe. Justus Liebigs Ann. Chem. **175**, 230—251 (1875)

Miescher, F.: Die Spermatozoen einiger Wirbeltiere. Verh. Naturf. Ges. (Basel) **6**, 138—153 (1874)

Miller, R. L., Adamczyk, D. L.: Inosine 5′-monophosphate dehydrogenase from sarcoma 180 cells—substrate and inhibitor specificity. Biochem. Pharmacol. **25**, 883—888 (1976)

Minkowski, O.: Über den Einfluß der Leberextirpation auf den Stoffwechsel. Arch. exp. Path. Pharmak. **21**, 41—52 (1886)

Needham, J.: Biochemistry and Morphogensis. Cambridge: Univ. Pr. 1942

Nelson, D. M.: Unpublished observations 1976

Noronha, J. M., Aboobaker, V. S.: Studies on the folate compounds of human blood. Arch. Biochem. Biophys. **101**, 445—447 (1963)

Örström, Å., Örström, M., Krebs, H. A.: The formation of hypoxanthine in pigeon liver. Biochem. J. **33**, 990—994 (1939)

Oró, J., Kimball, A. P.: Synthesis of purines under possible primitive earth conditions. II. Purine intermediates from hydrogen cyanide. Arch. Biochem. Biophys. **96**, 293—313 (1962)

Pfleiderer, W.: Über den Abbau von Harnsäure mit Wasser unter Druck. Chem. Ber. **92**, 2468—2477 (1959)

Piccard, J.: Über Protamin, Guanin und Sarkin als Bestandteile des Lachssperma. Ber. dtsch. chem. Ges. **7**, 1714—1719 (1874)

Remy, C. N., Remy, W. T., Buchanan, J. M.: Biosynthesis of purines. VIII. Enzymatic synthesis and utilization of α-5-phosphoribosylpyrophosphate. J. biol. Chem. **217**, 885—895 (1955a)

Remy, C. N., Remy, W. T., Buchanan, J. M.: Biosynthesis of purines. VIII. Enzymatic synthesis and utilization of α-5-phosphoribosylpyrophosphate. J. biol. Chem. **217**, 885—895 (1955b)

Renzo, E. C., De: Chemistry and biochemistry of xanthine oxidase. Advanc. Enzymol. **17**, 293—328 (1956)

Richter, E., Taylor, Jr., E. C.: Eine neue Synthese von Purinen. Angew. Chem. **67**, 303 (1955a)

Richter, E., Taylor, Jr., E. C.: Eine neue Synthese von Purinen. Angew. Chem. **67**, 303 (1955b)

Ringertz, H. G.: Crystal structure of purines. In: Purines Theory and Experiment, pp. 61—71. Jerusalem: Israeli Acad. of Sci. 1972

Robins, R. K.: Potential purine antagonists. I. Synthesis of some 4,6-substituted pyrazolo-[3,4-d]pyrimidines. J. Amer. chem. Soc. **78**, 784—790 (1956)

Rundles, R. W., Elion, G. B., Hitchings, G. H.: Allopurinol in the treatment of gout and secondary hyperuricemia. Bull. rheum. Dis. **16**, 400—403 (1966)

Rundles, R. W., Wyngaarden, J. B., Hitchings, G. H., Elion, G. B.: Drugs and uric acid. Ann. Rev. Pharmacol. **9**, 345—362 (1969)

Sarasin, J., Wegmann, E.: Synthèse de l'hétéroxanthine à partir d'un dérivé de l'imidazol. Helv. chim. Acta **7**, 713—719 (1924)

Scheele, K. W.: Examen chemicum calculi. Urinarii Opuscula **2**, 73—79 (1776)

Scherer, P.: Über einen im thierischen Organismus vorkommenden, dem Xanthicoxyd verwandten Körper. Justus Liebigs Ann. Chem. **73**, 328—334 (1850)

Schulman, M. P., Buchanan, J. M.: Mechanism of hypoxanthine synthesis from glycine, formate and 4-amino,5-imidazolecarboxamide. Fed. Proc. **10**, 244—245 (1951)

Seegmiller, J. E., Grayzel, A. L., Laster, L., Liddle, L.: Uric acid production in gout. J. clin. Invest. **40**, 1304—1314 (1961)

Shannon, J. S., Letham, D. S.: Regulators of cell division in plant tissues. IV. The mass spectra of cytokinins and other 6-aminopurines. N.Z. Jl. Sci. **9**, 833—842 (1966)

Shaw, E.: A new synthesis of the purines adenine, hypoxanthine, xanthine and isoguanine. J. biol. Chem. **185**, 439—447 (1950)

Shemin, D., Rittenberg, D.: On the utilization of glycine for uric acid synthesis in man. J. biol. Chem. **167**, 875—876 (1947)

Sonne,J.C., Buchanan,J.M., Delluva,A.M.: Biological precursors of uric acid carbon. J. biol. Chem. **166**, 395—396 (1946)

Sonne,J.C., Buchanan,J.M., Delluva,A.M.: Biological precursors of uric acid. I. The role of lactate, acetate, and formate in the synthesis of the ureide groups of uric acid. J. biol. Chem. **173**, 69—98 (1948)

Sonne,J.C., Lin,I., Buchanan,J.M.: The role of N^{15} glycine, glutamine, aspartate, and glutamate in hypoxanthine synthesis. J. Amer. chem. Soc. **75**, 1516—1517 (1953)

Sonne,J.C., Lin,I., Buchanan,J.M.: Biosynthesis of the purines. IX. Precursors of the nitrogen atoms of the purine ring. J. biol. Chem. **220**, 369—378 (1956)

Spector,T.: Inhibition of urate production by allopurinol. Biochem. Pharmacol. (in press) (1977)

Spector,T., Johns,D.G.: Stoichiometric inhibition of reduced xanthine oxidase by hydroxypyra-zolo[3,4-d]pyrimidines. J. biol. Chem. **245**, 5079—5085 (1970)

Stetten,Jr.,D.: The pool of miscible uric acid in normal and gouty man. J. Mt. Sinai Hosp. **17**, 149—158 (1950)

Stetten,M.R., Fox,Jr.,C.L.: An amine formed by bacteria during sulfonamide bacteriostasis. J. biol. Chem. **161**, 333—349 (1945)

Stirpe,F., Della Corte,E.: Regulation of xanthine dehydrogenase in chick liver. Effect of starvation and of administration of purines and purine nucleotides. Biochem. J. **94**, 309—313 (1965)

Stokstad,E.L.R.: Isolation of a nucleotide essential for the growth of Lactobacillus casei. J. biol. Chem. **139**, 475—476 (1941)

Taylor,E.C., Cheng,C.C.: Purine chemistry. VI. Convenient one-step synthesis of hypoxanthine. Tetrahedron Lett. **12**, 9—11 (1959)

Taylor,E.C., McKillop,A.: The Chemistry of Cyclic Enaminonitriles and o-Aminonitriles, Vol.7. New York: Interscience 1970

Tesar,C., Rittenberg,D.: The metabolism of L-histidine. J. biol. Chem. **170**, 35—53 (1947)

Tuttle,J., Krenitsky,T.A.: Evidence for two types of mammalian xanthine oxidases. Fed. Proc. **36**, 776 (1977)

Unger,B.: Das Guanin und seine Verbindungen. Justus Liebigs Ann. Chem. **59**, 58—68 (1846)

Westerfeld,W.W., Richert,D.A.: Liver and intestinal xanthine oxidases in relation to diet. J. biol. Chem. **192**, 35—48 (1951)

Wiener,H.: Über synthetische Bildung der Harnsäure im Tierkörper. Beitr. chem. Physiol. Path. **2**, 42—85 (1902)

Windaus,A., Langenbeck,W.: Über die 4(5)-Nitro-imidazole-5(4)-carbonsäure. Ber. dtsch. chem. Ges. **56**, 683—686 (1923)

Winkler,K.C., Haan,P.G., De: On the action of sulfanilamide. XII. A set of noncompetitive sulfanilamide antagonists for *Escherichia coli*. Arch. Biochem. **18**, 97—107 (1948)

Wöhler,F., Liebig,J.: Untersuchungen über die Natur der Harnsäure. Ann. Pharm. **26**, 241—338 (1838 a)

Wöhler,F., Liebig,J.: Über Marcet's Xanthic-Oxyd. Annl. Pharm. **26**, 340—345 (1838 b)

Woods,D.D.: Biochemical significance of the competition between p-aminobenzoic acid and the sulphonamides. Ann. N.Y. Acad. Sci. **52**, 1199—1211 (1950)

Wyngaarden,J.B., Kelley,W.N.: In; Stanbury,J.B., Wyngaarden,J.B., Fredrickson,D.S. (Eds.): The Metabolic Basis of Inherited Disease, 3rd Ed., pp.889—968. New York: McGraw-Hill 1972

Wyngaarden,J.B., Stetten,Jr., D.: Uricolysis in normal man. J. biol. Chem. **203**, 9—21 (1953)

CHAPTER 2

Regulation of Purine Biosynthesis De Novo

E. W. HOLMES, JR.

A. Introduction

Hyperuricemia can result from an increase in the rate of purine biosynthesis de novo, a decrease in the renal clearance of uric acid, or a combination of these two processes. The relative contribution of each of these processes to the development of hyperuricemia varies with the subpopulation under study. This might be expected, since gout is a clinical disorder of diverse etiologies. Some referral centers have reported that as many as 75% of their patients with gout exhibit increased rates of purine biosynthesis as judged from isotopic incorporation techniques (GUTMAN et al., 1958; SEEGMILLER et al., 1961). However, the experience in other centers suggests that only 15–25% of their patients with primary gout develop hyperuricemia due to an increase in the rate of purine biosynthesis (WATTS et al., 1976). While the prevalence of purine overproduction in the general gouty population is not known, it appears that a significant proportion of these patients develop hyperuricemia due to an increase in the rate of purine biosynthesis de novo. Because of this association, the mechanisms responsible for the regulation of purine biosynthesis have been the subject of numerous studies.

Before discussing these regulatory processes, it may be helpful to review the pathway of purine biosynthesis and urate production. (For a more indepth discussion of this topic the reader is referred to the first chapter in this volume.) Figure 1 illustrates the terminal portion of this pathway. In man the final excretory product of purine metabolism is uric acid, since uricase activity has been lost during the course of evolution. Uric acid is formed from the purine bases, xanthine and hypoxanthine, in a reaction catalyzed by xanthine oxidase. These purine bases are obtained from two sources: catabolism of dietary nucleic acids and catabolism of endogenous purine ribonucleotides. Figure 2 depicts two sources of endogenous purine ribonucleotides: catabolism of nucleic acid and de novo synthesis. The entire pathway of purine biosynthesis de novo is shown in Figure 3. Phosphoribosylamine (PRA) is the product of the first reaction unique to this pathway, and the factors which determine its rate of synthesis play an important role in the control of purine biosynthesis (see below). Carbon and nitrogen atoms derived from amino acids, "formyl" groups, and bicarbonate are added to PRA in nine subsequent enzymatic reactions to form the parent purine ribonucleotide, inosine-5'-monophosphate (IMP). There is no branch point in the pathway leading from PRA to IMP. However, once IMP is formed several routes of metabolism are available to this nucleotide. Continuing the synthetic route, IMP can be metabolized to either adenosine 5'-monophosphate (AMP) or guanosine 5'-monophosphate (GMP), and these nucleotide monophosphates can

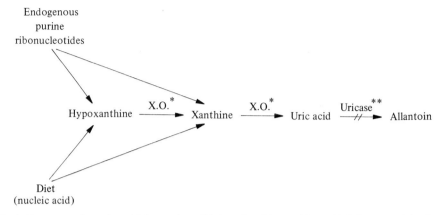

Fig. 1. Precursors for uric acid formation. *X.O. = Xanthine oxidase; **Uricase Activity is not detectable in human tissues in vivo

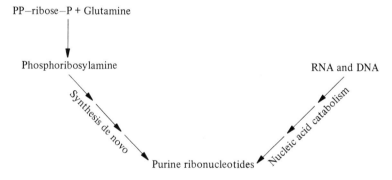

Fig. 2. Precursors of endogenous purine ribonucleotide

be further phosphorylated to di- and triphosphates. In the catabolic route, IMP is dephosphorylated to inosine with subsequent phosphorolysis of inosine to hypoxanthine (Fig. 4). Hypoxanthine is either phosphoribosylated to IMP in a reaction of the salvage pathway catalyzed by hypoxanthine-guanine phosphoribosyltransferase (HPRT) or oxidized to xanthine and uric acid by xanthine oxidase (Fig. 4). The interconversion between the purine ribonucleotides, catabolism of nucleotides, and reutilization of the purine bases are the subjects of the next three chapters in this volume. The remainder of this chapter will review the factors which are currently thought to be important in the control of PRA synthesis and subsequent IMP production.

B. Rate-Limiting Step

There are several reasons for hypothesizing that PRA formation is rate-limiting for purine biosynthesis de novo: (1) PRA is the product of the first reaction unique to purine biosynthesis, and there are no branch points in the pathway between PRA

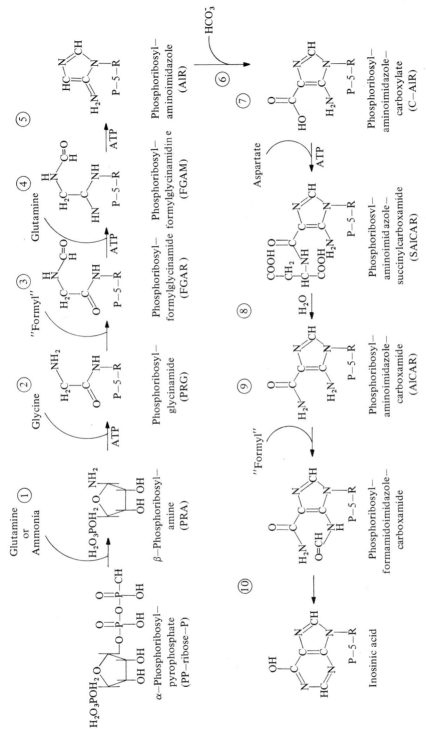

Fig.3. Reactions and intermediates in the pathway of purine biosynthesis de novo

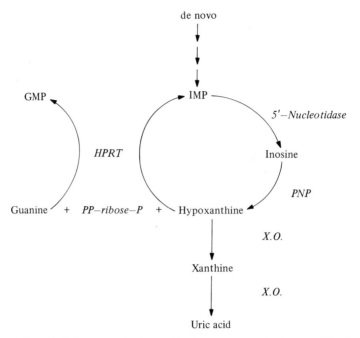

Fig. 4. Interrelationship between purine biosynthesis de novo, purine base reutilization, and uric acid formation

and IMP. Thus, the reaction which controls PRA formation is suitably located to control the entire pathway of purine biosynthesis. (2) In the absence of genetic deletions or chemical blocks of enzymatic reactions the intermediates between PRA and IMP do not accumulate in mammalian cells (BROCKMAN and ANDERSON, 1963; BROCKMAN and CHUMLEY, 1965). Although the experiments cited above were not performed with human cells, the limited data available from studies with human cells are in agreement with these observations. For example, formylglycinamide ribonucleotide (FGAR), the product of the third reaction in the pathway (Fig. 3), does not accumulate in human cells in the absence of a specific inhibitor of FGAR amidotransferase (ROSENBLOOM et al., 1968). Likewise, the product of the fifth reaction, aminoimidazole ribonucleotide, probably does not accumulate in significant quantities, since this could be detected by the appearance of a pink, red, or purple pigment in the cells (SMIRNOV et al., 1967). (3) The activity of glutamine phosphoribosylpyrophosphate (PP-ribose-P) amidotransferase (Fig. 5), the enzyme which catalyzes PRA synthesis, is greater in cells with an increased demand for purines. In extracts from hepatic tumors (KATUNUMA and WEBER, 1974), erythroleukemic cells (REEM and FRIEND, 1975), and human lymphoblasts (HOLMES, unpublished observations), the activity of PP-ribose-P amidotransferase is increased when compared to the activity of this enzyme found in extracts from the nontransformed counterpart of these cells. Derepression of PP-ribose-P amidotransferase has been demonstrated in bacteria when cells are grown in media with limited availability of purines (NIERLICH and MAGASANIK, 1963; MOMOSE et al., 1966). (4) There are many experiments

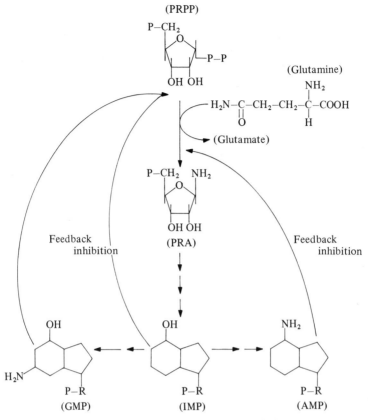

Fig. 5. Role of PP-ribose-P amidotransferase in purine biosynthesis de novo

which indicate that PP-ribose-P may be limiting for purine biosynthesis de novo. Since PP-ribose-P is a substrate for PP-ribose-P amidotransferase (Fig. 5), PRA synthesis would be directly influenced by the availability or concentration of PP-ribose-P. (5) Likewise, there are data which suggest that glutamine availability may be limiting for purine biosynthesis de novo under certain circumstances. This could also be explained by an effect on PP-ribose-P amidotransferase activity and PRA synthesis. (6) PRA synthesis is controlled by the end products of the de novo pathway, purine ribonucleotides. When cells are incubated with purines the rate of purine biosynthesis de novo is reduced, and there is no accumulation of the intermediates in the de novo pathway (WYNGAARDEN et al., 1958). If the source of preformed purine is a nucleoside, such as 6-methylmercaptopurine ribonucleoside (6-MMPR), that is only metabolized to a nucleoside monophosphate, the inhibition of purine biosynthesis de novo is associated with an increase in the concentration of PP-ribose-P (PATERSON and WANG, 1970). This suggests that the block in purine biosynthesis is secondary to inhibition of PP-ribose-P amidotransferase with a resultant decrease in PRA formation (Fig. 5). Direct studies document that human PP-ribose-P amidotransferase is sensitive to feedback inhibition by naturally occurring purine ribonucleotides, such as IMP, AMP, and GMP. The only other enzyme of the de novo pathway which exhibits feedback inhibition is FGAR amidotransferase (reaction 4, Fig. 3), but the concentration of nucleotide required to obtain inhibition is thought to be too high to be of physiologic significance (HOWARD and APPEL, 1968). In addition, FGAR does not accumulate in cells in which purine biosynthesis has been inhibited by the administration of preformed purines (WYNGAARDEN et al., 1958). Thus, the inhibitory effect of nucleotides on purine biosynthesis appears to be exerted at the level of PRA formation. (7) Two cell lines, one yeast (NAGY, 1971) and one mammalian (HENDERSON et al., 1967), have been reported to synthesize purines at an excessive rate due to an alteration in the kinetic properties of PP-ribose-P amidotransferase. In addition, three patients with purine overproduction and increased activity of PP-ribose-P amidotransferase have been described (MARCOLONGO et al., 1974). If confirmed, these data provide strong evidence that the activity of the enzyme catalyzing PRA synthesis is rate-limiting for purine biosynthesis.

The seven points listed above support the hypothesis that PRA synthesis is regulated, and its rate of formation is an important determinant of the rate of purine biosynthesis de novo. This chapter will be restricted to the factors which control PRA synthesis; however, other potential mechanisms for the regulation of purine biosynthesis may be operative. For example, the control of PP-ribose-P synthesis and its utilization in reactions other than PRA formation are clearly important determinants of the rate purine biosynthesis de novo. These topics will not be covered in detail here but will be presented in Chapters 3 and 7.

C. Enzymatic Activities Leading to PRA Synthesis

The preceding discussion has outlined the reasons for assuming that the rate of PRA formation may be limiting for purine biosynthesis. One approach to understanding the control of PRA synthesis is to examine the regulatory properties of the enzyme(s) which catalyzes its formation. In addition to glutamine PP-ribose-P amidotransferase (reaction 1, Table 1), two other activities have been reported to catalyze the synthesis of PRA: PP-ribose-P aminotransferase (reaction 2, Table 1) and ribose-5-phosphate aminotransferase (reaction 3, Table 1) (REEM, 1968; REEM, 1972; REEM, 1974a).

Recent studies have characterized these reactions in a eukaryotic cell line (FELDMAN and TAYLOR, 1975; HOLMES et al., 1976). Extracts from wild-type cells contained all three activities, while a mutant deficient in both PP-ribose-P amidotransferase and PP-ribose-P aminotransferase activities was shown to be auxotrophic for purines (HOLMES et al., 1976). Extracts from the mutant cells exhibited ribose-5-phos-

Table 1. Reactions leading to the synthesis of phosphoribosylamine

PP-ribose-P Amidotransferase	
Glutamine + PP-ribose-P $\longrightarrow$ PRA + PPi + Glutamate	(Reaction #1)
PP-ribose-P Aminotransferase	
NH_3 + PP-ribose-P $\longrightarrow$ PRA + PPi	(Reaction #2)
Ribose-5-phosphate Aminotransferase	
NH_3 + ATP + Ribose-5-phosphate $\longrightarrow$ PRA + PPi + AMP	(Reaction #3)

phate aminotransferase activity comparable to that in extracts from wild-type cells, yet the mutant cells remained auxotrophic even when supplemented with ammonia. Both groups of investigators concluded that ribose-5-phosphate aminotransferase does not play a significant role in PRA and purine biosynthesis in this eukaryotic cell.

The studies of HOLMES et al. establish a role for PP-ribose-P amidotransferase, PP-ribose-P aminotransferase, or both activities in PRA synthesis. The relative contribution of the amidotransferase and aminotransferase activities to purine synthesis in man has not been clearly delineated, but a recent report suggested that 30–60% of the nitrogen used for PRA synthesis might be supplied directly by ammonia (SPERLING et al., 1973). This interpretation is supported by experiments with cultured cells which demonstrate that ammonia, as well as glutamine, can be used for PRA synthesis (HENDERSON, 1963; REEM, 1974b; KING et al., 1977).

It is not clear at this time whether the PP-ribose-P amidotransferase and PP-ribose-P aminotransferase activities are enzymatic functions of one protein or two distinct proteins. The observation that the general category of enzymes called amidotransferases have the potential to use ammonia as well as glutamine for substrate (PRUSINER and STADTMAN, 1973), and in particular, highly purified chicken liver PP-ribose-P amidotransferase uses ammonia as well as glutamine for PRA synthesis (HARTMAN, 1963), suggests that the amidotransferase and aminotransferase activities may be enzymatic functions of the same protein. Additional support for this conclusion can be found in studies with human tissues. In extracts from human placenta the ratio of PP-ribose-P amidotransferase to PP-ribose-P aminotransferase activity is constant in all subcellular fractions, and the two activities coelute and cosediment with a constant specific activity ratio in gel filtration, ion exchange, and sedimentation velocity experiments (KING and HOLMES, 1977). The concurrent loss of both activities in a eukaryotic cell line auxotrophic for purines (HOLMES et al., 1976) and the simultaneous return of both activities in a revertant of this mutant (TAYLOR et al., 1976) further support the hypothesis that the amidotransferase and aminotransferase are enzymatic functions of the same protein.

In contrast to these findings, studies with human lymphoblasts indicate that the PP-ribose-P amidotransferase and PP-ribose-P aminotransferase activities can be separated by gel filtration chromatography (REEM, 1974a). On the one hand, this observation might suggest that the PP-ribose-P amidotransferase and PP-ribose-P aminotransferase activities were enzymatic functions of two distinct proteins, but this is not the only interpretation of these data. It has also been suggested that the aminotransferase activity may be a subunit of the amidotransferase, and dissociation of the native enzyme, amidotransferase, leads to the formation of a smaller aminotransferase (REEM, 1974a). This explanation is supported by the demonstration that several other enzymes of the amidotransferase category are composed of aminotransferase subunits (PRUSINER and STADTMAN, 1973). If this latter hypothesis were accepted, all of the data could be accomodated by the following explanation: one protein, PP-ribose-P amidotransferase, functions either as an amidotransferase or aminotransferase depending on the available nitrogen source. Although this is an unresolved question at the present time, we will accept the hypothesis that one protein catalyzes PRA synthesis in eukaryotic cells and refer to this enzyme as PP-ribose-P amidotransferase during the remainder of this discussion.

D. Properties of Human PP-ribose-P Amidotransferase

Table 2 lists some of the kinetic properties of human PP-ribose-P amidotransferase. The range of $S_{0.5}$ values for PP-ribose-P is 0.1–0.48 mM (WOOD and SEEGMILLER, 1973; HOLMES et al., 1973a; REEM, 1974a). Although the PP-ribose-P concentration is not known in human liver, a major site of purine synthesis, the concentration in human red blood cells (0.002–0.007 mM), white blood cells (0.005 mM), and fibroblasts (0.013 mM) has been determined (KELLEY et al., 1970a, b; FOX and KELLEY, 1971; BECKER, 1976a; BROSH et al., 1976). In rodent liver the concentration is estimated to range from 0.01 to 0.015 mM (CLIFFORD et al., 1972; LALANNE and HENDERSON, 1975). In cells obtained from patients with a deficiency of hypoxanthine-guanine phosphoribosyltransferase (HPRT) or overactivity of PP-ribose-P synthetase, the concentration of PP-ribose-P is increased two to 20 fold (FOX and KELLEY, 1971; BECKER, 1976a). Thus, it appears that the concentration of PP-ribose-P in normal cells is below the apparent K_m of amidotransferase for this substrate. This enzyme may not be saturated with PP-ribose-P, even in pathologic states where the PP-ribose-P concentration is markedly increased. Consequently, an increase or decrease in the concentration of PP-ribose-P could lead to an alteration in PRA and purine synthesis.

The effect of PP-ribose-P concentration on the activity of amidotransferase is more complex than might be appreciated from the preceding discussion. Since the substrate-velocity plot for PP-ribose-P is sigmoidal (WOOD and SEEGMILLER, 1973; HOLMES et al., 1973a; KOVARSKY et al., 1977), there is not a hyperbolic relationship between enzyme activity and PP-ribose-P concentration. As a consequence, relatively small changes in the concentration of PP-ribose-P can produce relatively large changes in the activity of amidotransferase. This allosteric property of amidotransferase provides a sensitive mechanism for altering the rate of PRA synthesis in response to small changes in the concentration of PP-ribose-P.

The $S_{0.5}$ of human PP-ribose-P amidotransferase for glutamine is also included in Table 2. The apparent K_m for glutamine ranges from 1.0 to 1.6 mM (WOOD and SEEGMILLER, 1973; HOLMES et al., 1973a; REEM, 1974a). In contrast to the results obtained with PP-ribose-P, the substrate-velocity plot for glutamine is hyperbolic under all conditions studied, and there is no evidence for cooperativity in the binding of this substrate (WOOD and SEEGMILLER, 1973; HOLMES et al., 1973a, KING and HOLMES, 1977).

The concentration of glutamine in human liver is not known, but the concentration in plasma ranges from 0.5 to 0.7 mM (SEGAL and WYNGAARDEN, 1955; YU et al.,

Table 2. Kinetic properties of human PP-ribose-P amidotransferase

Substrate	k_m or $S_{0.5}$	Hill coefficient
PP-ribose-P	0.1–0.48 mM	1.8–2.7[a]
Glutamine	1.0–1.6 mM	1.0
Ammonia	2.0–3.8 mM	1.4

[a] A value of 1.8 is obtained in the absence of phosphate, and this falls to 1.0 in the presence of 50 mM phosphate.

1969; PAGLIARA and GOODMAN, 1969). In rodent liver the glutamine concentration has been reported to vary from less than 1 mM to greater than 7 mM (WILLIAMSON et al., 1967; WALSER et al., 1973; BERGMEYER, 1974). This range of glutamine concentrations extends below the K_m of human PP-ribose-P amidotransferase for this substrate. If a similar range of glutamine concentrations were found in human liver, as well as in other cells, alterations in the concentration of this amino acid could lead to changes in PRA and purine synthesis.

As pointed out earlier, there is evidence to suggest that a significant proportion of the nitrogen used for PRA synthesis in man is derived directly from ammonia (SPERLING et al., 1973). Table 2 also lists the kinetic properties of human PP-ribose-P amidotransferase which concern NH_3 utilization (REEM, 1974a; KING and HOLMES, 1977). The intracellular concentration of NH_3 in human liver is not known, but the concentration of total ammonia (NH_3 plus NH_4^+) in rodent liver is approximately 0.7 mM (BROSNAN, 1976). Of the total ammonia approximately 1/75 will be present as NH_3 at pH 7.4. Unlike glutamine, NH_3 demonstrates cooperativity in its binding (Hill coefficient, Table 2) (KING and HOLMES, 1977), and this allosteric property provides a mechanism by which the enzyme may efficiently utilize NH_3 when the concentration of this substrate is considerably below the $S_{0.5}$. Furthermore, if the enzyme is saturated with glutamine, PRA synthesis can be increased even further when NH_3 is included in the assay (KING and HOLMES, 1977). Thus, the kinetic properties of amidotransferase suggest that this enzyme may use NH_3 as a substrate at relatively low concentrations and in the presence of saturating concentrations of glutamine.

Amidotransferase activity is not only controlled by the availability of its substrates, but the concentrations of purine ribonucleotides also regulate the activity of this enzyme. The first direct demonstration of feedback inhibition of PP-ribose-P amidotransferase was reported in 1959 with an enzyme preparation obtained from pigeon liver (WYNGAARDEN and ASHTON, 1959). Subsequent studies have demonstrated that the human enzyme is also sensitive to feedback inhibition by purine ribonucleotides (WOOD and SEEGMILLER, 1973; HOLMES et al., 1973a, b; REEM, 1974a). The purine nucleoside monophosphate is a more potent inhibitor than the diphosphate, and the diphosphate is a more potent inhibitor than the triphosphate (HOLMES et al., 1973a). As originally noted with pigeon liver amidotransferase (CASKEY et al., 1964), the combination of a 6-hydroxy (GMP or IMP) and a 6-amino (AMP) purine ribonucleotide produces synergistic inhibition of the human enzyme (HOLMES et al., 1973a). Synergistic inhibition suggests an interaction between nucleotide binding sites, and this has been confirmed in other studies by demonstrating cooperativity in nucleotide binding (KOVARSKY et al., 1977).

Several lines of evidence suggest an allosteric mechanism for the feedback inhibition produced by purine ribonucleotides. In partially purified preparations of the human (HOLMES et al., 1973a), as well as the pigeon liver (CASKEY et al., 1964) enzyme, inhibition by nucleotides may be lost while catalytic activity is preserved. This suggests that the purine ribonucleotides bind at a site topologically distinct from the catalytic site. In addition, purine ribonucleotides produce a qualitative change in the kinetics of the reaction catalyzed by amidotransferase (HOLMES et al., 1973a). As shown in Figure 6, the inhibition produced by purine ribonucleotides is associated with a shift from a hyperbolic to a sigmoidal substrate-velocity plot for

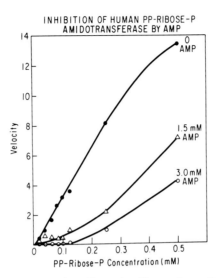

Fig. 6. Effect of PP-ribose-P and purine ribonucleotide on the activity of human PP-ribose-P amidotransferase

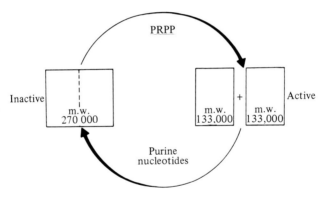

Fig. 7. Model for control of human PP-ribose-P amidotransferase by PP-ribose-P and purine ribonucleotides

PP-ribose-P. This is a common property of many allosteric enzymes, and it indicates an interaction between the nucleotide and catalytic sites of the enzyme. The importance of this interaction in the control of PRA synthesis can be readily appreciated from Figure 6. When the concentration of purine ribonucleotide is increased there is an abrupt decrease in enzyme activity. On the other hand, the inhibition produced by purine ribonucleotide can be overcome by increasing the concentration of PP-ribose-P.

The molecular basis for these opposing actions of PP-ribose-P and purine ribonucleotides has been elucidated by other studies (HOLMES et al., 1973 b). Two forms of human PP-ribose-P amidotransferase have been identified: a small form with a molecular weight of 133000 and a large form with a molecular weight of 270000. The small form is converted to the large form by incubation with purine ribonucleotides, and the large form is converted to the small form by incubation with PP-ribose-P. Furthermore, catalytic activity is closely correlated with the amount of amidotransferase present in the small form relative to that in the large form. A model illustrating these findings is shown in Figure 7. With increments in the concentration of PP-ribose-P, there is shift from the large catalytically inactive to the small catalytically active form of the enzyme; with increments in the concentration of purine ribonucleotide, there is a shift from the active to the inactive form. This model provides a molecular basis for explaining the opposing actions of PP-ribose-P and purine ribonucleotides on PRA synthesis. It may also explain how alterations in the concentrations of PP-ribose-P and purine ribonucleotides produce changes in the rate of purine biosynthesis de novo.

E. Studies with Intact Cells

The preceding section has reviewed in vitro studies pertaining to the regulatory properties of the enzyme which catalyzes PRA synthesis. The next section will review studies relating to the control of PRA and purine synthesis in intact cells. Before presenting these data, it may be helpful to explain the methods which have been used to assess the rate of PRA and purine biosynthesis de novo in intact cells. Due to the lability of PRA this compound cannot be directly quantified in extracts from cells. However, the third intermediate of the pathway, formylglycinamide ribonucleotide (FGAR), is stable, and it accumulates within the cell when the fourth reaction of the de novo pathway is blocked with the glutamine analogue azaserine (Fig. 3). The concentration of azaserine employed in these studies selectively blocks the fourth but not the first reaction in the de novo pathway. FGAR production is quantified by introducing a radiolabel into this compound at the second (^{14}C-glycine) or the third reaction (^{14}C-formate). Assuming that FGAR production is dependent on the rate of PRA synthesis, the FGAR assay is a reasonable approximation of the rate of PRA synthesis within the cell. Another method commonly used for assessing the rate of purine biosynthesis de novo is quantification of the rate of incorporation of one of the above isotopes into nucleic acids, nucleotides, nucleosides, and bases. The latter method has the advantage of not introducing a block in the pathway and interrupting the synthesis of purine ribonucleotides, which might produce feedback inhibition.

Our understanding of the control of purine biosynthesis in human cells has been aided by the identification of several inherited disorders of purine metabolism in man. With the appreciation of abnormalities in specific enzymatic reactions, it has been possible to better define the importance of certain metabolites in the regulation of this pathway. For example, the description of HPRT deficiency in patients with the Lesch-Nyhan Syndrome played a critical role in establishing the importance of PP-ribose-P in the control of purine biosynthesis (SEEGMILLER et al., 1967; ROSENBLOOM et al., 1968). The concentration of PP-ribose-P is increased four to five fold in skin fibroblasts from these patients, and the cells exhibit increased rates of purine biosynthesis de novo (ROSENBLOOM et al., 1968). Numerous reports have confirmed that PP-ribose-P concentrations are elevated in erythrocytes, white blood cells, lymphoblasts, neural cells, and hepatic cells which are deficient in HPRT catalytic activity (these studies are reviewed in Chapter 3). In those cells capable of synthesizing purines de novo, the deficiency of HPRT is associated with an increase in the rate of purine biosynthesis. Thus, these observations establish a direct correlation between the concentration of PP-ribose-P and the rate of purine biosynthesis de novo. The mechanism responsible for the increase in PP-ribose-P concentration in HPRT deficient cells is less clear, however. ROSENBLOOM et al. demonstrated that PP-ribose-P was generated at a normal rate in these cells and proposed that the increased concentration was the result of decreased utilization in the HPRT reaction (Fig. 4). Subsequently, increased activity of PP-ribose-P synthetase has been described in cells deficient in HPRT, and it has been proposed that increased activity of this enzyme leads to increased production of PP-ribose-P (REEM, 1975; MARTIN and MALER, 1976). The relative importance of each of these mechanisms remains to be clarified in future studies.

The correlation between PP-ribose-P concentration and the rate of purine biosynthesis has been confirmed in patients with other inherited abnormalities of purine metabolism. Cells from individuals with increased activity of PP-ribose-P synthetase have increased concentrations of PP-ribose-P and exhibit increased rates of purine biosynthesis de novo (SPERLING et al., 1972; BECKER, 1973). In these individuals overactivity of PP-ribose-P synthetase is the primary defect, and there is no associated decrease in HPRT activity. In addition to this mutation, fibroblast cell lines from two patients have been reported to have increased PP-ribose-P concentrations and increased rates of purine biosynthesis de novo with normal activities of PP-ribose-P synthetase and HPRT (BECKER, 1976 a). These cells had increased concentrations of ribose-5-phosphate, and it was postulated that the increased availability of this substrate led to increased synthesis of PP-ribose-P.

The concentration of PP-ribose-P within the cell can be increased by other means as well. Following the incubation of human fibroblasts and leukocytes with methylene blue, the concentration of PP-ribose-P is increased (BROSH et al., 1976), and the rate of purine biosynthesis de novo is also accelerated (KELLEY et al., 1970b; BROSH et al., 1976). It has been demonstrated that incubation of human erythrocytes with methylene blue stimulates the oxidative pentose pathway and increases the production of ribose-5-phosphate (HERSHKO et al., 1969). The increase in ribose-5-phosphate may lead to an increase in PP-ribose-P synthesis under appropriate conditions. However, the physiologic importance of an increase in ribose-5-phosphate concentration in purine overproduction has been questioned, since this effect of methylene blue can only be demonstrated at high concentrations of inorganic phosphate (HERSHKO et al., 1969). Furthermore, in experiments with patients the administration of methylene blue does not lead to an increase in the erythrocyte concentration of PP-ribose-P (FOX and KELLEY, 1971).

In addition to methylene blue, the intracellular concentration of PP-ribose-P can be increased in human leukocytes by incubation of the cells with inorganic phosphate (BROSH et al., 1976). In these studies the increase in PP-ribose-P concentration was associated with an acceleration in the rate of purine biosynthesis de novo. Thus, these data provide further documentation of the correlation between PP-ribose-P concentration and the rate of purine biosynthesis.

The converse of the above findings can also be demonstrated. When the PP-ribose-P concentration is reduced, there is a concomitant reduction in the rate of purine biosynthesis de novo. Many studies have demonstrated that cells incubated with purine bases, or analogs of these bases, decrease their rate of purine biosynthesis in association with a decrease in the concentration of PP-ribose-P (Fox and KELLEY, 1971). However, these studies are somewhat difficult to interpret, since incubation with purine bases also leads to an increase in the concentration of purine ribonucleotides, and this could result in an increase in feedback inhibition of PP-ribose-P amidotransferase. In an attempt to avoid this ambiguity, human fibroblasts have been incubated with pyrimidine bases. This maneuver also produces a concomitant reduction in the concentration of PP-ribose-P and the rate of purine biosynthesis (KELLEY et al., 1970). However, human PP-ribose-P amidotransferase is sensitive to inhibition by pyrimidine nucleotides, as well as purine ribonucleotides (HOLMES et al., 1973a).

The data presented in the preceding paragraphs document a direct correlation between the rate of purine biosynthesis and the intracellular concentration of PP-ribose-P under a variety of genetic and metabolic conditions in human cells. These results indicate that the concentration of PP-ribose-P is limiting for PRA and purine biosynthesis under the conditions studied and suggest that amidotransferase may not be saturated with this substrate. This conclusion is supported by the in vitro kinetic data obtained with human PP-ribose-P amidotransferase and the kinetic properties of amidotransferase assessed intracellularly in EHRLICH ascites tumor cells (BAGNARA et al., 1974a).

While the observations described above clearly indicate a role for PP-ribose-P in the control of purine biosynthesis, other studies suggest that additional factors may be important in the regulation of this pathway. For example, the decrease in purine biosynthesis which results from incubation of cells with purine bases could be the result of a decrease in the concentration of PP-ribose-P or an increase in the concentration of purine ribonucleosides with resultant feedback inhibition. As already pointed out, it is difficult to determine the relative importance of each of these mechanisms in mediating the inhibitory effect of purine bases. In fact, it may be a combination of both mechanisms that leads to the decrease in purine biosynthesis following incubation of cells with purine bases. This dual effect of purine bases can be avoided by incubating cells with a purine nucleoside that is not catabolized to a purine base but is phosphorylated to a purine ribonucleotide. Under these conditions, it is possible to study the effect of an increase in the concentration of purine ribonucleotide without a concomitant decrease in the concentration of PP-ribose-P. 6-Methylmercaptopurine ribonucleoside (6-MMPR), an adenosine analogue, is suitable for such experiments, since phosphorolysis has not been demonstrated but phosphorylation has (CALDWELL et al., 1966; HENDERSON et al., 1967; HERSHFIELD and SEEGMILLER, 1976). Following the incubation of EHRLICH ascites tumor cells (HENDERSON, 1963b), human fibroblasts (HENDERSON et al., 1968; ROSENBLOOM et al., 1968), and human lymphoblasts (HERSHFIELD and SEEGMILLER, 1976) with 6-MMPR, purine biosynthesis is markedly inhibited. If this decrease in purine synthesis were the result of feedback inhibition of PP-ribose-P amidotransferase by 6-methylmercaptopurine ribonucleotide, one would anticipate that the concentration of PP-ribose-P might increase, while the concentration of adenine and guanine nucleotides might fall. In cells exposed to 6-MMPR the concentration of PP-ribose-P is elevated as much as 20 fold (PATERSON and WANG, 1970), and the concentrations of adenine and guanine nucleotides are decreased (SCHOLAR et al., 1972). The increase in PP-ribose-P concentration is particularly important, because it localizes the point of inhibition to the reaction catalyzed by amidotransferase, and it dissociates the inhibition produced by purines from a decrease in the concentration of PP-ribose-P. Thus, these experiments with intact cells demonstrate a role for feedback inhibition of PP-ribose-P amidotransferase by purine ribonucleotides in the control of this pathway.

Regulation of purine biosynthesis by the mechanism of feedback inhibition can also be demonstrated by studying mutant cells in which there is an alteration in the kinetic properties of PP-ribose-P amidotransferase, rendering it less sensitive to inhibition by purine ribonucleotides. Cells from such a mutant should synthesize purines at an excessive rate when the medium is supplemented with a source of preformed purines. To date, a feedback-resistant amidotransferase has not been identified in human cells, but a mutant derived from an EHRLICH ascites line has been shown to synthesize purines at an accelerated rate when incubated with gua-nine and 6-MMPR (HENDERSON et al., 1967). Purine transport, nucleotide synthesis, and catabolism were all normal in the mutant cells. Although direct quantification of amidotransferase activity in the presence of purine ribonucleotides was not per-formed, the authors concluded that the mechanism responsible for purine overpro-duction in these cells was resistance of amidotransferase to feedback inhibition by purine ribonucleotides. A mutant of S. pombe has also been reported to synthesize purines at an excessive rate in the presence of 8-azaguanine, and in this case the genetic locus responsible for the abnormality in purine metabolism mapped very close to that for PP-ribose-P amidotransferase (HESLOT et al., 1966; NAGY, 1971). In addition, direct assay of PP-ribose-P amidotransferase in extracts from the mutant cells demonstrated that this enzyme was less sensitive to inhibition by IMP and GMP (NAGY, 1970). Thus, these studies with mutant cells provide further support for the physiologic importance of feedback inhibition of amidotransferase in the regula-tion of purine biosynthesis.

In experiments cited thus far, alterations in the concentration of PP-ribose-P, purine ribonucleotide, or both compounds provide an adequate explanation for observed changes in the rate of purine biosynthesis. However, in other studies it is more difficult to be certain of the mechanism responsible for the observed changes in purine synthesis. For example, incubation of human fibroblasts with inosine leads to a reduction in the rate of purine biosynthesis in both normal and HPRT-deficient cells (BECKER, 1976b). PP-ribose-P concentration is increased in both cell lines fol-lowing incubation with inosine, probably as a consequence of the increase in ribose-5-phosphate production from ribose-1-phosphate upon phosphorolysis of inosine. In normal cells incubated with inosine, there is also an increase in the intracellular concentration of purine ribonucleotide, and this may explain the observed reduction in purine synthesis. However, in HPRT deficient cells the concentration of purine ribonucleotide is not detectably increased, yet there is a small decrease in the rate of purine biosynthesis. While it is possible that a small increase in nucleotide concen-tration was not detected in the HPRT-deficient cells due to current technology, the results of this study leave open the possibility that factors other than PP-ribose-P and purine ribonucleotide concentration may play a role in the regulation of purine biosynthesis. Studies with EHRLICH ascites tumor cells have also demonstrated that multiple mechanisms may exist for the regulation of purine biosynthesis (BAGNARA et al., 1974 b).

Another factor which may be important in the control of purine biosynthesis is the availability of a nitrogen source for PRA synthesis. This has proved to be a difficult hypothesis to test in tissue culture experiments for several reasons. First, the human cells most often grown in culture, fibroblasts and lymphoblasts, do not synthesize appreciable amounts of glutamine; consequently, it is not possible to determine with these cells whether the "normal" intracellular concentration of glutamine is limiting for PRA and purine biosynthesis. Second, fibroblasts and lymphoblasts are not capable of synthesizing urea, and in the absence of this pathway it is difficult to interpret the effects of variation in the extracellular concentration of ammonia on purine biosynthesis. Third, no genetic abnormalities in nitrogen metabolism that lead to an alteration in glutamine or ammonia concentration have been identified in eukaryotic cells presently available for culture. Hopefully these problems can be overcome when the methodology for growing hepatocytes has advanced sufficiently to permit studies with these cells. Evaluation of purine biosynthesis in hepatocytes from normal subjects as well as patients with increased glutamine and ammonia concentrations may shed some light on the role of these nitrogen sources in the control of purine biosynthesis.

Alterations in glutamine and ammonia concentration may influence the rate of purine biosynthesis through factors other than nitrogen availability. For example, reduction of the glutamine concentration has been reported to reduce the availability of PP-ribose-P in human lymphoblasts (SKAPER et al., 1976).

After considering the studies reviewed in this section, one is led to the conclusion that both the concentration of PP-ribose-P and purine ribonucleotide are important determinants of the rate of purine biosynthesis de novo in human cells. The effect of these two factors on purine synthesis may be explained at the molecular level by their opposing actions on PP-ribose-P amidotransferase activity. The role of other factors, such as glutamine and ammonia availability in the control of purine biosynthesis, are less well defined, and their importance will have to be established in future experiments.

F. Studies In Vivo

Our current understanding of the control of purine biosynthesis at the enzymatic and cellular levels owes a great deal to observations originally made in patients with disorders of purine metabolism. It is difficult to single out any one study, but the identification of the enzymatic defect in patients with the Lesch-Nyhan Syndrome has probably done more than any other to enhance our understanding of the control of purine biosynthesis in man (SEEGMILLER et al., 1967). The flagrant overproduction of uric acid in these patients is the consequence of a deficiency in HPRT catalytic activity (Fig.4). The increase in purine biosynthesis de novo observed in these patients is associated with an increase in the intracellular concentration of PP-ribose-P (ROSENBLOOM et al., 1968). The correlation between the concentration of PP-ribose-P and the rate of purine biosynthesis has been confirmed on numerous occasions in other patients with HPRT deficiency, and this observation is one of the strongest arguments in support of the hypothesis that the concentration of PP-ribose-P is important in the control of purine biosynthesis in vivo. Additional support for this hypothesis has been provided by studies in another group of gouty patients who exhibited excessive rates of purine biosynthesis and elevated intracellular concentrations of PP-ribose-P due to an increase in the activity of PP-ribose-P synthetase (SPERLING et al., 1972; BECKER et al., 1973). (The reader is referred to Chapters 3 and 4 of this volume for a more detailed discussion of these enzymatic abnormalities).

The association between PP-ribose-P concentration and purine overproduction is well established in patients with a deficiency of HPRT and increased activity of PP-ribose-P synthetase. Less well understood is the relationship between PP-ribose-P concentration and purine metabolism in other subtypes of gout. It has been suggested that individuals with glucose-6-phosphatase deficiency, Type I glycogen storage disease, synthesize purines at an excessive rate because of increased production of ribose-5-phosphate and PP-ribose-P via increased metabolism of glucose-6-phosphate by the hexose monophosphate shunt (HOWELL, 1968). This hypothesis is supported by the demonstration that human fibroblasts, which contain increased concentrations of ribose-5-phosphate, have increased concentrations of PP-ribose-P and exhibit increased rates of purine biosynthesis de novo (BECKER, 1976a). Although elevated concentrations of PP-ribose-P were not found in erythrocytes from individuals with glucose-6-phosphatase deficiency (GREENE and SEEGMILLER, 1969), other tissues may contain increased concentrations of this metabolite, since there is a poor correlation between PP-ribose-P concentration in erythrocytes and other cells (EMMERSON and WYNGAARDEN, 1969; BECKER, 1976a).

A similar mechanism has also been proposed to explain the association between hyperuricemia and increased activity of glutathione reductase (LANG, 1970). In these individuals, it has been suggested that the increased activity of glutathione reductase leads to increased production of NADP, with a resultant stimulation of the hexose monophosphate shunt. However, in the latter group of patients it was not shown that these individuals overproduce purines, nor that the increase in glutathione reductase activity was primary rather than secondary to dietary factors, which are known to alter the activity of this enzyme (BEUTLER, 1966).

There is another clinical situation that suggests that purine overproduction is associated with an increase in the concentration of PP-ribose-P. When 2-ethylamino-1,3,4-thiadiazole (EA-TDA) is administered to patients, there is a striking increase in the rate of purine biosynthesis de novo (SEEGMILLER et al., 1963). Since EA-TDA produces a marked increase in mouse hepatocyte concentration of PP-ribose-P (LALANE and HENDERSON, 1975), it has been suggested that this may be the mechanism by which EA-TDA increases the rate of purine biosynthesis in man.

While the data obtained from patients with inherited disorders of purine metabolism and drug-induced purine overproduction indicate that the concentration of PP-ribose-P plays an important role in the control of purine biosynthesis, it has been more difficult to unambiguously demonstrate feedback inhibition by nucleotides in the control of purine biosynthesis in patients. As discussed in the section on studies with intact cells, the administration of purine bases, or analogues such as allopurinol, may produce a decrease in purine biosynthesis for two reasons; it is difficult to distinguish between the relative importance of these two mechanisms. With cells grown in culture it is possible to separate the effect of PP-ribose-P depletion from that of an increase in the concentration of purine ribonucleotide by administering a nucleoside analogue, 6-MMPR, which is metabolized only to a nucleotide. Similar studies have not been performed in man because of the toxicity produced by this drug (HENDERSON, 1972), but in mice the rate of purine biosynthesis is reduced following the administration of 6-MMPR (HENDERSON and MERCER, 1966).

There has been no description of a mutant form of PP-ribose-P amidotransferase that is less sensitive to feedback inhibition in patients with gout. Originally, it was proposed that resistance to feedback inhibition might be the mechanism responsible for the increased rate of purine biosynthesis observed in fibroblasts from two patients with gout (HENDERSON et al., 1968), but more recent studies have shown that the primary defect in one of these patients was increased activity of PP-ribose-P synthetase (BECKER et al., 1973). Increased activity of PP-ribose-P amidotransferase has been noted in WBC lysates from three patients with gout (MARCOLONGO et al., 1974), but the mechanism responsible for this increase in activity has not been determined. Future studies into the kinetic properties of amidotransferase from these patients and other gouty subjects may provide examples of a feedback-resistant mutant. One might predict that a feedback resistant mutant may be found, since two eukaryotic cell lines with such a mutation of amidotransferase overproduce purines (HENDERSON et al., 1967; NAGY, 1970).

There are data which indirectly suggest that glutamine and/or ammonia availability may be limiting for purine biosynthesis in man. In normal subjects on a purine-free diet, a six- to eight-fold increase in nitrogen intake results in a three-to four-fold increase in the daily excretion of uric acid (CALLOWAY and MARGEN, 1968; BOWERING et al., 1970). In the study of BOWERING et al. uric acid turnover was also quantified, and the increase in nitrogen intake and uric acid excretion was associated with 200% increase in uric acid turnover. These results suggested that the increase in uric acid excretion was a consequence of an increase in the rate of purine biosynthesis. Isotope-incorporation studies have confirmed this by demonstrating a 45% increase in [^{15}N]glycine labeling of uric acid when nitrogen intake was doubled in one normal and one gouty subject (BIEN et al., 1953). The mechanism responsible for this increase in purine biosynthesis has not been established, but it has been suggested that the increase in nitrogen intake leads to an increase in glutamine and/or ammonia availability. This hypothesis is supported by the demonstration of increased uric acid excretion in patients receiving glutamine or ammonia (BORSOOK and KEIGHLEY, 1935). However, these studies have been criticized because potential changes in the renal clearance of uric acid were not evaluated. Isotope incorporation techniques have not been utilized in man to evaluate purine biosynthesis following the administration of glutamine or ammonia, but in rodents [^{14}C]glycine incorporation into purine is accelerated 1.7–2.5 fold by the administration of glutamine and ammonia (FEIGELSON and FEIGELSON, 1966). Additional studies are needed to determine whether gouty subjects differ from normal individuals with respect to the influence of nitrogen metabolism on purine biosynthesis. As originally suggested by BENEDICT et al., gouty man may retain more of his evolutionary uricotelic vestige than his nongouty counterpart (BENEDICT et al., 1952).

G. Conclusion

This chapter has reviewed studies performed with isolated enzyme systems, with cells grown in culture, and in patients with disorders of purine metabolism. Based on the data obtained from these studies, it seems justified to conclude that the concentration of PP-ribose-P and purine ribonucleotides are important determinants of the rate of purine biosynthesis in human cells. These compounds exert opposing influences on this pathway: an increase in the concentration of PP-ribose-P leads to an increase in the rate of purine biosynthesis, while an increase in the concentration of purine ribonucleotide leads to a decrease in the rate of purine biosynthesis. The molecular basis for these opposing actions of PP-ribose-P and purine ribonucleotides may be explained by their allosteric effects on human PP-ribose-P amidotransferase. Thus, those factors which control PP-ribose-P amidotransferase activity and PRA production appear to be important in the control of purine biosynthesis. Data were also reviewed that suggested that glutamine or ammonia availability may be limiting for purine biosynthesis under certain conditions. Future studies may identify additional factors which alter the rate of PRA synthesis, and these may in turn prove to be important in the control of purine biosynthesis.

References

Bagnara,A.S., Brox,L.W., Henderson,J.F.: Kinetics of amidophosphoribosyltransferase in intact tumor cells. Biochim. biophys. Acta (Amst.) **350**, 171—182 (1974a)

Bagnara,A.S., Letter,A.A., Henderson,J.F.: Multiple mechanisms of regulation of purine biosynthesis de novo in intact tumor cells. Biochim. biophys. Acta (Amst.) **374**, 259—270 (1974b)

Becker,M.A.: Patterns of phosphoribosylpyrophosphate and ribose-5-phosphate concentration and generation in fibroblasts from patients with gout and purine overproduction. J. clin. Invest. **57**, 308—318 (1976a)

Becker,M.A.: Regulation of purine nucleotide synthesis. Effects of inosine on normal and hypoxanthine-guanine phosphoribosyltransferase deficient fibroblasts. Biochim. biophys. Acta (Amst.) **435**, 132—144 (1976b)

Becker,M.A., Meyer,L.J., Wood,A.W., Seegmiller,J.E.: Purine overproduction in man associated with increased phosphoribosylpyrophosphate synthetase activity. Science **179**, 1123—1126 (1973)

Benedict,J.D., Roche,M., Yu,T.-F., Bein,E.J., Gutman,A.B., Stetten,D., Jr.: Incorporation of glycine nitrogen into uric acid in normal and gouty man. Metabolism **1**, 3—12 (1952)

Bergmeyer,H.U.: Methods of Enzymatic Analysis, 2nd Ed. New York: Acad. Pr. 1974

Beutler,E.: Effect of riboflavin compounds on glutathione reductase activity. In vivo and in vitro studies. J. clin. Invest. **48**, 1957—1966 (1966)

Bien,E.J., Yu,T.-F., Benedict,J.O., Gutman,A.B., Stetten,D., Jr.: The relation of dietary nitrogen consumption to the rate of uric acid synthesis in normal and gouty man. J. clin. Invest. **32**, 778—780 (1953)

Borsook,H., Keighley,G.L.: The "continuing" metabolism of nitrogen in animals. Proc. roy. Soc. **B 118**, 488—521 (1935)

Bowering,J., Calloway,D.H., Margen,S., Kaufman,N.A.: Dietary protein level and uric acid metabolism in normal man. J. Nutr. **100**, 249—261 (1970)

Brockman,R.W., Anderson,E.P.: Biochemistry of cancer. Ann. Rev. Biochem. **32**, 463—512 (1963)

Brockman,R.W., Chumley,S.W.: Inhibition of formylglycinamide ribonucleotide synthesis in neoplastic cells by purines and analogs. Biochem. Biophys. Acta **95**, 365—379 (1965)

Brosh,S., Boer,P., Kupper,B., Vries,A. de, Sperling,O.: De novo synthesis of purine nucleotides in human peripheral blood leukocytes. J. Clin. Invest. **58**, 289—297 (1976)

Brosnan,J.T.: Factors affecting intracellular ammonia concentrations in liver. In: Grisolia,S., Bagvena,R., Mayor,F. (Eds.): The Urea Cycle. New York: John Wiley and Sons 1976

Caldwell,I.C., Henderson,J.F., Paterson,A.R.P.: The enzymatic formation of 6-methylmercaptopurine ribonucleoside phosphate. Canad. J. Biochem. **44**, 229—245 (1966)

Calloway,D.H., Margen,S.: Human response to diets very high in protein. Fed. Proc. **27**, 725a (1968)

Caskey, C. T., Ashton, D. M., Wyngaarden, J. B.: The enzymology of feedback inhibition of glutamine phosphoribosylpyrophosphate amidotransferase by purine ribonucleotides. J. biol. Chem. **239**, 2570—2579 (1964)

Clifford, A. S., Riumallo, J. A., Baliga, B. S.: Liver nucleotide metabolism in relation to amino acid supply. Biochim. biophys. Acta (Amst.) **277**, 443—458 (1972)

Emmerson, B. T., Wyngaarden, J. B.: Purine metabolism in heterozygous carriers of hypoxanthine-guanine phosphoribosyltransferase deficiency. Science **166**, 1533—1535 (1969)

Feigelson, M., Feigelson, P.: Relationships between hepatic enzyme induction, glutamate formation and purine nucleotide biosynthesis in gluco-corticoid action. J. biol. Chem. **241**, 5819—5826 (1966)

Feldman, R. I., Taylor, M W.: Purine mutants of mammalian cell lines. II. Identification of a phosphoribosylpyrophosphate amidotransferase deficient mutant of Chinese hamster lung cells. Biochem. Genet. **13**, 227—234 (1975)

Fox, I. H., Kelley, W. N.: Phosphoribosylpyrophosphate in man: biochemical and clinical significance. Ann. intern. Med. **74**, 424—433 (1971)

Greene, M. L., Seegmiller, J. E.: Elevated erythrocyte phosphoribosylpyrophosphate in x-linked uric acid: Importance of PRPP concentration in the regulation of human purine biosynthesis. J. clin. Invest. **48**, 32 a (1969)

Gutman, A. B., Yu, T.-F., Black, H.: Incorporation of glycine-1-C^{14} and glycine-N^{15} into uric acid in normal and gouty subjects. Amer. J. Med. **25**, 917—932 (1958)

Hartman, S. C.: Phosphoribosylpyrophosphate amidotransferase: purification and general catalytic properties. J. biol. Chem. **238**, 3024—3035 (1963)

Henderson, J. F.: Dual effects of ammonium chloride on purine biosynthesis de novo in Ehrlich ascites tumor cells in vitro. Biochim. biophys. Acta (Amst.) **76**, 173—180 (1963 a).

Henderson, J. F.: Feedback inhibition of purine biosynthesis in ascites tumor cells by purine analogs. Biochem. Pharmacol. **12**, 551—556 (1963 b)

Henderson, J. F.: Pathological abnormalities of purine biosynthesis de novo. In: Regulation of Purine Biosynthesis de Novo. Monograph 170, p. 254. Washington, D.C. (1972)

Henderson, J. F., Caldwell, I. C., Paterson, A. R. P.: Decreased feedback inhibition in a 6-methyl-mercaptopurine ribonucleoside resistant tumor. Cancer Res. **27**, 1773—1778 (1967)

Henderson, J. F., Mercer, N. J. H.: Feedback inhibition of purine biosynthesis de novo in mouse tissue in vivo. Nature (Lond.) **212**, 507—508 (1966)

Henderson, J. F., Rosenbloom, F. M., Kelley, W. N., Seegmiller, J. E.: Variations in purine metabolism of cultured skin fibroblast from patients with gout. J. clin. Invest. **47**, 1511—1516 (1968)

Hershfield, M. S., Seegmiller, J. E.: Regulation of de novo purine biosynthesis in human lymphoblasts. J. biol. Chem. **251**, 7348—7354 (1976)

Hershfield, M. S., Seegmiller, J. E.: Regulation of de novo purine synthesis in human lymphoblasts. Advanc. exp. Med. (in press) (1977)

Hershko, A., Razin, A., Mager, J.: Regulation of the synthesis of 5-phosphoribosyl-1-pyrophosphate in intact red blood cells and in cell free preparations. Biochim. biophys. Acta (Amst.) **184**, 64—76 (1969)

Heslot, H., Nagy, M., Whitehead, E.: Recherches genetiques et biochimiques sur la premier enzyme de la biosynthese des purine chez le Schizosaccharomyces. C.R. Acad. Sci. (Paris) [D] **263**, 57—58 (1966)

Holmes, E. W., King, G. L., Leyva, A., Singer, S. C.: A purine auxotroph deficient in phosphoribosylpyrophosphate amidotransferase and phosphoribosylpyrophosphate aminotransferase activities with normal activity of ribose-5-phosphate aminotransferase. Proc. natl. Acad. Sci. (Wash.) **73**, (7), 2458—2461 (1976)

Holmes, E. W., McDonald, J. A., McCord, J. M., Wyngaarden, J. B., Kelley, W. N.: Human glutamine phosphoribosylpyrophosphate amidotransferase: kinetic and regulatory properties. J. biol. Chem. **248**, 144—150 (1973 a)

Holmes, E. W., Wyngaarden, J. B., Kelley, W. N.: Human glutamine phosphoribosylpyrophosphate amidotransferase: two molecular forms interconvertible by purine ribonucleotides and phosphoribosylpyrophosphate. J. biol. Chem. **248**, 6035—6040 (1973 b)

Howard, W. J., Appel, S. H.: Control of purine biosynthesis: FGAR amidotransferase. Clin. Res. **16**, 344 (1968)

Howell, R. R.: Hyperuricemia in childhood. Fed. Proc. **27**, 1078 (1968)

Katunuma, N., Weber, G.: Glutamine phosphoribosylpyrophosphate amidotransferase: Increased activity in hepatomas. FEBS Letters **49**, 53—56 (1974)

Kelley, W. N., Fox, I. H., Wyngaarden, J. B.: Regulation of purine biosynthesis in cultured human cells. I. Effects of orotic acid. Biochim. biophys. Acta (Amst.) **215**, 512—516 (1970a)

Kelley, W. N., Fox, I. H., Wyngaarden, J. B.: Essential role of phosphoribosylpyrophosphate in regulation of purine biosynthesis in cultured human fibroblasts. Clin. Res. **18**, 457 (1970b)

King, G. L., Holmes, E. W.: Comparison of NH_3 and glutamine utilization by human PP-ribose-P amidotransferase. Fed. Proc. (abstracts 1977)

King, G. L., Meade, J. C., Holmes, E. W.: Demonstration of NH_3 utilization in the first reaction of purine biosynthesis de novo. Clin. Res. **25**, 32A (1977)

Kovarsky, J., Evans, M., Holmes, E. W.: Regulation of human amidophosphoribosyltransferase: interaction of orthophosphate, PP-ribose-P and purine ribonucleotides. Canad. J. Biochem. (in press)

Lalane, M., Henderson, J. F.: Effects of hormones and drugs on phosphoribosylpyrophosphate concentrations in mouse liver. Canad. J. Biochem. **53**, 394—399 (1975)

Lang, W. K.: Association between glutathione reductase variants and plasma uric acid concentration in a Negro population. Amer. J. hum. Genet. **22**, 14a—15a (1970)

Marcolongo, R., Micheli, V., Pompucci, G., Marinello, E.: Comportaments della glutamina-fosforibosilpirosfato amidotransferasi in pazienti affetti da gotta primativa. Reumatismo **26**, 223—229 (1974)

Martin, D. W., Jr., Maler, B. A.: Phosphoribosylpyrophosphate synthetase is elevated in fibroblasts from patients with the Lesch-Nyhan syndrome. Science **193**, 408—411 (1976)

Momose, H., Nishikawa, H., Shies, L.: Regulation of purine nucleotide synthesis in Bacillus subtilis. J. biol. Chem. **59**, 325 (1966)

Nagy, M.: Regulation of the biosynthesis of purine nucleotides in Schizosaccharomyces pombe. I. Properties of the phosphoribosylpyrophosphate: glutamine amidotransferase of the wild strain and of a mutant desensitized towards feedback modifiers. Biochem. biophys. Acta (Amst.) **198**, 471—481 (1971)

Nierlich, D. P., Magasanik, B.: Control by repression of purine biosynthetic enzymes in aerogenes. Fed. Proc. **22**, 476 (1963)

Pagliara, A. S., Goodman, A. D.: Elevation of plasma glutamate in gout, its possible role in the pathogenesis of hyperuricemia. New Engl. J. Med. **281**, 767—770 (1969)

Paterson, A. R. P., Wang, M. C.: Mechanism of the growth inhibition potentiation arising from combinations of 6-mercaptopurine with 6-methylmercaptopurine ribonucleoside. Cancer Res. **30**, 2379—2387 (1970)

Prusiner, S., Stadtman, E. R.: The Enzymes of Glutamine Metabolism. New York-London: Acad. Pr. 1973

Reem, G. H.: Enzymatic synthesis of 5'-phosphoribosylamine from ribose 5-phosphate and ammonia, on alternate first step in purine biosynthesis. J. biol. Chem. **243**, 5695—5701 (1968)

Reem, G. H.: De novo purine biosynthesis by two pathways in Burkitt lymphoma cells and in human spleen. J. clin. Invest. **51**, 1058—1062 (1972)

Reem, G. H.: Enzymatic synthesis of phosphoribosylamine in human cells. J. biol. Chem. **249**, 1696—1703 (1974a)

Reem, G. H.: Pharmacologic regulation of the early steps of purine biosynthesis in Burkitt lymphoma cells and in Ehrlich ascites tumor cells. J. Pharmacol. exp. Ther. **191**, 1—9 (1974b)

Reem, G.: Phosphoribosylpyrophosphate overproduction; a new metabolic abnormality in the Lesch-Nyhan syndrome. Science **190**, 1098—1099 (1975)

Reem, G. H., Friend, C.: Purine metabolism in murine virus-induced erythroleukemic cells during differentiation in vitro. Proc. nat. Acad. Sci. (Wash.) **72**, 1630—1634 (1975)

Rosenbloom, F. M., Henderson, J. F., Caldwell, I. C., Kelley, W. N., Seegmiller, J. E.: Biochemical bases of accelerated purine biosynthesis de novo in human fibroblasts lacking hypoxanthine-guanine phosphoribosyltransferase. J. biol. Chem. **243**, 1166—1173 (1968)

Scholar, E. M., Brown, P. R., Parks, R. E., Jr.: Synergistic effect of 6-mercaptopurine and 6-methylmercaptopurine ribonucleoside on the levels of adenine nucleotides of sarcoma 180 cells. Cancer Res. **32**, 259—269 (1972)

Seegmiller, J. E., Grayzel, A. I., Laster, L., Liddle, L.: Uric acid production in gout. J. clin. Invest. **40**, 1304—1314 (1961)

Seegmiller,J.E., Grayzel,A.I., Liddle,L.: The effect of 2-ethylamino-1,3,4-thiadiazole on the in-
corporation of glycine into urinary purines and uric acid in man. Metabolism **12**, 507—515
(1963)
Seegmiller,J.E., Rosenbloom,R.M., Kelley,W.N.: An enzyme defect associated with a sex-linked
human neurological disorder and excessive purine synthesis. Science **155**, 1682—1684 (1967)
Segal,S., Wyngaarden,J.B.: Plasma glutamine and oxypurine content in patients with gout. Proc.
Soc. exp. Biol. (N.Y.) **88**, 342—345 (1955)
Skaper,S.D., Willis,R.C., Seegmiller,J.E.: Intracellular 5-phosphoribosyl-1-pyrophosphate: Decreased availability during glutamine limitation. Science **193**, 587—588 (1976)
Smirnov,M.N., Smirnov,V.N., Budowsky,E.I., Inge-Vechtomov,S.G., Serebrjakov,N.C.: Red
pigment of adenine deficient yeast *Saccharomyces cerevisiae*. Biochem. Biophys. Res. Com-
mun. **27**, 299—304 (1967)
Sperling,O., Boer,P., Persky-Brosh,S.: Altered kinetic property of erythrocyte phosphoribo-
sylpyrophosphate synthetase in excessive purine production. Rev. europ. Etud. clin. Biol. **17**,
703—706 (1972)
Sperling,O., Wyngaarden,J.B., Starmer,C.F.: The kinetics of intramolecular distribution of ^{15}N
in uric acid after administration of [^{15}N]glycine. J. clin. Invest. **52**, 2468—2485 (1973)
Taylor,M.W., Ling,L., Pipkorn,J.: Coordinate effect of mutation on PRPP amidotransferase and
PRPP aminotransferase activities in Chinese hamster lung cells. In vitro, abstract (1976)
Walser,M., Lung,P., Roderman,N.B.: Synthesis of essential amino acids from their α-keto ana-
logues by perfused rat liver and muscle. J. clin. Invest. **52**, 2865—2877 (1973)
Watts,R.W.E.: (Chairman of panel discussion "Hyperuricemia as a Risk Factor.") Second Inter-
national Symposium on Purine Metabolism in Man. Baden (Austria), June 20—26, 1976
Williamson,D.H., Lopes-Vieira,O., Walker,B.: Concentration of free glucogenic amino acids in
livers of rats subjected to various metabolic stresses. Biochem. J. **104**, 497—502 (1967)
Wood,A.W., Seegmiller,J.E.: Properties of 5-phosphoribosyl-1-pyrophosphate amidotransferase
from human lymphoblasts. J. biol. Chem. **248**, 138—143 (1973)
Wyngaarden,J.B., Ashton,D.M.: The regulation of activity of phosphoribosylpyrophosphate
amidotransferase by purine ribonucleotides: a potential feedback control of purine biosynthesis. J. biol. Chem. **234**, 1492—1496 (1959)
Wyngaarden,J.B., Silberman,H.R., Sadler,J.H.: Feedback mechanisms influencing purine ribotide synthesis. Ann. N.Y. Acad. Sci. **75**, 45—60 (1958)
Yü,T.-F., Adler,M., Bobrow,E.: Plasma and urinary amino acids in primary gout, with special
reference to glutamine. J. clin. Invest. **48**, 885—894 (1969)

CHAPTER 3

Purine Salvage Enzymes

W.J.ARNOLD

A. Introduction

The purine phosphoribosyltransferases, hypoxanthine-guanine phosphoribo-syltransferase (HGPRT, E.C. 2.4.2.8.) and adenine phosphoribosyltransferase (APRT, 2.4.2.7.) catalyze the transfer of the ribose-5-phosphate (R-5-P) moiety of 5'-phosphoribosyl-1-pyrophosphate (PP-ribose-P) to the purine bases hypoxanthine, guanine, and adenine to form the corresponding nucleotides inosine-5'-monophosphate (IMP), guanosine-5'-monophosphate (GMP), and adenosine-5'-monophosphate (AMP), respectively (KORNBERG et al., 1955; KORN et al., 1955). The direct conversion of hypoxanthine to IMP was first demonstrated in pigeon liver extracts by WILLIAMS and BUCHANAN (1953), while KORNBERG et al. (1955) were the first to actually define the precise enzymatic nature of the purine phosphoribosyltransferase. Subsequent studies revealed that HGPRT and APRT activity increased in rapidly dividing normal and neoplastic tissue (MURRAY, 1966a; MURRAY, 1967a). HGPRT and APRT were thought to function solely as "purine salvage enzymes" that supplied GMP and AMP as precursors of nucleic acids to rapidly dividing tissues or to tissues without the capacity to synthetize purines de novo (ROSENBLOOM et al., 1967). No major role in control of purine metabolism or other physiologic or biochemical processes was envisioned (KORNBERG, 1957).

However, as in other instances in modern molecular biology, insight into the true role and importance of HGPRT and APRT has been obtained by the discovery of individuals with an inherited deficiency of the activity of these enzymes. In 1964, LESCH and NYHAN described two brothers with marked hyperuricemia and hyperuricosuria associated with a bizarre neurobehavioral disorder (LESCH and NYHAN, 1964). In 1967, SEEGMILLER et al. discovered the virtually complete absence of HGPRT activity in erythrocytes from patients with the Lesch-Nyhan syndrome (SEEGMILLER et al., 1967). In the ensuing 10 years, intensive investigations of HGPRT and its role in the pathogenesis of the metabolic and clinical features of the Lesch-Nyhan syndrome has produced a virtual explosion in our understanding of not only the relationship of HGPRT activity to the regulation of purine metabolism but also to the importance of HGPRT in the maturation and function of the nervous system. The recent description of a male child with a complete deficiency of APRT activity associated with 2,8-dioxyadenine renal calculi promises to supply exciting new insights into the physiologic and biochemical importance of APRT activity (CARTIER et al., 1974; DEBRAY et al., 1976; VAN ACKER et al., 1976). In view of the pivotal importance of the inherited deficiencies of HGPRT and APRT activity, this chapter will examine both the purine salvage enzymes in direct relationship to our knowledge of their importance in the pathogenesis of their related illnesses.

B. Normal Hypoxanthine-Guanine Phosphoribosyltransferase (HGPRT)

I. Assay Methods and Kinetic Properties

HGPRT activity has been found in every human tissue, with the highest activity in the brain, particularly the basal ganglia (ROSENBLOOM et al., 1967a; KRENITSKY, 1969a). In mammals HGPRT activity is located predominantly in the cytosol, while in bacteria HGPRT activity is found in the periplasmic space loosely associated with the membrane (GUTENSOHN and GUROFF, 1972; HOCHSTADT-OZER and STADTMAN, 1971).

HGPRT activity has been assayed in vitro by a wide variety of methods both in intact cells and cell lysates. Assays of HGPRT activity in intact cells may be a useful screening technique, particularly in the prenatal diagnosis of the Lesch-Nyhan syndrome; however, the technique would not readily allow the determination of kinetic constants and has the disadvantage of assuming that adequate membrane transport of purines occurs in all situations (DE BRUYN et al., 1976). Radiochemical assays of HGPRT activity in dialyzed cell lysates allow exact adjustments of substrates and cofactor to assure optimum activity. The various procedures differ primarily in the way the radioactive mononucleotide product is separated from the radioactive purine base substrate. This has been done by high voltage electrophoresis on paper or cellulose acetate (KELLEY et al., 1967a; KIZAKI and SAKURADA, 1976). This method allows direct identification with short wavelength UV light of the nucleotide product and substrate by their comigration with appropriate standards. In addition, potential alternate metabolites of the nucleotide product, such as nucleosides, can also be readily identified. Other techniques that have been used include ion exchange chromatography, precipitation with lanthanum chloride, and binding to DEAE-cellulose paper discs or polyethyleneimine-cellulose-coated glass-fiber filters (NYHAN et al., 1967; BAKAY et al., 1969; BAKHRU-KISHORE and KELLEY, 1976; ATKINSON and MURRAY, 1965; DE BRUYN et al., 1974; SCHMIDT et al., 1976). Erythrocytes are the ideal tissue source, since venipuncture is relatively simple and the level of erythrocyte HGPRT enzyme activity is higher than in any other tissue except the central nervous system (KELLEY, 1972a). In addition, other enzymes for which guanine, hypoxanthine, GMP, or IMP may be substrates, such as guanase, xanthine oxidase, and 5′-nucleotidase, are absent from the mature erythrocyte. HGPRT activity can be readily assayed in crude lysates, which contain 5′-nucleotidase or xanthine oxidase, by the inclusion of inhibitors of these enzymes in the HGPRT reaction mixture. HGPRT has been successfully assayed in fibroblast lysate, which contain 5′-nucleotidase, by the inclusion of thymidine triphosphate at a final concentration of 3.3 mM in the reaction mixture (MURRAY and FRIEDRICHS, 1969; KELLEY and MEADE, 1971). Inhibition of xanthine oxidase by inclusion of allopurinol [4-hydroxypyrozolo(3,4-d)pyrimidine]—(final concentration of 0.25 μM in the reaction mixture)—has permitted the assay of HGPRT activity in rat intestinal homogenates (YIP and BALIS, 1976).

The kinetic analysis of HGPRT from a variety of sources has been reported. These include human erythrocytes, developing mouse liver, Ehrlich ascites tumor cells, rat brain, bacteria (E. Coli and lacto Bacillus casei), Plasmodium chabaudi, Chinese hamster brain, and brewer's yeast (MURRAY, 1966a; MURRAY, 1967a; HENDERSON, 1968; KRENITSKY et al., 1969a; KRENITSKY and PAPAIOANNOU, 1969; HENDERSON, 1968b; MURRAY, 1966b; MILLER et al., 1972; MARTIN and YOUNG,

1972; KRENITSKY et al., 1970; WALTER and KONIGK, 1974; OLSEN MILMAN, 1974a; MILLER and BIEBER, 1968). In humans a single protein species is catalytically active not only with the purine bases hypoxanthine and guanine but also catalyzes the formation of xanthylic acid (XMP) from xanthine (KELLEY et al., 1967b). However, in *E. Coli* at least two different protein species exist, one with an affinity for hypoxanthine and the other towards guanine and xanthine (MILLER et al., 1972; MARTIN and YOUNG, 1972; KRENITSKY et al., 1970). The natural purine bases guanine and hypoxanthine as well as an analogue of the latter, 6-mercaptopurine (6-MP), are the best substrates for the enzyme. Other substrates include allopurinol, 8-azaguanine, and 6-thioguanine (KRENITSKY, 1969; BROCKMAN, 1965). However, azathioprine, adenine, uric acid, and uracil are not substrates for this enzyme. In general, the enzyme effectively binds substances with an oxo- or thio-group in position 6, while the imidazole portion of the ring is important but not solely sufficient for binding (KRENITSKY, 1969). As mentioned above, the human HGPRT enzyme is capable of catalyzing the conversion of xanthine to XMP but with such a low velocity that it is of doubtful significance in vivo (KRENITSKY et al., 1969a; KELLEY et al., 1967b).

The nonpurine substrate PP-ribose-P is the sole compound capable of donating the ribose-5-P moiety to the HGPRT-catalyzed reaction. Magnesium is a required cofactor for the HGPRT reaction, with maximal enzyme activity at concentrations of magnesium ranging from 5 mM to 20 mM (KRENITSKY, 1969). Kinetic analysis has revealed that at fixed concentrations of magnesium and PP-ribose-P the human HGPRT enzyme exhibits classic hyperbolic kinetics when the concentration of the purine bases guanine or hypoxanthine is varied (HENDERSON et al., 1968a; KRENITSKY, 1969; KRENITSKY et al., 1969a). Double reciprocal plots have shown an apparent K_m of 1.8–4 μM for guanine, 2.4–9.9 μM for hypoxanthine, and 2.4 μM for PP-ribose-P with either hypoxanthine or guanine as the purine substrate (KRENITSKY, 1969). Analysis of the reaction mechanism of HGPRT has revealed a marked dependency on the concentration of magnesium relative to PP-ribose-P (HENDERSON, 1968a; KRENITSKY et al., 1969a). With varying magnesium and PP-ribose-P concentrations and constant purine base, classic hyperbolic kinetics are obtained except at low ratios of magnesium to PP-ribose-P (KRENITSKY, 1969). In this instance, further increasing the concentration of PP-ribose-P reveals sigmoidal kinetics. In all instances the PP-ribose-P binds first to the enzyme, but with magnesium in moderate excess the enzyme then binds the purine base and forms a ternary complex. The product (nucleotide) is released first then the pyrophosphate. However, at large excess of magnesium the binding of PP-ribose-P is immediately followed by the release of pyrophosphate with the formation of an enzyme-ribosylphosphate intermediate. The purine base then adds to the enzyme, and the nucleotide product is released.

Purine nucleotides, pyrophosphate (PPi), and sulfhydryl-binding agents are inhibitors of the HGPRT enzyme reaction. As would be expected, the mononucleotide products of the reaction, GMP and IMP, are effective inhibitors (HENDERSON et al., 1968a; KRENITSKY et al., 1969a; VAN ACKER et al., 1976; HENDERSON, 1968b; MURRAY, 1966b). Both GMP and IMP inhibit the enzyme competitively with respect to PP-ribose-P and noncompetitively with respect to guanine and hypoxanthine. GMP and its di- and triphosphate derivatives are more effective inhibitors (Ki GMP– 0.014 mM) than is inosinic acid (Ki 0.14 mM). However, since the intracellular concentrations of these nucleotides is very low, the physiologic role of end-product inhibition in regulation of the HGPRT enzyme reaction is of doubtful significance. PPi is an effective inhibitor of the HGPRT enzyme reaction (HENDERSON et al., 1968a; KRENITSKY et al., 1969a). However, the inhibitory properties of PPi are directly related to the concentration of magnesium in the reaction mixture (KRENITSKY et al., 1969a). Lower magnesium concentrations (0.5 mM) enhance PPi-mediated inhibition, while at 5 mM magnesium concentration PPi-mediated inhibition is abolished. The sulfhydryl-binding agents p-chloromercuribenzoate (p-CMB) and N-ethylmaleimide at concentrations of 0.25 mM inactive the HGPRT enzyme (KRENITSKY et al., 1969a; MILLER et al., 1972). The inhibition produced by p-CMB can be blocked by reincubation of the human HGPRT enzyme with Mg PP-ribose-P but not with purine bases, nucleotides, or PPi (KRENITSKY et al., 1969a). The bacterial HGPRT enzyme is also inhibited by p-CMB, and this inhibition can be reversed with either dithiothreitol or β-mercaptoethanol (MILLER et al., 1972).

II. Physical Properties

As mentioned above, in mammalian tissues the HGPRT enzyme activity appears to reside in a single protein species. However, in *E. Coli* nucleotide synthesis from guanine, xanthine, and hypoxanthine is catalyzed by two distinct protein species separable by DEAE-cellulose or Ecteola-cellulose chromatography and isoelectric focusing but not by Sephadex G-100 chromatography (MILLER et al., 1972; MARTIN and YOUNG, 1972; KRENITSKY et al., 1970). One enzyme species with an isoelectric point (pI) of pH 5.8 displays preferential activity towards hypoxanthine, while the other enzymatic species has pI of 5.50 and preferentially binds guanine and xanthine (K_m of 0.037 mM for guanine, K_m of 0.33 M for PP-ribose-P) (MILLER et al., 1972). This latter enzyme species binds xanthine four times and hypoxanthine 67 times less effectively than guanine. This and other kinetic data from *E. Coli* suggest that the purine salvage mechanisms are strikingly different from the mammalian system.

While two to five isozymes for HGPRT have been observed with the enzyme from mammalian species, these differently charged species of the HGPRT enzyme protein are of unknown physiologic significance. The number of HGPRT isozymes detected appears to result at least in part from the tissue source and the technique utilized to study the enzyme. Isoelectric focusing has been the most frequently used technique in the study of HGPRT isozymes. Using this technique to study HGPRT from human erythrocytes, DAVIES and DEAN (1971) found three isozymes (pI, 7.5, 6.5, and 6.0); ARNOLD and KELLEY (1971) noted three isozymes (pI 6.01 ± 0.09, 5.8 ± 0.06, and 5.65 ± 0.06); and DER KALOUSTIAN et al. (1973) found three isozymes (pI 6.00, 5.8, and 5.71). However, only two peaks of HGPRT activity were found by RUBIN et al. when human hemolysate was analyzed by DEAE-cellulose chromatography, while BAKAY and NYHAN distinguished four isozymes of HGPRT in human hemolysate using polyacrylamide gel disc electrophoresis (RUBIN et al., 1971; BAKAY and NYHAN, 1971). Studies in the rat have shown two isozymes of HGPRT activity in hemolysate by isoelectric focusing (pI 5.90 and 5.80), while DEAE-cellulose chromatography of partially purified rat brain revealed at least three isozymes (DER KALOUSTIAN et al., 1973; GUTENSOHN and GUROFF, 1972). Also, three isozymes of HGPRT activity have been found by isoelectric focusing in Chinese hamster brain (pI 6.55, 6.43, and 6.24) and liver (pI 6.70, 6.49, and 6.33) (OLSEN and MILMAN, 1974a).

Although seemingly incongruous, these studies document the certainty of the existence of multiple isozymes for HGPRT activity. Several lines of evidence suggest that the observed isozymes of HGPRT activity result from a nongenetic, posttranslational alteration of a single HGPRT protein species (ARNOLD and KELLEY, 1971; KELLEY and ARNOLD, 1973). Firstly, the single mutation event resulting in the Lesch-Nyhan syndrome is associated with the virtually complete absence of HGPRT activity in all tissues of the body (ROSENBLOOM et al., 1967a). Therefore, it seems unlikely that there are multiple genes coding for the enzyme. Secondly, in at least one study reporting isozymes for human HGPRT, hemolysate was obtained only from male donors (ARNOLD and KELLEY, 1971). Since it is known that the gene coding for the synthesis of HGPRT is located on the x-chromosome, this study suggests that multiple alleles cannot account for the isozymes. Thirdly, instability of the pI's of the HGPRT isozymes to storage has been found and suggests that the variation in charge is not a result of stable differences in the primary amino acid sequences of the isozymes (DAVIES and DEAN, 1971; ARNOLD and KELLEY, 1971). Fourthly, although a detailed kinetic study of each HGPRT isozyme has not been performed, in one report the activity of each of the three isozymes of human HGPRT from hemolysate was found to be similar towards guanine, hypoxanthine, and PP-ribose-P, and all three isozymes exhibited similar degrees of inhibition with a 10-fold excess of PP-ribose-P (ARNOLD and KELLEY, 1971). Finally, the native molecular weight and subunit composition (by Sephadex G-100 chromatography and SDS-polyacrylamide gel electrophoresis, respectively) as well as the net charge (urea polyacrylamide gel electrophoresis) of the three isozymes was found to be identical (ARNOLD and KELLEY, 1971).

The exact nature of the posttranslational alteration of the HGPRT protein responsible for the isozymes remains unknown. Differential sialation appears to be unlikely. Most likely the isozymes result from differential amidation phosphorylation, or some other modification that occurs during the aging of the HGPRT enzyme protein (ARNOLD and KELLEY, 1971).

The subunit structure of highly purified HGPRT has been examined by several groups. ARNOLD and KELLEY (1971) reported the purification of HGPRT to apparent homogeneity from human erythrocytes. In this study, human HGPRT was estimated to have a molecular weight of 68000 and a Stokes radius of 36 A by Sephadex G-100 chromatography. This data agreed well with a previous estimation of $60000 \pm 10\%$ for the molecular weight of a partially purified preparation of human erythrocyte HGPRT (KRENITSKY, 1969). Further analysis by SDS polyacrylamide gel electrophoresis of highly purified human erythrocyte HGPRT in the presence of B-mercaptoethanol suggested that the enzyme was a dimer composed of two subunits of identical molecular weight, 34500 (ARNOLD and KELLEY, 1971). Subsequently, three studies of highly purified HGPRT from mammalian tissues have indicated that HGPRT may be a trimer rather than a dimer. In the first study HGPRT was purified from Chinese hamster brain, liver, and V 79 tissue culture cells (OLSEN and MILMAN, 1974a). The native molecular weight was estimated to be between 78000 and 85000, as determined by Sephadex G-100 chromatography and acrylamide gel electrophoresis. SDS polyacrylamide gel electrophoresis demonstrated a single species of molecular weight 25000, thus suggesting that the native HGPRT enzyme was a trimer. The same investigators also reported that purified human erythrocyte HGPRT had physical properties nearly identical to the Chinese hamster HGPRT enzyme (OLSEN and MILMAN, 1974b). In the third study HGPRT was purified to apparent homogeneity from mouse liver (HUGHES et al., 1975). These investigators estimated the native molecular weight of HGPRT to be 80000 ± 4000 and also found the most likely structure of the native HGPRT to be a trimer with a subunit molecular weight of 27000 ± 1000. Recently, an additional study has appeared that suggests that the results of the above studies can be reconciled by hypothesizing that selective partial degradation of the 34500 molecular weight HGPRT subunit can result in a subunit of molecular weight 26500 (STRAUSS, 1975).

III. Role in Cellular Transport of Purines

The entrance of the purine bases hypoxanthine and guanine into cells may potentially be accomplished by one of three mechanisms: (1) group translocation, i.e., purine cellular transport in association with further metabolism by HGPRT; (2) carrier-mediated transport, i.e., purine cellular transport mediated by specific membrane protein distinct from any metabolic event; (3) simple diffusion (ALFORD and BARNES, 1976). In *E. Coli* and *B. Subtilis* the transport of hypoxanthine appears to be mediated by a group translocation involving HGPRT that is loosely associated with the membrane in the periplasmic space (HOCHSTADT-OZER and STADTMAN, 1971; BERLIN and STADTMAN, 1966). However, in mammalian cells the transport of hypoxanthine occurs by the carrier-mediated mechanism independently of HGPRT activity (ALFORD and BARNES, 1976; ZYLKA and PLAGEMANN, 1975). In Chinese hamster cells, the rate of hypoxanthine uptake in wild-type and mutant cell lines was similar despite a 100- to 5000-fold reduction in the HGPRT activity of the mutant cell lines. Also, inhibiton of hypoxanthine uptake with p-chloromercuriphenylsulfonate occurred with no effect on HGPRT activity. These observations are extended by the report of chlorpromazine-mediated inhibition of hypoxanthine transport in human skin epithelial cells with no effect on HGPRT activity (DYBING, 1974). In a brief report concerning HGPRT activity and hypoxanthine uptake by human erythrocytes, transport of hypoxanthine occurred independently of the amount of HGPRT bound to the red cell membrane (GUTENSOHN, 1975). Therefore, the studies available in the literature clearly show that purine base transport in bacterial and mammalian cells differs markedly. Apparently a group translocation mechanism involving HGPRT predominates in bacteria, while a carrier-mediated transport apart from phosphoribosylation is the major mechanism in mammalian cells.

C. Clinical Syndromes Associated with a Deficiency of HGPRT

Two distinct clinical syndromes are associated with a deficiency of HGPRT activity. The Lesch-Nyhan syndrome is a bizarre x-linked neurobehavioral disorder characterized biochemically by hyperuricemia, hyperuricosuria, and a virtually complete deficiency of HGPRT activity (SEEGMILLER et al., 1967). In 1967, following the description of HGPRT deficiency in the Lesch-Nyhan syndrome, a group of adult gouty patients with severe tophaceous gout, hyperuricemia, and hyperuricosuria, but without a characteristic neurobehavioral syndrome, were described to have an x-linked partial deficiency of HGPRT activity (KELLEY et al., 1967a).

I. Lesch-Nyhan Syndrome

Following the initial description of the clinical manifestations of the Lesch-Nyhan syndrome and its association with HGPRT deficiency, almost 100 cases have appeared in the literature (DIZMANG and CHEATHAM, 1970; THORPE, 1971; CRAWHALL et al., 1972; NYHAN, 1972; SEEGMILLER, 1976). The incidence of the Lesch-Nyhan Syndrome has been estimated to be 1 in 380000 live births (CRAWHALL et al., 1972). With a few notable exceptions, the clinical features have been remarkably constant (GEERDINK et al., 1973; TOYO-OKA et al., 1975). Few if any abnormalities are noted at birth, and usually the development of the child is reported as normal until 2–3 months of age. The first suggestion of abnormal development is the inability to perform simple motor functions such as rolling over or sitting. Also, hypo- or hypertonia may be the initial manifestation of the severe neurologic dysfunction that will ensue. In retrospect, parents often recall the appearance of yellowish-orange crystals in the diaper, which only later are appreciated as the initial manifestations of the hyperuricosuria present from birth. With advancing age the neurologic dysfunction becomes more obvious and is characterized by spasticity, choreoathetosis, growth, and mental retardation. The severe spasticity is manifest as a "scissors gait" due to adductor spasm and leads to an inability to sit or walk unaided; it may contribute to the frequent finding of hip dislocation. Choreoathetosis produces not only abnormal movement and posture of the trunk and extremities, but also leads to marked difficulty in speech. Indeed, several investigators have noted that these children may perform poorly on intelligence testing not because they are truly mentally deficient but as a consequence of their marked motor and speech impediments (CRAWHALL et al., 1972; NYHAN, 1973; SEEGMILLER, 1976). Although no reproducible abnormalities of bony structure or development have been noted in these patients, the majority are smaller in stature than would be expected (SKYLER et al., 1974). The growth retardation is not associated with abnormalities of thyroid or pituitary function (SKYLER et al., 1974).

The most striking and variable component of the neurologic syndrome is the unusual aggressive behavioral disorder displayed by these patients. The aggression most prominently takes the form of self-mutilation but also can be manifested as hostile actions, both physical and verbal, against lovedones as well as health care professionals. These aggressive tendencies may appear at any age, and, once present, they often wax and wane unpredictably. Patients will uncontrollably bite their fingers or lips, batter their heads or knees against beds or walls, and if left unrestrained, hurl themselves from bed or chair. These actions are usually accompanied by an apparent high level of anxiety and are performed even though they are painful. Patients welcome the use of physical restraints or other protective measures (helmets, knee pads, heavy mittens) to prevent the uncontrollable tendency to self-mutilate. Indeed, patients usually display their highest anxiety levels when they are about to be unrestrained. Aggressive tendencies towards others often take the form of vile epithets but also include physical combativeness. Most health care personnel involved with these children soon learn to remove their glasses prior to approaching an unrestrained patient.

While the neurobehavioral manifestations of the Lesch-Nyhan syndrome are the most prominent part of this disorder, the clinical manifestations of hyperuricemia and hyperuricosuria are frequently those that lead to the discovery of HGPRT deficiency. As mentioned above, the appearance of yellow-orange crystalline deposits on the diapers may be noted from birth and is a reflection of the marked increase in the synthesis of uric acid and consequent hyperuricosuria (LESCH and NYHAN, 1964). Therefore, these children are susceptible to all the clinical manifestations of the gouty diathesis, including gouty arthritis, uric acid lithiasis, urate nephropathy, and tophi (NYHAN, 1972; NYHAN, 1973; SEEGMILLER, 1976). While uric acid lithiasis accompanied by flank pain and hematuria may be the most common manifestation, urate nephropathy produces the major morbidity and is most frequently the cause of early mortality (NYHAN, 1973). Other inconstant clinical manifestations include vomiting, which may be a result of, or through dehydration contribute to, uric acid lithiasis and grand mal seizures of uncertain etiology (NYHAN, 1973).

The most consistent abnormality detected by clinical laboratory analysis of patients with the Lesch-Nyhan syndrome is the marked elevation of urinary uric acid content, which is a reflection of the "flamboyant" overproduction of uric acid (KELLEY, 1972b). In infants and young children the serum urate is not infrequently normal despite the marked hyperuricosuria. This is most likely due to the kidney's enhanced ability to excrete uric acid prior to age 2. Therefore, while the majority of patients with the Lesch-Nyhan syndrome will display hyperuricemia, the measurement of urinary uric acid content is of prime importance in establishing the presence of uric acid overproduction (KELLEY, 1972b). This judgement may be made by determining the ratio of uric acid (mg-%) and creatinine (mg-%) in a spot urine sample rather than necessitating the laborious and often incomplete collection of a 24-h urine sample (KAUFMAN et al., 1968). Most patients with the Lesch-Nyhan syndrome will have a ratio of uric acid (mg-%) to creatinine (mg-%) greater than 2 while normals will be less than 1.

A megaloblastic anemia unresponsive to Vitamin B_{12} and folic acid has been reported with the Lesch-Nyhan syndrome (VAN DER ZEE, 1968).

1. Characteristics of the Mutant HGPRT in Patients with the Lesch-Nyhan Syndrome

Following the initial description of a virtually complete deficiency of HGPRT activity in erythrocytes from patients with the Lesch-Nyhan syndrome, investigators have attempted to elucidate not only the precise genetic and biochemical nature of the HGPRT deficiency but also the relationship between deficiency of HGPRT activity and the bizarre neurobehavioral disorder and overproduction of uric acid characteristic of patients with the Lesch-Nyhan syndrome. Evidence for striking heterogeneity of the mutations that may result in a deficiency of HGPRT activity has been obtained. In addition, these studies have indicated an important role for HGPRT activity in the regulation of purine biosynthesis and central nervous system function. The following discussion will focus on the genetic and biochemical characteristics of the HGPRT deficiency and its relationship to neurologic dysfunction in patients with the Lesch-Nyhan syndrome, while the relationship between HGPRT deficiency and the accelerated de novo purine biosynthesis will be covered elsewhere in this volume (see Chapter 7).

Initial studies of HGPRT in tissues from patients with the Lesch-Nyhan syndrome failed to reveal detectable enzyme activity in either hemolysate ((< 1.0 n mole/mg of protein/h), liver (< 1.0 n mole/mg of protein/h), or brain (< 4.0 n moles/mg of protein/h) (SEEGMILLER et al., 1967; KELLEY, 1968a). However, in 1970 FUJIMOTO and SEEGMILLER reported that low levels of HGPRT activity were present in tissue culture fibroblasts derived from four patients with the Lesch-Nyhan syndrome. This observation was confirmed by KELLEY and MEADE (1971) in tissue culture fibroblasts from 11 patients with the Lesch-Nyhan syndrome. These investigators also excluded the participation of trace amounts of HGPRT activity from fetal calf serum, mycoplasma infection, or other phosphoribosyltransferases in the PP-ribose-P dependent synthesis of GMP from guanine. It has been recently documented that mycoplasmal contamination of tissue culture fibroblasts can lead to the presence of HGPRT activity, thus requiring repeated culturing of spent media as done by KELLEY and MEADE (1971) or electrophoretic characterization of HGPRT activity when low levels of HGPRT activity are being studied (STANBRIDGE and TISCHFIELD, 1975). In addition, with the group of 11 cell strains derived from patients with the Lesch-Nyhan syndrome, at least three phenotypes could be distinguished on the basis of product inhibition by IMP or GMP and thermal stability at $57°$ C. This study provided the first evidence for genetic heterogeneity of the mutant HGPRT found in patients with the Lesch-Nyhan syndrome and indicated that in this group of patients the mutation(s) responsible for the HGPRT deficiency most likely was located on the gene coding for the synthesis of HGPRT. Other investigators have also confirmed the presence of low levels of HGPRT in tissue culture fibroblasts derived from patients with the Lesch-Nyhan syndrome (WOOD and PINSKY, 1973; RICCARDI and LITTLEFIELD, 1972; BENKE et al., 1973a). In these studies, low levels of HGPRT activity in tissue culture fibroblasts were detected either by direct assay of HGPRT activity or by assessment of H^3-hypoxanthine uptake into acid-precipitable nucleic acids using radioautography.

Although initially erythrocyte HGPRT activity was undetectable when fresh hemolysate was examined, low levels of HGPRT activity could be found (MIZUNO et al., 1970; SORENSON, 1970; ARNOLD et al., 1972). Using the technique of erythrocyte fractionation on density gradients, evidence for instability of the mutant HGPRT activity in older arythrocytes from three of five patients was found, and this provided further evidence for genetic heterogeneity (ARNOLD et al., 1972). Perhaps the most striking illustration of both the genetic heterogeneity and the nature of the mutation in patients with the Lesch-Nyhan syndrome was the report of a "K_m mutant" of the HGPRT enzyme by MACDONALD and KELLEY (1971). These investigators studied the HGPRT activity present in hemolysate from a patient using the classical concentrations of purine base (0.1 mM) and Mg PP-ribose-P (1.0 mM); low levels of HGPRT were detectable (0.2% of normal). However, in the presence of a 10-fold excess of Mg PP-ribose-P (10 mM) virtually normal maximal velocity of nucleotide synthesis was observed with hypoxanthine as substrate. This mutant HGPRT enzyme had an apparent K_m of 0.18 mM for hypoxanthine and 2.8 mM for Mg PP-ribose-P. Subsequently, an additional patient who also most likely represents a K_m mutant of HGPRT activity has been reported (BENKE et al., 1973b).

Other studies have noted an apparent activation of the mutant HGPRT enzyme activity in vivo or in vitro and add support to the hypothesis that an altered HGPRT enzyme protein is present in patients with the Lesch-Nyhan syndrome. The relationship between cell density and HGPRT activity has been noted in tissue culture fibroblasts derived from patients with the Lesch-Nyhan syndrome, with maximal HGPRT activity evident during exponential growth (KELLEY and MEADE, 1971; WOOD and PINSKY, 1973). RICCARDI and LITTLEFIELD (1972) noted the gradual development of aminopterin resistance in Lesch-Nyhan tissue culture fibroblasts. This was associated with an increase in cellular uptake of H^3-hypoxanthine and a doubling of assayable HGPRT activity. Increasing the magnesium concentration to 20 mM in media has been reported to increase apparent HGPRT activity and sensitize fibroblasts from patients with the Lesch-Nyhan syndrome to 8-azaguanine (BENKE et al., 1973a). BAKAY and NYHAN (1972) reported that mixing of normal hemolysate and Lesch-Nyhan hemolysate followed either by Sephadex column chromatography or polyacrylamide gel electrophoresis resulted in an apparent activation of mutant HGPRT activity. Activation of erythrocyte HGPRT activity in patients with the Lesch-Nyhan syndrome has been observed in vivo. When patients were maintained on a diet essentially free of purines for 14–17 days, erythrocyte HGPRT activity rose 60–300%. Restoration of purine intake by dietary adenine-supplementation resulted in a prompt decrease in HGPRT activity to undetectable levels (ARNOLD and KELLEY, 1973).

Another approach to the elucidation of the nature of the mutation(s) responsible for the virtually complete deficiency of HGPRT has been to examine tissues from patients with the Lesch-Nyhan syndrome for antigenic material that is immunologically cross-reactive (CRM) with normal HGPRT enzyme protein. These studies have again indicated a striking heterogeneity in that either the presence (CRM-positive) or absence (CRM-negative) of CRM may be found in tissues from patients with the Lesch-Nyhan syndrome. Using antisera prepared against highly purified human erythrocyte HGPRT initial studies noted the presence of CRM in erythrocytes from 18 different patients with the Lesch-Nyhan syndrome (ARNOLD et al., 1972; RUBIN et al., 1971; MULLER and STEMBERGER, 1974). Normal amounts of CRM were detected in these studies not only by the ability of hemolysates from patients with the Lesch-Nyhan syndrome to remove antibodies that catalytically inactivate normal HGPRT but also by immunodiffusion and immunoelectrophoresis. However, subsequent studies using similar techniques but perhaps more monospecific anti-HGPRT serum have failed to support these early observations and suggest that most patients with the Lesch-Nyhan syndrome are CRM-negative (UPCHURCH et al., 1975; GHANGAS and MILMAN, 1975; BAKAY et al., 1976). UPCHURCH et al. (1975) utilized purified anti-HGPRT serum to examine hemolysates from 10 patients with the Lesch-Nyhan syndrome. Nine of the patients, including three who previously were reported to be CRM-positive, were found to contain less than 3% of normal CRM. The one patient with the Lesch-Nyhan syndrome found to be CRM-positive was the patient with the K_m mutant for HGPRT activity described by MACDONALD and KELLEY (1971). Therefore, it now appears that tissues from most patients with the Lesch-Nyhan syndrome are CRM-negative.

In summary, these studies indicate marked heterogeneity of the mutations responsible for a deficiency of HGPRT activity in patients with the Lesch-Nyhan syndrome. As cited above, considerable biochemical evidence suggests that a low level of HGPRT activity is present in erythrocytes and fibroblasts from patients with the Lesch-Nyhan syndrome. However, recent immunochemical data indicates that in the majority of patients with the Lesch-Nyhan syndrome no immunologically detectable HGPRT enzyme protein is present. Therefore, while the former suggests that a mutation(s) on the structural gene(s) responsible for the synthesis of HGPRT is the basic genetic abnormality in patients with the Lesch-Nyhan syndrome, the latter raises the possibility of a quantitatively abnormal synthesis of HGPRT enzyme protein due to a mutation(s) on the gene(s) responsible for the regulation of HGPRT synthesis. Although this controversy cannot be resolved at present, it is possible that both types of mutations ("structural" and "regulator") do occur or, alternatively, that an abnormally labile HGPRT is present. Studies in HGPRT-deficient Chinese hamster cell lines obtained by mutagenesis indicate both the occurrence of CRM-positive and CRM-negative HGPRT activity deficient cell lines and the increased susceptibility of the mutant HGPRT enzyme protein to degradation (BEAUDET et al., 1973). In addition, the degradation rate of missense mutant HGPRT molecules has been reported to be 3–17.5-fold faster than the normal HGPRT enzyme protein (CAPECCHI et al., 1974).

2. Inheritance of HGPRT

All available evidence indicates that HGPRT is inherited in an x-linked recessive fashion (KELLEY et al., 1969). Pedigree analysis of families with the Lesch-Nyhan syndrome strongly supports an x-linked recessive inheritance pattern; however, since patients with the Lesch-Nyhan syndrome do not reproduce, the crucial test of an absence of male-to-male inheritance has not been met. However, pedigree analysis of families of patients with the partial deficiency of HGPRT activity clearly demonstrates the pattern of x-linked recessive inheritance (KELLEY et al., 1969; Fox et al., 1975).

The most convincing data indicating that the gene coding for the synthesis of HGPRT is located on the x-chromosome has come from autoradiographic studies of fibroblasts from patients with the Lesch-Nyhan syndrome and maternal obligate heterozygotes. ROSENBLOOM et al. (1967b) first demonstrated that fibroblasts derived from patients with the Lesch-Nyhan syndrome failed to incorporate H^3-hypoxanthine into acid precipitable nucleic acids. However, obligate heterozygotes demonstrated two populations of cells: one which failed to incorporate H^3-hypoxanthine (40% of total cells) and another which did so normally (60% of total cells). This study both confirmed the x-linked inheritance of HGPRT and provided a striking illustration of the random inactivation of the x-chromosome as predicted by the Lyon hypothesis (LYON, 1961). It has also been shown that the genes for HGPRT and glucose-6-phosphate dehydrogenase are linked in Chinese hamster cells (ROSENSTRAUS and CHOSIN, 1975). Recent studies have shown that insertion of a normal x-chromosome into HGPRT deficient cells results in the restoration of HGPRT activity (MC BRIDGE and OZER, 1973).

The determination of the x-linked inheritance pattern for HGPRT and the availability of tissue culture media that can select positive and negative cells for HGPRT provided the initial approach to screening of individuals for heterozygosity for

HGPRT deficiency (LITTLEFIELD, 1964; MIGEON, 1969; FELIX and DEMARS, 1971). Subsequently, GARTLER et al. (1971) described heterozygote detection based on assay of HGPRT and APRT activity in hair follicles obtained from individuals at risk. Since the hair follicle is derived from a single cell, heterozygotes are found to have mosaicism of hair follicle HGPRT activity. Other authors have subsequently confirmed this finding and documented its usefulness (SILVERS et al., 1972; FRANCKE et al., 1973; DE BRUYN et al., 1974).

Prenatal diagnosis of the Lesch-Nyhan syndrome by ammiocentesis and HGPRT activity determination has been demonstrated (BOYLE et al., 1970). Also, recently developed microassay techniques for HGPRT activity in single cells greatly facilitates this diagnosis without the delay incurred by culturing of cells prior to assay (DE BRUYN et al., 1976).

3. Pathogenesis of the Neurobehavioral Disorder

In contrast to the relationship between HGPRT deficiency and the overproduction of uric acid in patients with the Lesch-Nyhan syndrome, very little is known of the role of HGPRT deficiency in the pathogenesis of the neurobehavioral abnormalities in these patients. The finding that patients with a partial deficiency of HGPRT have relatively mild, if any, neurologic abnormalities suggests that the neurobehavioral abnormalities are in some way related to the virtually complete deficiency of HGPRT (KELLEY et al., 1969). Histologic examination of the central nervous system at autopsy has failed to reveal any consistent pathologic alterations. Most often no significant findings have been noted at autopsy (HOEFNAGEL et al., 1965; CRUSSI et al., 1969).

The possibility that certain metabolic consequences of HGPRT deficiency might mediate the pathogenesis of the neurobehavioral disorder have been studied. While abnormal levels of uric acid and oxypurines are present in the cerebrospinal fluid of patients with the Lesch-Nyhan syndrome, the lack of response to allopurinol therapy from birth and the presence of equally high uric acid and oxypurine levels in patients with partial deficiency without neurologic disease suggest that these compounds are not involved (ROSENBLOOM et al., 1967a). While folic acid and adenine have been shown to enhance the growth of tissue culture fibroblasts from patients with the Lesch-Nyhan syndrome, no demonstrable benefit to the neurobehavioral disorder occurred when they were administered to patients (SCHULMAN et al., 1971; BENKE et al., 1973c). Guanine nucleotide synthesis in tissue culture fibroblasts from patients with the Lesch-Nyhan syndrome is dependent on the glutamine concentration of the media, suggesting that glutamine may be depleted in vivo (RAIVIO and SEEGMILLER, 1973). Finally, the CNS toxicity of methylxanthines have been studied in vivo in a rabbit and rat model system (NYHAN, 1973). Administration of caffeine and theophylline to rabbits produces self-multilatory behavior (MORGAN et al., 1970). Since theophylline is more effective in this respect and because of its well-defined capacity to inhibit phosphodiesterase, it has been suggested that cAMP may play a role in the genesis of self-mutilation (NYHAN, 1973).

Recently, several important observations have been made which relate the neurobehavioral manifestations of the Lesch-Nyhan syndrome to disordered adrenergic function and serotonin metabolism. ROCKSON et al. have demonstrated elevated plasma levels of dopamine β-hydroxylase (DBH) in six patients with the classic Lesch-Nyhan syndrome (ROCKSON et al., 1974). In contrast, four patients with a partial deficiency of HGPRT activity and three patients with cerebral palsy and normal HGPRT activity had normal levels of plasma DBH. SKAPER and SEEGMILLER subsequently reported diminished activity of monoamine oxidase (MAO) in mutagenized and spontaneously HGPRT-deficient cultured rat glioma cells (SKAPER and SEEGMILLER, 1976). These cell lines were shown to have biochemic abnormalities identical to those present in tissue culture fibroblasts derived from patients with the Lesch-Nyhan syndrome (WOOD et al., 1973). The diminished monoamine oxidase activity in these cells results in a reduced capacity to oxidatively deaminate serotonin and tryptamine. The abnormalities of DBH and MAO activities associated with a complete deficiency of HGPRT strongly suggest that the neurobehavioral abnormalities of the Lesch-Nyhan syndrome may be related to excess liberation of catecholamines from sympathetic nerve terminals or excessive levels of serotonin, respectively. In light of the latter possibility, it is puzzling that attempts to elevate brain serotonin levels by administration of 5-hydroxytryptamine to patients with the Lesch-Nyhan syndrome have been successful in ameliorating self-mutilatory tendencies (MIZUNO and YUGARI, 1974).

4. Secondary Metabolic and Enzymatic Abnormalities

While the x-linked recessive inheritance of a complete deficiency of HGPRT activity is the primary mutational event in patients with the Lesch-Nyhan syndrome, a variety of other metabolic and enzymatic abnormalities have been demonstrated in these patients. These associated abnormalities appear not to be due to a separate genetic abnormality but as a secondary consequence of the primary genetic defect.

The concentration of PP-ribose-P is elevated as much as 10-fold in erythrocytes and fibroblasts from patients with the Lesch-Nyhan syndrome (ROSENBLOOM et al., 1968; GREENE et al., 1970; FOX and KELLEY, 1971). Since the rate of the first reaction of purine biosynthesis de novo is related to the availability of PP-ribose-P, elevated intracellular concentrations of this compound are responsible for the accelerated activity of the de novo pathway in patients with the Lesch-Nyhan syndrome (KELLEY et al., 1970).

Elevated intracellular concentration of PP-ribose-P in patients with the Lesch-Nyhan syndrome may result from increased production of PP-ribose-P by the enzyme PP-ribose-P synthetase or by decreased utilization due to the complete deficiency of HGPRT activity. Initial studies suggested that the latter was the case and found no evidence for elevated production of PP-ribose-P in cells from patients with the Lesch-Nyhan syndrome (ROSENBLOOM et al., 1968). However, recent studies point to the possibility that an elevated activity of PP-ribose-P synthetase may be present both in mutagenized HGPRT-deficient cultured rat hepatoma (HTC) cells and human lymphoblasts as well as lymphocytes and fibroblasts from patients with the Lesch-Nyhan syndrome (GRAF et al., 1976; REEM, 1975; MARTIN and MALER, 1976). These studies report that the increase of PP-ribose-P seen in HGPRT-deficient cells is due to the present of an increased amount ot PP-ribose-P synthetase enzyme protein. As a result, it has been suggested that the genetic material responsible for synthesis of the HGPRT enzyme protein has an additional function, e.g., regulation of the gene responsible for the synthesis of PP-ribose-P synthetase. Thus, it has been hypothesized that a mutation(s) resulting in a deficiency of HGPRT activity may also result in an increased synthesis of PP-ribose-P synthetase enzyme, which then is the primary cause of elevated intracellular concentrations of PP-ribose-P in patients with the Lesch-Nyhan syndrome (MARTIN and MALER, 1976).

In addition to an apparently central role in the development of accelerated purine biosynthesis de novo in patients with the Lesch-Nyhan syndrome, the elevated intracellular concentration of PP-ribose-P may also be related to the presence of increased APRT activity in erythrocytes and fibroblasts from patients with the Lesch-Nyhan syndrome. Since the initial description of a two- to three-fold increase in the specific activity of APRT in erythrocytes from patients with the Lesch-Nyhan syndrome, other investigators have consistently documented this finding (SEEG-MILLER et al., 1967; KELLEY, 1968; GREENE et al., 1970; RUBIN et al., 1969). The increase in the specific activity of APRT has been attributed to substrate stabilization by PP-ribose-P (GREENE et al., 1970). Several lines of evidence support this hypothesis. Firstly, APRT enzyme activity is protected by PP-ribose-P against thermal denaturation in vitro (GREENE et al., 1970). Secondly, the APRT enzyme from patients with the Lesch-Nyhan syndrome is more stable to heat in vitro than is the enzyme in normal subjects (KELLEY et al., 1969). Thirdly, the half-life of erythrocyte APRT activity determined by fractionation of erythrocytes by age is prolonged in patients with the Lesch-Nyhan syndrome, thereby suggesting that the APRT enzyme is stabilized in vivo (KELLEY et al., 1970). Fourthly, immunochemical structural and kinetic analysis of the APRT enzyme from patients with the Lesch-Nyhan syndrome fails to show any difference from the normal APRT enzyme (YIP et al., 1973; BASHKIN, 1973).

In contrast, the elevated specific activity of another phosphoribosyltransferase enzyme, orotate phosphoribosyltransferase (OPRT), as well as the next enzyme in the pathway, orotidine, 5'-decarboxylase in erythrocytes from patients with the Lesch-Nyhan syndrome does not appear to be related to substrate stabilization by PP-ribose-P. A 2–10-fold increase in the specific activity of ODC and OPRT has been found in erythrocytes from patients with the Lesch-Nyhan syndrome (BEARD-MORE et al., 1973). However, the specific activity of ODC and OPRT was normal in leukocytes obtained from the same patients. The exact mechanism of the elevated ODC and OPRT specific activity remains to be elucidated.

PEHLKE et al. (1972) have reported an elevation of inosinic acid dehydrogenase (IMP-DH) in erythrocytes but not leukocytes or skeletal muscle from patients with the Lesch-Nyhan syndrome. The elevated activity of IMP-DH may be of physiologic significance in the generation of adequate levels of GMP. While the exact mechanism of the elevated specific activity of IMP-DH remains unknown, studies have suggested that it may be due both to the absence of a dialyzable inhibitor of the enzyme, which is normally present in erythrocytes, as well as stabilization of the enzyme in circulating erythrocytes in vivo. A subsequent preliminary report suggests that the inhibitor may be 2,3-diphosphoglyceric acid (LOMMEN et al., 1974).

The transport of purines into cells from patients with the Lesch-Nyhan syndrome has been studied by BENKE et al. (1973d). This study utilized cultured human fibroblasts from normals and patients with the Lesch-Nyhan syndrome and suggested that HGPRT regulates hypoxanthine transport in these cells. Uptake of hypoxanthine was found to be virtually eliminated in HGPRT-deficient cells as judged by retention of radioactivity in the cells following incubation with C^{14}-hypoxanthine. However, as observed by ALFORD and BARNES, the magnitude of entry of hypoxanthine into cells will be greatly underestimated in the absence of HGPRT, since free hypoxanthine can readily reequilibrate with the media while in the presence of HGPRT, the mononucleotide will be formed and is much less readily diffusible (ALFORD and BARNES, 1976). Therefore, at the present time any conclusions regarding the effect of HGPRT deficiency on the cellular transport of purines must be considered tentative.

The absence of HGPRT activity in patients with the Lesch-Nyhan syndrome results in an alteration of the metabolism of certain drugs that are analogs of the natural purine substrate of HGPRT. The metabolic abnormalities of these agents in patients with the Lesch-Nyhan syndrome is not only of interest from the standpoint of pharmacogenetics but also may be of therapeutic importance in selected instances. The purine analog azathioprine is a potent chemotherapeutic agent used in the treatment of malignant and diffuse inflammatory diseases. Although its precise mechanism of action in these situations is unknown, this agent has been shown to produce a diminished rate of purine synthesis de novo when administered to individuals with normal HGPRT activity (SORENSON, 1966). However, when given to patients with the Lesch-Nyhan syndrome no decrease in de novo purine synthesis is observed (KELLEY et al., 1967c). This suggests that these purine analogs must first be converted to their ribonucleotide derivative by HGPRT in order to produce a decrease in purine biosynthesis de novo.

Allopurinol (4-hydroxypyrazolo 3,4-d pyrimidine) produces a decrease in uric acid synthesis by two mechanisms: (1) As a free base, allopurinol and its metabolic product oxipurinol directly inhibit xanthine oxidase; (2) Allopurinol administration also results in a decrease in the rate of purine biosynthesis de novo (RUNDLES, 1966). The first action of allopurinol occurs unrelated to the presence or absence of HGPRT activity. However, the latter effect of a decrease in purine biosynthesis de novo requires the presence of HGPRT enzyme activity and is also accompanied by a decrease in the erythrocyte concentration of PP-ribose-P (KELLEY et al., 1968b; FOX et al., 1970; KELLEY et al., 1969). When given to patients with the Lesch-Nyhan syndrome, allopurinol is an effective antihyperuricemic agent but does not produce a decrease in the rate of purine biosynthesis de novo as judged by the total 24-h excretion of oxypurines.

This inherited variation in drug metabolism consequent to the deficiency of HGPRT has also supplied a valuable in vitro chemical selection technique for HGPRT negative cells in culture. When tissue culture fibroblasts derived from patients with the Lesch-Nyhan syndrome are grown in media containing the purine analog 8-azaguanine, no cell death ensues. However, 8-azaguanine is highly toxic to cells with normal HGPRT activity (LITTLEFIELD, 1964; FELIX and DEMARS, 1971). In contrast, when HGPRT-deficient cells are grown in the presence of aminopterin, an inhibitor of purine de novo synthesis, cell death results despite supplementation of the media with hypoxanthine and thymidine. However, when cells with normal HGPRT activity are grown in HAT (hypoxanthine-aminopterin-thymidine), media normal cell growth results despite inhibition of purine synthesis de novo, since HGPRT can provide IMP synthesis from hypoxanthine in the absence of activity of the de novo synthetic pathway (RICCARDI and LITTLEFIELD, 1972).

II. Partial Deficiency of HGPRT

With the availability of a sensitive radiochemical assay for HGPRT and the knowledge of the relationship between HGPRT activity and uric acid metabolism derived from studies of patients with the Lesch-Nyhan syndrome, KELLEY et al. (1967c) surveyed adult gouty patients and found a subgroup of patients with an x-linked partial deficiency of HGPRT activity. In the initial report of five patients erythrocyte HGPRT activity varied between 1% and 10% of normal activity. Subsequently patients with partial HGPRT deficiency have been noted to have from 0.03% to 39% of normal erythrocyte HGPRT activity (KELLEY et al., 1967a; KELLEY et al., 1969; Fox et al., 1975). Clinically, all affected individuals are males who present severe gouty arthritis early in their third or fourth decades, often accompanied by tophi and renal stones (KELLEY et al., 1969; KOGUT et al., 1970; YÜ et al., 1972; EMMERSON and THOMPSON, 1973). Patients with a partial HGPRT deficiency comprise less than 1% of the total adult gouty population. In direct contrast to patients with the Lesch-Nyhan syndrome, no consistent neurobehavioral abnormalities have been reported in patients with partial HGPRT deficiency; however, varied types of neurologic impairment, such as seizures, spinocerebellar degeneration, and mild mental retardation, have been noted (Fox et al., 1975; EMMERSON and THOMPSON, 1973). The presence of neurobehavioral abnormalities in patients with a partial HGPRT deficiency is not related to the level of HGPRT activity in erythrocytes (EMMERSON and THOMPSON, 1973).

The hyperuricemia seen in patients with a partial deficiency of HGPRT is due to accelerated purine biosynthesis de novo with overproduction of uric acid (KELLEY et al., 1969; KOGUT et al., 1970; EMMERSON and THOMPSON, 1973). The resulting hyperuricosuria often leads to the development of renal stones if untreated and occasionally to chronic renal insufficiency (KELLEY et al., 1969).

1. Characteristics of the Mutant HGPRT Enzyme in Patients with a Partial Deficiency of HGPRT Activity

Patients with the clinical syndrome of partial HGPRT deficiency have been shown to have from 0.5% to 50% of normal HGPRT activity in erythrocytes, fibroblasts, leukocytes, and rectal mucosa (KELLEY et al., 1967a; KELLEY et al., 1969; Fox et al., 1975; KOGUT et al., 1970; YÜ et al., 1972; EMMERSON and THOMPSON, 1973). Enzymatic analysis of HGPRT activity present in the central nervous system has not been reported in patients with a partial deficiency of HGPRT activity.

The total HGPRT activity present in patients with the partial HGPRT deficiency differs widely between families but is similar in affected individuals within the same family (KELLEY, 1972). This observation provided the first suggestion of significant genetic heterogeneity of the mutation(s) producing the partial deficiency. Subsequent detailed kinetic, electrophoretic, and structural analysis have confirmed the heterogeneity of the mutation(s) producing the partial deficiency. Kinetic analysis of mutant HGPRT activity in patients with a partial deficiency has revealed both normal and altered apparent affinity (K_m) for the substrates PP-ribose-P, guanine, and hypoxanthine (BAKAY et al., 1972; Fox et al., 1975). In addition, a change from hyperbolic to sigmoidal kinetics in the presence of the inhibitor GMP has been noted in one patient with a partial HGPRT deficiency (Fox et al., 1975). Electrophoresis of mutant HGPRT from patients with partial HGPRT deficiency has revealed an abnormal anodally migratory component both by starch gel electrophoresis and polyacrylamide gel electrophoresis (BAKAY et al., 1972; KELLEY et al., 1969). Isoelectric focusing has been used to demonstrate abnormal HGPRT enzyme forms in four patients with partial HGPRT deficiency (FOX et al., 1975; FOX and LACROIX, in press). Variable thermal stability of mutant HGPRT activity in vitro has been described in several families with a partial deficiency of HGPRT activity (KELLEY et al., 1969).

No highly purified preparations of mutant HGPRT from patients with the partial deficiency have been reported. Therefore, detailed structural analysis has not been performed. In one case the molecular weight of the native mutant HGPRT present in hemolysate of a patient with the partial deficiency has been estimated to be 48000 by gel filtration and sedimentation on sucrose density gradients (FOX et al., 1975).

Most likely, the partial deficiency of HGPRT activity is the result of a mutation(s) on the gene responsible for the coding of the HGPRT enzyme protein and results in the synthesis of a catalytically defective HGPRT enzyme molecule. All available evidence indicates a marked heterogeneity of the mutation(s) responsible for the partial HGPRT deficiency. However, in the single study published to date, antisera specific for normal HGPRT failed to document the presence of immunologically detectable enzyme protein in four patients with a partial HGPRT deficiency (UP-CHURCH et al., 1975). Since the sensitivity of the immunologic technique utilized could not determine, the presence of less than 3% normal CRM—and all four patients had less than 0.4% of normal HGPRT activity—it is possible that a small amount of CRM was present. Additional immunologic studies on patients with a partial HGPRT deficiency and higher levels of HGPRT activity should clarify this observation.

2. Inheritance of Partial HGPRT Deficiency

The partial deficiency of HGPRT activity is also inherited as an x-linked recessive trait (KELLEY et al., 1969; EMMERSON and THOMPSON, 1973). Only males have been described with the characteristic clinical syndrome associated with a partial deficiency of HGPRT activity. No male-to-male transmission of this defect has been demonstrated. Two populations of cells, HGPRT positive and HGPRT negative, can be demonstrated in heterozygotes for partial HGPRT deficiency by autoradiography of tissue culture fibroblasts (KELLEY et al., 1969). In contrast to heterozygotes for the Lesch-Nyhan syndrome, heterozygotes for the partial deficiency may have levels of HGPRT activity as low as 20% of normal in erythrocyte hemolysate (FOX et al., 1975; EMMERSON and THOMPSON, 1973; EMMERSON et al., 1972). This finding has been documented in two heterozygotes for the partial deficiency to be due to the presence of two populations of erythrocytes in peripheral blood, one with normal HGPRT activity and one with markedly reduced HGPRT activity, while heterozygotes for the complete deficiency have only erythrocytes with normal HGPRT activity (JOHNSON et al., 1976). In addition, electrophoretic analysis of erythrocyte HGPRT activity from heterozygote females for the partial HGPRT deficiency demonstrated two peaks of HGPRT activity, one of which closely corresponded to the migration of normal HGPRT and another which moved further anodally (BAKAY et al., 1972; FOX et al., 1976). In addition, heterozygotes for the partial deficiency even in the absence of hyperuricemia may have an accelerated rate of purine synthesis de novo as judged by the incorporation of C^{14}-glycine into urinary uric acid and 24-h urinary excretion of uric acid (EMMERSON and WYNGAARDEN, 1969).

3. Secondary Metabolic and Enzymatic Abnormalities

Patients with a partial deficiency of HGPRT and heterozygotes both have elevated intracellular concentrations of PP-ribose-P in proportion to the severity of the enzyme deficiency (FOX et al., 1975; FOX and KELLEY, 1971; HERSHKO et al., 1968; GORDON et al., 1974). Heterozygotes for the partial HGPRT deficiency also have elevations of intracellular PP-ribose-P in proportion to the reduction of HGPRT activity.

Erythrocyte APRT activity is elevated in most patients with the partial HGPRT deficiency and in the erythrocytes of some heterozygotes for partial HGPRT deficiency (KELLEY et al., 1969; FOX et al., 1975; GORDON et al., 1974). In the latter case, the level of APRT activity is correlated with the intracellular concentration of PP-ribose-P and suggests that the elevated APRT activity is related to substrate stabilization by PP-ribose-P (GREENE et al., 1970).

An elevated level of orotate phosphoribosyltransferase and orotidine 5'-phosphate decarboxylase in erythrocytes from a patient with partial HGPRT deficiency has been reported (FOX et al., 1975).

D. Normal Adenine Phosphoribosyltransferase (APRT)

I. Assay Methods and Kinetic Properties

Adenine phosphoribosyltransferase (APRT, E.C. 2.4.2.7.) catalyzes the transfer of the ribose-5-P moiety from PP-ribose-P to the N-9 position of the purine base adenine to form adenylic acid (AMP). The APRT enzyme activity exists unbound in the cytosol except in bacteria, where it is located in the periplasmic space in loose association with the membrane (HOCHSTADT-OZER and STADTMAN, 1971). APRT enzyme activity has been assayed by a variety of spectrophotometric and radiochemical methods. The latter are differentiated largely by the technique used to separate the radioactive substrate from the product. These techniques include high voltage electrophoresis on paper, ascending chromatography on thin-layer cellulose, filtration over DEAE cellulose filter discs, Butanol extraction of C^{14}-AMP, anion-exchange chromatography, and electrophoresis on polyacrylamide gel and cellulose acetate (THOMAS et al., 1973; HOCHSTADT-OZER and STADTMAN, 1971; MURRAY and WONG, 1967; HORI and HENDERSON, 1966a; BERLIN and STADTMAN, 1966; BAKAY et al., 1969; KIZAKI and SAKURADA, 1976).

Kinetic analysis and substrate and inhibitor profiles of APRT have been performed in crude or highly purified preparations from human erythrocytes, rat liver, monkey liver, Ehrlich ascites tumor cells, Salmonella typhimurium, Bacillus subtilis, E. Coli, and yeast. The APRT enzyme is active over a broad pH range (THOMAS et al., 1973; HORI and HENDERSON, 1966a; KENIMER et al., 1975). The APRT enzyme from humans is most active with the 6-NH_2 purine, adenine; however, significant nucleotide formation from 2,6-diaminopurine and 4-amino-5-imidazolecarboxamide (AIC) has also been noted (THOMAS et al., 1973). Highly purified APRT from *E. Coli* does not catalyze nucleotide formation from AIC (HOCHSTADT-OZER and STADTMAN, 1971). Human erythrocyte APRT activity purified to homogeneity shows no activity with hypoxanthine, guanine, or adenosine and minimal activity with 6-mercaptopurine as substrate (THOMAS et al., 1973). The apparent affinity constant (K_m) of the APRT enzyme for the purine base adenine has varied from 1.4×10^{-4} M for the human erythrocyte APRT enzyme to 9×10^{-7} M for the APRT enzyme from Ehrlich ascites tumor cells (SRIVASTAVA and BEUTLER, 1971; HORI and HENDERSON, 1966b).

PP-ribose-P is the only effective donor of the ribose-5-phosphate moiety studied to date (GADD and HENDERSON, 1970). The APRT enzyme is inactive with ribose-5-phosphate or ribose 1,5-diphosphate as substrate. A detailed study of the binding of PP-ribose-P and other sugar mono- and diphosphates to APRT enzyme from Ehrlich ascites cells revealed that the distance between 1-pyrophosphoryl and 5-phosphoryl moieties of PP-ribose-P was the most important requirement for the binding of PP-ribose-P. Human APRT has a K_m of 6×10^{-6} for PP-ribose-P, while HGPRT has a K_m of 2×10^{-4} M (HENDERSON, 1968). This suggests that HGPRT competes poorly if at all with APRT for available PP-ribose-P.

The enzyme activity of purified preparations of APRT exhibit an absolute requirement for divalent cations (HOCHSTADT-OZER and STADTMAN, 1971; SRIVASTAVA and BEUTLER, 1971; FLAKS et al., 1957). Magnesium has been shown to the be most effective metal cofactor; however, manganese (Mn^{+2}), calcium (Ca^{+2}), cobalt (Co^{+2}), nickel (Ni^{+2}), and zinc (Zn^{+2}) will also support enzyme activity in order of decreasing effectiveness (HORI and HENDERSON, 1966a). Maximal APRT enzyme activity is achieved when magnesium is at approximately twice the concentration of PP-ribose-P, while concentrations of Mg^{+2} higher than 1 mM inhibit enzyme activity (HOCHSTADT-OZER and STADTMAN, 1971; HORI and HENDERSON, 1966a).

Several studies have indicated that the reaction mechanism of AMP synthesis by APRT is an ordered sequential mechanism in which Mg PP-ribose-P and then adenine bind to the enzyme (E) with the formation of a ternary complex, adenine-E-PP-ribose-P (SRIVASTAVA and BEUTLER, 1971; BERLIN, 1969; GADD and HENDERSON, 1969). Apparently via an intramolecular transition the intermediate ternary complex PPi-E-AMP is formed with the subsequent orderly release of PPi then AMP. Kinetic data supporting this analysis include linear double-reciprocal plots of initial velocity with variable PP-ribose-P and constant adenine and vice versa, and competitive product inhibition by AMP versus PP-ribose-P (BERLIN, 1969). Inhibition by AMP and PPi is noncompetitive with adenine and inhibition by PPi is noncompetitive with PP-ribose-P. These data indicate that only AMP and PP-ribose-P share a binding site on the same enzyme form, while the noncompetitive kinetics imply that AMP and PPi do not add to the same site as PP-ribose-P. Protection of APRT enzyme protein from thermal denaturation (40° for 10 min) by Mg^{+2}-PP-ribose-P, AMP and Mg^{+2} + PPi but not adenine or PPi alone has been offered as support for this hypothesized reaction mechanism (SRIVASTAVA and BEUTLER, 1971).

Nucleotides, metal ions, and sulfhydryl-binding agents have been demonstrated to effectively inhibit APRT enzyme activity. In Ehrlich ascites tumor cells the nucleotides AMP, adenosine diphosphate (ADP), adenosine triphosphate (ATP), and guanosine monophosphate (GMP) were shown to be competitive inhibitors versus PP-ribose-P (K_m=7.5, 21.9, 39.5, and 118 µm, respectively) (MURRAY, 1966a). Later studies in the same system demonstrated that a variety of 6-oxopurine nucleotides, including GDP, GTP, IMP, IDP, ITP, and XMP, were also effective inhibitors of APRT with guanylate being the most effective (HENDERSON et al., 1969; HENDERSON et al., 1972). Inhibition of APRT by guanylate is interesting in that in the presence of guanylate, double-reciprocal plots of initial velocity become nonlinear, and low concentrations of guanylate stimulated enzyme activity. A pH-dependent stimulation of APRT enzyme activity by ATP has also been noted (MURRAY and WONG, 1967; HORI et al., 1967). Other workers in bacterial systems have also noted the inhibitory effectiveness of 6-amino and 6-oxonucleotides on APRT activity and have proposed the term hetergeneous pool inhibition to describe the apparent low specificity for the interation of the nucleotides at the PP-ribose-P binding site of the enzyme (HOCHSTADT-OZER and STADTMAN, 1971). In view of the metabolic interconvertibility of the nucleotides, this type of nonspecific inhibition of APRT permits control of the size of the entire nucleotide pool rather than the level of one specific nucleotide. This type of nonspecific nucleotide inhibition of APRT contrasts sharply with the relative specificity of nucleotide inhibition patterns for human HGPRT, which is not inhibited by AMP (KRENITSKY, 1969).

APRT enzyme activity is also inhibited by a variety of monovalent ions. Sodium (Na^+) has been found to be an inhibitor of APRT from human and bacterial sources (HOCHSTADT-OZER and STADTMAN, 1971; SRIVASTAVA and BEUTLER, 1971; BERLIN, 1969). Potassium does not inhibit enzyme activity. Inhibition mediated by Na^+ can be reversed by increasing concentrations of magnesium (SRIVASTAVA and BEUTLER, 1971; BERLIN, 1969). Careful analysis of the mechanism of APRT inhibition by Na^+ suggests that the inhibition is produced by an interaction of Na^+ and Mg^{+2} at a site on the enzyme, potentially at the binding site for the Mg^{+2} chelated-pyrophosphoryl moiety of Mg^{+2}-PP-ribose-P (BERLIN, 1969). Also, anions such as sulfate succinate and citrate have been shown to produce 30–80% inhibition of APRT activity at 0.03 M concentration (SRIVASTAVA and BEUTLER, 1971; HORI and HENDERSON, 1966b).

Depending on the source of APRT enzyme, divalent metal ions and sulfhydryl binding agents have been shown to produce variable inhibition of APRT activity. Mercuric (Hg^{+2}) ion at concentrations as low as 10^{-5} M have been shown to produce essentially complete inhibition of APRT enzyme activity from several sources (HOCHSTADT-OZER and STADTMAN, 1971; HORI and HENDERSON, 1966a; SRIVASTAVA and BEUTLER, 1971). Sodium iodoacetate (0.1 mM) and p-choromercuribenzoate (p-CMB) (1.0 mM) are also effective inhibitors; however, p-CMB has no effect on the APRT enzyme from monkey liver (KRENITSKY et al., 1969b). N-ethylmaleimide, sodium arsenite, and sodium arsenate have no effect on APRT enzyme activity. Quantitative binding studies with p-CMB and amino acid analysis of a homogeneous preparation of APRT from rat liver indicate the presence of 3.6–3.3 mol of sulfhydryl or cysteic acid per enzyme molecule, respectively (KENIMER et al., 1975). B-mercaptoethanol and Mg2-PP-ribose-P have been shown to protect the APRT enzyme from inactivation by Hg^{+2} and p-CMB, respectively (HOCHSTADT-OZER and STADTMAN, 1971; GADD and HENDERSON, 1969).

In addition to the classic time, temperature, and Mg^{+2}-dependent generation of AMP by APRT from adenine and PP-ribose-P, an initial non-Mg^{+2}-dependent "burst synthesis" of AMP at 0° C has been described using a homogeneous preparation of APRT in the presence of adenine and PP-ribose-P (THOMAS et al., 1973; KENIMER et al., 1975). A similar burst synthesis of GMP at 0° has also been noted using a crude preparation of HGPRT (KRENITSKY, 1967). The site of the burst synthesis on the APRT enzyme can be dissected from the site responsible for the Mg^{+2}-dependent AMP synthesis by a differential inhibitor sensitivity to Hg^{+2} and p-CMB (KENIMER et al., 1975).

II. Physical Properties

The structure and physical characteristics of APRT have been studied in highly purified preparations of the enzyme from Ehrlich ascites tumor cells, *B. subtilis*, human erythrocytes, *E. Coli*, and rat liver. A remarkable variability of the molecular weight of APRT has been noted. In *B. subtilis* and *E. Coli*, the native molecular weight of APRT was noted to be 45000 and 40000 daltons, respectively (BERLIN, 1969; HOCHSTADT-OZER and STADTMAN, 1971). However, in *E. Coli* two less prominent molecular species of APRT enzyme with molecular weights of 28000 and 19000 were also noted. APRT from rat liver was estimated to have a molecular weight of approximately 20000 (KENIMER et al., 1975). The native molecular weight of a 33000-fold purified preparation of APRT from erythrocytes was noted to be 34000 daltons (Stokes radius–24.9 Å; $S_{20, w}$ –3.35); however, species of APRT with molecular weights of 69000 and 21000 were also noted (THOMAS et al., 1973). In this study the highly purified APRT activity was found to have a subunit molecular weight of approximately 11000, suggesting thereby that human erythrocyte APRT may exist ordinarily as a trimer but the enzyme is also active as a hexamer and a dimer. In contrast, no subunit structure was noted for the highly purified APRT from rat liver (KENIMER et al., 1975).

Normal human APRT and APRT from patients with the Lesch-Nyhan syndrome exist as a single electrophoretic species when examined on polyacrylamide gel (BAKAY et al., 1969). Also, isoelectric focusing of APRT from human erythrocytes and Ehrlich ascites tumor cells has revealed only a single species with an estimated pI of 4.85 and 5.1, respectively (THOMAS et al., 1973; HORI and HENDERSON, 1966a). Recently, isoelectric focusing of human erythrocyte APRT has revealed two differently charged species (FOX et al., in press). The pI of the major peak was 4.50. A minor peak at pI, 4.7, was consistently present and was 8–10% of the height of the major peak.

III. Role in Cellular Transport of Purines

The transport of adenine in *B. subtilis* appears to occur via a group translocation mechanism involving APRT (BERLIN and STADTMAN, 1966). Incubation of resting cell suspensions with $8\text{-}C^{14}$ adenine results in a rapid, stepwise uptake of radioactivity with over 95% of the intracellular label present in the nucleotide form. The direct participation of APRT in the uptake of $8\text{-}C^{14}$ adenine is suggested by the ability of nucleotide inhibitors of APRT to produce a decrease in uptake. Also, the uptake of different, but related purines to adenine was proportional to the relative activity of the APRT enzyme with respect to the same purines. In addition, in studies of $8\text{-}C^{14}$

adenine uptake by membrane vesicles from *E. Coli*, a decrease in APRT activity associated with the vesicles produced a corresponding decrease in purine uptake (HOCHSTADT-OZER and STADTMAN, 1971). Studies in mammalian systems have also demonstrated a specific saturable transport for purine bases, including adenine. In both rabbit polymorphonuclear leukocytes and human erythrocytes, addition of adenosine inhibits the uptake of adenine from the media (HAWKINS and BERLIN, 1969; PLANET and FOX, 1976). The adenosine inhibition of adenine uptake that is mediated by an inhibition of phosphoribosylpyrophosphate synthesis with lowering of intracellular PP-ribose-P concentrations also suggests the importance of the APRT enzyme in adenine uptake.

E. Clinic Syndromes Associated with a Deficiency of APRT

I. Partial Deficiency of APRT

The first patient with a partial deficiency of APRT was described by KELLEY et al. in 1968 (KELLEY et al., 1968b). Since then, individuals from 10 different families have been demonstrated to have a level of erythrocyte APRT activity greater than two standard deviations below normal (Fox et al., in press; DELBARRE et al., 1974; EMMERSON et al., 1975). The incidence in the population of a partial APRT deficiency has been estimated to be 0.4%, 0.9%, and 1% in three separate studies (SRIVASTAVA et al., 1972; Fox et al., in press; EMMERSON et al., 1976). Although pedigree data is incomplete in most cases, analysis of the pattern of APRT deficiency in published pedigrees suggests an autosomal mode of inheritance (KELLEY et al., 1968b; DELBARRE et al., 1974; EMMERSON et al., 1975). This is supported by the assignment of the locus for APRT to the long arm of chromosome 16 or chromosome 8 (TISCHFIELD and RUDDLE, 1974; KOZAK et al., 1975). Nonetheless, an inborn genetic basis for the partial APRT deficiency has not been established in all cases. The demonstration of elevated levels of APRT activity in newborns and patients with megaloblastic anemia and reticulocytosis illustrates that APRT activity may be secondarily altered (Fox et al., 1976).

No characteristic clinical syndrome has been found in association with a partial deficiency of APRT. While hyperuricemia, gouty arthritis, and renal calculi are commonly found in propositi, this may reflect the propensity of the investigators to perform APRT enzyme assay in populations with a high incidence of these clinical features. When the propositi are excluded, pedigree analysis reveals that partial APRT deficiency and hyperuricemia are discordant (Fox et al., 1973). No neurologic abnormalities have been noted in patients with partial APRT deficiency.

1. Characteristics of the APRT Enzyme in Patients with a Partial Deficiency

The specific activity of APRT in dialyzed hemolysates from normal individuals varies between 20 and 30 nmol AMP/mg protein/h in different laboratories. All subjects with a partial deficiency of APRT have less that 50% of normal enzyme activity in erythrocytes, with most patients having less than 40% normal APRT activity. While several hypothesis have been proposed to clarify this finding, no definite explanation has emerged (Fox et al., in press; KELLEY et al., 1968b). Of note is the recent demonstration that spontaneous mutations at the APRT locus in cultured Chinese hamster cells result in either the presence of 35% of normal or no detectable APRT activity (JONES and SARGENT, 1974). Although readily detectable in hemolysate, the partial APRT deficiency has usually not been found in other tissues from the same individual. Recently, however, four of seven patients with partial APRT deficiency have also been shown to have a deficiency of leukocyte APRT ranging from 30 to 45% of normal activity (Fox et al., in press). In addition, one patient had a depression of APRT activity in rectal mucosa below the normal range.

Kinetic analysis of the APRT activity present in erythrocytes from patients with a partial APRT deficiency has been performed by several authors (Fox et al., in press; EMMERSON et al., 1975; HENDERSON et al., 1968b). Not unexpectedly, the residual APRT enzyme activity has been indistinguishable from normal APRT activity when analyzed for substrate affinity, end-product inhibition, and reaction mechanism. In addition, the residual APRT enzyme activity has had normal thermal stability and in most instances a normal half-life in circulating erythrocytes. However, these latter two parameters are not always concordant, as recently demonstrated in two patients whose residual APRT activity was found to have normal thermal stability but an abnormally short half-life in circulating erythrocytes (Fox et al., in press). This may be due to an abnormal degradation of the APRT activity in aging erythrocytes (YIP et al., 1974).

No consistent alteration of the physical characteristics of the residual APRT enzyme activity has been described (Fox et al., in press). The Stokes radius of the residual APRT activity present in hemolysate was determined by chromatography on Sephadex G-100 and found to be normal (24.8 ± 0.2 A) (Fox et al., in press). Isoelectric focusing has recently been employed to analyze the residual APRT activity in hemolysates from seven patients with a partial APRT deficiency (Fox et al., in press). This sensitive technique has demonstrated a potentially significant variation in the isoelectric point of a minor component of the residual APRT activity in six of the seven patients. While in normal individuals this minor component comprises only 8–10% of the total APRT activity, it may constitute as much as 25% of the residual APRT activity in patients with a partial deficiency.

2. Metabolic Abnormalities Associated with a Partial APRT Deficiency

Although a partial deficiency of APRT may be sporadically associated with abnormalities of triglyceride and cholesterol metabolism, no consistent relationship has been noted (Fox et al., in press; KELLEY et al., 1968b; EMMERSON et al., 1975). Most investigations have centered on the association of a partial deficiency of APRT with abnormalities of purine metabolism. As mentioned above, although hyperuricemia is commonly noted in the index case with partial APRT deficiency, the two traits segregate independently. In most instances a partial deficiency of APRT has not been associated with an abnormality of purine metabolism. Erythrocytes from patients with partial APRT deficiency have a normal concentration of PP-ribose-P and ATP (Fox et al., 1973). The 24-h excretion of uric acid and the urinary uric acid-to-creatinine ratio have been found to be normal. Although of uncertain significance, two patients with partial APRT deficiency had an abnormally high increase in urinary oxypurine excretion following fructose administration (Fox et al., in press).

Whether this represents an altered regulation of the nucleotide pool associated with the partial APRT deficiency or simply an expansion of the nucleotide pool susceptible to degradation remains to be clarified.

II. Complete Deficiency of APRT Activity

Several patients with a complete deficiency of APRT activity have now been described (CARTIER et al., 1974; DEBRAY et al., 1976; VAN ACKER et al., 1976). Analysis of APRT enzyme activity in hemolysate from the first patient revealed that both parents and a maternal grandfather had a partial deficiency of APRT, while the propositus had an essentially undetectable level of APRT activity (0.002 nmol/mg hemoglobin/h).

Recurrent renal lithiasis was the primary clinical manifestation of complete APRT deficiency in this patient. Beginning at age $2^1/_2$ years, this young male experienced recurrent episodes of renal lithiasis associated with flank pain and hematuria. Minimal hyperuricemia and hyperuricaciduria were also noted. Initially, the stones were incorrectly identified as uric acid. However, reanalysis of ultraviolet, infrared, and x-ray spectra determined the true composition as 2,8-dioxyadenine.

Preliminary metabolic studies in a second patient with a clinical presentation similar to the first revealed elevated levels of adenine in the plasma and urine which remained increased on a purine-free diet (VAN ACKER et al., 1976). The association of a complete deficiency of APRT with elevated levels of adenine and the occurrence of 2,8-dioxyadenine renal stones has focused new attention on the metabolic significance of APRT. Normally, very little adenine (1.1–8.0 mg/day) is excreted in the urine, and plasma adenine levels are normally low (3.7–11.4 μm) (KELLEY and WYNGAARDEN, 1970; WEISSMAN et al., 1957). Since in man there has been to date no direct metabolic source of adenine described, the role of APRT in adenine salvage appeared to be minimal. The association of a complete deficiency of APRT with 2,8-dioxyadenine not only illustrates the importance of APRT in adenine salvage but also raises the important question as to the endogenous mechanism for the formation of adenine. Clearly, more cases of APRT deficiency will be described as populations of patients with "uric acid" stones are carefully analyzed both retrospectively and prospectively for the presence of 2,8-dioxyadenine stones.

References

Acker, K. J. Van, Simmonds, A. H., Cameron, J. S.: Complete deficiency of adenine phosphoribosyltransferase (APRT): Report of a family. J. Clin. Chem. Clin. Biochem. **14**, 277—282 (1976)

Alford, B. L., Barnes, E. M.: Hypoxanthine transport by cultured chinese hamster lung fibroblasts. J. biol. Chem. **251**, 4823—4827 (1976)

Arnold, W. J., Kelley, W. N.: Human hypoxanthine-guanine phosphoribosyltransferase. J. biol. Chem. **246**, 7398—7404 (1971)

Arnold, W. J., Kelley, W. N.: Dietary-induced variation of hypoxanthineguanine phosphoribosyltransferase activity in patients with the Lesch-Nyhan syndrome. J. clin. Invest. **52**, 970—973 (1973)

Arnold, W. J., Meade, J. C., Kelley, W. N.: Hypoxanthine-guanine phosphoribosyltransferase: characteristics of the mutant enzyme in erythrocytes from patients with the Lesch-Nyhan syndrome. J. clin. Invest. **51**, 1805—1812 (1972)

Atkinson, M. R., Murray, A. W.: Inhibition of purine phosphoribosyltransferase of Ehrlich ascites tumor cells by 6-mercaptopurine. Biochem. J. **94**, 64—70 (1965)

Bakay, B., Becker, M. A., Nyhan, W. L.: Reaction of antibody to normal human hypoxanthine-phosphoribosyltransferase with products of mutant genes. Arch. Biochem. Biophys. **177**, 415—426 (1976)

Bakay, B., Nyhan, W. L.: The separation of adenine and hypoxanthine-guanine phosphoribosyltransferase isoenzymes by disc gel electrophoresis. Biochem. Genet. **5**, 81—90 (1971)

Bakay, B., Nyhan, W. L.: Activation of variants of hypoxanthine-guanine phosphoribosyltransferase by the normal enzyme. Proc. nat. Acad. Sci. (Wash.) **69**, 2523—2527 (1972)

Bakay, B., Nyhan, W. L., Fawcett, N., Kogut, M. D.: Isoenzymes of hypoxanthineguanine phosphoribosyltransferase in a family with partial deficiency of the enzyme. Biochem. Genet. **7**, 73—85 (1972)

Bakay, B., Telfer, M. A., Nyhan, W. L.: Assay of hypoxanthine-guanine and adenine phosphoribosyltransferases. A simple screeningtest for the Lesch-Nyhan syndrome and related disorders of purine metabolism. Biochem. Med. **3**, 230—235 (1969)

Bakhru-Kishore, R., Kelley, S.: A rapid method for hypoxanthine-guanine phosphoribosyltransferase in blood. Clin. chim. Acta **70**, 149—152 (1976)

Bashkin, P., Sperling, O., Schmidt, R., Szeinberg, A.: Erythrocyte adenine phosphoribosyltransferase in the Lesch-Nyhan syndrome. Israel J. med. Sci. **9**, 1554—1558 (1973)

Beardmore, T. D., Meade, J. C., Kelley, W. N.: Increased activity of two enzymes of pyrimidine biosynthesis de novo in erythrocytes from patients with the Lesch-Nyhan syndrome. J. Lab. clin. Med. **81**, 43—52 (1973)

Beaudet, A. L., Roufa, D. J., Caskey, C. T.: Mutations affecting the structure of hypoxanthine-guanine phosphoribosyltransferase in cultured chinese hamster cells. Proc. nat. Acad. Sci. (Wash.) **70**, 320—324 (1973)

Benke, P. J., Hebert, A., Herrick, N.: In vitro effects of magnesium ions on mutant cells from patients with the Lesch-Nyhan syndrome. New Engl. J. Med. **289**, 446—450 (1973 a)

Benke, P. J., Herrick, N., Hebert, A.: Hypoxanthine-guanine phosphoribosyltransferase variant associated with accelerated purine synthesis. J. clin. Invest. **52**, 2234—2240 (1973 b)

Benke, P. J., Herrick, N., Smitten, L., Aradine, C., Laessig, R., Wolcott, G. J.: Adenine and folic acid in the Lesch-Nyhan syndrome. Pediat. Res. **7**, 729—738 (1973 c)

Benke, P. J., Herrick, N., Hebert, A.: Transport of hypoxanthine if fibroblasts with normal and mutant hypoxanthine-guanine phosphoribosyltransferase. Biochem. Med. **8**, 309—323 (1973 d)

Berlin, R. D.: Adenylate pyrophosphorylase: purification reaction sequence and inhibition by sodium ion. Arch. Biochem. Biophys. **134**, 120—129 (1969)

Berlin, R. D., Stadtman, E. R.: A possible role of purine nucleotide phosphorylases in the regulation of purine uptake by *Bacillus subtilis*. J. biol. Chem. **241**, 2679—2686 (1966)

Boyle, J. A., Raivio, K. O., Astrin, K. H., Schulman, J. D., Graf, M. L., Seegmiller, J. E., Jacobsen, C. B.: Lesch-Nyhan syndrome: prevention control by prenatal diagnosis. Science **169**, 688—689 (1970)

Brockman, R. W.: Resistance to purine antagonists in experimental leukemia systems. Cancer Res. **25**, 1596—1605 (1965)

Bruyn, C. H. M. M. de, Oei, T. L., Ter Harr, B. G. A.: Studies on hair roots for carrier detection in hypoxanthine-guanine phosphoribosyltransferase deficiency. Clin. Genet. **5**, 449—454 (1974)

Bruyn, C. H. M. M. de, Oei, T. L., Hosli, P.: Quantitative radiochemical enzyme assays in single cells: purine phosphoribosyltransferase activities in cultured fibroblasts. Biochem. Biophys. Res. Commun. **68**(2), 483—488 (1976)

Capecchi, M. R., Capecchi, N. E., Hughes, S. H., Wahl, G. M.: Selective degradation of abnormal proteins in mammalian tissue culture cells. Proc. nat. Acad. Sci. (Wash.) **71**, 4732—4736 (1974)

Cartier, M. P., Hamet, M., Hamburger, J.: Une nouvele maladie metabolique le deficit complete en adenine phosphoribosyltransferase avec lithiase de 2,8-dihydroxyadenine. C.R. Acad. Sci. (Paris) D **279**, 883—886 (1974)

Crawhall, J. C., Henderson, J. F., Kelley, W. N.: Diagnosis and treatment of the Lesch-Nyhan syndrome. Pediat. Res. **6**, 504—513 (1972)

Crussi, F. G., Robertson, D. M., Hiscox, J. L.: The pathological condition of the Lesch-Nyhan syndrome. Amer. J. Dis. Child. **118**, 501—506 (1969)

Davies,M.R., Dean,B.M.: The heterogeneity of IMP: pyrophosphate phosphoribosyltransferase and purine nucleoside phosphorylase by isoelectric focusing. FEBS. Letters **18**, 283—286 (1971)

Debray,H., Cartier,P., Temstet,A., Cendron,J.: Child's urinary lithiasis revealing a complete deficit in adenine phosphoribosyltransferase. Pediat. Res. **10**, 762—766 (1976)

Delbarre,F., Auscher,C., Amor,B., Gery,A. de, Cartier,P., Hamet,M.: Gout with adenine phosphoribosyltransferase deficiency. Biomedicine **21**, 82—85 (1974)

Demars,R., Sarto,G., Felix,J.S.: Lesch-Nyhan mutation: prenatal detection with aminiotic fluid cells. Science **164**, 1303—1305 (1969)

Der Kaloustian,V.M., Awdeh,Z.L., Hallal,R.T., Wakid,N.W.: Analysis of human hypoxanthine-guanine phosphoribosyltransferase isozymes by isoelectric focusing in polyacrylamide gel. Biochem. Genet. **9**, 91—95 (1973)

Dizmang,L.H., Cheatham,C.F.: The Lesch-Nyhan syndrome. Amer. J. Psychiat. **127**, 671—685 (1970)

Dybing,E.: Chlorpromazine and purine transport in cultured human skin epithelial cells. Acta Pharmacol. Toxicol. **35**, 42—48 (1974)

Emmerson,B.T., Gordon,R.B., Thompson,L.: Adenine phosphoribosyltransferase deficiency: its inheritance and occurrence in a female with gout and renal disease. Aust. N.Z.J. Med. **5**, 440—446 (1975)

Emmerson,B.T., Johnson,L.A., Gordon,R.B.: Incidence of APRT deficiency. J. Clin. Chem. Clin. Biochem. **14**, 285—290 (1976)

Emmerson,B.T., Thompson,L.: The spectrum of hypoxanthine-guanine phosphoribosyltransferase deficiency. Quart. J. Med. **42**, 423—440 (1973)

Emmerson,B.T., Thompson,C.J., Wallace,D.C.: Partial deficiency of hypoxanthine-guanine phosphoribosyltransferase: intermediate enzyme deficiency in heterozygote red cells. Ann. intern. Med. **76**, 285—287 (1972)

Emmerson,B.T., Wyngaarden,J.B.: Purine metabolism in heterozygous carriers of hypoxanthine-guanine phosphoribosyltransferase deficiency. Science **164**, 1533—1535 (1969)

Felix,J.S., Demars,R.: Detection of females heterozygous for the Lesch-Nyhan mutation by 8-azaguanine-resistant growth of cultured fibroblasts. J. Lab. clin. Med. **77**, 596—604 (1971)

Flaks,J.G., Erwin,M.J., Buchanan,J.M.: Biosynthesis of the purines. XVI. The synthesis of adenosine 5′-phosphate and 5 amino-4-imidazolecarboxamide ribotide by a nucleotide phosphorylase. J. biol. Chem. **228**, 201—213 (1957)

Fox,I.H., Dotten,D.A., Marchant,P.J., Lacroix,S.: Acquired increases of human erythrocyte purine enzymes. Metabolism **25**, 571—582 (1976)

Fox,I.H., Dwosh,I.L., Marchant,P.J., Lacroix,S., Moore,M.R., Omura,S., Wyhofsky,V.: Hypoxanthine-guanine phosphoribosyltransferase. Characterization of a mutant in a patient with gout. J. clin. Invest. **56**, 1239—1249 (1975)

Fox,I.H., Kelley,W.N.: Phosphoribosylpyrophosphate in man: biochemical and clinical significance. Ann. intern. Med. **74**, 424—433 (1971)

Fox,I.H., Lacroix,S.: Electrophoretic variation in the partial deficiency of hypoxanthine-guanine phosphoribosyltransferase. Biochem. Genet. (in press) (1977)

Fox,I.H., Lacroix,S., Planet,G., Moore,M.: Partial deficiency of adenine phosphoribosyltransferase in man. Medicine (in press) (1977)

Fox,I.H., Marchant,P.J., Lacroix,S.: Hypoxanthine-guanine phosphoribosyltransferase: mosaicism in the peripheral erythrocytes of a heterozygote for a normal and mutant enzyme. Biochem. Genet. **14**, 587—593 (1976)

Fox,I.H., Meade,J.C., Kelley,W.N.: Adenine phosphoribosyltransferase deficiency in man. Amer. J. Med. **55**, 614—619 (1973)

Fox,I.H., Wyngaarden,J.B., Kelley,W.N.: Depletion of erythrocyte phosphoribosylpyrophosphate in man. New Engl. J. Med. **283**, 1177—1182 (1970)

Francke,U., Bakay,B., Nyhan,W.L.: Detection of heterozygous carriers of the Lesch-Nyhan syndrome by electrophoresis of hair root lysates. J. Pediat. **82**, 472—478 (1973)

Gadd,R.E.A., Henderson,J.F.: Inhibition of adenine phosphoribosyltransferase by pyrophosphate. Biochem. biophys. Acta **191**, 735—737 (1969)

Gadd,R.E.A., Henderson,J.F.: Studies of the binding of phosphoribosylpyrophosphate to adenine phosphoribosyltransferase. J. biol. Chem. **245**, 2979—2984 (1970)

Gartler, S. M., Scott, R. C., Goldstein, J. L., Campbell, B.: Lesch-Nyhan syndrome: rapid detection of heterozygotes by use of hair follicles. Science **172**, 572—574 (1971)

Geerdink, R. A., Vries, W. H. M. de, Willemse, J., Oei, T. L., Bruyn, C. H. M. M. de: An atypical case of hypoxanthine-guanine phosphoribosyltransferase deficiency (Lesch-Nyhan syndrome). Clin. Genet. **4**, 348—352 (1973)

Ghangas, G. S., Milman, G.: Radioimmune determination of hypoxanthine phosphoribosyltransferase crossreacting material in erythrocytes of Lesch-Nyhan patients. Proc. nats. Acad. Sci. (Wash.) **72**, 4147—4150 (1975)

Gordon, R. B., Thompson, L., Emmerson, B. T.: Erythrocyte phosphoribosylpyrophosphate concentrations in heterozygotes for hypoxanthine-guanine phosphoribosyltransferase deficiency. Metabolism **23**, 921—927 (1974)

Graf, L. H., Mc Roberts, J. A., Harrison, T. M., Martin, D. W.: Increased PRPP synthetase activity in cultured rat hepatoma cells containing mutations in the hypoxanthine-guanine phosphoribosyltransferase. J. Cell. Physiol. **88**, 331—342 (1976)

Greene, M. L., Boyles, J. R., Seegmiller, J. E.: Substrate stabilization: genetically controlled reciprocal relationship of two human enzymes. Science **167**, 887—889 (1970)

Gutensohn, W.: Hypoxanthine phosphoribosyltransferase and hypoxanthine uptake in human erythrocytes. Hoppe-Seylers Z. physiol. Chem. **356**, 1105—1112 (1975)

Gutensohn, W., Guroff, G.: Hypoxanthine-guanine phosphoribosyltransferase from rat brain (purification, kinetic properties, development, and distribution). J. Neurochem. **19**, 2139—2150 (1972)

Hawkins, R. A., Berlin, R. D.: Purine transport in polymorphonuclear leukocytes. Biochem. Biophys. Acta **173**, 324—337 (1969)

Henderson, J. F.: Kinetic properties of hypoxanthine-guanine and adenine phosphoribosyltransferases. Fed. Proc. **27**(4), 1053—1054 (1968)

Henderson, J. F., Brox, L. W., Kelley, W. N.: Kinetic studies of hypoxanthineguanine phosphoribosyltransferase. J. biol. Chem. **243**, 2514—2522 (1968a)

Henderson, J. F., Gadd, R. E. A., Palser, H. M., Hori, M.: Mechanisms of inhibition of adenine phosphoribosyltransferase by adenine nucleosides and nucleotides. Canad. J. Biochem. **48**, 573—579 (1969)

Henderson, J. F., Hori, M., Palser, H. M., Gadd, R. E. A.: Kinetic studies of inhibition of adenine phosphoribosyltransferase by guanylate. Biochem. biophys. Acta **268**, 70—76 (1972)

Henderson, J. F., Miller, H. R., Kelley, W. N., Rosenbloom, F. M., Seegmiller, J. E.: Kinetic studies of mutant human erythrocyte adenine phosphoribosyltransferases. Canad. J. Biochem. **46**, 703—706 (1968b)

Hershko, A., Hershko, C., Mager, J.: Increased formation of 5-phosphoribosyl-1-pyrophosphate in red blood cells of some gouty patients. Israel J. Med. Sci. **4**, 939—943 (1968)

Hochstadt-Ozer, J., Stadtman, E. R.: The regulation of purine utilization in bacteria. J. biol. Chem. **246**, 5312—5320 (1971)

Hoefnagel, D., Andrew, E. D., Mireault, N. G., Berndt, W. O.: Hereditary choreoathetosis, self mutilation, and hyperuricemia in young males. New Engl. J. Med. **273**, 130—135 (1965)

Hori, M., Gadd, R. E. A., Henderson, J. F.: Inhibition and stimulation of adenine phosphoribosyltransferase by purine nucleotides. Biochem. Biophys. Acta. Commun. **28**, 616—620 (1967)

Hori, M., Henderson, J. F.: Purification and properties of adenylate pyrophosphorylase from Ehrlich ascites tumor cells. J. biol. Chem. **241**, 1406—1411 (1966a)

Hori, M., Henderson, J. F.: Kinetic studies of adenine phosphoribosyltransferase. J. biol. Chem. **241**, 3404—3408 (1966b)

Hughes, S. H., Wahl, G. M., Capecchi, M. R.: Purification and characterization of mouse hypoxanthine-guanine phosphoribosyltransferase. J. biol. Chem. **250**, 120—126 (1975)

Johnson, L. A., Gordon, R. B., Emmerson, B. T.: Two populations of heterozygote erythrocytes in moderate hypoxanthine-guanine phosphoribosyltransferase deficiency. Nature (Lond.) **64**, 172—174 (1976)

Jones, G. E., Sargent, P. A.: Mutants of cultured chinese hamster cells deficient in adenine phosphoribosyltransferase. Cell **2**, 43—48 (1974)

Kaufman, J. M., Greene, M. L., Seegmiller, J. E.: Urine uric acid to creatinine ratio: screening test for disorders of purine metabolism. J. Pediat. **73**, 583—587 (1968)

Kelley, W. N.: Hypoxanthine-guanine phosphoribosyltransferase deficiency in the Lesch-Nyhan syndrome and gout. Fed. Proc. **27**, 1047—1052 (1968)

Kelley,W.N.: Biochemistry of the x-linked uric aciduria-enzyme defect and its genetic variants. Arch. intern. Med. **130**, 199—206 (1972a)

Kelley,W.N.: The Lesch-Nyhan Syndrome in the Metabolic Basis of Inherited Disease, 3rd Ed., pp. 969—991. In: Stanbury,J.B., Wyngaarden,J.B., Fredrickson,D.S. (Eds.). New York: McGraw-Hill 1972

Kelley,W.N., Arnold,W.J.: Human hypoxanthine-guanine phosphoribosyltransferase: studies on the normal and mutant forms of the enzyme. Fed. Proc. **32**, 1656—1659 (1973)

Kelley,W.N., Fox,I.H., Wyngaarden,J.B.: Regulation of purine biosynthesis in cultured human cells. Biochem. biophys. Acta **215**, 512—516 (1970)

Kelley,W.N., Greene,M.L., Rosenbloom,F.M., Henderson,J.F., Seegmiller,J.E.: Hypoxanthine-guanine phosphoribosyltransferase deficiency in gout. Ann. intern. Med. **70**, 155—205 (1969)

Kelley,W.N., Levy,R.I., Rosenbloom,F.M., Henderson,J.F., Seegmiller,J.E.: Adenine phosphoribosyltransferase deficiency: a previously undescribed genetic defect in man. J. clin. Invest. **47**, 2281—2289 (1968b)

Kelley,W.N., Meade,J.C.: Studies on hypoxanthine-guanine phosphoribosyltransferase in fibroblasts from patients with the Lesch-Nyhan syndrome. J. biol. Chem. **246**, 2953—2958 (1971)

Kelley,W.N., Rosenbloom,F.M., Henderson,J.F., Seegmiller,J.E.: A specific enzyme defect in gout associated with overproduction of uric acid. Proc. nat. Acad. Sci. (Wash.) **57**, 1735—1739 (1967a)

Kelley,W.N., Rosenbloom,F.M., Henderson,J.F., Seegmiller,J.E.: Xanthine phosphoribosyltransferase in man: relationship to hypoxanthine-guanine phosphoribosyltransferase. Biochem. Biophys. Res. Commun. **28**, 34—345 (1967b)

Kelley,W.N., Rosenbloom,F.M., Seegmiller,J.E.: The effects of azathioprine on purine synthesis in clinical disorders of purine metabolism. J. clin. Invest. **46**, 1518—1529 (1967c)

Kelley,W.N., Rosenbloom,F.M., Miller,J., Seegmiller,J.E.: An enzymatic basis for variation in response to allopurinol therapy hypoxanthine-guanine phosphoribosyltransferase deficiency. New. Engl. J. Med. **278**, 287—293 (1968a)

Kelley,W.N., Wyngaarden,J.B.: Effect of dietary purine restriction allopurinol and oxypurinol on urinary excretion of ultraviolet absorbing compounds. Clin. Chem. **16**, 707—713 (1970)

Kenimer,J.G., Young,L.G., Groth,D.P.: Purification and properties of rat liver adenine phosphoribosyltransferase. Biochem. biophys. Acta **384**, 87—101 (1975)

Kizaki,H., Sakurada,T.: A micro-assay method for hypoxanthine-guanine and adenine phosphoribosyltransferase. Anal. Biochem. **72**, 49—56 (1976)

Kogut,M.D., Donnell,G.N., Nyhan,W.L., Sweetman,L.: Disorder of purine metabolism due to partial deficiency of hypoxanthine-guanine phosphoribosyltransferase. Amer. J. Med. **48**, 148—162 (1970)

Korn,E.D., Remy,C.N., Wasileyko,A.C., Buchanan,J.M.: Biosynthesis of nucleotides from bases by partially purified enzymes. J. biol. Chem. **217**, 875—883 (1955)

Kornberg,A.: In: McElroy,W.D., Glass,B. (Eds.): The Chemical Basis of Heredity, p. 579. Baltimore: Johns Hopkins Press 1957

Kornberg,A., Lieberman,I., Simms,E.S.: Enzymatic synthesis of purine nucleotides. J. biol. Chem. **215**, 417—427 (1955)

Kozak,C., Nichols,E., Ruddle,F.H.: Gene linkage analysis in the mouse by somatic cell hybridization: assignment of adenine phosphoribosyltransferase to chromosome 8 and α-galactosidase to the x-chromosome. Som. Cell Genet. **1**, 371—375 (1975)

Krenitsky,T.A.: Tissue distribution of purine ribosyl- and phosphoribosyltransferases in the Rhesus monkey. Biochim. biophys. Acta (Amst.) **179**, 506—509 (1969)

Krenitsky,T.A., Neil,S.M., Elion,G.B., Hitchings,G.H.: Adenine phosphoribosyltransferase from monkey liver. J. biol. Chem. **244**, 4779—4787 (1969b)

Krenitsky,T.A., Neil,S.M., Miller,R.L.: Guanine and xanthine phosphoribosyltransferase activities of Lactobacillus casei and *Escherichia coli*. J. biol. Chem. **245**, 2605—2611 (1970)

Krenitsky,T.A., Papaioannou,R.: Human hypoxanthine phosphoribosyltransferase: II. Kinetics and chemical modification. J. biol. Chem. **244**, 1271—1277 (1969)

Krenitsky,T.A., Papaioannou,R., Elion,G.B.: Human hypoxanthine phosphoribosyltransferase: I. Purification, properties, and specificity. J. biol. Chem. **244**, 1263—1270 (1969a)

Lesch,M., Nyhan,W.L.: A familial disorder of uric acid metabolism and central nervous system function. Amer. J. Med. **36**, 561—570 (1964)

Littlefield, J. W. L.: Selection of hybrids from matings of fibroblasts in vitro and their presumed recombinants. Science **145**, 709—710 (1964)

Lommen, E. J. P., Abreu, R. A. de, Trijbels, J. M. F., Schretlen, E. D. A. M.: The IMP dehydrogenose catalyzed reaction in erythrocytes of normal individuals and patients with hypoxanthine-guanine phosphoribosyltransferase deficiency. Acta paediat. scand. **63**, 140—142 (1974)

Lyon, M. F.: Gene action on the x-chromosome of the mouse (Mus musculus L.). Nature (Lond.) **190**, 372—373 (1961)

MacDonald, J. A., Kelley, W. N.: Lesch-Nyhan syndrome: altered kinetic properties of mutant enzyme. Science **171**, 689—691 (1971)

Mc Bride, O. W., Ozer, H. L.: Transfer of genetic information by purified metaphase chromosomes. Proc. nat. Acad. Sci. (Wash.) **70**, 1258—1262 (1973)

Martin, D. W., Maler, B. A.: Phosphoribosylpyrophosphate synthetase is elevated in fibroblasts from patients with the Lesch-Nyhan syndrome. Science **192**, 408—410 (1976)

Martin, W. R., Young, R. R.: Inosine and guanine phosphoribosyltransferase in Escherichia Coli. Biochem. Biophys. Res. Commun. **48**, 1641—1648 (1972)

Migeon, B. R.: X-linked hypoxanthine-guanine phosphoribosyltransferase deficiency: detection of heterozygotes by selective medium. Biochem. Genet. **4**, 377—383 (1969)

Miller, R. L., Bieber, A. L.: Purification and properties of inosine monophosphate: pyrophosphate phosphoribosyltransferase from brewer's yeast. Biochemistry **7**, 1420—1426 (1968)

Miller, G. L., Ramsey, G. A., Krenitsky, T. A., Elion, G. B.: Guanine phosphoribosyltransferase from Escherichia Coli, specificity and properties. Biochemistry **11**, 4723—4731 (1972)

Mizuno, T. M., Segawa, M., Kurumada, T., Maruyama, H., Onosawa, J.: Clinical and therapeutic aspects of the Lesch-Nyhan syndrome in Japanese children. Neuropaediatrie **2**, 38—52 (1970)

Mizuno, T., Yugari, Y.: Self-mutilation in the Lesch-Nyhan syndrome. Lancet **1974 I**, 761

Morgon, L. L., Schneiderman, N., Nyhan, W. L.: Theophylline: induction of self-biting in rabbits. Psychon. Sci. **19**, 37—38 (1970)

Muller, M. M., Stemberger, H.: Immunologic studies of hypoxanthine-guanine phosphoribosyltransferase in Lesch-Nyhan syndrome. Advanc. exp. med. Biol. [A] **41**, 187—194 (1974)

Murray, A. W.: Purine-phosphoribosyltransferase activities in rat and mouse tissues and in Ehrlich ascites-tumor cells. Biochem. J. **100**, 664—670 (1966a)

Murray, A. W.: Inhibition of purine phosphoribosyltransferase from Ehrlich ascites-tumor cells by purine nucleotides. Biochem. J. **100**, 671—674 (1966b)

Murray, A. W.: The activities and kinetic properties of purine phosphoribosyltransferases in developing mouse liver. Biochem. J. **104**, 675—678 (1967)

Murray, A. W., Friedrichs, B.: Inhibition of 5'-nucleotidase from Ehrlich ascites-tumour cells by nucleoside triphosphates. Biochem. J. **111**, 83—89 (1969)

Murray, A. W., Wong, P. C. L.: Stimulation of adenine phosphoribosyltransferase by adenosine triphosphate and other nucleoside triphosphates. Biochem. J. **104**, 669—674 (1967)

Nyhan, W. L.: Clinical features of the Lesch-Nyhan syndrome. Arch. intern. Med. **130**, 186—192 (1972)

Nyhan, W. L.: The Lesch-Nyhan syndrome. Ann. Rev. Med. **24**, 41—60 (1973)

Nyhan, W. L., Pesek, J., Sweetman, L., Carpenter, D. G., Carter, C. H.: Genetics of an x-linked disorder of uric acid metabolism and cerebral function. Pediat. Res. **1**, 5—13 (1967)

Olsen, A. S., Milman, G.: Chinese hamster hypoxanthine-guanine phosphoribosyltransferase. J. biol. Chem. **249**, 4030—4037 (1974a)

Olsen, A. S., Milman, G.: Subunit molecular weight of human hypoxanthineguanine phosphoribosyltransferase. J. biol. Chem. **249**, 4038—4040 (1974b)

Pehlke, D. M., Mc Donald, J. A., Holmes, E. W., Kelley, W. N.: Inosinic acid dehydrogenase activity in the Lesch-Nyhan syndrome. J. clin. Invest. **51**, 1398—1404 (1972)

Planet, G., Fox, I. H.: Inhibition of phosphoribosylpyrophosphate synthesis by purine nucleosides in human erythrocytes. J. biol. Chem. **251**, 5839—5844 (1976)

Raivio, K. O., Seegmiller, J. E.: Role of glutamine in purine synthesis and in guanine nucleotide formation in normal fibroblasts deficient in hypoxanthine phosphoribosyltransferase activity. Biochem. biophys. Acta **299**, 283—292 (1973)

Reem, G. H.: Phosphoribosylpyrophosphate overproduction, a new metabolic abnormality in the Lesch-Nyhan syndrome. Science **190**, 1098—1099 (1975)

Riccardi, V. M., Littlefield, J. W.: Adaptation in Lesch-Nyhan cells exposed to aminopterin. Exp. Cell Res. **74**, 417—422 (1972)

Rockson, S., Stone, R., Van der Weyden, M., Kelley, W. N.: Lesch-Nyhan syndrome: evidence for abnormal adrenergic function. Science **186**, 934—935 (1974)

Rosenbloom, F. M., Kelley, W. N., Henderson, J. F., Seegmiller, J. E.: Lyon hypothesis and x-linked disease. Lancet **1967 II** b, 305

Rosenbloom, F. M., Henderson, J. F., Caldwell, I. C., Kelley, W. N., Seegmiller, J. E.: Biochemical basis of accelerated purine biosynthesis de novo in human fibroblasts lacking hypoxanthine-guanine phosphoribosyltransferase. J. biol. Chem. **243**, 1166—1173 (1968)

Rosenbloom, F. M., Kelley, W. N., Miller, J., Henderson, J. F., Seegmiller, J. E.: Inherited disorder of purine metabolism: correlation between central nervous system dysfunction and biochemical defects. J. Amer. med. Ass. **202**, 175—177 (1967 a)

Rosenstraus, M., Chosin, L. A.: Isolation of mammalian cell mutants deficient in glucose-6-phosphate dehydrogenase activity: linkage to hypoxanthine phosphoribosyltransferase. Proc. nat. Acad. Sci. (Wash.) **72**, 493—497 (1975)

Rubin, C. S., Balis, M. E., Piomelli, S., Berman, P. H., Dancis, J.: Elevated AMP pyrophosphorylase activity in congenital IMP pyrophosphorylase deficiency (Lesch-Nyhan disease). J. Lab. clin. Med. **74**, 732—741 (1969)

Rubin, C. S., Dancis, J., Yip, L. C., Nowinski, R. C., Balis, M. E.: Purification of IMP: pyrophosphate phosphoribosyltransferase, catalytically incomplete enzymes in Lesch-Nyhan disease. Proc. nat. Acad. Sci. (Wash.) **68**, 1461—1464 (1971)

Rundles, R. W.: Metabolic effects of allopurinol and alloxanthine. Ann. rheum. Dis. **25**, 615—620 (1966)

Schmidt, R., Foret, M., Reichert, U.: Improved microscale assay for purine phosphoryltransferase activities. Clin. Chem. **22** (1), 67—69 (1976)

Schulman, J. D., Greene, M. L., Fujimoto, W. Y., Seegmiller, J. E.: Adenine therapy for Lesch-Nyhan syndrome. Pediat. Res. **5**, 77—82 (1971)

Seegmiller, J. E.: Inherited deficiency of hypoxanthine-guanine phosphoribosyltransferase in x-linked uric aciduria. Advan. hum. Genet. **6**, 57—98 (1976)

Seegmiller, J. E., Rosenbloom, F. M., Kelley, W. N.: An enzyme defect associated with a sex-linked human neurological disorder and excessive purine synthesis. Science **155**, 1682—1684 (1967)

Silvers, P. N., Cox, R. P., Balis, M. E., Dancis, J.: Detection of the heterozygote in Lesch-Nyhan disease by hair-root analysis. New Engl. J. Med. **286**, 390—394 (1972)

Skaper, S. D., Seegmiller, J. E.: Hypoxanthine-guanine phosphoribosyltransferase mutant glioma cells: diminished monoamine oxidase activity. Science **194**, 1171—1173 (1976)

Skyler, J. S., Neelon, F. A., Arnold, W. J., Kelley, W. N., Lebovitz, H. E.: Growth retardation in the Lesch-Nyhan syndrome. Acta Endocr. **75**, 3—10 (1974)

Sorenson, L. B.: Suppression of the shunt pathway in primary gout by azathioprine. Proc. nat. Acad. Sci. (Wash.) **55**, 571—575 (1966)

Sorenson, L. B.: Mechanism of excessive purine biosynthesis in hypoxanthineguanine phosphoribosyltransferase deficiency. J. clin. Invest. **49**, 968 (1970)

Srivastava, S. K., Beutler, E.: Purification and kinetic studies of adenine phosphoribosyltransferase. Arch. biochem. Biophys. **142**, 426—434 (1971)

Srivastava, S. K., Villacorte, D., Beutler, E.: Correlation between adenylate metabolizing enzymes and adenine nucleotide levels of erythrocytes during blood storage in various media. Transfusion **12**, 190—195 (1972)

Stanbridge, E. J., Tischfield, J. A.: Appearance of hypoxanthine-guanine phosphoribosyltransferase activity as a consequence of mycoplasma contamination. Nature (Lond.) **256**, 329—330 (1975)

Strauss, M.: Determination of the subunit molecular weight of hypoxanthineguanine phosphoribosyltransferase from human erythrocytes by recovery of enzyme activity from sodium dodecyl sulphate gels. Biochem. biophys. Acta **410**, 426—430 (1975)

Thomas, C. B., Arnold, W. J., Kelley, W. N.: Human adenine phosphoribosyltransferase. J. biol. Chem. **248**, 2529—2535 (1973)

Thorpe, W. P.: The Lesch-Nyhan syndrome. Enzyme **12**, 129—142 (1971)

Tischfield, J. A., Ruddle, F. H.: Assignment of the gene for adenine phosphoribosyltransferase to human chromosome 16 by mouse-human somatic cell hybridization. Proc. nat. Acad. Sci. (Wash.) **71**, 45—49 (1974)

Toyo-Oka, T., Hanaoka, F., Akaoka, I., Yamada, M.: X-linked hypoxanthineguanine phosphoribosyltransferase deficiency without neurologic disorders. A report of a family. Clin. Genet. **7**, 181—185 (1975)

Upchurch, K. S., Leyva, A., Arnold, W. J., Holmes, E. W., Kelley, W. N.: Hypoxanthine phosphoribosyltransferase deficiency: association of reduced catalytic activity with reduced levels of immunologically detectable enzyme protein. Proc. nat. Acad. Sci. (Wash.) **72**, 4142—4146 (1975)

Van der Zee, S. P. M., Monnens, L. A. H., Schretlen, E. D. A. M.: Hereditary disorder of purine metabolism with cerebral affection and megaloglastic anemia. Ned. T. Geneesk. **112**, 1475—1479 (1968)

Walter, R. D., Konigk, E.: Hypoxanthine-guanine phosphoribosyltransferase and adenine phosphoribosyltransferase from Plasmodium chabaudi-purification, and properties. Tropenmed. Parasitol. **25**, 227—235 (1974)

Weissman, B., Bronberg, P. A., Gutman, A. B.: The purine bases of human urine: Semiquantitative estimation and isotope incorporation. J. biol. Chem. **224**, 423 (1957)

Williams, W. J., Buchanan, J. M.: Biosynthesis of Purines. V. Conversion of hypoxanthine to inosinic acid by liver enzymes. J. biol. Chem. **203**, 583—593 (1953)

Wood, S., Pinsky, L.: Lesch-Nyhan mutation: the influence of population density on purine phosphoribosyltransferase activities and exogenous purine utilization in monolayer cultures of skin fibroblasts. J. Cell. Physiol. **80**, 33—40 (1973)

Wood, A. W., Becker, M. A., Minna, J. D., Seegmiller, J. E.: Purine metabolism in normal and thioguanine-resistant neuroblastoma. Proc. nat. Acad. Sci. (Wash.) **70**, 3880—3883 (1973)

Yip, L. C., Balis, M. E.: A rapid and simple assay for inosinic acid: pyrophosphate phosphoribosyltransferase in the presence of xanthine oxidase and vice versa. Anal. Biochem. **71**, 14—23 (1976)

Yip, L. C., Dancis, J., Balis, M. E.: Immunochemical studies of AMP: pyrophosphate phosphoribosyltransferase from normal and Lesch-Nyhan subjects. Biochem. biophys. Acta **293**, 359—369 (1973)

Yip, L. C., Dancis, J., Mathieson, B., Balis, M. E.: Age-induced changes in adenosine monophosphate: pyrophosphate phosphoribosyltransferase and inosine monophosphate: pyrophosphate phosphoribosyltransferase from normal and Lesch-Nyhan erythrocytes. Biochemistry **13**, 2558—2561 (1974)

Yü, T. F., Balis, M. E., Krenitsky, T. A., Dancis, J., Silvers, D. N., Elion, G. B., Glutman, A. B.: Rarity of x-linked partial hypoxanthine-guanine phosphoribosyltransferase deficiency in a large gouty population. Ann. intern. Med. **76**, 255—264 (1972)

Zylka, J. M., Plagemann, P. G. W.: Purine and pyrimidine transport by cultured Novikoff Cells. J. biol. Chem. **250**, 5756—5767 (1975)

Purine Nucleotide Interconversions

J. F. HENDERSON

A. Pathways of Purine Nucleotide Interconversion

The various reactions of purine ribonucleotide synthesis result in the formation of adenylate, inosinate, and guanylate; xanthylate may also be formed, but this seems to be a quantitatively minor process in most mammalian cells. These purine ribonucleoside monophosphates can be metabolized in several different ways; these processes can in general be classified as (1) phosphorylation and subsequent metabolism of di- and triphosphates, (2) dephosphorylation, and (3) interconversion.

In most mammalian cells, the major route of anabolism of newly synthesized adenylate and guanylate is phosphorylation to form ADP and GDP; these in turn can be converted to the corresponding triphosphates. In rare instances, inosinate can also be phosphorylated to di- and triphosphates, although in most cells it is not metabolized by this route. ADP and GDP can be reduced to the corresponding 2'-deoxyribonucleotides, dADP, and dGDP; the latter are readily converted to the deoxyribonucleoside mono- and triphosphates. Purine ribonucleoside triphosphates can be converted into various coenzymes, and both ribo- and deoxyribonucleoside triphosphates can be incorporated into nucleic acids.

Just as phosphorylation is a major route of anabolism of purine ribonucleoside monophosphates, so is dephosphorylation an important reaction in their catabolism. Adenylate, inosinate, guanylate, and xanthylate all can be dephosphorylated to the corresponding ribonucleosides, though in intact mammalian cells these compounds are not all dephosphorylated at equal rates. Little is known about the dephosphorylation of adenylosuccinate in mammalian systems.

The reactions just described do not involve alteration of the purine base moiety of the purine nucleotides but mostly involve adenine and guanine nucleotides. Another set of reactions, however, exists to convert these nucleotide purines one into another; these are generally known as "purine nucleotide interconversions." These pathways are shown in Figure 1.

Through the reactions of purine nucleotide interconversion, adenylate and guanylate can be converted to inosinate, and inosinate can be converted to both adenylate and guanylate. Adenylosuccinate is an intermediate in the formation of adenylate from inosinate, and xanthylate is an intermediate in the formation of guanylate from inosinate. Two amino acids are required: aspartate donates its amino group in the formation of adenylate; and glutamine donates its amide group in the conversion of xanthylate to guanylate. In addition to aspartate, the conversion of inosinate to adenylosuccinate requires GTP as energy source, whereas ATP is energy source for the synthesis of guanylate from xanthylate and glutamine. Finally, the oxidation of

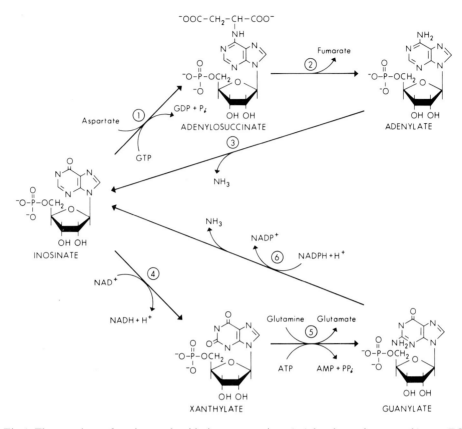

Fig. 1. The reactions of purine nucleotide interconversion. *1*, Adenylosuccinate synthetase, EC 6.3.4.4; *2*, Adenylosuccinate lyase, EC 4.3.2.2; *3*, Adenylate deaminase, EC 3.5.5.4; *4*, Inosinate dehydrogenase, EC 1.2.1.14; *5*, Guanylate synthetase, EC 6.3.5.2; *6*, Guanylate reductase, EC 1.6.6.8

inosinate to xanthylate requires NAD^+, and the reductive deamination of guanylate to inosinate requires NADPH. The deamination of adenylate to inosinate is purely hydrolytic and requires no coenzyme. Further general descriptions of these pathways and of the individual enzymes involved may be found in various reviews (HARTMAN, 1970; GOTS, 1971; ZIELKLE and SUELTER, 1971; SANWAL et al., 1971; LOWENSTEIN, 1972; HENDERSON and PATERSON, 1973).

The pathways shown in Figure 1 constitute the major routes of purine nucleotide interconversion in mammalian cells (at least so far as is presently known). It should be pointed out, however, that other pathways do exist by which such interconversions can be accomplished; these are either quantitatively minor pathways in mammalian cells or are found only in microorganisms.

Adenylate can at least potentially be converted to inosinate via the following pathway:

adenylate → adenosine → inosine → hypoxanthine → inosinate .

Although GREEN and ISHII (1972) proposed that this might be an important pathway in mammalian cells, subsequent studies (BROX and HENDERSON, 1976) have demonstrated that it is quantitatively a minor route in several different cell types. However, this pathway is of considerable importance in some microorganisms, especially those that lack adenylate deaminase.

A second alternative pathway of interconversion is related to the pathway of histidine biosynthesis; the relevant reactions may be shown as follows:

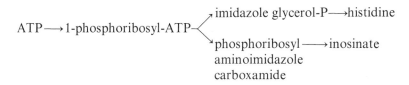

This process usually is considered to occur only in microorganisms; however, it is not certain that histidine is an essential amino acid for adult humans (LaDu, 1972), and hence some human cells may also synthesize histidine via this pathway.

Finally, the metabolism of S-adenosylmethionine may provide yet another alternative pathway of interconversion:

ATP———→S-adenosyl———→S-adenosyl———→adenosine———→adenylate
       methionine   homocysteine   │

    inosinate←———— –hypoxanthine←——inosine

The quantitative importance of these reactions has not yet been evaluated.

The alternative pathways of purine nucleotide interconversion that have just been described will not be discussed further, either because they have been little studied in mammalian cells, or because they are not believed to be quantitatively important in the purine metabolism of mammalian cells.

This chapter, then, will focus on the reactions of Figure 1 and will concentrate on their operation in intact mammalian cells, rather than on the properties of the six individual enzymes that catalyze these reactions. Among the questions that will be discussed here are the following. How are the reactions of purine nucleotide interconversion regulated in intact cells? What are the relative rates of the individual reactions in intact cells of different types? Do these reactions operate as cycles or as unidirectional processes? What are the functions of the pathways of purine nucleotide interconversion? Can these reactions be inhibited by drugs?

B. Regulation of Enzymes of Purine Nucleotide Interconversion in Intact Mammalian Cells

Factors that potentially may regulate the reactions of purine nucleotide interconversion in intact cells include (1) enzyme amount and subcellular localization, (2) substrate concentrations, (3) alternative pathways of metabolism of substrates, and (4) effects of other metabolites. Each will be discussed in turn.

I. Enzyme Amount and Localization

In no single mammalian cell have the amounts or total activities of all six of the reactions of purine nucleotide interconversion been measured. In a few cases the total activities of two or three of these enzymes have been compared, and these data are shown in Table 1. In all of the tissues studied, the activity of adenylate deaminase is greater than those of the other enzymes measured.

Tissue and species differences in the distribution of adenylate deaminase activity have been studied in considerable detail (reviewed by Lee, 1960; Zielkle and Suelter, 1971), and limited studies have been conducted with respect to inosinate dehydrogenase (Saccoccia and Miech, 1969) and adenylosuccinate lyase (Barnes and Bishop, 1975). The other enzymes have been measured in only a few mammalian tissues, and guanylate reductase in only one.

Several isozymes of adenylate deaminase have been separated, and it is known that the occurrence of these varies from one tissue to another (Ogasawara et al., 1975a; Raggi et al., 1975). Isozymes of the other enzymes of purine nucleotide interconversion have not been identified.

Changes in the total activity, physical properties, and isozyme pattern of adenylate deaminase during embryonic and postnatal development have been studied (Kluge and Wieczorek, 1968; Ogasawara et al., 1975b; Kaletha, 1975), as have changes due to exercise (Winder et al., 1974) and diet (Turner and Fern, 1974). The other enzymes have not yet been studied with respect to such factors.

Table 1. Relative actives of enzymes of purine nucleotide interconversion (Units are those of the original authors)

Tissue	Enzyme			Reference
	Adenylate deaminase	Adenylosuccinate synthetase	Adenylosuccinate lyase	
Rat red quadriceps muscle	70	0.94	[a]	Winder et al. (1974)
Rat white quadriceps muscle	85	0.66	[a]	Winder et al. (1974)
Rat soleus muscle	33	0.72	[a]	Winder et al. (1974)
Rat skeletal muscle	157	0.46	0.38	Schultz and Lowenstein (1976)
Rat brain	5.2	0.036	0.18	Schultz and Lowenstein (1976)
Rat kidney cortex	14.9	1.27	1.38	Bogusky et al. (1976)
	Adenylate deaminase	Inosinate dehydrogenase		
Rat brain	9	0.3		Santos et al., (1968)

[a] Not measured.

Finally, some information is available regarding the intracellular localization of two of the enzymes of purine nucleotide interconversion. There is some difference of opinion regarding the localization of adenylate deaminase, and this may indeed vary with the tissue studied and methods used. The preponderance of evidence seems to point to adenylate deaminase activity in several cell fractions, with most being particulate; this subject has been reviewed briefly by WEIL-MALHERBE (1975). Inosinate dehydrogenase is largely localized in the microsomal fraction of chicken liver (NAGATA et al., 1969), and although this enzyme activity can be found in the soluble fraction of Sarcoma 180 cells (ANDERSON and SARTORELLI, 1968) and rat liver (JACKSON et al., 1975), its intracellular localization in mammalian cells really has not been systematically studied.

Although all of the factors just mentioned have potential relevance to the operation of the reactions of purine nucleotide interconversion in intact cells and tissues, this point unfortunately has not yet been studied directly. In addition, our information is far from complete regarding these factors. Until we have more information and until such studies are carried out using intact cells and not just cell extracts, one must be very cautious in inferring any possible physiologic significance from the experimental results so far published (HENDERSON et al., 1977).

II. Substrate Concentrations

The first step in assessing the real role of substrate concentration in the regulation of a metabolic pathway in intact cells, is to compare known intracellular concentrations of substrates with the Michaelis constants reported for the appropriate enzymes. This is somewhat difficult to do in a meaningful way in the case of purine nucleotide interconversion, because the concentrations of the purine ribonucleoside monophosphate substrates are very low and are quite difficult to measure accurately; many published values either are suspect or are clearly too high due to breakdown of ATP and GTP during sample preparation.

However, Table 2 presents the best values determined or estimated in the author's laboratory for the concentrations of purine ribonucleoside monophosphates

Table 2. Substrate concentrations and Michaelis constants

Enzyme	Substrate	Substrate conc.[a] (µM)	Michaelis constant[b] (µM)
Inosinate dehydrogenase	Inosinate	30	20
Adenylosuccinate synthetase	Inosinate	30	30
Adenylosuccinate lyase	Adenylosuccinate	4	10
Adenylate deaminase	Adenylate	60	1400[c]
Guanylate synthetase	Xanthylate	4	3.6
Guanylate reductase	Guanylate	8	7[d]

[a] From HENDERSON et al., 1977.
[b] From HENDERSON and PATERSON, 1973.
[c] Varies widely, depending on assay conditions.
[d] From SPECTOR, 1975.

in Ehrlich ascites tumor cells incubated in vitro and in cultured mouse lymphoma L 5178 Y cells (HENDERSON et al., 1977); the degree to which these values are representative of normal mammalian cells in vivo is not known. The Michaelis constants reported for the enzymes of purine nucleotide interconversion are also presented.

It is seen that the concentration of inosinate is approximately the same as the Michaelis constants for the two enzymes that utilize it, adenylosuccinate synthetase and inosinate dehydrogenase. Likewise, the concentrations of guanylate and xanthylate are approximately the same as the Michaelis constants for guanylate reductase and guanylate synthetase, respectively. In contrast, the concentrations of adenylosuccinate and adenylate are appreciably lower than the Michaelis constants of adenylosuccinate lyase and adenylate deaminase, respectively.

Because of the numerous other factors that regulate enzyme velocities in intact cells, it is imprudent to draw too many conclusions about the operation of purine nucleotide interconversion in intact cells from the data of Table 2. It is far more informative to study the effect on enzyme rate in cells of increasing or decreasing intracellular substrate concentrations. In the case of the purine ribonucleoside monophosphate substrates, unfortunately, this is not easy to accomplish; because of the impermeability of cells to nucleotides, their concentrations cannot simply be manipulated by adding them to cell suspensions or injecting them into animals.

Three types of approaches have been made to this problem. One has been to compare apparent activities (SNYDER et al., 1972) of some of the enzymes of purine nucleotide interconversion when cells were incubated in vitro with high and low concentrations of purine bases (especially hypoxanthine), when nucleotide formation from these bases was rapid. Whether the use of high purine base concentrations leads to an increase in the intracellular concentration of inosinate or simply in an increased rate of its synthesis really is not known.

However, in Ehrlich ascites tumor cells incubated in vitro, relatively more inosinate was converted to adenine nucleotides when cells were incubated with 100 µM hypoxanthine than when incubated with 5 µM hypoxanthine; thus, the ratio of radioactivity in adenine nucleotides to that in guanine nucleotides changed from 2.8:1–6.2:1 (CRABTREE and HENDERSON, 1971a; CRABTREE, 1970). However, this ratio was 10.2 when human platelets were incubated with 1.9 µM hypoxanthine but 7.6 when platelets were incubated with 15.7 µM hypoxanthine (RIVARD et al., 1975). In addition, the deamination of adenylate in Ehrlich ascites tumor cells was affected by the concentration of adenine with which the cells were incubated (CRABTREE and HENDERSON, 1971a; CRABTREE, 1970).

A second approach has been to use drugs to block either adenylosuccinate synthetase or inosinate dehydrogenase, and then to determine whether the amount of inosinate metabolized via the uninhibited pathway would increase. Thus, when hadacidin was used to inhibit the conversion of inosinate to adenylosuccinate either in Ehrlich ascites tumor cells (CRABTREE and HENDERSON, 1971a) or in cultured skin fibroblasts (RAIVIO and SEEGMILLER, 1973a), an increased metabolism of inosinate via inosinate dehydrogenase was detected. When tumor cells in vivo were treated with hadacidin, intracellular concentrations of guanine nucleotides increased, again suggesting that inosinate synthesized de novo was being dehydrogenated at an increased rate (SMITH and HENDERSON, 1976). However, in cells in which inosinate dehydrogenase was inhibited with mycophenolic acid, no increase in the apparent activity of adenylosuccinate synthetase was noted (SNYDER et al., 1972; SMITH et al., 1974; SMITH and HENDERSON, 1976); however, this drug does have some side effects that complicate interpretation of these results.

The third approach has been to induce the rapid breakdown of ATP in Ehrlich ascites tumor cells by means of inhibitors of energy metabolism, such as 2-deoxyglucose and 2,4-dinitrophenol; as a result, the rates of synthesis of adenylate and inosinate are greatly increased, and intracellular concentrations of these nucleotides increase at least transiently. The results of these experiments show that there was a good correlation between the rate of deamination of adenylate and the rate of its formation; however, there was no correlation between rate of deamination and adenylate concentrations (LOMAX et al., 1975).

Inosinate dehydrogenase activity also increased with increasing rates of inosinate production during ATP breakdown but seemed to be saturated at high inosinate concentrations; however, these results did not seem to be directly related to the reported Michaelis constant for this enzyme (LOMAX et al., 1975).

All of the results just discussed led to the tentative conclusion that the rates of at least some of the reactions of purine nucleotide interconversion are greatly influenced by the rate of synthesis of their purine ribonucleoside monophosphate substrates but not necessarily by the actual intracellular concentrations of these substrates.

In contrast to the somewhat equivocal results regarding purine ribonucleoside monophosphate concentrations in the regulation of purine nucleotide interconversion, there is clear evidence that concentrations of aspartate and glutamine influence the rates of the adenylosuccinate synthetase and guanylate synthetase reactions, respectively. Thus, the addition of either of these amino acids to Ehrlich ascites tumor cells (CRABTREE and HENDERSON, 1971a, b) or cultured skin fibroblasts (RAIVIO and SEEGMILLER, 1973b) incubated in an amino-acid-free medium considerably increased the conversion of inosinate to adenine and guanine nucleotides. Asparagine can replace aspartate, apparently because of intracellular deamidation (HENDERSON et al., 1975; RAIVIO and SEEGMILLER, 1973b); even the addition of glutamine alone stimulates the adenylosuccinate synthetase reaction due to its conversion to aspartate in cells (HENDERSON, 1963).

Addition of aspartate, through its stimulation of adenylosuccinate synthetase, decreases the extent of inosinate breakdown to inosine and hypoxanthine (CRABTREE and HENDERSON, 1971b; HENDERSON et al., 1975). Similarly, the addition of glutamine stimulates guanylate synthetase activity and decreases the extent of catabolism of xanthylate to xanthosine and xanthine in Ehrlich ascites tumor cells (CRABTREE and HENDERSON, 1971a, b) and in rabbit erythrocytes (HERSHKO et al., 1967). In the former system, the concentration of xanthylate increased very considerably when glutamine was omitted from the medium and ATP breakdown was induced using 2,4-dinitrophenol (LOMAX et al., 1975).

The possibility that concentrations of NAD^+ and of NADPH might regulate rates of inosinate dehydrogenase and guanylate reductase, respectively, in intact cells has not been investigated.

ATP and GTP are substrates of guanylate synthetase and adenylosuccinate synthetase, respectively. Studies with hadacidin-treated tumor cells in vivo showed that decreases in ATP concentrations did not affect guanine nucleotide concentrations;

hence, these experiments gave no indication of a decreased rate of the guanylate synthetase reaction. In the same system, lowered GTP concentrations (to ∞10% of normal) caused by mycophenolic acid treatment did cause a small (11%) apparent inhibition of adenylosuccinate synthetase activity and a 17% decrease in adenine nucleotide concentrations (SMITH and HENDERSON, 1976). However, lowering of GTP concentration to less than 10% of normal in cultured lymphoma L 5178 Y cells by the use of mycophenolic acid (LOWE et al., 1977) or to ∞30% of normal in cultured neuroblastoma cells (CASS et al., 1977) did not produce any appreciable change in ATP concentration. Thus, neither purine nucleoside triphosphate appears to be limiting for the processes of purine nucleotide interconversion in intact cells.

III. Alternative Pathways of Substrate Metabolism

Another factor that at least potentially may be involved in the regulation of purine nucleotide interconversion is the metabolism of the purine ribonucleoside monophosphates by alternative pathways of metabolism. In particular, these substrates can be removed both by phosphorylation to ribonucleoside di- and triphosphates and by dephosphorylation to ribonucleosides.

Although phosphorylation is an important route of metabolism of adenylate and guanylate, xanthylate and adenylosuccinate are not converted to diphosphate derivatives, and inosinate appears to be phosphorylated only in human erythrocytes (FRASER et al., 1975). Quantitative studies of Ehrlich ascites tumor cells incubated with radioactive adenine have shown that the relative rates of phosphorylation and deamination of adenylate are 70:1; guanylate is also predominantly metabolized by phosphorylation (SNYDER and HENDERSON, 1973a). Similar observations have been made using other types of cells, and it seems quite possible that rapid phosphorylation of adenylate is an important factor in the regulation of adenylate deaminase activity in intact cells.

Rates of nucleotide dephosphorylation are quite low in cells incubated in rich media but increase when adenylosuccinate synthetase and guanylate synthetase activities are limited by lack of aspartate and glutamine, respectively, or when these enzymes are inhibited by hadacidin or diazo-oxo-norleucine, respectively; this has been observed in rabbit erythrocytes (HERSHKO et al., 1967), Ehrlich ascites tumor cells (CRABTREE and HENDERSON, 1971a, b), and skin fibroblasts (RAIVIO and SEEGMILLER, 1973a, b).

The rate of dephosphorylation is especially important when ATP catabolism is accelerated, e.g., by incubation of cells with 2-deoxyglucose. In Ehrlich ascites tumor cells the increased adenylate so formed is predominantly deaminated, and less than 20% is dephosphorylated (LOMAX and HENDERSON, 1973). However, this percentage is greater in some other cell types, and dephosphorylation may under some circumstances be masked by rephosphorylation via adenosine kinase (EC 2.7.1.20). When inosinate synthesis is rapidly increased during accelerated ATP catabolism in Ehrlich ascites tumor cells, most of the inosinate so formed is dephosphorylated rather than dehydrogenated (LOMAX et al., 1975). Dephosphorylation is markedly retarded, however, under anaerobic conditions.

IV. Effects of Other Metabolites

Numerous studies of the individual enzymes of purine nucleotide interconversion in cell extracts or in partially purified preparations have shown that they can be inhibited or stimulated by various metabolites, particularly purine ribonucleotides themselves. On the basis of these enzyme studies various hypotheses have been elaborated regarding the operation of the pathways of purine nucleotide interconversion in intact mammalian cells. Space does not permit a detailed review or discussion of this literature, but several reviews are available (GOTS, 1971; SANWAL et al., 1971; LOWENSTEIN, 1972; HENDERSON and PATERSON, 1973).

In the last few years it has become possible to evaluate hypothesis regarding the regulation of purine nucleotide interconversion by purine ribonucleotides by means of appropriate experiments using intact mammalian cells; these studies will be reviewed here. Most of this work has employed Ehrlich ascites tumor cells incubated in vitro under conditions in which intracellular concentrations of adenine or guanine nucleotides could be either elevated or lowered. The extent to which the results of such studies are applicable to other types of cells remains to be determined.

A general comment should perhaps be made regarding studies in which purine nucleotide concentrations are elevated by incubation of cells with adenine or guanine. These are of course converted to purine ribonucleoside monophosphates, and it is sometimes implicitly assumed that the concentrations of these monophosphates are greatly increased in such experiments; in fact, however, the monophosphates are rapidly phosphorylated to the di- and triphosphates. Although the concentration of mono- and diphosphates are elevated somewhat, their absolute concentrations remain quite low. The concentrations of ATP and GTP increase most in such experiments.

In cells in which the concentration of GTP was elevated, inhibition of inosinate dehydrogenase activity could be clearly demonstrated; the degree of inhibition increased with increasing GTP concentration (SNYDER and HENDERSON, 1973b). It is of interest that inhibition of inosinate dehydrogenase was also observed in experiments in which either RNA synthesis or both RNA and DNA synthesis was inhibited by actinomycin D or daunomycin; such cells contained elevated concentrations of both ATP and GTP, presumably because purine nucleotides were not being used for nucleic acid synthesis (SNYDER and HENDERSON, 1974). Elevation of ATP concentrations alone had little or no effect on inosinate dehydrogenase activity in intact cells.

Other experiments have been conducted in which ATP and GTP concentrations both were lowered together, and in such cells the activity of inosinate dehydrogenase was considerably increased (BARANKIEWICZ and HENDERSON, 1977). Unfortunately, for technical reasons it was not possible to study this question in cells in which GTP concentrations alone were lowered.

Neither elevation nor lowering of ATP or GTP concentrations had any demonstrable effect on the apparent activity of adenylosuccinate synthetase in Ehrlich ascites tumor cells (SNYDER and HENDERSON, 1973b, 1974; BARANKIEWICZ and HENDERSON, 1977).

The apparent activities of both guanylate reductase and of adenylate deaminase are quite low in cells incubated in vitro, and hence it is difficult to accurately measure

changes in their activities. However, neither elevation nor lowering in intracellular
ATP or GTP concentrations appeared to have any appreciable effect on guanylate
reductase activity. Adenylate deaminase activity was slightly ($< 11\%$) decreased in
cells containing elevated GTP concentrations, whereas changes in ATP concentrations had no detectable effect (SNYDER and HENDERSON, 1973b). Lowering ATP and
GTP concentrations had no effect on either reaction (BARANKIEWICZ and HENDER-
SON, 1977).

In another study using Ehrlich ascites tumor cells, the rate of deamination of
adenylate was greatly accelerated by inducing ATP breakdown by incubating cells
with 2-deoxyglucose (LOMAX et al., 1975). Attempts were made to distinguish between the role of increased substrate availability and that of lowered ATP concentration in the observed acceleration of adenylate deaminase activity; it was concluded
that there was no evidence for regulation of the enzyme by ATP under these conditions.

Few studies have been reported of the possible regulation of purine nucleotide
interconversion by purine ribonucleotides in intact cells other than mouse tumor
cells. However, in studies using cultured lymphoblasts, HERSHFIELD and SEEG-
MILLER (1976) provided presumptive evidence for inhibition of adenylosuccinate synthetase by adenine nucleotides and for inhibition of inosinate dehydrogenase by
guanine nucleotides.

C. Functions of the Reactions of Purine Nucleotide Interconversion in Mammalian Cells

The pathways of purine nucleotide interconversion that are shown in Figure 1 can
have several different functions. Firstly, they can serve in the net biosynthesis of ATP
and GTP from a variety of purine bases and via the de novo pathway. A second
function has been proposed which is somewhat related to the first, namely to keep
the concentrations of adenine nucleotides and guanine nucleotides in "balance" by
permitting the conversion of one type of nucleotide to the other. Thirdly, some of the
reactions of purine nucleotide interconversion can participate in the breakdown of
ATP and GTP, and perhaps also of nucleotides formed upon the breakdown of
nucleic acids. Finally, it has been suggested that the cycle of reactions that intercon-
vert adenylate and inosinate play a role in the deamination of amino acids and
perhaps also in the regulation of glycolysis and the tricarboxylic acid cycle. Each of
these functions will be discussed in turn.

I. Biosynthesis of ATP and GTP

ATP and GTP are of course required for both RNA and coenzyme synthesis, and
dATP and dGTP for DNA synthesis. Thus, the needs of cells for purine nucleotides
will depend on rates of cell growth, rates of RNA turnover unrelated to cell division,
and on rates of coenzyme synthesis and turnover. Although nucleic acid synthesis
utilizes roughly equal amounts of adenine and guanine nucleotides, the concentration of free adenine and guanine nucleotides are not equal. Even in some rapidly

dividing cultured cells, guanine nucleotides do not exceed 20% of the total free purine nucleotides (e.g., SNYDER et al., 1973), and in many cell types guanine nucleotides comprise only 5–10%, or even less (see MANDEL, 1964).

The rates of the different reactions of purine nucleotide interconversion in the biosynthesis of ATP and GTP will depend on the total cellular requirements for these nucleotides, on the relative rates of the different processes of adenylate, inosinate, and guanylate synthesis, on the relative amounts of the different enzymes that actually are present, as well as on the various aspects of their regulation that have already been discussed.

Cultured cells and many mammalian cells in vivo ordinarily depend predominantly on purine biosynthesis de novo, and hence inosinate is the quantitatively most important purine ribonucleotide that is synthesized. The relative utilization of the different purine bases and of adenosine in different cells in vivo is not known for certain, although there is reason to believe that the conversion of hypoxanthine to inosinate is quantitatively important in some tissues (SORENSEN, 1970; MURRAY, 1971; SMITH and HENDERSON, 1976). In these cases the biosynthetic needs of the cells are achieved by the reactions leading from inosinate to adenylate and to guanylate. It is of interest, however, that the ratio of adenylate synthesis from inosinate to guanylate synthesis from inosinate varies in different types of cells; this ratio is approximately 2 in human leukocytes (SHAPIRA et al., 1961; HENDERSON et al., 1974) and in cultured lymphoblasts (SNYDER et al., 1973), 5 in Ehrlich ascites tumor cells incubated in vitro (SNYDER and HENDERSON, 1973a), and 10 in mouse brain slices in vitro (WONG and HENDERSON, 1972). These ratios are not proportional either to the relative concentrations of free adenine and guanine nucleotides in these cells, or to their relative needs for adenine and guanine nucleotides for nucleic acid synthesis. In rabbit reticulocytes this ratio is 4 (COOK and VIBERT, 1966), whereas in mature rabbit erythrocytes it is 8 (LOWY et al., 1961); in human erythrocytes inosinate is converted neither to adenylate nor to guanylate (e.g., HENDERSON et al., 1974).

There is only indirect evidence for the utilization of guanine for nucleotide synthesis in mammalian tissues in vivo (ROSENBLOOM et al., 1967). However, numerous studies using radioactive guanine (e.g., CRABTREE and HENDERSON, 1971a; SNYDER and HENDERSON, 1973a; SNYDER et al., 1973; HENDERSON et al., 1974; COOK and VIBERT, 1966; LOWY et al., 1961) have shown that guanylate is predominantly phosphorylated to GDP and GTP and that only small amounts (∞1–5% or less) are reductively deaminated to inosinate.

There is even less evidence for the utilization of adenine by mammalian cells in vivo than for guanine, although there is some evidence for the utilization of adenosine (LERNER and LOWY, 1974). Studies with radioactive adenine (see references above) indicate that adenylate is predominantly phosphorylated and that only small amounts are deaminated to inosinate. In apparent contradiction to such results, some cultured cells can utilize adenine for growth when purine biosynthesis de novo is blocked and no other purines are present in the medium (WARNICK et al., 1973; BROX, personal communication).

For the purposes of biosynthesis of ATP and GTP, therefore, the reactions of purine nucleotide interconversion appear to operate predominantly as undirectional processes from one or another purine ribonucleoside monophosphate to adenylate and guanylate. The pathways starting from inosinate seem to be most important in many mammalian cells, although slow rates of interconversion starting with guanylate and adenylate can be detected.

II. Balance Between ATP and GTP Concentrations

It has been proposed that the adenylate deaminase and guanylate reductase reactions serve to keep the concentrations of adenine and guanine ribonucleotides in "balance" should their relative concentrations deviate from normal. Thus, should the concentration of ATP or of GTP become elevated relative to the other, the rate of conversion of adenylate or guanylate to inosinate would become accelerated. In fact, there is no evidence that this occurs in mammalian cells. It has already been noted that the concentrations of these nucleotides are not equal, and that their relative concentration varies from one cell type to another. In the few experimental studies that have been conducted on this point (SNYDER and HENDERSON, 1973a; LOMAX et al., 1975; LOWE and HENDERSON, unpublished observations), elevated concentrations of ATP or GTP seem to be stable and not converted one to another at accelerated rates.

III. Catabolism of Adenine and Guanine Nucleotides

It seems certain that an important function of adenylate deaminase is in the catabolism of adenine nucleotides. Thus, although some types of cells (e.g., brain) appear predominantly to dephosphorylate adenylate to adenosine (DEUTICKE et al., 1966; MATTHIAS and BUSCH, 1969; WONG and HENDERSON, 1972), other cells predominantly deaminate adenylate to inosinate; the latter may then be dephosphorylated to inosine. Deamination of adenylate, for example, is the predominant pathway in Ehrlich ascites tumor cells incubated with inhibitors of energy metabolism (LOMAX and HENDERSON, 1973; LOMAX et al., 1975) and in skeletal muscle (see LOWENSTEIN, 1972). It is of some interest that some of the inosinate formed during the course of ATP breakdown in Ehrlich ascites tumor cells is in fact converted to guanine nucleotides via the other reactions of purine nucleotide interconversion (LOMAX and HENDERSON, 1973). However, this does not lead to net increases in guanine nucleotides in as much as the use of energy inhibitors also leads to GTP breakdown (LOMAX et al., 1975).

In rabbit erythrocytes, GTP turnover in vitro occurred predominantly via deamination of guanylate to inosinate; most of the latter was dephosphorylated, and some was converted to xanthylate and then dephosphorylated. In addition, some guanylate was dephosphorylated directly (HERSHKO et al., 1967). This is the best documented example of the role of guanylate reductase in mammalian cells. In Ehrlich ascites tumor cells, the breakdown of GTP proceeds almost entirely by way of dephosphorylation of guanylate; guanylate reductase activity remains very low (LOMAX et al., 1975).

IV. Deamination of Amino Acids

LOWENSTEIN (1972) and his collaborators have proposed that one part of the system of purine nucleotide interconversion may play a role in the deamination of amino acids in mammalian tissues in vivo and also possibly in the regulation of glycolysis and the tricarboxylic acid cycle. This proposal concerns only the reactions involved in the interconversion of adenylate and inosinate, and LOWENSTEIN has termed these reactions "the purine nucleotide cycle"; this is a somewhat unfortunate term, as the particular nucleotides involved are not specified, and there are in fact several other cycles of purine nucleotide metabolism besides this one.

The purine nucleotide cycle hypothesis says that (1) adenylate is deaminated to inosinate and ammonia; (2) amino groups are transferred to oxaloacetate by transamination to form aspartate; (3) aspartate reacts with inosinate to form adenylosuccinate; (4) fumarate is released and adenylate is formed; and the cycle starts over again. In addition to the role of such a cycle in the deamination of amino acids, the utilization of oxaloacetate and release of fumarate have obvious implications for the operation of the tricarboxylic acid cycle. Finally, this cycle affects the concentration of adenylate, which is an activator of phosphofructokinase (EC 2.7.1.11), and hence might contribute to the regulation of glycolysis (TORNHEIM and LOWENSTEIN, 1975). It has also been shown recently that fructose bisphosphate is an inhibitor of adenylosuccinate synthetase (OGAWA et al., 1976).

Although the operation of the purine nucleotide cycle has been demonstrated in suitably fortified *extracts* of muscle (TORNHEIM and LOWENSTEIN, 1972), kidney (BOGUSKY et al., 1976), brain (SCHULTZ and LOWENSTEIN, 1976) and liver (MOSS and McGIVAN, 1975), this cycle has not yet been demonstrated in intact mammalian tissues. Attempts to demonstrate such a cycle in intact Ehrlich ascites tumor cells (CRABTREE and HENDERSON, 1971a) and intact skin fibroblasts (RAIVIO and SEEGMILLER, 1973a) were negative. However, a major objection to the purine nucleotide cycle hypothesis is that some of the conditions used in its demonstration in cell extracts—particularly the premise of rather high concentrations of adenylate—do not seem physiologically realistic. Although this proposal is intriguing, it remains a hypothesis until such time as it can be demonstrated in intact cells and tissues.

D. Effects of Drugs on the Reactions of Purine Nucleotide Interconversion

Some of the reactions of purine nucleotide interconversion can be inhibited by drugs, and such inhibition can lead to inhibition of growth of tumors and cultured cells. A very brief discussion of this topic will be presented here. For the most part, literature citations will be to reviews.

The drugs that inhibit purine nucleotide interconversion may be divided into four main classes: (1) purine derivatives and analogs, including 6-thiopurines, 6-halopurines, and 6-aminopurines; (2) imidazole ribonucleoside derivatives; (3) amino acid analogs; and (4) others.

The ribonucleoside monophosphates of 6-mercatopurine, 6-thioguanine, and 6-chloropurine inhibit inosinate dehydrogenase and guanylate reductase activities in cell extracts, and 6-mercaptopurine ribonucleotide also inhibits adenylosuccinate synthetase and adenylosuccinate lyase activities. There is some evidence that 6-mercaptopurine ribonucletide may interfere with the conversion of inosinate to adenylate in intact cells, and that 6-chloropurine ribonucleotide interferes with the conversion of inosinate to guanylate in tumor cells (BALIS, 1968; HENDERSON and PATERSON, 1973; PATERSON and TIDD, 1975).

Two 6-aminopurine nucleoside analogs, psicofuranine and decoyinine, inhibit guanylate synthetase in bacteria without being phosphorylated; however, they have little or no effect in mammalian systems (NICHOL, 1975). In intact tumor cells, a nucleotide derivative of 1-aminoguanosine inhibits inosinate dehydrogenase activity (SMITH et al., 1974).

Imidazole ribonucleoside derivatives that inhibit purine ribonucleotide interconversion include virazole (or ribavirin) and bredinin. Virazole is known to inhibit inosinate dehydrogenase activity both in intact cells and in extracts (LOWE et al., 1977). Bredinin inhibits the conversion of inosinate to guanylate in intact cells, but its enzymatic site of action is not yet precisely defined (SAKAGUCHI et al., 1975).

Amino acid analogs include the aspartate analogs hadacidin and alanosine, which inhibit adenylosuccinate synthetase (BALIS, 1968), and the glutamine analog diazo-oxo-norleucine, which inhibits guanylate synthetase (BALIS, 1968; BENNETT, 1975). The use of these drugs has been described above.

Mycophenolic acid falls in a class by itself, as it is not obviously an analog of either inosinate or NAD^+, yet is a potent inhibitor of inosinate dehydrogenase both in cells and in extracts (NICHOL, 1975).

In conclusion, much remains to be learned regarding the operation of the reactions of purine nucleotide interconversion in intact mammalian cells and tissues. Several of the enzymes involved have not been studied in much detail in mammalian systems, and studies using intact cells have employed mainly just three types of mammalian cells. It is especially necessary to distinguish the different functions of the pathways of purine nucleotide interconversion, and to study each in appropriate experimental systems.

Acknowledgement. The preparation of this review and the original work described were supported by the National Cancer Institute of Canada.

References

Anderson, J. H., Sartorelli, A. C.: Inosinic acid dehydrogenase of Sarcoma 180 cells. J. biol. Chem. **243**, 4762—4768 (1968)

Balis, M. E.: Antagonists and nucleic acids, pp. 38—70. Amsterdam: North-Holland Publ. Co. 1968

Barankiewicz, J., Henderson, J. F.: Effect of lowered intracellular ATP and GTP concentrations on purine ribonucleotide synthesis and interconversion. Canad. J. Biochem. **55**, 257—262 (1977)

Barnes, L. B., Bishop, S. H.: Adenylosuccinate lyase from human erythrocytes. Int. J. Biochem. **6**, 497—503 (1975)

Bennett, L. L., Jr.: Glutamine antagonists. In: Handbook of Experimental Pharmacology, Vol. 38, Part 2, Sartorelli, A. C., Johns, D. G. (eds.): Antineoplastic and Immunosuppressive Agents, pp. 484—538. Berlin-Heidelberg-New York: Springer 1975

Bogusky, R. T., Lowenstein, L. M., Lowenstein, J. M.: The purine nucleotide cycle. A pathway for ammonia production in the rat kidney. J. clin. Invest. **58**, 326—335 (1976)

Brox, L. W., Henderson, J. F.: The "adenosine cycle" is not a significant route of purine metabolism in mammalian cells. Canad. J. Biochem. **54**, 200—202 (1976)

Cass,C.E., Lowe,J.K., Manchak,J.M., Henderson,J.F.: Biological effects of inhibition of guanine nucleotides by mycophenolic acid in cultured neuroblastoma cells. Cancer Research **37**, 3314—3320 (1977)

Cook,J.L., Vibert,M.: The utilization of purines and their ribosyl derivatives for the formation of adenosine triphosphate and guanosine triphosphate in the rabbit reticulocyte. J. biol. Chem. **241**, 158—160 (1966)

Crabtree,G.W.: Studies on the control of purine nucleotide metabolism in Ehrlich ascites tumor cells in vitro. Ph.D. Thesis, University of Alberta, 1970

Crabtree,G.W., Henderson,J.F.: Rate limiting steps in the interconversion of purine ribonucleotides in Ehrlich ascites tumor cells in vitro. Cancer Res. **31**, 985—991 (1971a)

Crabtree,G.W., Henderson,J.F.: Pathways of purine ribonucleotide catabolism in Ehrlich ascites tumor cells in vitro. Canad. J. Biochem. **49**, 959—963 (1971b)

Deuticke,B., Gerlach,E., Dierkermann,R.: Abbau freier Nucleotide in Herz, Skelettmuskel, Gehirn und Leber der Ratte bei Sauerstoffmangel. Pflügers Arch. ges. Physiol. **292**, 239—254 (1966)

Fraser,J.H., Meyers,H., Henderson,J.F., Brox,L.W., McCoy,E.E.: Individual variation in inosine triphosphate accumulation in human erythrocytes. Clin. Biochem. **8**, 353—364 (1975)

Gots,J.S.: Regulation of purine and pyrimidine metabolism. In: Vogel,H.J. (Ed.): Metabolic Pathways, 3rd Ed., Vol. 5, pp. 225—255. New York: Academic Press 1971

Green,H., Ishii,K.: On the existence of a guanine nucleotide trap, the role of adenosine kinase and a possible cause of excessive purine production in mammalian cells. J. Cell Sci. **11**, 173—177 (1972)

Hartman,S.C.: Purines and pyrimidines. In: Greenberg,D.M. (Ed.): Metabolic Pathways, 3rd Ed., Vol.4, pp. 1—64. New York: Academic Press 1970

Henderson,J.F.: Dual effects of ammonium chloride on purine biosynthesis de novo in Ehrlich ascites tumor cells in vitro. Biochim. biophys. Acta (Amst.) **76**, 173—180 (1963)

Henderson,J.F., Bagnara,A.S., Crabtree,G.W., Lomax,C.A., Shantz,G.D., Snyder,F.F.: Regulation of enzymes of purine metabolism in intact tumor cells. Advanc. Enzyme Regul. **13**, 37—64 (1975)

Henderson,J.F., Fraser,J.H., McCoy,E.E.: Methods for the study of purine metabolism in human cells. Clin. Biochem. **7**, 339—358 (1974)

Henderson,J.F., Lowe,J.K., Barankiewicz,G.: Purine and pyrimidine metabolism: pathways, pitfalls and perturbations. In: Purine and Pyrimidine Metabolism. Ciba Foundation Symposium, No. 48 (1977) pp. 3—14

Henderson,J.F., Paterson,A.R.P.: Nucleotide Metabolism, pp. 136—151. New York: Academic Press 1973

Hershfield,M.S., Seegmiller,J.E.: Gout and the regulation of purine biosynthesis. Horiz. Biochem. Biophys. **2**, 134—162 (1976)

Hershko,A., Razin,A., Shoshani,T., Mager,J.: Turnover of purine nucleotides in rabbit erythrocytes. II. Studies in vitro. Biochim. biophys. Acta (Amst.) **149**, 59—73 (1967).

Jackson,R.C., Weber,G., Morris,H.P.: IMP dehydrogenase, an enzyme linked with proliferation and malignancy. Nature (Lond.) **256**, 331—333 (1975)

Kluge,H., Wieczorek,V.: Die Aktivitäten von Adenylsäure- und Adenosinedesaminase in Hirnregionen von Ratten verschiedener Altersstufen. Acta biol. med. germ. **21**, 271—278 (1968)

Kaletha,K.: Changes of the heat sensibility of AMP-deaminase from rat skeletal muscle in the course of postnatal development. Int. J. Biochem. **6**, 471—474 (1975)

LaDu,B.N.: Histidinemia. In: Stanbury,J.B., Wyngaarden,J.B., Fredrickson,D.S. (Eds.): The Metabolic Basis of Inherited Disease, 3rd Ed., pp. 338—350. New York: McGraw-Hill 1972

Lee,Y.P.: Adenylic deaminase. In: Boyer,P.D., Lardy,H., Myrbäck,K. (Eds.): The Enzymes, 2nd Ed., Vol.4, pp. 279—283. New York: Academic Press 1960

Lerner,M.H., Lowy,B.A.: The formation of adenosine in rabbit liver and its possible role as a direct precursor of erythrocyte adenine nucleotides. J. biol. Chem. **249**, 959—967 (1974)

Lomax,C.A., Bagnara,A.S., Henderson,J.F.: Studies on the regulation of purine nucleotide catabolism. Canad. J. Biochem. **53**, 231—241 (1975)

Lomax,C.A., Henderson,J.F.: Adenosine formation and metabolism during adenosine triphosphate catabolism in Ehrlich ascites tumor cells. Cancer Res. **33**, 2825—2829 (1973)

Lowe, J. K., Brox, L., Henderson, J. F.: Consequences of inhibition of guanine nucleotide synthesis by mycophenolic acid and virazole. Cancer Res. **37**, 736—743 (1977)

Lowenstein, J. M.: Ammonia production in muscle and other tissues: the purine nucleotide cycle. Physiol. Rev. **52**, 382—414 (1972)

Lowy, B. A., Williams, M. K., London, I. M.: The utilization of purines and their ribosyl derivatives for the formation of adenosine triphosphate and guanosine triphosphate in the mature rabbit erythrocyte. J. biol. Chem. **236**, 1439—1441 (1961)

Mandel, P.: Free nucleotides in animal tissues. Progr. Nucl. Acid. Res. Mol. Biol. **3**, 299—334 (1964)

Matthias, R., Busch, E.: Abbau der Purinnucleotide in ischämischen Gehirn- und Muskelgeweben von Kaninchen. Hoppe-Seylers Z. physiol. Chem. **350**, 1410—1414 (1969)

Moss, K. M., McGivan, J. D.: Characteristics of aspartate deamination by the purine nucleotide cycle in the cytosol fraction of rat liver. Biochemistry **150**, 275—283 (1975)

Murray, A. W.: The biological significance of purine salvage. Ann. Rev. Biochem. **40**, 811—826 (1971)

Nagata, K., Mitsui, A., Tsushima, K.: Intracellular localization of inosine-5'-phosphate dehydrogenase in chicken liver. Biochim. biophys. Acta (Amst.) **177**, 680—682 (1969)

Nichol, C. A.: Antibiotics resembling adenosine: tubercidin, toyocomycin, sangivamycin, formycin, psicofuranine, and decoyinine. In: Handbook of Experimental Pharmacology, Vol. 38, Part 2, Sartorelli, A. C.; Johns, D. G. (eds.): Antineoplastic and Immunosuppressive Agents, pp. 434—457. Berlin-Heidelberg-New York: Springer 1975

Ogasawara, N., Goto, H., Watanabe, T.: Isozymes of rat AMP deaminase. Biochim. biophys. Acta (Amst.) **403**, 530—537 (1975a)

Ogasawara, N., Goto, H., Watanabe, T.: Isozymes of rat brain AMP deaminase: developmental changes and characterizations of five forms. FEBS Letters **58**, 245—248 (1975b)

Ogawa, H., Shiraki, H., Nakagawa, H.: Study on the regulatory role of fructose-1,6-diphosphate in the formation of AMP in rat skeletal muscle. A mechanism for synchronization of glycolysis and the purine nucleotide cycle. Biochem. Biophys. Res. Commun. **68**, 524—528 (1976)

Paterson, A. R. P., Tidd, D. M.: 6-Thiopurines. In: Handbook of Experimental Pharmacology, Vol. 38, Part 2, Sartorelli, A. C., Johns, D. G. (eds.): Antineoplastic and Immunosuppressive Agents, Vol. XXXVIII, Part 2, pp. 384—403. Berlin-Heidelberg-New York: Springer 1975

Raggi, A., Bergamini, C., Ronca, G.: Isozymes of AMP deaminase in red and white skeletal muscles. FEBS Letters **58**, 19—23 (1975)

Raivio, K. O., Seegmiller, J. G.: Adenine, hypoxanthine and guanine metabolism in fibroblasts from normal individuals and from patients with hypoxanthine phosphoribosyltransferase deficiency. Biochim. Biophys. Acta **299**, 273—282 (1973a)

Raivio, K. O., Seegmiller, J. E.: Role of glutamine in purine synthesis and in guanine nucleotide formation in normal fibroblasts and in fibroblasts deficient in hypoxanthine phosphoribosyltransferase activity. Biochim. biophys. Acta (Amst.) **299**, 283—292 (1976b)

Rivard, G. E., McLaren, J. D., Brunst, R. F.: Incorporation of hypoxanthine into adenine and guanine nucleotides by human platelets. Biochim. biophys. Acta (Amst.) **381**, 144—156 (1975)

Rosenbloom, F. M., Kelley, W. N., Miller, J., Henderson, J. F., Seegmiller, J. E.: Inherited disorder of purine metabolism: correlation between central nervous system dysfunction and the biochemical defects. J. Amer. med. Ass. **202**, 175—177 (1967)

Saccoccia, P. A., Jr., Miech, R. P.: Inosinic acid dehydrogenase in mammalian tissues. Molec. Pharmacol. **5**, 26—29 (1969)

Sakaguchi, K., Tsujino, M., Yoshizawa, M., Mizuno, K., Hayano, K.: Action of Bredinin on mammalian cells. Cancer Res. **35**, 1643—1648 (1975)

Santos, J. N., Hempstead, K. W., Kopp, L. E., Miech, R. P.: Nucleotide metabolism in rat brain. J. Neurochem. **15**, 367—376 (1968)

Sanwal, B. D., Kapoor, M., Duckworth, H. W.: The regulation of branched and converging pathways. Curr. Top. Cell Regul. **3**, 1—115 (1971)

Schultz, V., Lowenstein, J. M.: Purine nucleotide cycle. Evidence for the occurrence of the cycle in brain. J. biol. Chem. **251**, 485—492 (1976)

Shapira, J., Bornstein, I., Wells, W., Winzler, R. J.: Metabolism of human leukocytes in vitro. IV. Incorporation and interconversion of adenine and guanine. Cancer Res. **21**, 265—270 (1961)

Smith,C.M., Fontenelle,L.J., Muzik,H., Paterson,A.R.P., Unger,H., Brox,L.W.: Inhibition of inosinate dehydrogenase activity in Ehrlich ascites tumor cells in vitro. Biochem. Pharmacol. **23**, 2727—2735 (1974)

Smith,C.M., Henderson,J.F.: Relative importance of alternative pathways of purine nucleotide biosynthesis in Ehrlich ascites tumor cells in vivo. Canad. J. Biochem. **54**, 341—349 (1976)

Snyder,F.F., Henderson,J.F.: A kinetic analysis of purine nucleotide synthesis and interconversion in intact Ehrlich ascites tumor cells. J. Cell Physiol. **82**, 349—361 (1973a)

Snyder,F.F., Henderson,J.F.: Effects of elevated intracellular ATP and GTP concentrations on purine ribonucleotide synthesis and interconversions. Canad. J. Biochem. **51**, 943—948 (1973b)

Snyder,F.F., Henderson,J.F.: Effects of actinomycin D on purine ribonucleotide metabolism in Ehrlich ascites tumor cells in vitro. Canad. J. Biochem. **52**, 263—267 (1974)

Snyder,F.F., Henderson,J.F., Cook,D.A.: Inhibition of purine metabolism—computer-assisted analysis of drug effects. Biochem. Pharmacol. **21**, 2351—2357 (1972)

Snyder,F.F., Henderson,J.F., Kim,S.C., Paterson,A.R.P., Brox,L.W.: Purine nucleotide metabolism and nucleotide pool sizes in synchronized lymphoma L5178Y cells. Cancer Res. **33**, 2425—2430 (1973)

Sorensen,L.B.: Mechanism of excessive purine biosynthesis in hypoxanthine-guanine phosphoribosyltransferase deficiency. J. clin. Invest. **49**, 968—978 (1970)

Spector,T.: Studies with GMP synthetase from Ehrlich ascites cells—purification, properties, and interactions with nucleotide analogs. J. biol. Chem. **250**, 7372—7376 (1975)

Tornheim,K., Lowenstein,J.M.: The Purine Nucleotide Cycle. The production of ammonia from aspartate by extracts of rat skeletal muscle. J. biol. Chem. **247**, 162—169 (1972)

Tornheim,K., Lowenstein,J.M.: Purine nucleotide cycle. 5. Control of phosphofructokinase and glycolytic oscillations in muscle extracts. J. biol. Chem. **250**, 6304 (1975)

Turner,L.V., Fern,E.B.: Changes in activity of rat muscle AMP deaminase in relation to proportion of dietary protein. Brit. J. Nutr. **32**, 539—548 (1974)

Warnick,C.T., Kim,S.C., Paterson,A.R.P.: Inhibition of purine biosynthesis de novo in cultured L5178Y cells by methylthioinosine. Biochem. Pharmacol. **22**, 2777—2779 (1973)

Weil-Malherbe,H.: The subcellular distribution of rat brain adenylate deaminase and its association with neurosteinin. J. Neurochem. **24**, 801—804 (1975)

Winder,W.W., Terjung,R.L., Baldwin,K.M., Holloszy,J.O.: Effect of exercise on AMP deaminase and adenylosuccinase in rat skeletal muscle. Amer. J. Physiol. **227**, 1411—1414 (1974)

Wong,P.C.L., Henderson,J.F.: Purine ribonucleotide biosynthesis, interconversion and catabolism in mouse brain in vitro. Biochem. Pharmacol. **129**, 1085—1090 (1972)

Zielkle,C.L., Suelter,C.H.: Purine, purine nucleoside and purine nucleotide aminohydrolases. In: Boyer,P.D. (Ed.): The Enzymes, 3rd Ed., Vol.4, pp. 47—78. New York: Academic Press 1971

CHAPTER 5

Degradation of Purine Nucleotides

I.H.Fox

A. Introduction

Purine nucleotides have a vital role in metabolism. Therefore, the maintenance of a constant nucleotide composition of the cell is essential for normal function. Purine nucleotides are synthesized by purine biosynthesis de novo, by salvage pathways and nucleoside kinases, and by degradation of nucleic acids. The use of nucleotides occurs in nucleic acid synthesis, in various reactions of intermediary metabolism and in the degradation to the inert product uric acid. Regulated activity of these many pathways by synthesizing and degrading nucleotides appears to be critical.

In this article the pathways of purine nucleotide degradation will be discussed. Recent evidence has suggested that this catabolic reaction sequence can abruptly increase its activity, leading to a cascade of nucleotide degradation to end products. This phenomenon, together with the current discovery of inborn errors of purine catabolism associated with immune function disorders, has focused attention on the importance of nucleotide degradation pathways to man.

B. Reactions of Purine Nucleotide Degradation

Purine nucleoside monophosphates are degraded to purine end products by means of a final common pathway (Fig. 1). AMP, IMP, XMP, and GMP are dephosphorylated to form the ribonucleoside derivatives. Specific 5'-phosphomonesterase (E.C.3.1.3.5.) and nonspecific alkaline phosphatase (E.C.3.13.2.) hydrolyze AMP, IMP, XMP, and GMP to adenosine, inosine, xanthosine, and guanosine, respectively. These enzymes are mainly localized to the microsomal cell fractions with highest specific activities in the plasma membrane (DRUMMOND and YAMAMOTO, 1971; FOX and MARCHANT, 1976; SONG and BODANSKY, 1966; WIDNELL, 1972). The major inhibitor is the nucleotide pool (DRUMMOND and YAMAMOTO, 1971; FOX and MARCHANT, 1976a; MURRAY and FRIEDRICHS, 1969). In particular, human 5'-nucleotidase and alkaline phosphatase are inhibited by ATP and inorganic phosphate, respectively (FOX and MARCHANT, 1976a). The purine ribonucleosides inosine, xanthosine, and guanosine are converted to purine bases and ribose-1-phosphate by a nucleoside phosphorylase enzyme (E.C.2.4.4.1). Although adenosine has not been regarded as a substrate for this enzyme, recent evidence suggests that it could be (ZIMMERMAN et al., 1970), and that there could be a distinctive adenosine phosphorylase (DIVEKAR, 1976). In mammalian tissues, adenine nucleotide catabolism proceeds mainly through IMP and inosine (LOMAX and HENDERSON, 1973; LOMAX et al., 1975). Adenosine is deaminated to inosine in a number of mammalian tissues by adenosine

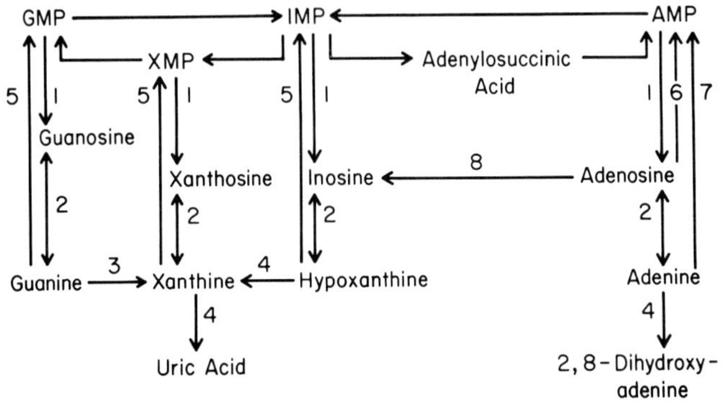

Fig. 1. Final common pathway for purine nucleotide degradation. AMP, IMP, XMP, and GMP are initially dephosphorylated by 5′-nucleotidase and nonspecific phosphatases (1). The resultant nucleosides inosine, xanthosine or guanosine are degraded by purine nucleoside phosphorylase (2) to hypoxanthine, xanthine, or guanine (2). Although evidence suggests that adenosine is converted to adenine by a similar pathway (2), this remains a controversial point and requires clarification. Adenosine is converted to inosine by adenosine deaminase (8). Guanine is degraded to xanthine by guanine deaminase (3). Hypoxanthine is converted to xanthine and xanthine is converted to uric acid by xanthine oxidase (4). When adenine accumulates to excess, it may be degraded by this enzyme (4) to 2,8-dihydroxyadenine. Nucleoside degradation products may be converted back to nucleotides. GMP, XMP, or IMP are formed from guanine, xanthine, or hypoxanthine by hypoxanthine-guanine phosphoribosyltransferase (5). AMP is synthesized from adenosine by adenosine kinase (6) or from adenine by adenine phosphoribosyltransferase (7)

deaminase (E.C.3.5.4.6.). The catabolism of AMP to inosine may be the most important degradation pathway, since adenine nucleotides comprise a substantial proportion of the nucleotide pool with ATP forming approximately 60% of the total nucleoside triphosphate pool (LOWRY et al., 1964; LOWRY et al., 1971). Guanine is deaminated to xanthine by guanine deaminase (E.C.3.5.4.3). Hypoxanthine and xanthine are converted to uric acid by xanthine oxidase (E.C.1.2.3.2.) located primarily in the liver and jejunum of mammals. These catabolic pathways are interrupted by reactions which allow the resynthesis of nucleotides. Adenosine kinase (E.C.2.7.1.20) catalyzes the conversion of adenosine to AMP, while hypoxanthine-guanine phosphoribosyltransferase (E.C.2.4.2.8) converts hypoxanthine, xanthine, or guanine to IMP, XMP, or GMP, respectively. Adenine phosphoribosyltransferase (E.C.2.4.2.7) catalyzes the formation of AMP from adenine. Any excess adenine is converted by xanthine oxidase to 2,8-dihydroxyadenine (DEBRAY et al., 1976). This catabolic pathway also degrades 2′-deoxyribonucleotides, which are substrates for this reaction sequence.

The precursor substrates of the final common pathway of purine nucleotide degradation are formed from different sources (Fig. 2):

(1) Dietary nucleoproteins are degraded in the small intestinal lumen by pancreatic nucleases and phosphodiesterases and then by nucleotidases and phosphatases. The resultant purine nucleosides and bases are absorbed from the intestinal lumen and may enter the catabolic pathways.

(2) The degradation of nucleic acids to nucleoside monophosphates in cells occurs by ribonuclease a and b, deoxyribonuclease I and II and phosphodiesterase.

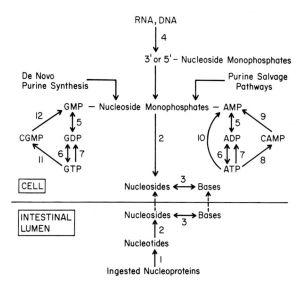

Fig. 2. Precursor substrates for purine nucleotide degradation. There are different ways by which precursor substrates of purine catabolism are formed. Ingested nucleoproteins are digested by pancreatic nucleases and phosphodiesterases (1) to nucleotides and then are degraded by nucleotidases and phosphatases (2) to nucleosides. Nucleosides are directly absorbed or are converted by purine nucleoside phosphorylase (3) to bases which are then absorbed. Nucleic acids are degraded by ribonuclease a and b, deoxyribonuclease I and II, and phosphodiesterase to 3′- or 5′-nucleoside monophosphates (4). Both 2′-oxy and 2′-deoxy derivatives are formed. GTP may be converted to CGMP by guanylate cyclase (11) or to GDP by reactions of intermediary metabolism (7), nucleoside diphosphatase (7) or nucleoside diphosphate kinases (6). GMP is ultimately formed from GDP by nucleoside monophosphate kinases (5) or from CGMP by phosphodiesterase (12). ATP is ultimately converted to AMP by a similar series of reactions (6,7,5 or 8,9). In addition, ATP is directly converted to AMP by reactions of intermediary metabolism (10) or nucleotide pyrophosphatase (10)

(3) The purine salvage pathways and purine biosynthesis de novo form nucleotides which may be substrates of this pathway.

(4) Finally, cyclic nucleotides and nucleoside diphosphate and triphosphate derivatives are converted to nucleoside monophosphate derivatives. In some instances there is direct laboratory evidence for the conversion of these precursors to purine end products using radiochemical tracer compounds (COULSON, 1976; CRABTREE and HENDERSON, 1971; LOMAX and HENDERSON, 1973; LOMAX et al., 1975; WONG and HENDERSON, 1972).

C. Properties of Purine Catabolic Enzymes

I. 5′-Nucleotidase (E.C.3.1.3.5) and Other Phosphatases

This enzyme and nonspecific phosphatase catalyze the following reactions:

$$\text{Nucleoside Monophosphate} + H_2O \rightarrow \text{Nucleoside} + Pi.$$

Table 1. Inhibition of human placental microsomal 5'-nucleotidase (From Fox and Marchant, 1976)

Compound	Apparent K_i mM	K_i Slope mM
GMP	0.1	
Allopurinol ribonucleotide		0.01
ADP		0.02
GDP	0.2	
UDP	0.2	
CDP	0.7	
NAD	0.2	
ATP		0.05
GTP		0.12
TTP	3.0	
UTP	0.2	
CTP	0.5	
XTP	0.8	
Adenosine	0.4	
Inosine	3.0	
Cytidine	5.0	
NaF	6.0	
P_i	42.0	

Although 5'-nucleotidase from vertebrate tissue, snake venom, yeast bacteria, and seminal fluid have been studied (Drummond and Yamamoto, 1971), only recently is there information about a human enzyme (Fox and Marchant, 1976; Fox and Marchant, 1976a). Placental microsomal 5'-nucleotidase was partially purified and found to have seven electrophoretic variants ranging from pH 5.44 to 6.70. These had the same kinetic characteristics. Electrophoretic variants similar to those observed in placenta have been found by isofocusing of crude extracts of human leukocytes and cultured diploid fibroblasts (Lacroix et al., unpublished observations). The variants appeared to be composed of different proportions of a heavy, medium, and light molecular weight forms. The medium and light molecular weight variants were interconvertible and had molecular weights of 86 500 and 43 500, respectively. These multiple electrophoretic forms of 5'-nucleotidase appeared to represent pseudoiso-zymes based on different states of aggregation of a common primary sequence. The enzyme was activated by $MgCl_2$ and had the pH optimum shifted from 9.8 to a plateau from 7.4 to 9.8 with this ion. With AMP as 100, the relative substrate activity was CMP, 122; NMN, 74; GMP, 68; IMP, 63; XMP, 28; and UDP-glucose, 68. Kinetic studies using AMP and $MgCl_2$ suggested sequential binding with a Michaelis constant of 14 μM for AMP and 3 μM for $MgCl_2$ (Fox and Marchant, 1976a). The Michaelis constant for GMP and CMP ranged from 33 to 67 μM and 170 to 250 μM, respectively. A large number of nucleoside mono-, di-, and triphosphates inhibited the enzyme (Table 1). ATP or ADP was the competitive inhibitor when AMP was the substrate with a K_i of 54 or 20 μM (Figs. 3, 4). Allopurinol ribonucleotide, a competitive inhibitor with AMP, had a K_i of 10 μM, while GTP, a noncompetitive inhibitor, had a K_i slope of 120 μM. Placental nonspecific phosphatases also

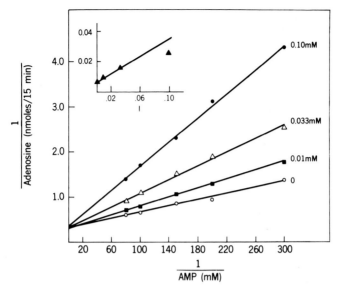

Fig. 3. Inhibition of 5′-nucleotidase by ADP. This is a double reciprocal plot of nucleotide inhibition studies with variable AMP concentration and fixed ADP concentrations ranging from 0 mM to 0.10 mM using partially purified human placental microsomal 5′-nucleotidase. MgCl$_2$ concentration was 5 mM. Inset shows a secondary plot of the slope versus ADP (I) concentration in mM. The K_i slope was 20 μM

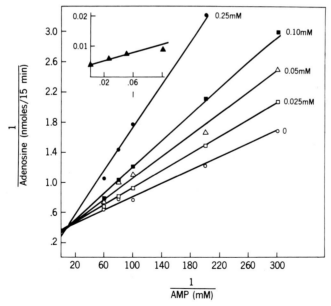

Fig. 4. Inhibition of 5′-nucleotidase by ATP. This is a double reciprocal plot of nucleotide inhibition studies with variable AMP concentration and fixed ATP concentrations ranging from 0 mM to 0.25 mM using partially purified human placental microsomal 5′-nucleotidase. MgCl$_2$ was 5 mM. Inset shows a secondary plot of the slope versus ATP (I) concentration in mM. The K_i slope was 54 μM

Table 2. Comparison of nucleotide 5′-phosphomonoesterase activity of two human placental microsomal enzymes (From Fox and Marchant, 1976)

	5′-Nucleotidase	Alkaline phosphatase
K_mAMP	12 μM	400 μM
Mg 5 mM-% stimulation	134	19
% Maximum activity at pH 7.4	90	18
Substrate specificity	5′-Nucleoside monophosphate	Any phosphorylated compound
K_i (apparent) P_i	42 mM	0.6 mM
Inhibition by	Nucleotides	Any phosphorylated compound

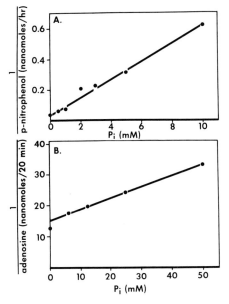

Fig. 5. Inhibitory effects of inorganic phosphate (P_i). This is a plot of variable P_i concentration versus the reciprocal of the velocity using partially purified human placental microsomal enzymes. The apparent K_i for P_i was 0.6 mM for alkaline phosphatase (A) and 42 mM for 5′-nucleotidase (B)

had phosphomonoesterase activity which was substantially different from 5′-nucleotidase (Table 2) (Fox and Marchant, 1976a). One very important difference between these enzymes was related to the effects of inorganic phosphate. The apparent K_i for Pi for alkaline phosphatase was 0.6 mM—well within the physiologie range. This was not the case for 5′-nucleotidase (Fig. 5). These observations suggest that 5′-nucleotidase and alkaline phosphatase may be inhibited by ATP and Pi respectively under normal intracellular conditions and that AMP may be preferentially hydrolyzed by 5′-nucleotidase.

There is a great deal of literature on 5′-nucleotidase from tissues other than man. Four distinctive subcellular types of 5′-nucleotidase have been delineated in rat liver homogenate (SOLYOM and TRAMS, 1972). The plasma membrane enzyme had a pH optimum of 9.0, was stimulated by Mg^{2+}, and had a K_m of 30 μM for AMP. Microsomal 5'-nucleotidase had a pH optimum between 7.0 and 7.4, was not stimulated by Mg, and had a K_m of 10 μM. Lysosomal membrane 5'-nucleotidase had pH optimum of 6.5 and was inhibited by L(+) tartrate, while the cytoplasmic enzyme had a pH optimum between 6.2 and 6.9, was dependent on Mg^{2+}, and had a K_m of 6.8 mM. Morphologic and functional chemical studies have presented convincing data that the plasma membrane form of 5'-nucleotidase is localized to the external surface (BROWNLEE and HEATH, 1975; CERCIGNANI et al., 1974; DEPIERRE and KARNOVSKY, 1974; FARQUHAR et al., 1974; NEWLY et al., 1975; WIDNELL, 1972; WOO and MANERY, 1975). Inhibition of ecto-5'-nucleotidase but not non-specific phosphatase by concanavalin A was reversible by treatment with α-methyl-D-glucoside or α-methyl-D-mannoside (STEFANOVIC et al., 1975). It was unclear whether concanavalin A was bound to 5'-nucleotidase itself or to an adjacent membrane site. However, partially purified 5'-nucleotidase from many different rat tissues were 92–96% inhibited by concanavalin A (REIMER and WIDNELL, 1975). There is evidence to suggest that the plasmalemmal membrane protein 5'-nucleotidase is preferentially coded for by membranebound polyribosomes in the mouse liver (BERGERON et al., 1975).

Plasma membrane 5'-nucleotidase was found to be a lipoprotein containing a phospholipid (HUANG and KEENAN, 1972; NAKAMURA, 1976; WIDNELL and UNKELESS, 1968). In one instance, sphingomyelin has been found (WIDNELL and UNKELESS, 1968). However, active mouse liver plasma membrane 5'-nucleotidase was present without detectable amount of phospholipids but stained positively for glycoprotein (EVANS and GURD, 1973). Estimates of the molecular weight of 5'-nucleotidase by gel filtration or sucrose gradient ultracentrifugation have ranged from 52000 to 235000 (EVANS and GURD, 1973; IPATA, 1968; LISOWSKI, 1966; MURRAY and FRIEDRICHS, 1969; NEU, 1967; TANAKA et al., 1973). Smaller forms of 5'-nucleotidase have molecular weights from 10000 to 33000 (DRUMMOND and YAMAMOTO, 1971; MURRAY and FRIEDRICHS, 1969). Multiple electrophoretic forms of 5'-nucleotidase have been described (CENTER and BEHAL, 1966; HARDONK and DE BOER, 1968; HARDONK and KOUDSTAAL, 1968; SCOTT, 1965). However, it has been unclear whether these forms of enzymes represent different subcellular fractions or contamination with non-specific phosphatase activity. Molecular weight variants of mammalian nucleotidase have also been observed (EVANS and GURD, 1973; HUANG and KEENAN, 1972; MURRAY and FRIEDRICHS, 1969; PLETSCH and COFFEY, 1972; TANAKA et al., 1973; WIDNELL and UNKELESS, 1968). These have been attributed either to a degradation of the enzyme (WIDNELL and UNKELESS, 1968), a separate enzyme (HUANG and KEENAN, 1972), or a dimer and monomer form (EVANS and GURD, 1973). Different forms of nucleotidase during the sporulating cycle of Bacillus subtilis have 3'-nucleotidase and 5'-nucleotidase activity (FELICIOLI et al., 1973).

In general, substrate specificities have included ribose and 2'-deoxyribose compounds, an inability to hydrolyze 2'- and 3'-nucleotides with the exception of rat liver lysosomes, nucleoside monophosphate derivatives, and with few exceptions, an inability to hydrolyze UDP-glucose (DRUMMOND and YAMAMOTO, 1971; NEU, 1967a; NEU, 1968). The pH optima of 5'-nucleotidase from different sources vary. A double pH optimum, with an alkaline pH peak appearing in the presence of magnesium, has been found with bull seminal plasma (LEVIN and BODANSKY, 1966), bovine cerebral cortex (TANAKA et al., 1973), mammalian liver plasma membrane (EVANS and GURD, 1973; SONG and BODANSKY, 1966; SONG and BODANSKY, 1967), and bovine fat globule membranes (HUANG and KEENAN, 1972). The K_m for nucleoside monophosphates ranged from 3 to 2500 µM (BURGER and LOWENSTEIN, 1975; CERCIGNANI et al., 1974; EDWARDS and MAGUIRE, 1970; FELICIOLI et al., 1973; HUANG and KEENAN, 1972; NAKAMURA, 1976; NEWLY et al., 1975; SONG and BODANSKY, 1967; TANAKA et al., 1973a; WIDNELL and UNKELESS, 1968), with 10–100 µM being the most commonly observed values. Many forms of 5'-nucleotidase were activated by divalent cations with the K_m of Mg^{2+} ranging from 15 µM for bovine cerebral cortex to 3000 µM for rat cerebellum (BOSMANN and PIKE, 1971; CENTER and BEHAL, 1966; CERCIGNANI et al., 1974; DRUMMOND and YAMAMOTO, 1971; HUANG and KEENAN, 1972; LEVIN and BODANSKY, 1967; SONG and BODANSKY, 1967; TANAKA et al., 1973; TANAKA et al., 1973a). Nucleosides inhibited 5'-nucleotidase from yeast (DRUMMOND and YAMAMOTO, 1971), bull seminal plasma (LEVIN and BODANSKY, 1966), rat cerebellum (BOSMANN and PIKE, 1971), bovine pituitary (LISKOWSKI, 1966), and cerebral cortex (TANAKA et al., 1973). Inorganic phosphate was not an inhibitor of 5'-nucleotidase from sheep brain (IPATA, 1968) or Escherichia coli (NEU, 1967). Inhibition with nucleoside triphosphates was competitive (BOSMANN and PIKE, 1971; FELICIOLI et al., 1973; MURRAY and FRIEDRICHS, 1969), noncompetitive (CERCIGNANI et al., 1974; MURRAY and FRIEDRICHS, 1969) and sigmoidal (BOSMANN and PIKE, 1971; IPATA, 1968). Sigmoid inhibitory kinetics (IPATA, 1968) could not be confirmed (BURGER and LOWENSTEIN, 1975). The K_i or $I_{0.5}$ has ranged from 10^{-7} to 10^{-3} M, depending on the enzyme source. The wide variability of the regulatory characteristics may be related to a different subcellular localization of the 5'-nucleotidases studied.

A 5'-nucleotidase that preferentially hydrolyzes IMP and GMP was originally described in the supernatant fraction of chicken liver (ITOH et al., 1967). Although the importance of this form of 5'-nucleotidase has not been clear, it has been found that the supernatant 5'-nucleotidase may contain up to 27% of the total activity of beef thyroid gland (MATSUZAKI et al., 1973). Chicken liver cytosol 5'-nucleotidase has been purified to homogeneity (NAITO and TSUSHIMA, 1976). It was found to be a tetramer with a native molecular weight of 205000 and a subunit molecular weight of 51000. The pH optimum was 6.5 and Mg^{2+} was required for activity. The relative activity (using IMP as 100) was GMP 96, XMP 43, AMP 13, and UMP 10. The Michaelis constants were IMP 0.31 mM, GMP 0.53 mM, and AMP 18 mM.

Other microsomal enzymes hydrolyze nucleoside diphosphates and triphosphates. Nucleoside diphosphatase (E.C.3.6.1.6) catalyzes the following reaction:

$$\text{Nucleoside Diphosphate} + H_2O \rightarrow \text{Nucleoside Monophosphate} + P_i.$$

It has been localized to the inner surface of the rat liver microsomal membranes, enclosing the microsomal vesicles (KURIYAMA, 1972). The pig liver and chicken liver enzyme were predominately located in the microsomal fraction (PINSLEY and SCRUTON, 1973). Although rat liver microsomes have nucleoside diphosphatase activities with ADP, CDP, GDP, UDP, and IDP (ERNSTER and JONES, 1962), the purified enzyme from pig liver and other sources only degraded UDP, IDP, and GDP. It had only a slight activity with CDP and no activity with ADP or TDP (PINSLEY and

SCRUTON, 1973). The molecular weight of the pig liver enzyme was 155000, while rat liver and bovine liver were 100000. Nonlinear allosteric kinetics with linearity being restored by ATP were observed with the hydrolysis of all nucleotide substrates by pig liver nucleotide diphosphatases (PINSLEY and SCRUTON, 1973). Nucleotide pyrophosphatase (E.C.3.6.1.9) is a glycoprotein and catalyzes the following reaction:

$$\text{Dinucleotide} + H_2O \rightarrow 2 \text{ Mononucleotides}.$$

It is localized to the external surface of the plasma membrane and to the endoplasmic reticulum (BACHORIK and DIETRICH, 1972; BISCHOFF et al., 1975; BISCHOFF et al., 1976; EVANS, 1974). Its molecular weight is 30000–137000 (BISCHOFF et al., 1975; EVANS, 1974). This enzyme is thought to account for rapid degradation of nucleotides, such as ATP, UDP-galactose, and NAD, by perfused livers (EVANS, 1974). Besides hydrolyzing p-nitrophenyl-thymidine-5′-monophosphate, nucleotide pyrophosphatase hydrolyzes the pyrophosphate bond of nucleotides, yielding a nucleoside 5′-monophosphate (BISCHOFF et al., 1975). Other cleavage products were glucose-1-phosphate with UDP-glucose and PP_i with ATP or UTP as substrates. The relative activity of the enzyme was as follows: UDP-glucose, 60; NAD, 27; NADH, 40; UTP, 7; and ATP, 4.5 (BISCHOFF et al., 1975). These was no detectable hydrolysis of ADP, AMP, or CAMP (BACHORIK and DIETRICH, 1972). The enzyme is inhibited by various nucleotides by a competitive mechanism, sodium fluoride and EDTA (BACHORIK and DIETRICH, 1972; BISCHOFF et al., 1975). There may be many other specific nucleotide hydrolyzing enzymes. For example, in a study of the enzyme nucleoside triphosphate pyrophosphohydrolase (E.C.3.6.1.19), which catalyzes the degradation of ITP to IMP, an inverse relationship was found between enzyme activity and ITP concentrations in human erythrocytes (SODER et al., 1976). In addition, ribosomes, uncharged t-RNA, and microsomal wash protein factor from rat liver will degrade GTP to guanine (GRUMMT and SPECKBACHER, 1975).

II. Purine Nucleoside Phosphorylase (E.C.2.4.4.1)

This enzyme catalyzes the following reactions:

$$\text{Nucleoside (Base + Ribose)} + P_i \rightleftharpoons \text{Base + Ribose-1-P}$$

The normal purine nucleoside phosphorylase enzyme has been extensively characterized. The structural gene for this enzyme maps on chromosome 14 (GEORGE and FRANCKE, 1976). The human enzyme is widely distributed in many tissues (EDWARDS et al., 1971), but only the erythrocyte enzyme has been crystallized with a 7300-fold purification and a specific activity of 96 μmoles/min/mg protein (AGARWAL and PARKS, 1969). The pH optimum for the reaction was 6.5–8.0. The molecular weight was 81000 (AGARWAL and PARKS, 1969) to 84000 (GEORGE and FRANCKE, 1976). Six variants were observed by isoelectric focusing with pI values from 5.85 to 6.25 (AGARWAL et al., 1975). The substrate K_m values for these variants were similar (AGARWAL et al., 1975). These values ranged from 13–30 μM for nucleosides or bases, including inosine, deoxyinosine, guanosine, deoxyguanosine, guanine, and hypoxanthine. All six variants displayed substrate activation with inosine and deoxyinosine at concentrations above 0.2 mM (AGARWAL et al., 1975). These variants were studied carefully by starch gel electrophorus and appeared to represent a secondary modification of primary isozymic form of the enzyme (EDWARDS et al., 1971). Three rare variant alleles have been found. The four-banded isozyme pattern exhibited by fibroblast and hair follicle cell extracts from individuals with a variant hemolysate pattern suggest that nucleoside phosphorylase is a trimer (EDWARDS et al., 1971). Kinetic analysis was consistent with an ordered Bi-Bi reaction mechanism with the nucleoside the first substrate to add to the enzyme and the purine base the last product to leave the enzyme surface (KIM et al., 1968). Both ribose-1-phosphate and deoxyribose-1-phosphate served as sugar donor. The K_i of ribose-1-phosphate and inorganic phosphate were estimated to be 0.15 mM and 0.32 mM, respectively (KIM et al., 1968). Certain purine analogs were substrates or inhibitors for the enzyme. The K_i values for 6-mercaptopurine and 6-thioguanine were approximately 0.1 mM, while the values for allopurinol and oxipurinol were considerably higher (KRENITSKY et al., 1968). Adenine was bound poorly to the enzyme and adenosine was not degraded by the enzyme (KRENITSKY et al., 1968). Recently, adenine has been shown to be converted to adenosine at a rate similar to the conversion of hypoxanthine to inosine (ZIMMERMAN et al., 1970). However, the K_m for adenine was higher than that for hypoxanthine.

The purine nucleoside phosphorylase has been characterized from other sources. A crystalline preparation from chicken liver had an $S_{20}w$ of 5.45 S, demonstrated substrate activation with inosine, and had a kinetic mechanism consistent with a random Bi-Bi reaction (MURAKAMI and TSUSHIMA, 1975). A homogeneous preparation of rabbit liver purine nucleoside phosphorylase had native and monomeric molecular weight of 46000 and 39000, respectively, and K_m's as follows: inorganic phosphate, 15.4 mM; guanosine, 0.02 mM; and ribose-1-phosphate, 0.13 mM (LEWIS and GLANTZ, 1976). Xanthine was a poor substrate and adenosine was not phosphorylyzed. A homogeneous preparation of calf spleen purine nucleoside phosphorylase had a native molecular weight of 84600 ± 3000 and a subunit molecular weight of 28000 (EDWARDS et al., 1973). Chinese hamster purine nucleoside phosphorylase had a native molecular weight of 84600 ± 3000 and a subunit molecular ular weight, which in the native form behaved as a mixture of dimers of 68000 molecular weight and trimers of 89000 molecular weight (MILMAN et al., 1976). The Michaelis constants were 20 µM for both hypoxanthine and guanine, 35 µM for guanosine, 50 µM for inosine, and 200 µM for both ribose-1-phosphate and phosphate. The enzyme from Salmonella typhimurium or *Escherichia coli* had a native molecular weight of 138000–141000; a subunit molecular weight of 23500; and K_m for inosine, deoxyinosine, and phosphate ion of 0.05 µM, 0.05 µM, and 0.37 mM, respectively (ROBERTSON and HOFFEE, 1973; JENSEN and NYGAARD, 1975). Purine nucleoside phosphorylase has been localized histochemically to the cytoplasm and nucleus of blood vessels (RUBIO et al., 1972), but there is data to suggest that there may be a membrane-bound form of the enzyme (LI and HOCHSTADT, 1976).

III. Adenosine Deaminase (E.C.3.5.4.6)

This enzyme catalyzes the following reaction:

$$\text{Adenosine} + H_2O \rightarrow \text{Inosine} + NH_3.$$

Adenosine deaminase has been carefully characterized in many tissues. The structural gene for the catalytic subunit of this enzyme has been mapped on chromosome 20 (CREAGAN et al., 1973). In human erythrocytes, multiple electrophoretic forms have been distinguished and have been related to a polymorphism based upon two major autosomal alleles ADA^1 and ADA^2 (HOPKINSON et al., 1969). Isofocusing of an ADA^{1-2} human hemolysate demostrated three major peaks and one minor peak of between pH 4.70 and 5.06 (OSBORNE and SPENCER, 1973). A study of the highly pure erythrocyte enzyme has suggested that these electrophoretically different forms are maintained and are the result of posttranslational modification of a single polypeptide chain (SCHRADER et al., 1976; DADDONA and KELLEY, 1977). The erythrocyte enzyme has been purified to homogeneity using different forms of affinity chromatography (SCHRADER et al., 1976; ROSSI et al., 1975; DADDONA and KELLEY, 1977) and had a molecular weight of 36000–38000 (SCHRADER et al., 1976; DADDONA and KELLEY, 1977) and contained carbohydrates (DADDONA and KELLEY, 1977). Amino acid composition was consistant with a minimum molecular weight of 35700 (DADDONA and KELLEY, 1977). Multiple molecular weight and electrophoretic forms of the enzyme have been observed in other human tissues (EDWARDS et al., 1971; AKEDO et al., 1972; NISHIHARA et al., 1972; HIRSCHHORN et al., 1973; VAN DER WEYDEN et al., 1974; HIRSCHHORN, 1975; VAN DER WEYDEN and KELLEY, 1976a), but the catalytic activity appears to be under control of a single genetic locus (AKEDO et al., 1972; NISHIHARA et al., 1972; HIRSCHHORN et al., 1973; VAN DER WEYDEN et al., 1974; HIRSCHHORN, 1975; VAN DER WEYDEN and KELLEY, 1976a). The relative distribution of adenosine deaminase in the cell cytosol between three molecular weight species of 36000, 114000, and 298000 (VAN DER WEYDEN and KELLEY, 1976a) depended on the quantity of conversion factor, a polypeptide of molecular weight 200000 (AKEDO et al., 1972; NISHIHARA et al., 1972; VAN DER WEYDEN and KELLEY, 1976a). The small form was present in erythrocytes and predominated in tissue preparations having a high specific activity and no conversion factor activity (e.g., from stomach and spleen) (VAN DER WEYDEN and KELLEY, 1976a). The large form of adenosine deaminase was found in those tissues with a lower specific activity and abundant conversion factor activity as was evident in kidney and lung tissues (VAN DER WEYDEN and KELLEY, 1976a). A particulate form of adenosine deaminase has also been demonstrated to comprise at least a small percentage of adenosine deaminase assayable in cell homogenates (VAN DER WEYDEN and KELLEY, 1976a; TRAMS and LAUTER, 1975) and may not have a major role in deaminating exogenous adenosine in whole-cell studies (TRAMS and LAUTER, 1975). Although the different molecular weight forms of adenosine deaminase were composed of multiple isoenzymes, these were not tissue specific (VAN DER WEYDEN and KELLEY, 1976a).

Human adenosine deaminase had a pH optimum at about pH 7.0–7.4 (AKEDO et al., 1972; VAN DER WEYDEN and KELLEY, 1976a), although the intermediate form of the enzyme had a pH optimum of 5.5. The K_m for adenosine ranged from 45 μM to 150 μM (OSBORNE and SPENCER, 1973; DADDONA and KELLEY, 1977; AKEDO et al., 1972; VAN DER WEYDEN and KELLEY, 1976a; TRAMS and LAUTER, 1975) without any difference found for the electrophoretic and molecular weight variants (OSBORNE and SPENCER, 1973; VAN DER WEYDEN and KELLEY, 1976a). The K_i for inosine is from 60 to 700 μM (VAN DER WEYDEN and KELLEY, 1976; DADDONA and KELLEY, 1977). Many adenosine analogs are excellent substrates and inhibitors of the erythrocyte enzyme (PARKS, 1975). Coformycin was the most potent inhibitor with a K_i of 0.01 µM.

Adenosine deaminase has also been extensively characterized in other tissues. Calf intestinal mucosa had a pH optimum of 7, an isoelectric pH of 4.85 (BRADY and O'CONNELL, 1962), and K_m values as follows: adenosine, 35 µM; deoxyadenosine, 23 µM; cordycepin, 23 µM; 2,6-diaminopurine riboside, 32 µM (CODDINGTON, 1965). It was inhibited with K_i values as follows: N-methydeoxyadenine, 3.4 µM; deoxyguanosine, 93 µM; and 8-azaguanine, 280 µM (CODDINGTON, 1965). A homogeneous preparation from calf spleen had an $S_{20}w$ of 2.73 S, a molecular weight of 32 500 by gel filtration and 33 000 by amino acid analysis, and was found to contain glucosamine and galactosamine (PFROGNER, 1967; PFROGNER, 1967a). The pH optimum was 6.3 and the K_m for adenosine was 400 µM. The K_m for deoxyadenosine was 143 µM (PFROGNER, 1967). The calf serum form had an $S_{20}w$ of 3.9 S, two major and two minor electrophoretic peaks, a pH optimum from 6.5 to 8.5 and a K_m of 33 µM (CORY et al., 1967). Similar properties were evident for homogeneous bovine placental adenosine deaminase which had a $S_{20}w$ of 4.3 S, a molecular weight of 35 500, but only one protein band and two sulfhydryl groups per mole of enzyme (SIM and MAGUIRE, 1971; MAGUIRE and SIM, 1971). This enzyme catalyzed the hydrolytic removal of amino, chloro, hydroxylamino, methoxy, and methoxyamino substituents from the 6 position of purine ribonucleosides (MAGUIRE and SIM, 1971). Both a bond-forming component dependent on steric factors, and a bond-stretching component dependent on the electronegativity of the leaving group appeared to be involved in the rate-determining formation of a transition complex (MAGUIRE and SIM, 1971). Chicken egg yolk contained an adenosine deaminase with a pH optimum at 6.5, a K_m for adenosine of 66 µM, a molecular weight of 14 000, and a substrate specificity that included deoxyadenosine, cytidine, and guanosine (DE BOECK et al., 1975). Other hen enzymes had similar properties, with molecular weights varying from 30 000 to 110 000 (DE BOECK et al., 1975). Recent studies of rabbit adenosine deaminase have shown similar features to the human enzyme. A large form of adenosine deaminase of molecular weight 260 000 was present in intestine, liver, and spleen, while the vermiform appendix and brain possessed only small adenosine deaminase of molecular weight 34 000 (PIGGOTT and BRADY, 1976).

The adenosine deaminase enzyme has been studied in patients with severe combined immunodeficiency disease. The mutant enzyme had 0.5% of normal activity in splenic tissue from one patient (VAN DER WEYDEN et al., 1974). This mutant adenosine deaminase had an $S_{20}w$ of 7.4 S and a molecular weight of 115 000, corresponding to an intermediate form. Another form of this enzyme had a higher molecular weight and was at the bottom of the sucrose gradient (VAN DER WEYDEN et al., 1974; VAN DER WEYDEN and KELLEY, 1976). The substrate specificity, pH optimum, K_m for adenosine of 130 µM, or K_i for inosine of 1.6 mM of the adenosine deaminase from this patient were comparable to the normal corresponding molecular form (VAN DER WEYDEN and KELLEY, 1976). The hemolysate from another patient was found to inhibit adenosine deaminase partially purified from a normal individual, suggesting the production of an adenosine deaminase inhibitor (TROTTA et al., 1976). Cultured skin fibroblasts have been useful for the study of mutant adenosine deaminase, although the uptake of adenosine deaminase from the culture medium and mycoplasma may introduce artifacts. Cells from two different patients showed less than 1% and 10% of normal activity (CHEN et al., 1975). In the latter case, the pH optimum and the K_m were similar to the normal values. This mutant enzyme was resistant to heat inactivation and migrated more quickly to the anode than the normal enzyme during electrophoresis. The fibroblasts from four immunodeficient patients were similarily found to have about 20% of normal enzyme activity, a normal K_m for adenosine of 65 µM, increased electrophoretic motility, and increased heat stability (HIRSCHHORN et al., 1976). This mutant enzyme had a molecular weight of about 260000. Immunochemical studies of adenosine deaminase in combined immunodeficiency disease have demonstrated one enzyme with a greater amount of immunoreactive activity than catalytically active enzymes (CARSON et al., 1976) and one enzyme with an equivalent amount of immunoreactive and catalytically active enzyme (DADDONA et al., 1976). Although tissue and erythrocyte forms of adenosine deaminase were deficient, conversion factor activity was normal (HIRSCHHORN et al., 1973; HIRSCHHORN, 1975).

IV. Guanine Deaminase (E.C.3.5.4.3)

This enzyme catalyzes the following reaction:

$$\text{Guanine} + H_2O \rightarrow \text{Xanthine} + NH_3$$

Guanine deaminase has been extensively characterized in rabbit, mouse, and rat tissue, but virtually no data is available concerning the human enzyme. Rabbit liver guanine deaminase is the only species of this enzyme to be purified to homogeneity (LEWIS and GLANTZ, 1974; LEWIS and GLANTZ, 1975). The enzyme is a single polypeptide of 55000 which was irreversibly inactivated by p-chloromercuribenzoate. The pH optimum was 6.8 when guanine was a substrate. The K_m for guanine was 12.5 µM at pH 7.0, 333 µM for 8-azaguanine at pH 6.0 and 800 µM for 6-thioguanine at pH 7.0. GDP and GTP did not alter enzyme activity. The enzyme was competitively inhibited by aminoimidazolecarboxamide, its ribonucleotide derivative, or tetrahydrofolic acid with K_i values of 30.5, 258, or 568 µM, respectively. At saturating substrate concentrations, deuterium isotope enhanced the catalytic rate of the enzyme. Similar substrate K_m values were observed with a cruder rabbit liver enzyme (CURRIE et al., 1967).

Rodent brain and liver guanine deaminase have been studied in detail. The enzyme was in a 15000 g supernatant of rat liver, kidney, and spleen, but was also located in the light mitochondrial fraction of whole brain (KUMAR et al., 1967). Two enzyme forms, type A and B, were evident on DEAE ion exchange chromatography in the supernatant from rat brain (KUMAR et al., 1967) or liver (MANSOOR et al., 1963). In these tissues sigmoid kinetics and a $S_{0.5}$ from 5.3 to 6.6 µM were observed for guanine with the type A enzyme, while hyperbolic kinetics were evident for the type B enzyme (KUMAR et al., 1972; KUMAR et al., 1973). GTP activated the A enzyme and caused linear kinetics but had no effect on the B enzyme (JOSAN and KRISHMAN, 1968; KUMAR et al., 1972; KUMAR et al., 1973). The type A liver enzyme was also activated by 1 mM of $MgCl_2$ (JOSAN and KRISHMAN, 1968; KUMAR et al., 1973) but was inhibited by allantoin (KUMAR et al., 1973). In the mouse, all guanine deaminase was in the supernatant 15000 g fraction in liver, and 20% was in the particulate fraction of brain (KUMAR et al., 1972). There were two supernatant enzymes in the brain, one obeying sigmoidal kinetics and the other hyperbolic kinetics. The K_m for guanine was 5 μM and 66 μM, respectively. GTP, MgCl$_2$, or allantoin had little or no effects on mouse tissue guanine deaminase (KUMAR et al., 1973). Aminoimidazolecarboxamide was an inhibitor of guanine deaminase from mouse liver (MANDEL et al., 1957).

Guanine deaminase is regulated by dietary effects on enzyme activity and by a lipoprotein inhibitor located in the outer membrane of the heavy mitochondrial fraction (ALI et al., 1974). This inhibitor was evident in kidney, brain, and liver but not in rat spleen (KUMAR et al., 1967). Guanine deaminase increased 24–48 h following the feeding of guanine (SITARAMAYYA et al., 1974). This change was accompanied by an increased activity of the mitochondria inhibitor and was inhibited by ethionine, cyclohexamide, or actinomycin D (SITARAMAYYA et al., 1974). A second isoenzyme appeared in mouse liver during guanine feeding. Although this isoenzyme showed a sigmoidal response to increasing substrate concentration, it was not affected by GTP, allantoin, or Mg^{2+} (SITARAMAYYA et al., 1976).

Other observations were made using crude extracts of different tissues of man, mouse, rat, and guinea pig. A broad pH optimum from 6 to 9 was evident with guanine as the substrate in their liver and serum (GALANTI et al., 1975). The pH optimum was 6.0 when the substrate was azaguanine (GALANTI et al., 1976). The red blood cells of mouse and rat but not rabbit, sheep, or human contained guanine deaminase (FARKAS and SINGH, 1975). Rat erythrocytes had two activities on DEAE cellulose chromatography. One of these had a K_m of 4 μM and was neither activated by GTP nor inhibited by allantoin (FARKAS and SINGH, 1975).

V. Xanthine Oxidase (E.C.1.2.3.2)

This enzyme catalyzes the following reactions:

$$Hypoxanthine + H_2O + O_2 \rightarrow Xanthine + H_2O_2$$
$$Xanthine + H_2O + O_2 \rightarrow Uric\ Acid + H_2O_2$$

Xanthine oxidase has been extensively characterized in mammalian systems and has received recent review (WYNGAARDEN, 1972). It is found mainly in liver and small intestinal mucosa with significant trace activity in kidney, spleen, and heart muscle. This enzyme functions aerobically and anaerobically both as an oxidase with molecular oxygen and as a dehydrogenase with a variety of other electron acceptors, including methylene blue, cytochrome, and NAD. The underlying molecular basis for these two functions has been recently clarified (NAGLER and VARTANYAN, 1976; WAULD et al., 1975; WAULD and RAJAGOPALAN, 1976; WAULD and RAJAGOPALAN, 1976a). Rat liver xanthine dehydrogenase (type D) has been purified, and two types of oxidase enzymes (type O) have been derived from the type D by either heat or trypsin treatment (WAULD and RAJAGOPALAN, 1976). Type D enzyme can use NAD as an electron acceptor and NADH as an electron donor. The types D and O have distinctive affinities for DEAE cellulose and are inhibited differently by a type O-directed antiserum (WAULD and RAJAGOPALAN, 1976). Types D and O heated have a single polypeptide of 150000 and 28 reactive sulfhydrils, while type O trypsinized has a single major band with a molecular weight of 130000 and only eight reactive sulfhydrils (WAULD and RAJAGOPALAN, 1976 a). Native bovine milk xanthine oxidase has a molecular weight of about 300000 and a subunit molecular weight of 150000 (WAULD et al., 1975; NAGLER and VARTANYAN, 1976). Milk xanthine oxidase treated with pancreatin or other limited proteolytic enzymes forms three polypeptides with molecular weights 92000, 42000, and 20000 (WAULD et al., 1975; NAGLER and VARTANYAN, 1976). Only unproteolyzed preparations of type O rat liver enzyme and milk xanthine oxidase are converted to type D enzymes by treatment with dithiothreitol (WAULD and RAJAGOPALAN, 1976 a).

Xanthine oxidase is capable of functioning as an aldehyde oxidase, although aldehyde oxidase is known to possess an additional coenzyme Q-like quinone. However, the extent to which xanthine oxidase functions as an aldehyde oxidase in vivo is not known (WYNGAARDEN, 1972). There are definite kinetic differences in Michaelis-Menten constants for a variety of substrates of xanthine oxidase. In general, they are lower than those for aldehyde oxidase (KRENITSKY et al., 1972).

Bovine milk xanthine oxidase is a metalloflavoprotein which contains 2 mol of FAD, 2 mol of molybdenum, 8 mol of nonheme iron, and 8 mol of labile sulfide per 300000 molecular weight. These prosthetic groups appear to provide the basis for an internal electron transport chain. Although there are an even number of the prosthetic groups, there is evidence to suggest that the two FAD moieties of the enzyme are nonequivalent (KANDA and RAJAGOPALAN, 1972; KANDA et al., 1972). This indicates that it is not correct to assume that the even numbers can provide evidence for two identical and independent electron transport chains. Electrons are thought to be transported from molybdenum to iron sulfide to FAD and then finally to oxygen or anaerobically to an electron acceptor. The inhibitory action of allopurinol and oxipurinol appears to involve complex formation with molybdenum.

The enzyme has a wide substrate specificity. It hydrolyzes hypoxanthine to xanthine and xanthine to uric acid, 6-mercaptopurine to 6-thiouric acid, allopurinol to oxipurinol, and adenine to 2,8-dihydroxyadenine. It attacks a variety of other purines, pteridines, and aldehydes. The K_m for hypoxanthine or xanthine was 16 μM or 11 μM, respectively, for human liver enzyme (SMYTHE, 1976), 15 μM or 25 μM, respectively, for the mouse muscle enzyme (LALANNE and WILLEMOT, 1975), and 2 μM for xanthine with the rat liver enzyme (WAULD and RAJAGOPALAN, 1976). Alternative substrate K_m's for bovine liver xanthine oxidase range from as low as 20 μM for pteridine to as high as 2 mM for 3-dimethylxanthine (KRENITSKY et al., 1972). Human liver xanthine oxidase was inhibited by xanthine with a K_i of 9.3 μM when hypoxanthine was substrate and by uric acid 1.6 mM when xanthine was substrate (SMYTHE, 1976). The former value was close to its physiologic concentrations.

Xanthine oxidase is an inducible enzyme. Administration of RNA, hypoxanthine, ethylaminothiadiazole, or fructose to human subjects caused liver xanthine oxidase to increase from two to four times higher than the control group (MARCOLONGO et al., 1974). Hepatic (but not jejunal) xanthine oxidase was elevated in gouty patients who exhibited an overproduction of uric acid (MARCOLONGO et al., 1974). Rabbit liver xanthine oxidase increased five fold when dietary protein was increased from 8% to 23% of the diet (ROWE and WYNGAARDEN, 1966). Increased purine ingestion induced chicken liver xanthine dehydrogenase (WOODWARD et al., 1972), and vitamin E deficiency increased rabbit liver xanthine oxidase (CATIGNANI et al., 1974). In all rat hepatomas, xanthine oxidase was decreased two to 10 fold, a change which was accompanied by an increase of PP-ribose-P amidotransferase (PRAJDA and WEBER, 1975). This reprogramming of gene expression results in an imbalance that favors synthesis over catabolism. Dietary-induced deficiencies of iron or molybdenum led to a decrease of hepatic xanthine oxidase in experimental animals (BRAY, 1963).

D. Regulation of Purine Nucleotide Degradation

Evidence for complex regulation of nucleotide degradation has been obtained by studies designed to disrupt the usual mechanisms of control. Experiments have been performed in vivo and in vitro that lead to an increase of the degradation of purine nucleotides to catabolic intermediates and end products. Activation of nucleotide catabolism occurred in ascites tumor cells following incubation with 2-deoxyglucose or glucose (LOMAX and HENDERSON, 1973; LOMAX et al., 1975; McCOMB and YU-SHOK, 1964; OVERGAARD-HANSEN, 1965). There was a loss of high energy phosphate (primarily ATP), an increase of AMP levels, and a rise and later fall of IMP concentration, with a steady rise of inosine until it became a predominant compound absorbing at 250–260 nm (McCOMB and YUSHOK, 1964). The sudden diminution of

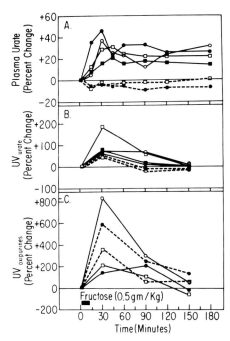

Fig. 6. Effect of fructose infusion on plasma urate and urinary excretion of uric acid and oxypurines. Results are expressed as percent change from the control value at time O. Solid lines indicate no allopurinol, and broken lines indicate pretreatment with allopurinol (Fox and KELLEY, 1972)

intracellular ATP concentration and the concomittant elevation of AMP and IMP levels appeared to be triggering factors for the activation of nucleotide degradation. Using radioactively labeled compounds and 2-deoxyglucose or 2,4-dinitrophenol, this degradation activation has recently been demonstrated for both adenine and guanine nucleotides (LOMAX et al., 1975).

The pathway of nucleotide degradation can be similarily activated in vivo in mammals. Fructose-induced hyperuricemia has provided a model for studying purine catabolism in man. The rapid infusion of fructose is followed in less than 60 min by an increase of serum uric acid, elevation of urinary uric acid and oxypurines, and the appearance of urinary inosine (Figs. 6 and 7) (FOX and KELLEY, 1972; NARINS et al., 1974; PERHEENTUPA and RAIVIO, 1967; RAIVIO et al., 1975; SIMKIN, 1972). In human liver there is a depletion of total adenine nucleotides (predominantly ATP) and inorganic phosphate within 30 min of a fructose infusion (BODE et al., 1973). Similar observations have been made in rat liver or kidney using fructose or glycerol (BURCH et al., 1970; MAENPAA et al., 1968; WOODS et al., 1970). Vigorous muscular exercise in man caused a rise of the serum uric acid (KNOCHEL et al., 1974; RAKESTRAW, 1921; SUTTON and FOX, 1975). Plasma and urinary oxypurine elevation was observed to accompany a diminution of vastus lateralis muscle ATP concentrations during a progressive cycle ergometer test of normal subjects (SUTTON and FOX,

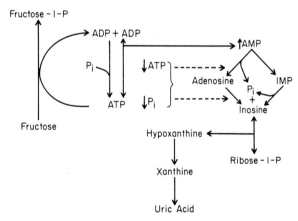

Fig. 7. Mechanism of fructose-induced purine nucleotide degradation. Fructose triggers the rapid breakdown of purine nucleotides to uric acid in the liver. The phosphorylation of fructose to fructose-1-phosphate causes ATP to be degraded to ADP. Fructose-1-P tends to accumulate and thus traps inorganic phosphate. ADP is converted back to ATP by the mitochondrial electron transport system that uses inorganic phosphate or by adenylate kinase. The latter reaction also forms AMP. The net result is a diminution of intracellular ATP and inorganic phosphate and a build-up of AMP. The elevated AMP concentration also leads to increased IMP concentration. Dephosphorylation by 5′-nucleotidase is triggered by the increased AMP and IMP concentration and possibly by decreasing ATP concentration. If AMP and IMP concentrations are high enough, then nonspecific phosphatase can be activated, a reaction which is released from inhibition by the decreasing inorganic phosphate concentrations. Once dephosphorylation is activated, there is a cascade of nucleotide degradation through the catabolic pathways, leading to increased synthesis of uric acid and accounting for hyperuricemia and the elevated urinary excretion of inosine, hypoxanthine, xanthine, and uric acid. Inhibition is indicated by dotted lines. Vertical arrows beside ATP, P_i, and AMP show changes caused by the fructose infusion

Table 3. Inhibition of human placental microsomal alkaline phosphatase (From Fox and Marchant, 1976)

Compound	Concentration (mM)	Percent inhibition
AMP	3.0	42
dAMP	3.0	26
2'-AMP	2.5	0
GMP	3.0	55
IMP	2.5	88
UMP	2.5	55
ADP	3.0	62
GDP	2.5	52
IDP	2.5	93
ATP	3.0	33
GTP	3.0	52
ITP	2.5	69
Glucose-6-P	2.5	41
Ribose-5-P	3.0	48
p-Nitrophenylphosphate	3.0	69
PP_i	3.0	99
P_i	4.0	100
D,L-phenylalanine	10.0	68
NaF	10.0	0

1975). These observations are compatible with an activation of purine nucleotide degradation during exercise. The basis for these profound metabolic changes appears to be the depletion of intracellular ATP and P_i with a triggering of ribonucleotide catabolism (Fig. 7) paralleling the in vitro alterations following 2-deoxyglucose. Although an increase of purine biosynthesis de novo has been observed following the administration of fructose (Raivio et al., 1975), these changes appear to be secondary to the diminution of intracellular nucleotides.

The critical, rate-limiting step of purine nucleotide degradation may be related to the dephosphorylation of nucleoside monophosphates. These reactions are catalyzed by 5'-nucleotidase, a low K_m enzyme; and nonspecific phosphatase, a high K_m enzyme (Table 2). Nucleoside diphosphates and triphosphates were inhibitors of 5'-nucleotidase with K_i values well below their intracellular concentrations (Figs. 3 and 4; Table 1). Although the K_m values of some 5'-nucleoside monophosphates for 5'-nucleotidase were similar to the physiologic concentrations, the nucleotide pool may normally inhibit this enzyme. In contrast, alkaline phosphatase is effectively inhibited by physiologic concentrations of inorganic phosphate (Fig. 5), but only high, nonphysiologic levels of nucleotides will produce the same effect (Table 3). The high K_m for this enzyme makes it unlikely to be active under normal conditions.

The regulation of the dephosphorylation of AMP and IMP has been examined in detail (Lomax et al., 1975) in Ehrlich ascites tumor cells and compared with previously published kinetic constants for 5'-nucleotidase derived from partially purified extracts of these cells (Murray and Friedrichs, 1969). During 2-deoxyglucose-induced purine catabolism, the concentrations of IMP reached 1000 μM, and AMP reached 400 μM as compared to their K_m values of 111 μM and 67 μM, respectively.

Concentrations of ATP declined to a minimum of 400 µM as compared to K_i values of 230 µM and 12 µM for the inhibition of the dephosphorylation of IMP and AMP, respectively. The high concentrations of IMP and AMP in the range of the K_m for alkaline phosphatase suggest that both 5'-nucleotidase and nonspecific phosphatases could have been active during this experiment. Thus, the rates of IMP and AMP formation and their concentrations appeared to be more important regulators of dephosphorylation than inhibition by ATP under the specific experimental conditions. Ineffective inhibition of alkaline phosphatase by nucleotides and a decline of inorganic phosphate concentrations may also have accounted for the apparent alkaline phosphatase activation. However, inorganic phosphate levels were not measured. It was also found (LOMAX et al., 1975) that 70% of the products formed during dinitrophenol-induced purine catabolism were nucleoside monophosphates, in contrast to the prominent dephosphorylation caused by 2-deoxyglucose. This accumulation of nucleoside monophosphates remained unexplained but could have been related to an alteration of intracellular inorganic phosphate, as well as to an inhibitory effect of the two-to-three-fold increase of ADP concentration which was observed (LOMAX et al., 1975).

Once nucleoside monophosphate compounds are dephosphorylated, the resultant products can enter the remainder of the pathway. In general, the other enzyme reactions appear to be controlled mainly by substrate concentration and are not regulated by nucleotides. The activity of purine nucleoside phosphorylase may be limited by the concentration of inorganic phosphate as well as by the intracellular levels of guanosine and inosine (PLANET and FOX, 1976). The inorganic phosphate released by the dephosphorylation reactions can be re-utilized for phosphorolysis of nucleosides if they are in the same compartment. Guanine nucleotide catabolism may be regulated at guanine deaminase by folate derivatives, aminoimidazolecarboxamide and its nucleotide, and on occasion by GTP and a protein inhibitor (ALI et al., 1974; CURRIE et al., 1967; JOSAN and KRISHMAN, 1968; KUMAR et al., 1967; KUMAR et al., 1972; KUMAR et al., 1973; LEWIS and GLANTZ, 1975; LEWIS and GLANTZ, 1974; MANDEL et al., 1957; MANSOOR et al., 1963; SITARAMAYYA et al., 1974; SITARAMAYYA et al., 1976). The deamination of guanine may be inhibited when purine biosynthesis de novo is active. The capacity to increase catabolism with an elevated substrate load is also controlled by the apparent induction of guanine deaminase and xanthine oxidase (CATIGNANI et al., 1974; MARCOLONGO et al., 1974; PRAJDA and WEBER, 1975; ROWE and WYNGAARDEN, 1966; SITARAMAYYA et al., 1974; SITARAMAYYA et al., 1976; WOODWARD et al., 1972).

The major regulatory mechanism of purine catabolism after dephosphorylation may be re-utilization pathways. Guanine, hypoxanthine, and xanthine may be resynthesized to their respective nucleotides by hypoxanthine-guanine phosphoribosyltransferase, while adenosine can be reconverted to AMP by adenosine kinase. Hypoxanthine-guanine phosphoribosyltransferase is regulated by the availability of intracellular PP-ribose-P and product inhibition. A role for this enzyme is suggested by its deficiency. There is an excessive synthesis of uric acid that results from an inability to re-utilize the substrate purine bases and an increase of purine biosynthesis de novo (KELLEY et al., 1967).

The re-utilization of adenosine depends on the relative activities of adenosine deaminase and adenosine kinase. The K_m values for adenosine deaminase are roughly an order of magnitude greater than those reported for adenosine kinase (MURRAY, 1968; ZIELKE and SUELTER, 1971). Therefore, a low concentration of adenosine will tend to favor re-utilization of adenosine by phosphorylation to AMP. Observations in Ehrlich ascites tumor cells demonstrated adenosine synthesis and rephosphorylation during normal cellular metabolism, although adenosine did not accumulate unless an adenosine deaminase inhibitor, coformycin, was present (LOMAX and HENDERSON, 1973). However, from these studies the dephosphorylation of AMP only accounted for 18% of degraded ATP (LOMAX and HENDERSON, 1973), indicating that adenosine synthesis was only a minor pathway when ATP concentrations were markedly reduced. However, adenosine rephosphorylation was an important route of adenosine metabolism when ATP concentrations were high (LOMAX and HENDERSON, 1973). Studies of both the stimulated and unstimulated lymphocytes suggested a dependence on adenosine deaminase activity for the metabolism of adenosine (SNYDER et al., 1976). In stimulated or unstimulated lymphocytes, phosphorylation occurred when adenosine had a concentration of less than 5 µM and 0.5 µM, respectively.

E. Inborn Errors of Purine Nucleotide Degradation

I. Adenosine Deaminase Deficiency

In 1972 a new disease was defined that associated an enzyme deficiency of purine metabolism with immune dysfunction (GIBLETT et al., 1972). The deficiency of adenosine deaminase was found in a group of patients with severe combined immunodeficiency disease. The genetic disease appeared to have an autosomal form of inheritance and was characterized by recurrent infections, diarrhea and malabsorption, failure to thrive and candidasis with absence of tonsils, adenoids, and thymus. Both cell- and antibody-mediated immunity were severely deficient (MEUWISSEN et al., 1975). X-rays demonstrated evidence of osteoporosis and small or absent thymus gland as well as a number of bony abnormalities. Pathologic evaluation revealed extreme thymic involution. A disorder of purine catabolism was suggested by elevated plasma adenosine concentrations and an increased quantity of adenine in the urine, plasma, and erythrocytes (MILLS et al., 1976). ATP concentrations were elevated in erythrocytes (AGARWAL et al., 1976) and lymphocytes (POLMAR et al., 1976), the latter being 10 times greater than the normal values. Therapy of this disorder has included bone marrow transplantation and normal erythrocyte transfusion (POLMAR et al., 1976). The favorable response to enzyme therapy suggested that a direct etiologic relationship existed between enzyme deficiency and immune dysfunction.

II. Purine Nucleoside Phosphorylase Deficiency

Purine nucleoside phosphorylase deficiency has been observed to occur with a disturbance of T-cell function (GIBLETT et al., 1975). The discovery of this new disease has emphasized the etiologic relationship between disorders of purine catabolism and immune function. Three patients had hypouricemia and hypouricosuria with excessive urinary excretion of inosine, guanosine, deoxyinosine, and deoxyguanosine (COHEN et al., 1976; WADMAN et al., 1976). On a low purine diet, the serum uric acid was 1.0 mg/dl, the urine uric acid 11 mg/24 h, and the urine nucleosides 1520 mg/24 h (COHEN et al., 1976). This overproduction of purine was accompanied by an elevation of erythrocyte phosphoribosylpyrophosphate concentrations (COHEN et al., 1976) to the level seen in the complete deficiency of hypoxanthine-guanine phosphoribosyltransferase (FOX and KELLEY, 1971). Recently, two brothers were observed with a less severe disease involving T-cell dysfunction, a serum uric acid of 2.5 mg/dl and 0.45% of normal erythrocyte purine nucleoside phosphorylase activity (EDWARDS et al., in preparation). This mutant enzyme was found to be structurally altered by virtue of a 10-fold increase in the K_m for inosine, an inability of inosine to protect against thermal inactivation, and an altered electrical change (FOX et al., 1977).

III. Xanthinuria

Xanthinuria is a rare disorder characterized by low concentration values of uric acid in the serum and urine and elevated urinary excretion of hypoxanthine and xanthine (WYNGAARDEN and KELLEY, 1976). This autosomal recessively inherited disease is associated with a gross deficiency of xanthine oxidase in the jejunal mucosa or liver. Xanthine stones, hypoxanthine, and xanthine deposits in the urine, and osteoarthritis have been observed in this disorder.

IV. Other Disorders

There are a number of other situations in which purine catabolism is altered. A 45–70-fold increase of erythrocyte adenosine deaminase has been observed in a kindred with hereditary hemolytic anemia (VALENTINE et al., 1977). This dominantly inherited, mild anemia is characterized by a decrease of erythrocyte adenine nucleotides to less than 50% of comparable reticulocyte-rich blood.

The surface 5'-phosphomonoesterase activity of peripheral lymphocytes was found to be significantly lower in patients with nonfamilial adult onset variable primary hypogammaglobulinemia than in non-hypogammaglobulinemic control subjects (JOHNSON et al., 1977). Whether this latter observation indicates a true identifiable clinical subgroup awaits further studies, including those experiments designed to distinguish 5'-nucleotidase from nonspecific phosphatase activity on the lymphocyte surface. A patient with hyperuricemia and gout exhibited a 20-fold increase in the conversion of adenine to hypoxanthine by his cultured skin fibroblasts (HENDERSON et al., 1968).

The complete deficiency of adenine phosphoribosyltransferase is characterized by excessive urinary excretion of adenine and 2,8-dihydroxyadenine and 2,8-dihydroxyadenine renal claculi (DEBRAY et al., 1976). In this disorder the accumulated adenine is not re-utilized and is converted to 2,8-dihydroxyadenine by xanthine oxidase (Fig. 2). The deficiency of hypoxanthine-guanine phosphoribosyltransferase is characterized by an inability to re-utilize hypoxanthine or guanine (KELLEY et al., 1967). The inability to re-utilize these compounds and the accelerated synthesis of IMP led to increased uric acid synthesis. There are other inherited and acquired disorders that can lead to increased purine nucleotide degradation as a result of increased substrate availability or decreased inhibition of these pathways (FOX, 1974).

F. Relationship of Purine Nucleotide Degradation to Immune Function

The discovery of the two enzyme deficiencies, adenosine deaminase and nucleoside phosphorylase, have provided the important clues for a role of purine nucleotide degradation in the regulation of immune function. The mechanism by which these enzyme deficiencies cause immunodeficiency disorders is not known. But it is clear that a block of the deamination of adenosine or the phosphorolysis of inosine and guanosine has profound immunologic effects. Two major lines of investigation have resulted from these observations: (1) studies delineating the biochemical and immunologic effects of excess purine nucleosides and (2) experiments evaluating purine nucleoside metabolism and its alteration in cells of the immune system during resting periods and during transformation.

Adenosine has been found to be cytotoxic to cultured fibroblasts, lymphocytes, and lymphosarcoma T-cells (BENKE and DITTMAR, 1976; GREEN and CHAN, 1973; ISCHII and GREEN, 1973; ULLMAN et al., 1976). In addition, the lymphocytoxic response directed against tumor cells (WOLBERG et al., 1975) and mitogen-mediated lymphoblastogenesis was inhibited by adenosine (CARSON and SEEGMILLER, 1976; FOX et al., 1975; HOVI et al., 1976). These inhibitory effects were potentiated by erythro-9-(2-hydroxyl-3-nonyl) adenine, an adenosine deaminase inhibitor.

These toxic effects have been related to a number of biochemical effects of adenosine. Adenosine and other purine nucleosides are capable of decreasing intracellular concentrations of PP-ribose-P (PLANET and FOX, 1976; SNYDER et al., 1976), an essential substrate for purine and pyrimidine nucleotide synthesis, by inhibiting the synthesis of PP-ribose-P (PLANET and FOX, 1976). A diminution of PP-ribose-P availability could have profound limiting effects on the formation of purine, pyrimidine, and pyridine compounds. Adenosine also increases intracellular cAMP concentrations by stimulation of adenylate cyclase (CLARK and SENEY, 1976; ZENSER, 1975; ZIMMERMAN et al., 1976) or by inhibition of certain cAMP-dependent nuclear protein kinases (HIRSCH and MARTELO, 1976). Since elevations of cAMP are associated with immunosuppressive and anti-inflammatory activity (BOURNE et al., 1974), it has been postulated that this effect of adenosine may cause immune system suppression. Recently, however, adenosine toxicity has been observed in specific mutants lacking adenylate cyclase, which indicates that the adenosine effect does not require cAMP (ULLMAN et al., 1976). There is evidence that adenosine may inhibit pyrimidine biosynthesis de novo, since orotic acid accumulates during adenosine toxicity, and the toxic effects can be reversed by uridine (SNYDER et al., 1976; BENKE and DITTMAR, 1976; GREEN and CHAN, 1973; ISCHII and GREEN, 1973; ULLMAN et al., 1976). The block by adenosine has been localized to orotate phosphoribosyltransferase in erythrocytes, peripheral circulating lymphocytes, and cultured fibroblasts. It appears to be related to decreased intracellular PP-ribose-P levels (PLANET and FOX, in preparation). Adenosine may also inhibit nucleic acid synthesis (BYNUM and VOLKIN, 1976; FOLTINOVA and KUZELA, 1976; PLANET and FOX, in preparation; VORNOVITSKAYA et al., 1975) and protein synthesis (BYNUM and VOLKIN, 1976). In cultured human fibroblasts and peripheral lymphocytes, the inhibitory effect of adenosine was related to a reduction of adenine nucleotide incorporation into nucleic acids, since incorporation of adenine into the nucleotide pool was almost normal

(PLANET and FOX, in preparation). Finally, the significance of the adenosine-induced elevation of adenine nucleotides is still unclear (GREEN and CHAN, 1973; ISCHII and GREEN, 1973). Such an elevation was observed in adenosine deaminase deficiency (AGARWAL et al., 1976; POLMAR et al., 1976). More work will be necessary to define which activity of adenosine is relevant to its cytotoxic effect. The toxic effects of inosine have been postulated to be related to its inhibition of adenosine deaminase (ULLMAN et al., 1976), thus leading to adenosine accumulation.

Besides documenting the toxic activity of adenosine toward cells of the immune system, metabolic studies have been performed in lymphocytes (SNYDER et al., 1976; HOVI et al., 1976) and macrophages (FISCHER et al., 1976). Transformation was accompanied by an adenosine deaminase increase up to ninefold in macrophages (FISCHER et al., 1976). This was associated with an increased activity of a 38000 molecular weight form of adenosine deaminase. A specific inhibitor of adenosine deaminase, erythro-9-(2-hydroxy-3-nonyl) adenine, inhibited the morphological changes associated with monocyte maturation as well as the accompanying acid phosphatase increase. Adenosine deaminase in mitogen-stimulated lymphocytes increased up to fourfold at 24–60 h (HOVI et al., 1976) and decreased to 44% of resting values at 72 h (SNYDER et al., 1976). In spite of a reduced adenosine deaminase activity in the latter situation, there was a 12-fold elevation of the rate of deamination in lymphocytes, suggesting an increased entry of adenosine into stimulated lymphocytes. Erythro-9-(2-hydroxy-3-nonyl) adenine or coformycin, another adenosine deaminase inhibitor, together with adenosine, inhibited mitogen-mediated blastogenesis of lymphocytes (CARSON and SEEGMILLER, 1976; FOX et al., 1975; HOVI et al., 1976; SNYDER et al., 1976). Thus, adenosine deaminase may have a role in monocyte to macrophage transformations and lymphocyte blastogenesis.

G. Other Relationships to Purine Nucleotide Degradation

The purine nucleoside intermediates have been implicated in other functions. Studies of the local regulation of coronary circulation have demonstrated an increased flow following the infusion of purine compounds (BERNE et al., 1971; MOIR and DOWNS, 1972; RUBIO and BERNE, 1969; RUBIO et al., 1969). Adenosine and its catabolic products have been detected during hypoxia in the coronary sinus blood. An elaborate hypothesis suggesting adenosine as an essential physiologic regulator of the coronary circulation has been proposed. The adenosine and other intermediates detected in sinus blood most likely result from the activation of purine catabolism.

The existence of "purinergic nerves" using purines as neurotransmitters has been proposed based on convincing data (BURNSTOCK, 1972). Evidence has suggested that adenosine itself has neurotransmitter properties which are inhibited by theophylline at a presumed adenosine receptor (BURNSTOCK, 1972; MARX, 1972; SATCHELL and MAGUIRE, 1975; WESTON, 1973). It seems possible that adenosine released from nerve endings originates from ATP, since the data suggests that both these substances may be effective neurotransmitters. Again, degradation of purine nucleotides appear to be involved.

The effects of adenosine on arteriolar vasodilatation and in synaptic transmission may not be separate distinctive functions. Since adenosine is known to elevate intracellular CAMP by a direct stimulation of adenylate cyclase on the cell membrane

(CLARK and SENEY, 1976; MARX, 1972; ZENSER, 1975; ZIMMERMAN et al., 1976), it is possible that these activities are mediated by this mechanism. There are a number of other effects of adenosine not reviewed in this article, which may be explainable on this basis. Thus, the "adenosine receptor" may be adenylate cyclase and the purine catabolic pathways may provide the regulated mechanism for synthesizing and degrading this purine nucleoside.

H. Conclusions

Purine nucleoside monophosphates are degraded to the end-product uric acid in man by a final common pathway involving dephosphorylation, phosphorolysis, deamination, and oxidation. The substrate for this pathway is provided by dietary nucleoproteins, nucleic acid degradation, purine salvage pathways, purine biosynthesis de novo, and degradation of cyclic nucleotides, nucleoside diphosphates, and triphosphates.

Purine nucleotide degradation to uric acid is a complexly regulated metabolic pathway. This has been studied in vivo and in vitro using models in which a cascade of nucleotide degradation is accompanied by decreasing intracellular ATP and inorganic phosphate concentrations. Fructose-induced hyperuricemia and exercise in man are models of this mechanism. The major rate-limiting step may be the dephosphorylation of nucleotides to nucleosides. This reaction appears to be regulated by substrate availability as well as the concentration of ATP and inorganic phosphate. Another important regulatory mechanism may be the ability to reuse some catabolic intermediates by the reactions of hypoxanthine-guanine or adenine phosphoribosyltransferases and adenosine kinase.

Inborn errors of purine nucleotide degradation have been the focus of intensive studies because of their relationship to immune dysfunction. Deficiency of adenosine deaminase is associated with T- and B-cell disorders, while deficiency of purine nucleoside phosphorylase is associated with T-cell disorders only. The basis for these diseases may possibly be related to the toxic effects of purine nucleosides and their complicated metabolic interactions. Other disorders of purine catabolism include xanthinuria and acquired abnormalities of the pathway.

A great deal is now known about purine nucleotide degradation, its complex regulation and the associated disorders. Continued investigation of these pathways seems essential and will probably yield important observations relevant to human biology and disease.

Acknowledgment. The author wishes to thank Gloria Spath for her excellent typing of the manuscript and for arranging the bibliography.

References

Agarwal, K. C., Agarwal, R. P., Stockler, J. D., Parks, Jr., R. E.: Purine nucleside phosphorylase. Microheterogeneity and comparison of kinetic behavior of the enzyme from several tissues and species. Biochemistry **14**, 79—84 (1975)

Agarwal, R. P., Crabtree, G. W., Parks Jr., R. E., Nelson, J. A., Keightly, R., Parkman, R., Rosen, F. S., Stern, R. C., Polmar, S. H.: Purine nucleoside metabolism in the erythrocytes of patients with adenosine deaminase deficiency and severe combined immunodeficiency. J. clin. Invest. **57**, 1025—1035 (1976)

Agarwal, R. P., Parks Jr., R. E.: Purine nucleoside phosphorylase from human erythrocytes: crystallization and some properties. J. biol. Chem. **244**, 644—647 (1969)

Akedo, H., Nishihara, H., Shinkai, K., Komatsu, K., Ishikawa, S.: Multiple forms of human adenosine deaminase I purification and characterization of two molecular species. Biochim. biophys. Acta (Amst.) **276**, 257—271 (1972)

Ali, S., Sitaramayya, A., Kumar, K. S., Krishnam, P. S.: Guanine deaminase inhibitor from rat livers: isolation and characterization. Biochem. J. **137**, 85—92 (1974)

Bachorik, P. S., Dietrich, L. S.: The purification and properties of detergent-solubilized rat liver nucleotide pyrophosphatase. J. biol. Chem. **247**, 5071—5078 (1972)

Benke, P. J., Dittmar, D.: Purine dysfunction in cells from patients with adenosine deaminase deficiency. Pediat. Res. **10**, 642—646 (1976)

Bergeron, J. J. M., Berridge, M. V., Evans, W. H. V.: Biogenesis of plasmalemmal glycoproteins. Intracellular site of synthesis of mouse liver plasmalemmal 5′-nucleotidase as determined by the subcellular location of messenger RNA coding for 5′-nucleotidase. Biochim. biophys. Acta (Amst.) **407**, 325—337 (1975)

Berne, R. M., Rubio, R., Dobson, J. O., Curnish, R. R.: Adenosine and adenine nucleotides as possible mediators of cardiac and skeletal muscle blood flow regulation. Circulat. Res. **28/29** (Suppl. 1), 115—119 (1971)

Bischoff, E., Tran-Thi, T., Decker, K. F. A.: Nucleotide pyrophosphatase of rat liver: a comparative study on the enzymes solubilized and purified from plasma membrane and endoplasmic reticulum. Europ. J. Biochem. **51**, 353—361 (1975)

Bischoff, I., Wilkening, J., Tran-Thi, T., Decker, K.: Differentiation of the nucleotide pyrophosphatases of rat liver plasma membrane and endoplasmic reticulum by enzymic iodination. Europ. J. Biochem. **62**, 279—283 (1976)

Bode, J. C., Zelder, O., Rumpelt, H. J., Wittkamp, U.: Depletion of liver adenosine phosphates and metabolic effects of intravenous infusion of fructose or sorbital in man and in the rat. Europ. J. clin. Invest. **3**, 436—441 (1973)

Bosmann, H. B., Pike, G.: Membrane marker enzymes: isolation, purification and properties of 5′-nucleotidase from rat cerebellum. Biochim. biophys. Acta (Amst.) **227**, 402—417 (1971)

Bourne, H. R., Lichtenstein, L. M., Melmon, K. L., Henney, C. S., Weinstein, Y., Shearer, G. M.: Modulation of inflammation and immunity by cyclic AMP. Science **184**, 19—28 (1974)

Brady, T. G., O'Connell, N.: A purification of adenosine deaminase from the superficial mucosa of calf intestine. Biochim. biophys. Acta (Amst.) **62**, 216—229 (1962)

Bray, R. C.: Xanthine oxidase. In: Boyer, P., Lardy, H., Myrbach, K. (Eds.): The Enzymes, 2nd Ed., p. 533. New York: Academic Press 1963

Brownlee, S. T., Heath, E. C.: An extracellular 5′-nucleotidase with both monoesterase and diesterase activity from micrococcus sodonensis. Arch. Biochem. Biophys. **166**, 1—7 (1975)

Burch, H. B., Lowry, O. H., Meinhardt, L., Max Jr., P., Chyu, K.: Effect of fructose, dihydroxyacetone, glycerol and glucose on metabolites and related compounds in liver and kidney. J. biol. Chem. **245**, 2092—2102 (1970)

Burger, R. M., Lowenstein, J. M.: 5′-nucleotidase from smooth muscle of small intestine and from brain. Inhibition of nucleotides. Biochemistry **14**, 2362—2366 (1975)

Burnstock, G.: Purinergic nerves. Pharmacol. Rev. **24**, 509—581 (1972)

Bynum, J. W., Volkin, E.: Wasting of 18 S ribosomal RNA by human myeloma cells cultured in adenosine. J. Cell Physiol. **88**, 197—206 (1976)

Carson, D. A., Goldblum, R., Keightley, R., Seegmiller, J. E.: Immunochemical analysis of adenosine deaminase in combined immunodeficiency disease. J. Clin. Chem. Clin. Biochem. **14**, 283 (1976)

Carson, D. A., Seegmiller, J. E.: Effect of adenosine deaminase inhibition upon human lymphocyte blastogenesis. J. clin. Invest. **57**, 274—282 (1976)

Catignani, G. L., Chytil, F., Darby, W. J.: Vitamin E deficiency: immunochemical evidence for increased accumulation of liver xanthine oxidase. Proc. nat. Acad. Sci. (Wash.) **71**, 1966—1968 (1974)

Center, M. S., Behal, F. J.: Calf intestinal 5′-nucleotidase. Arch. Biochem. Biophys. **114**, 414—421 (1966)

Cercignani, G., Serra, M. C., Fini, C., Natalini, P., Palmerini, C. A., Magni, G., Ipata, P. L.: Properties of 5′-nucleotidase from Bacillus cereus obtained by washing intact cells with water. Biochemistry **13**, 3628—3634 (1974)

Chen,S., Scott,R.C., Swedberg,R.K.: Heterogeneity for adenosine deaminase deficiency; expression of the enzyme in cultured skin fibroblasts and amniotic fluid cells. Amer. J. hum. Genet. **27**, 46—52 (1975)

Clark,R.B., Seney,M.N.: Regulation of adenylate cyclase from cultured human cell lines by adenosine. J. biol. Chem. **251**, 4239—4246 (1976)

Coddington,A.: Some substrates and inhibitors of adenosine deaminase. Biochim. biophys. Acta (Amst.) **99**, 442—451 (1965)

Cohen,A., Doyle,D., Martin,Jr.,D.W., Ammann,A.J.: Abnormal purine metabolism and purine overproduction in a patient deficient in purine nucleoside phosphorylase. New Engl. J. Med. **295**, 1449—1454 (1976)

Cory,J.G., Weinbaum,G., Suhadolnik,R.J.: Multiple forms of calf serum adenosine deaminase. Arch. Biochem. Biophys. **118**, 428—433 (1967)

Coulson,R.: Metabolism and excretion of exogenous adenosine 3′: 5′-monophosphate and guanosine 3′: 5′-monophosphate: studies in the isolated perfused kidney and in the intact rat. J. biol. Chem. **251**, 4958—4967 (1976)

Crabtree,G.W.C., Henderson,J.F.: Pathways of purine ribonucleotide catabolism in Ehrlich ascites tumor cells in vitro. Canad. J. Biochem. **49**, 959—963 (1971)

Creagan,R.P., Tischfield,J.A., Nichols,E.A., Ruddle,F.H.: Autosomal assignment of the gene for the form of adenosine deaminase which is deficient in patients with combined immunodeficiency syndrom. Lancet **1973 II**, 1449

Currie,R., Bergel,F., Bray,R.C.: Enzymes and cancer: preparation and some properties of guanase from rabbit liver. Biochem. J. **104**, 634—638 (1967)

Daddona,P., Kelley,W.N.: Human adenosine deaminase purification and subunit structure. J. biol. Chem. **252**, 110—115 (1977)

Daddona,P., Van der Weyden,M.B., Kelley,W.N.: Characterization of human adenosine deaminase. Clin. Res. **24**, 575 A (1976)

De Boeck,S., Rymen,T., Stockx,J.: Adenosine deaminase in chicken-egg yolk and its relation to homologous enzymes in liver and plasma of the adult hen. Europ. J. Biochem. **52**, 191—195 (1975)

Debray,H., Cartier,P., Temstet,A., Cendron,J.: Child's urinary lithiasis revealing a complete deficit in adenine phosphoribosyltransferase. Pediat. Res. **10**, 762—766 (1976)

Divekar,A.Y.: Adenosine phosphorylase activity as distinct from inosine-guanosine phosphorylase activity in sarcoma 180 cells and rat liver. Biochim. biophys. Acta (Amst.) **422**, 15—28 (1976)

Drummond,G.I., Yamamoto,M.: Nucleotide phosphomonoesterases: In: Boyer,P.D. (Ed.): The Enzymes, 3rd Ed., Vol.4, pp. 337. New York: Academic Press 1971

Edwards,M.J., Maguire,M.H.: Purification and properties of rat heart 5′-nucleotidase. Molec. Pharmacol. **6**, 641—648 (1970)

Edwards,N.L., Gelfand,E.W., Biggar,D., Fox,I.H.: Partial deficiency of purine nucleoside phosphorylase studies of pruine and pyrimidine metabolism. J. Lab. Clin. Med. (In press) (1978)

Edwards,Y.H., Edwards,P.A., Hopkinson,D.A.: A trimeric structure for mammalian purine nucleoside phosphorylase. FEBS Letters **32**, 235—237 (1973)

Edwards,Y.H., Hopkinson,D.A., Harris,H.: Inherited variants of human nucleoside phosphorylase. Ann. hum. Genet. **34**, 395—408 (1971)

Edwards,Y.H., Hopkinson,D.A., Harris,H.: Adenosine isozymes in human tissues. Ann. hum. Genet. **35**, 207—219 (1971a)

Ernster,L., Jones,L.C.: A study of the nucleoside: Tri- and diphosphate activities of rat liver microsomes. J. Cell Biol. **15**, 563—578 (1962)

Evans,W.H.: Nucleotide pyrophosphatase, a sialoglycoprotein located on the hepatocyte surface. Nature (Lond.) **250**, 391—394 (1974)

Evans,W.H., Gurd,J.W.: Properties of a 5′-nucleotidase purified from mouse liver plasma membranes. Biochem. J. **133**, 189—199 (1973)

Farkas,W.R., Singh,R.D.: Guanine aminohydrolase in rate and mouse red cells: a potent inhibitor of guanylation of tRNA. Biochem. Biophys. Acta **377**, 166—173 (1975)

Farquhar,M.G., Bergeron,J.J.M., Palade,G.E.: Cytochemistry of golgi fractions prepared from rat liver. J. Cell Biol. **60**, 8—25 (1974)

Felicioli,R.A., Senesi,S., Marmocchi,F., Falcon,G., Ipata,P.L.: Nucleoside phosphomonoesterases during growth cycle of Bacillus subtilis. Biochemistry **12**, 547—522 (1973)

Fischer,D., Van der Weyden,M.D., Snyderman,R., Kelley,W.N.: A role for adenosine deaminase in human monocyte maturation. J. clin. Invest. **58**, 399—407 (1976)

Foltinova,I., Kuzela,S.: Effect of nucleosides on the synthesis of nucleic acids and proteins in Ehrlich ascites carcinoma cells. Neoplasma **23**, 223—226 (1976)

Fox,I.H.: Human purine ribonucleotide catabolism clinical and biochemical significance. Nutr. Metab. **16**, 79—86 (1974)

Fox,I.H., Andres,C.M., Gelfand,E.W., Biggar,D.: Purine nucleoside phosphorylase deficiency: altered kinetic properties of a mutant enzyme. Science **197**, 1084—1086 (1977)

Fox,I.H., Kelley,W.N.: Phosphoribosylpyrophosphate in man: biochemical and clinical significance. Ann. intern. Med. **74**, 424—433 (1971)

Fox,I.H., Kelley,W.N.: Studies on the mechanism of fructose-induced hyperuricemia in man. Metabolism **21**, 713—721 (1972)

Fox,I.H., Keystone,E.C., Gladman,D.D., Moore,M., Cane,D.: Inhibition of mitogen mediated lymphocyte blastogenesis by adenosine. Immun. Commun. **4**, 419—427 (1975)

Fox,I.H., Marchant,P.J.: Human purine ribonucleotide catabolism: characterization of placental microsomal 5'-phosphomonoesterase. Can. J. Biochem. **54**, 462—469 (1976)

Fox,I.H., Marchant,P.J.: Purine catabolism in man: inhibition of 5'-phosphomonoesterase activities from placental microsomes. Canad. J. Biochem. **54**, 1055—1060 (1976a)

Galanti,B., Russo,M., Nardiello,S., Giusti,G.: Activation energy, relative substrate specificity and optimum pH of guanase from human, rat mouse and guinea pig sera and tissues. Enzyme **20**, 90—97 (1975)

Galanti,B., Russo,M., Nardiello,S., Giusti,G.: Further observations on the properties of serum and tissue guanase from man and some animal species. Enzyme **21**, 342—348 (1976)

George,D.L., Francke,U.: Gene dose effect: regional mapping of human nucleoside phosphorylase on chromosome 14. Science **194**, 851—852 (1976)

Giblett,E.R., Amman,A.J., Sandman,R., Wara,D.W., Diamond,L.K.: Nucleoside phosphorylase deficiency in a child with severely defective T-cell immunity and normal B-cell immunity. Lancet **1975I**, 1010—1013

Giblett,E.R., Anderson,J.E., Cohen,F., Pollara,B., Meuwissen,H.J.: Adenosine deaminase deficiency in two patients with severely impaired cellular immunity. Lancet **1972II**, 1067—1069

Green,H., Chan,T.: Pyrimidine starvation induced by adenosine in fibroblasts and lymphoid cells: role of adenosine deaminase. Science **182**, 836—837 (1973)

Grummt,F., Speckbacher,M.: GTP degradation to guanine catalyzed by ribosomal subunits and microsomal wash factors. Europ. J. Biochem. **57**, 579—585 (1975)

Hardonk,M.J., De Boer,H.G.A.: 5'-nucleotidase. III. Determinations of 5'-nucleotidase isozymes in tissues of rat and mouse. Histochimie **12**, 29—41 (1968)

Hardonk,M.J., Koudstaal,J.: 5'-nucleotidase. II. The significance of 5'-nucleotidase in the metabolism of nucleotides studied by histochemical and biochemical techniques. Histochimie **12**, 18—28 (1968)

Henderson,J.F., Rosenbloom,F.M., Kelley,W.N., Seegmiller,J.E.: Variations in purine metabolism of cultured skin fibroblasts. J. clin. Invest. **47**, 1511—1516 (1968)

Hirsch,J., Martelo,O.J.: Inhibition of nuclear protein kinases by adenosine analogues. Life Sci. **19**, 85—90 (1976)

Hirschhorn,R.: Conversion of human erythrocyte-adenosine deaminase activity to different tissue-specific isozymes: evidence for a common catalytic unit. J. clin. Invest. **55**, 661—667 (1975)

Hirschhorn,R., Bertatis,N., Rosen,F.S.: Characterization of residual enzyme activity in fibroblasts from patients with adenosine deaminase deficiency and combined immunodeficiency: evidence for a mutant enzyme. Proc. nat. Acad. Sci. (Wash.) **73**, 213—217 (1976)

Hirschhorn,R., Levytska,V., Pollara,B., Meuwissen,H.J.: Evidence for control of several different tissue-specific isoenzymes of adenosine deaminase by a single genetic locus. Nature (Lond.) New Biol. **246**, 200—202 (1973)

Hopkinson,D.A., Cook,P.J.L., Harris,H.: Further data on the adenosine deaminase (ADA) polymorphism and a report of a new phenotype. Ann. hum. Genet. **32**, 361—367 (1969)

Hovi,T., Smyth,J.F., Allison,A.C., Williams,S.C.: Role of adenosine deaminase in lymphocyte proliferation. Clin. exp. Immunol. **23**, 395—403 (1976)

Huang,C.M., Keenan,T.W.: Preparation and properties of 5'-nucleotidase from bovine milk fat globule membranes. Biochim. biophys. Acta (Amst.) **274**, 246—257 (1972)

Ipata,P.L.: Sheep brain 5'-nucleotidase. Some enzymatic properties and allosteric inhibition by nucleoside triphosphates. Biochemistry 7, 507—515 (1968)

Ischii,K., Green,H.: Lethality of adenosine for cultured mammalian cells by interference with pyrimidine biosynthesis. J. Cell Sci. **13**, 429—439 (1973)

Itoh,R., Mitsui,A., Tsushima,K.: 5'-nucleotidase of chicken liver. Biochim. biophys. Acta (Amst.) **146**, 151—159 (1967)

Jensen,K.F., Nygaard,P.: Purine nucleoside phosphorylase from Escherichia coli and Salmonella typhimurium. Europ. J. Biochem. **51**, 253—265 (1975)

Johnson,S.M., Asherson,G.L., Watts,R.W.E., North,M.E., Allsop,J., Webster,A.D.B.: Lymphocyte purine 5'-nucleotidase deficiency in primary hypogammaglobulinemia. Lancet **1977 I**, 168—170

Josan,V., Krishman,P.S.: Regulation of rat liver guanine amino hydrolase by GTP. Biochem. Biophys. Res. Commun. **31**, 299—302 (1968)

Kanda,M., Brady,F.O., Rajagopalan,K.V., Handler,P.: Studies on the dissociation of flavin adenine dinucleotide from metalloflavoproteins. J. biol. Chem. **247**, 765—770 (1972)

Kanda,M., Rajagopalan,K.V.: Nonequivalence of the flavin adenine dinucleotide moieties of chicken liver xanthine dehydrogenase. J. biol. Chem. **247**, 2177—2182 (1972)

Kelley,W.N., Rosenbloom,F.M., Henderson,J.F., Seegmiller,J.E.: A specific enzyme defect in gout associated with overproduction of uric acid. Proc. nat. Acad. Sci. (Wash.) **57**, 1735—1739 (1967)

Kim,B.K., Cha,S., Parks,Jr.,R.E.: Purine nucleoside phosphorylase from human erythrocytes. I. Kinetic analysis and substrate-binding studies. J. biol. Chem. **243**, 1771—1776 (1968)

Knochel,J.P., Dotin,L.N., Hamburger,R.: Heat stress, exercise and muscle injury: effects on urate metabolism and renal function. Ann. intern. Med. **81**, 321—328 (1974)

Krenitsky,T.A., Elion,G.B., Henderson,A.M., Hitchings,G.H.: Inhibition of human purine nucleoside phosphorylase: studies with intact erythrocytes and the purified enzyme. J. biol. Chem. **243**, 2876—2881 (1968)

Krenitsky,T.A., Neil,S.M., Elion,G.B., Hitchings,G.H.: A comparison of the specificities of xanthine oxidase and aldehyde oxidase. Arch. Biochem. Biophys. **150**, 585—599 (1972)

Kumar,S., Josan,V., Sanger,K.C.S., Tewari,K.K., Krishnan,P.S.: Studies on guanine deaminase and its inhibitors in rat tissues. Biochem. J. **102**, 691—704 (1967)

Kumar,K.S., Sitaramayya,A., Krishnan,P.S.: Guanine deaminase in rat liver and mouse liver and brain. Biochem. J. **128**, 1079—1088 (1972)

Kumar,K.S., Sitaramayya,A., Krishnan,P.S.: Modulation of guanine deaminase. Biochem. J. **131**, 683—687 (1973)

Kuriyama,Y.: Studies on microsomal nucleoside diphosphatase of rat hepatocytes. J. biol. Chem. **247**, 2979—2988 (1972)

Lacroix,S., Moore,M., Fox,I.H.: (unpublished observations)

Lalanne,M., Willemot,J.: Xanthine oxidase from mouse skeletal muscle purification and kinetic studies. Int. J. Biochem. **6**, 479—484 (1975)

Levin,S.J., Bodansky,O.: The double pH optimum of 5'-nucleotidase of bull seminal plasma. J. biol. Chem. **241**, 51—56 (1966)

Lewis,A.S., Glantz,M.D.: Rabbit liver guanine deaminase: chemical, physical, and kinetic properties. J. biol. Chem. **249**, 3862—3866 (1974)

Lewis,A.S., Glantz,M.D.: Isolation and purification of rabbit liver guanine deaminase. J. biol. Chem. **250**, 8220—8221 (1975)

Lewis,A.S., Glantz,M.D.: Monomeric purine nucleoside phosphorylase from rabbit liver: purification and characterization. J. biol. Chem. **251**, 407—413 (1976)

Li,C., Hochstadt,J.: Transport mechanisms in isolated plasma membranes: nucleoside processing by membrane vesicles from mouse fibroblast cells grown in defined medium. J. biol. Chem. **251**, 1175—1180 (1976)

Lisowski,J.: 5'-nucleotide phosphohydrolase from bovine pituitary gland. Biochim. biophys. Acta (Amst.) **113**, 321—331 (1966)

Lomax,C.A., Bagnara,A.S., Henderson,J.F.: Studies of regulation of purine nucleotide catabolism. Canad. J. Biochem. **53**, 231—241 (1975)

Lomax,C.A., Henderson,J.F.: Adenosine formation and metabolism during adenosine triphosphate catabolism in Ehrlich ascites tumor cells. Cancer Res. **33**, 2825—2829 (1973)

Lowry,O.H., Carter,J., Ward,J.B., Glaser,L.: The effects of carbon and nitrogen sources on the level of metabolic intermediates in *Escherichia coli*. J. biol. Chem. **246**, 6511—6521 (1971)

Lowry,O.H., Passonneau,J.V., Hasselberger,F.X., Schultz,D.W.: The relationship between substrates and enzymes of glycosine in brain. J. biol. Chem. **239**, 18—30 (1964)

Maenpaa,P.H., Raivio,K.O., Kekomaki,M.P.: Liver adenine nucleotides; fructose-induced depletion and its effect on protein synthesis. Science **161**, 1253—1255 (1968)

Maguire,M.H., Sim,M.K.: Studies on adenosine deaminase 2. specificity and mechanism of action of bovine placental adenosine deaminase. Europ. J. Biochem. **23**, 22—29 (1971)

Mandel,H.G., Way,J.L., Smith,P.K.: The effect of 4-amino-5-imidazolecarboxamide on the incorporation of purines into liver nucleic acids of the mouse. Biochim. biophys. Acta (Amst.) **23**, 402—404 (1957)

Mansoor,M., Kalyankar,G.D., Talwar,G.P.: Brain guanine deaminase: purification properties and regional distribution. Biochim. biophys. Acta (Amst.) **77**, 307—317 (1963)

Marcolongo,R., Marinello,E., Pompucci,G., Pagani,R.: The role of xanthine oxidase in hyperuricemic states. Arthr. and Rheum. **17**, 430—438 (1974)

Marx,J.L.: Cyclic AMP in brain: role in synaptic transmission. Science **178**, 1188—1190 (1972)

Matsuzaki,S., Pochet,R., Schell-Frederick,E.: A comparison of the subcellular distribution of 5'-nucleotidase, (Na^+-K^+)-ATP'ase and adenyl cyclase in beef thyroid gland. Biochim. biophys. Acta (Amst.) **313**, 329—337 (1973)

McComb,R.B., Yushok,W.D.: Metabolism of ascites tumor cells. IV. Enzymatic reaction involved in adenosine triphosphate degradation induced by 2-deoxyglucose. Cancer Res. **24**, 198—203 (1964)

Meuwissen,H.J., Pickering,R.J., Pollara,B., Porter,I.H.: Combined immunodeficiency disease and adenosine deaminase deficiency: a molecular defect. New York: Academic Press 1975

Mills,G.C., Schmalstieg,F.C., Trimmer,K.B., Goldman,A.S., Goldblum,R.M.: Purine metabolism in adenosine deaminase deficiency. Proc. nat. Acad. Sci. (Wash.) **73**, 2867—2871 (1976)

Milman,G., Anton,D.L., Weber,J.L.: Chinese hamster purine-nucleoside phosphorylase: purification, structural, and catalytic properties. Biochemistry **15**, 4967—4973 (1976)

Moir,T.W., Downs,T.D.: Myocardial reactive hyperemia: comparative effects of adenosine, ATP, ADP, AMP. Amer. J. Physiol. **222**, 1386—1390 (1972)

Murakami,K., Tsushima,K.: Crystallization and some properties of purine nucleoside phosphorylase from chicken liver. Biochim. biophys. Acta (Amst.) **384**, 390—398 (1975)

Murray,A.W.: Some properties of adenosine kinase from Ehrlich ascites tumour cells. Biochem. J. **106**, 549—555 (1968)

Murray,A.W., Friedrichs,B.: Inhibition of 5'-nucleotidase from Ehrlich ascites tumour cells by nucleoside triphosphates. Biochem. J. **111**, 83—89 (1969)

Nagler,L.G., Vartanyan,L.S.: Subunit structure of bovine milk xanthine oxidase: effect of limited cleavage by proteolytic enzymes on activity and structure. Biochim. biophys. Acta (Amst.) **427**, 78—90 (1976)

Naito,Y., Tsushima,K.: Cytosol 5'-nucleotidase from chicken liver. Biochim. biophys. Acta (Amst.) **438**, 159—168 (1976)

Nakamura,S.: Effect of sodium deoxycholate on 5'-nucleotidase. Biochim. biophys. Acta (Amst.) **426**, 339—347 (1976)

Narins,R.G., Weisberg,J.S., Meyers,A.R.: Effects of carbohydrate on uric acid metabolism. Metabolism **23**, 455—465 (1974)

Neu,H.C.: The 5'-nucleotidase of Escherichia coli. I. Purification and properties. J. biol. Chem. **242**, 3896—3904 (1967)

Neu,H.C.: The 5'-nucleotidase of Escherichia coli. II. Surface localization and purification of the E. coli 5'-nucleotidase inhibitor. J. biol. Chem. **242**, 3905—3911 (1967a)

Neu,H.C.: The 5'-nucleotidase (uridine diphosphate sugar hydrolases) of the enterobacteriacea. Biochemistry **7**, 3766—3773 (1968)

Newly,A.C., Luzio,J.P., Hales,C.N.: The properties and extracellular location of 5'-nucleotidase of the rat fat-cell plasma membrane. Biochem. J. **146**, 625—633 (1975)

Nishihara,H., Ishikawa,S., Shinkai,K., Akedo,H.: Multiple forms of human adenosine deaminase. II. Isolation and properties of a conversion factor from human lung. Biochim. biophys. Acta (Amst.) **302**, 429—442 (1972)

Osborne,W.R.A., Spencer,N.: Partial purification and properties of the common inherited forms of adenosine deaminase from human erythrocytes. Biochem. J. **133**, 117—123 (1973)

Overgaard-Hansen,K.: Metabolic regulation of the adenine nucleotide pool I. studies on the transient exhaustion of the adenine nucleotides by glucose in Ehrlich ascites tumor cells. Biochim. biophys. Acta (Amst.) **104**, 330—347 (1965)

Parks Jr.,R.E.: Discussion in Combined Immunodeficiency Disease and Adenosine Deaminase Deficiency: a Molecular Defect, pp. 195—199. In: Meuwissen,H.J., Pickering,R.J., Pollara,B., Porter,I.H. (Eds.). New York: Academic Press 1975

Perheentupa,J., Raivio,K.: Fructose-induced hyperuricemia. Lancet **1967 II**, 528—531

Pfrogner,N.: Adenosine deaminase from calf spleen. I. Purification. Arch. Biochem. Biophys. **119**, 141—146 (1967)

Pfrogner,N.: Adenosine deaminase from calf spleen. II. Chemical and enzymological properties. Arch. Biochem. Biophys. **119**, 147—154 (1967a)

Pierre,J.W. de, Karnovsky,M.L.: Ecto-enzyme of granulocytes: 5'-nucleotidase. Science **183**, 1096—1098 (1974)

Piggott,C.O., Brady,T.G.: Purification of multiple forms of adenosine deaminase from rabbit intestine. Biochim. biophys. Acta (Amst.) **429**, 600—607 (1976)

Pinsley,C.L., Scruton,M.C.: Nucleoside dephosphatase from pig liver, purification and some properties. Arch. Biochem. Biophys. **158**, 331—345 (1973)

Planet,G., Fox,I.H.: Inhibition of phosphoribosylpyrophosphate synthesis by purine nucleosides in human erythrocytes. J. biol. Chem. **251**, 5839—5844 (1976)

Planet,G., Fox,I.H.: Inhibition of pyrimidine nucleotide biosynthesis by purine nucleosides in human cells. (in preparation)

Pletsch,Q.A., Coffey,J.W.: Studies on 5'-nucleotidases of rat liver. Biochim. biophys. Acta (Amst.) **276**, 192—205 (1972)

Polmar,S.H., Stern,R.C., Schwartz,A.L., Wetzler,E.M., Chase,P.A., Hirschhorn,R.: Enzyme replacement therapy for adenosine deaminase deficiency and severe combined immunodeficiency. New Engl. J. Med. **295**, 1337—1343 (1976)

Prajda,N., Weber,G.: Malignant transformation linked inbalance: decreased xanthine oxidase activity in hepatomas. FEBS. Letters **59**, 245—249 (1975)

Raivio,K.O., Becker,M.A., Meyer,L.J., Greene,M.L., Nuki,G., Seegmiller,J.E.: Stimulation of human purine synthesis de novo by fructose infusion. Metabolism **24**, 861—869 (1975)

Rakestraw,N.W.: Chemical factors in fatigue. I. The effects of muscular exercise upon certain common blood constituents. J. biol. Chem. **47**, 565—591 (1921)

Reimer,B.L., Widnell,C.C.: The demonstration of a specific 5'-nucleotidase activity in rat tissues. Arch. Biochem. Biophys. **171**, 343—347 (1975)

Robertson,B.C., Hoffee,P.A.: Purification and properties of purine nucleoside phosphorylase from Salmonella typhimurium. J. biol. Chem. **248**, 2040—2043 (1973)

Rossi,C.A., Lucacchini,A., Montali,U., Ronca,G.: A general method of purification of adenosine deaminase by affinity chomatography. Int. J. Pept. Protein Res. **7**, 81—89 (1975)

Rowe,P.B., Wyngaarden,J.B.: The mechanism of dietary alterations in rat hepatic xanthine oxidase levels. J. biol. Chem. **241**, 5571—5576 (1966)

Rubio,R., Berne,R.M.: Release of adenosine by normal myocardium in dogs and its relationship to regulation of coronary resistance. Circulat. Res. **25**, 407—415 (1969)

Rubio,R., Berne,R.M., Katori,M.: Release of adenosine in reactive hyperemia of the dog heart. Amer. J. Physiol. **216**, 56—62 (1969)

Rubio,V.R., Weidmeier,T., Berne,R.M.: Nucleoside phosphorylase: location and role in the myocardial distribution of purines. Amer. J. Physiol. **222**, 550—555 (1972)

Satchell,D.G., Maguire,M.H.: Inhibitory effects of adenine nucleotide analogs on the isolated guinea pig taenia coli. J. Pharmacol. exp. Ther. **195**, 540—548 (1975)

Schrader,W.P., Stacy,A.R., Pollara,B.: Purification of human erythrocyte adenosine deaminase by affinity column chromatography. J. biol. Chem. **251**, 4026—4032 (1976)

Scott,T.G.: The distribution of 5'-nucleotidase in the brain of the mouse. J. Histochem. Cytochem. **13**, 657—667 (1965)

Sim,M.K., Maguire,M.H.: Studies on adenosine deaminase. I. Purification and some properties of bovine placental adenosine deaminase. Eur. J. Biochem. **23**, 17—21 (1971)

Simkin,P.A.: Hexose infusions in Cebus monkeys: effects on uric acid metabolism. Metabolism **21**, 1029—1036 (1972)

Sitaramayya,A., Ali,S., Kumar,K.S., Krishnan,P.S.: Induction of guanine deaminase and its inhibitor in rodent liver and brain. Biochem. J. **138**, 143—146 (1974)

Sitaramayya, A., Kumar, K. S., Krishnan, P. S.: Isoenzymicity in mouse liver guanine deaminase demonstrable under substrate stress. Biochem. Biophys. Res. Commun. **70**, 480—484 (1976)

Smythe, H. A.: Xanthine and uric acid as xanthine oxidase inhibitors. Arthr. and Rheum. **20**, 135—136 (1977)

Snyder, F. F., Mendelsohn, J., Seegmiller, J. E.: Adenosine metabolism in phytohemagglutinin-stimulated human lymphocytes. J. clin. Invest. **58**, 654—666 (1976)

Soder, C., Henderson, J. F., Zombor, G., McCoy, E. E., Verhoef, V., Morris, A. J.: Relationship between nucleoside triphosphate pyrophosphohyrolase activity and inosine triphosphate accumulation in human erythrocytes. Canad. J. Biochem. **54**, 843—847 (1976)

Solyom, A., Trams, E. G.: Enzyme markers in characterization of isolated plasma membranes. Enzyme **13**, 329—372 (1972)

Song, C. S., Bodansky, O.: Purification of 5'-nucleotidase from human liver. Biochem. J. **101**, 5c—6c (1966)

Song, C. S., Bodansky, D.: Subcellular localization and properties of 5'-nucleotidase in the rat liver. J. biol. Chem. **242**, 694—699 (1967)

Stefanovic, V., Mandel, P., Rosenberg, A.: Concanavalin A inhibition of ecto-5'-nucleotidase of intact cultured C6 glioma cells. J. biol. Chem. **250**, 7081—7083 (1975)

Sutton, J., Fox, I. H.: Alterations in purine metabolism during strenuous musclar exercise in man. Clin. Res. **23**, 639 A (1975)

Tanaka, R., Morita, H., Teruya, A.: Isolation and properties of 5'-nucleotidase from a membrane fraction of bovine cerebral cortex. Biochim. biophys. Acta (Amst.) **298**, 842—849 (1973)

Tanaka, R., Teruya, A., Morita, H.: Effects of divalent cations on 5'-mononucleotidase of bovine cerebral cortex. Canad. J. Biochem. **51**, 841—848 (1973a)

Trams, E. G., Lauter, C. J.: Adenosine deaminase of cultured brain cells. Biochem. J. **152**, 681—687 (1975)

Trotta, P. P., Smithwick, E. M., Balis, M. E.: A normal level of adenosine deaminase in red cell lysates of carriers and patients with severe combined immunodeficiency. Proc. nat. Acad. Sci. (Wash.) **73**, 104—108 (1976)

Ullman, B., Cohen, A., Martin Jr., D. W.: Characterization of a cell culture model for the study of adenosine deaminase and purine nucleoside phosphorylase-deficienct immunologic disease. Cell **9**, 205—211 (1976)

Valentine, W. N., Paglia, D. E., Tartaglia, A. P., Gilsanz, F.: Hereditary hemolytic anemia with increased red cell adenosine deaminase (45- to 70-fold) and decreased adenosine triphosphate. Science **195**, 783—785 (1977)

Van der Weyden, M. B., Buckley, R. H., Kelley, W. N.: Molecular form of adenosine deaminase in severe combined immunodeficiency. Biochem. Biophys. Res. Commun. **57**, 590—595 (1974)

Van der Weyden, M. B., Kelley, W. N.: Catalytic and physical characteristics of adenosine deaminase in severe combined immunodeficiency. J. clin. Chem. Clin. Biochem. **14**, 326—327 (1976)

Van der Weyden, M. B., Kelley, W. N.: Human adenosine deaminase: distribution and properties. J. biol. Chem. **251**, 5448—5456 (1976a)

Vornovitskaya, G. I., Ioannesyants, I. A., Borsenko, B. G., Shapot, V. S.: Effect of deoxyadenosine on the nucleic acids synthesis in malignant cells in the presence of an inhibitor of deaminase. Vaprosy Meditsinkoi **21**, 192—194 (1975)

Wadman, S. K., Bree, P. K. de, Van Gennip, A. H., Stoop, J. W., Zegers, B. J. M., Staal, G. E. J., Siegenbeck, L. H.: Urinary purine in patients with a severely defective T-cell immunity and a purine nucleoside phosphorylase deficiency in erythrocytes and lymphocytes. J. clin. Chem. Biochem. **14**, 326 (1976)

Wauld, W. R., Brady, F. O., Wiley, R. D., Rajagopalan, K. V.: A new purification procedure for bovine milk xanthine oxidase: effect of proteolysis on subunit structure. Arch. Biochem. Biophys. **169**, 695—701 (1975)

Wauld, W. R., Rajagopalan, K. V.: Purification and properties of the NAD$^+$-dependent (Type D) and O$_2$-dependent (Type O) forms of rat liver xanthine dehydrogenase. Arch. Biochem. Biophys. **172**, 354—364 (1976)

Wauld, W. R., Rajagopalan, K. V.: The mechanism of conversion of rat liver xanthine dehydrogenase from an NAD$^+$-dependent form (Type D) to an O$_2$-dependent form (Type O). Arch. Biochem. Biophys. **172**, 365—379 (1976a)

Weston, A. H.: Nerve-mediated inhibition of mechanical activity in rabbit duodenum and the effects of desentization to adenosine and several of its derivatives. Brit. J. Pharmacol. **48**, 302—308 (1973)

Widnell, C. C.: Cytochemical localization of 5'-nucleotidase in subcellular fractions isolated from rat liver. I. The origin of 5'-nucleotidase activity in microsomes. J. Cell Biol. **52**, 542—558 (1972)

Widnell, C. C., Unkeless, J. C.: Partial purification of a lipoprotein with 5'-nucleotidase activity from membrane of rat liver cells. Proc. nat. Acad. Sci. (Wash.) **61**, 1050—1057 (1968)

Wolberg, G., Zimmerman, T. P., Hiemstra, K., Winston, M., Chu, L.: Adenosine inhibition of lymphocyte-mediated cytolysis: possible role of cyclic adenosine monophosphate. Science **187**, 957—959 (1975)

Wong, P. L. C., Henderson, J. F.: Purine ribonucleotide biosynthesis, interconversion and catabolism in mouse brain in vitro. Biochem. J. **129**, 1085—1094 (1972)

Woo, Y., Manery, J. F.: 5'-nucleotidase: an ecto-enzyme of frog skeletal muscle. Biochim. Biophys. Acta (Wash.) **397**, 144—152 (1975)

Woods, H. F., Eggleston, L. V., Krebs, H. A.: The cause of hepatic accumulation of fructose-1-phosphate on fructose loading. Biochem. J. **119**, 501—510 (1970)

Woodward, N. D., Lee, P. C., Delapp, N. W., Fisher, J. R.: Induction of chicken liver xanthine dehydrogenase by purines. Arch. Biochem. Biophys. **153**, 537—542 (1972)

Wyngaarden, J. B.: Xanthinuria. In: Stanbury, J. B., Wyngaarden, J. B., Fredrickson, D. S. (Eds.): The Metabolic Basis of Inherited Disease, 3rd Ed. New York: McGraw-Hill 1972

Wyngaarden, J. B., Kelley, W. N.: Gout and Hyperuricemia. New York: Grune and Stratton 1976

Zenser, T. V.: Formation of adenosine 3', 5'-monophosphate from adenosine in mouse thymocytes. Biochem. Biophys. Acta **404**, 202—213 (1975)

Zielke, C. L., Suelter, C. H.: Purine, Purine Nucleoside, and Purine Nucleotide Aminohydrolases. In: Boyer, P. D. (Ed.); The Enzymes, 3rd Ed., Vol. 4, pp. 47—48. New York: Academic Press 1971

Zimmerman, M., Gersten, N., Miech, P. R.: Adenine and adenosine metabolism in liver. Proc. Amer. Ass. Cancer Res. **11**, 87 (1970)

Zimmerman, T. P., Rideout, J. L., Wolberg, G., Duncan, G. S., Elion, G. B.: 2-Fluoroadenosine 3': 5'-monophosphate: a metabolite of 2-fluoroadenosine in mouse cytoxic lymphocytes. J. biol. Chem. **251**, 6757—6766 (1976)

Interrelationship of Purine and Pyrimidine Metabolism

M. TATIBANA

A. Introduction

Purines and pyrimidines are found in equal amounts in nucleic acids, and the number far exceeds that present as free nucleotides and related low-molecular-weight compounds. Such being the case, cellular demands for synthesis of purines and pyrimidines would be almost equal. In fact, whole-body rates of pyrimidine synthesis de novo in man as estimated by WEISSMAN et al. (1962) are within the same order of magnitude with estimates of total purine production (SEEGMILLER et al., 1961). The question of specific control mechanisms that coordinate the synthesis of purines and pyrimidines is thus raised. Although a definitive answer awaits additional information, there is evidence of a mechanism by which purine and pyrimidine syntheses are coordinated through the intracellular level of 5-phosphoribosyl 1-pyrophosphate. Other possible mechanisms include those where key enzymes of the metabolism of purines or pyrimidines are regulated reciprocally by pyrimidine or purine derivatives. This type of regulation has been observed for certain enzyme reactions, although the physiologic significance remains unclear in most cases. This section deals with the following items: 1) such reciprocal control of activities of some key enzymes in the biosynthesis de novo, salvage synthesis, interconversion, and degradation of purine and pyrimidine nucleotides; 2) effects of exogenously administered natural or artificial purines or pyrimidines on the respective metabolism of pyrimidines or purines; 3) coordinate control of the purine and pyrimidine biosyntheses by phosphoribosyl pyrophosphate; 4) possible interference between purine and pyrimidine catabolism; 5) consideration of a possible interrelationship between purine and pyrimidine transport through membrane.

B. Control of Enzyme Activity by Pyrimidines in Purine Biosynthetic Pathways

Activities of key enzymes of the de novo purine nucleotide biosynthesis and of the salvage pathway do not appear to be significantly affected by pyrimidine nucleotides and related pyrimidine compounds. Results of studies on certain individual enzymes are described briefly.

I. Phosphoribosyl Pyrophosphate Amidotransferase

Phosphoribosyl pyrophosphate amidotransferase (E.C.2.4.2.14), the first and committed step unique to the de novo purine biosynthetic pathway, is inhibited in a cooperative or synergistic manner by purine nucleotides, such as AMP, GMP, and 6-mercaptopurine ribonucleotide, but does not appear to be significantly affected by pyrimidine nucleotides in pigeon liver (WYNGAARDEN and ASHTON, 1959; CASKEY et al., 1964), tumor cells (HILL and BENNETT, 1969), human placenta (HOLMES et al., 1973), and bacteria (NIERLICH and MAGASANIK, 1965; SHIIO and ISHII, 1969). Coordinated control of this step with certain other key reactions in nucleotide biosyntheses, through the intracellular level of phosphoribosyl pyrophosphate, is discussed later.

II. Adenylosuccinate Synthetase

Adenylosuccinate synthetase (E.C.6.3.4.4), which catalyzes the reaction at the branching point to the synthesis of AMP from inosinate (IMP), is subject to regulation by purine nucleotides, but effects of pyrimidine nucleotides have not been described (RUDOLF and FROMM, 1969; MUIRHEAD and BISHOP, 1974).

III. IMP Dehydrogenase

IMP dehydrogenase (E.C.1.2.1.14), the first enzyme in a branched pathway leading to the synthesis of GMP from IMP, is a potential site for the regulation of the synthesis. In fact, this enzyme in bacterial, fungal, and neoplastic mammalian cells is sensitive to inhibition by purine nucleotides such as xanthosine 5'-monophosphate, GMP, and AMP. Human IMP dehydrogenase is also inhibited by CMP, though the degree of inhibition (about 50% at a concentration of 5 mM) was much less marked than that observed with purine ribonucleotides (HOLMES et al., 1974).

The presence of guanine, guanosine, or adenosine in media for bacterial growth led to repression of the enzymes of purine ribonucleotide interconversion (for a review, HENDERSON and PATERSON, 1973). However, such effects have not been reported for pyrimidines.

IV. Adenosine Kinase

Adenosine kinase (E.C.2.7.1.20) is an important salvage enzyme for purine ribonucleotide biosynthesis. The enzyme in the extract of Ehrlich ascites cells utilizes ATP and other purine nucleoside triphosphates as well as some pyrimidine nucleoside triphosphates, such as CTP, UTP, and dTTP, as phosphate donors (MURRAY, 1968). The enzymatic activity is inhibited by purine nucleoside mono- and diphosphates in a competitive manner with respect to ATP but only very weakly by UMP, CMP, dUMP, or dCMP.

Pyrimidines or their derivatives do not appear to significantly affect the activity of adenine phosphoribosyltransferase (E.C.2.4.2.7) and hypoxanthine-guanine phosphoribosyltransferase (E.C.2.4.2.8).

C. Control of Enzyme Activity by Purines in Pyrimidine Biosynthetic Pathways

Activities of key enzymes in pyrimidine nucleotide biosynthesis are sensitive to regulation by purine nucleotides or related compounds. Although the physiologic

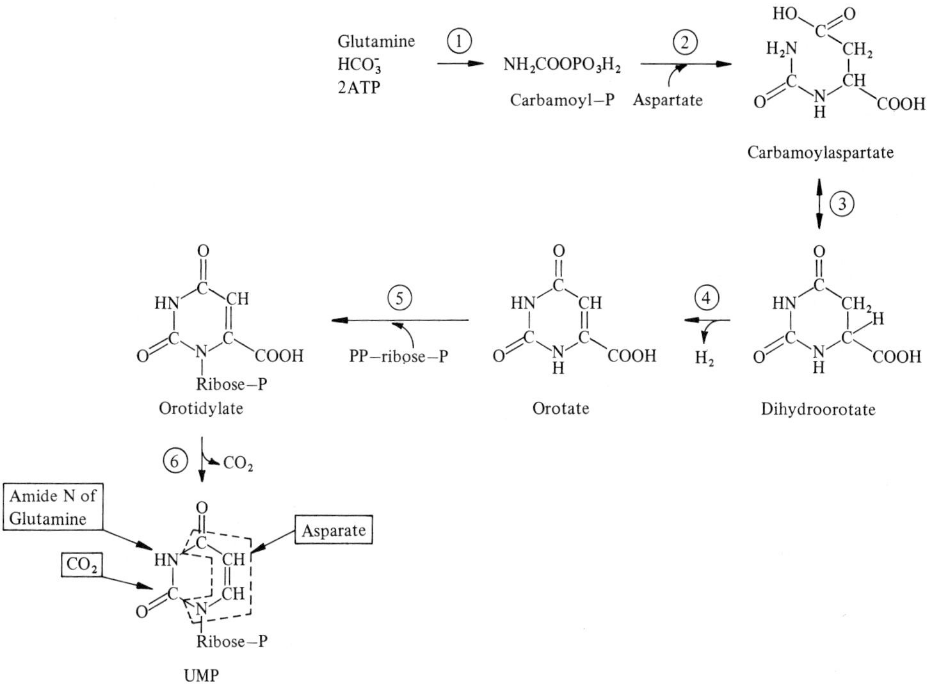

Glutamine ① NH₂COOPO₃H₂ ②
HCO₃⁻
2ATP

Carbamoyl–P Aspartate

Carbamoylaspartate

③

Orotidylate   PP–ribose–P   Orotate   Dihydroorotate

Ribose–P

⑤   ④   H₂

⑥ CO₂

Amide N of Glutamine

CO₂   Asparate

Ribose–P

UMP

Fig. 1. Reactions of uridylate biosynthesis de novo. Enzymes involved are: 1) glutamine-dependent carbamoyl-phosphate synthetase (E.C.2.7.2.9); 2) aspartate carbamoyltransferase (E.C.2.1.3.2); 3) dihydroorotase (E.C.3.5.2.3); 4) dihydroorotate dehydrogenase (E.C.1.3.3.1); 5) orotate phosphoribosyltransferase (E.C.2.4.2.10); 6) orotidylate decarboxylase (E.C.4.1.1.23)

role of all of the effects have not yet been established, it can be assumed that such may contribute to coordination of purine and pyrimidine biosyntheses. However, control by the energy charge of ATP-ADP-AMP system (ATKINSON and WALTON, 1967), to which several key enzymes in the pyrimidine pathways are sensitive, may be of limited significance in the coordinate control; variations in the energy charge do not necessarily lead to changes in the amount of total adenine nucleotides. The energy charge control may serve principally to maintain the balance between generation and utilization of high-energy phosphate bonds.

The enzymatic reactions leading to the synthesis of uridylate are illustrated in Figure 1. Recent advances in enzyme regulation of pyrimidine biosynthesis have been reviewed (BLAKLEY and VITOLS, 1968; O'DONOVAN and NEUHARD, 1970; JONES, 1971; KELLEY, 1972; TATIBANA and SHIGESADA, 1972).

I. Carbamoyl-Phosphate Synthetase II

Carbamoyl-phosphate synthetase II (glutamine-dependent, E.C.2.7.2.9) catalyzes the first step unique to the de novo pyrimidine biosynthesis (TATIBANA and ITO, 1967, 1969; HAGER and JONES, 1967a, b) and plays an important role in the control of this pathway (TATIBANA and ITO, 1967; ITO et al., 1970; LEVINE et al., 1971; TATIBANA and SHIGESADA, 1972b; SMITH et al., 1973; PAUSCH et al., 1975). The enzyme that is obtained from mouse spleen and rat liver is sensitive to allosteric inhibition by UTP, UDP, and other various pyrimidine ribo- and deoxyribonucleotides and to stimulation by phosphoribosyl pyrophosphate (TATIBANA and SHIGESADA, 1972a, c; MORI et al., 1975). Purine nucleotides such as ADP, GTP, and ITP are also moderately inhibitory. The relatively strong inhibition by ADP, which is competitive with regard to the substrate ATP, indicates the sensitivity of this enzyme to control by the energy

I. Escherichia coli

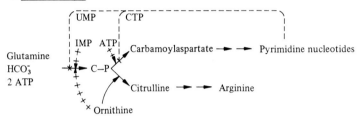

II. Neurospora, Saccharomyces

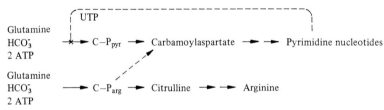

III. Ureotelic animals

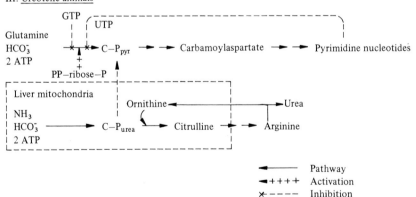

Fig. 2. Three distinct types of carbamoyl-phosphate metabolism and its regulation in nature. The schemes are confined only to those biological systems on which sufficient information is available and also to short-term regulation of considerable importance. C—P: carbamoyl-phosphate. C-P$_{pyr}$, C-P$_{arg}$, and C-P$_{urea}$ denote the pools of carbamoyl-phosphate specific for pyrimidine, arginine, and urea biosyntheses, respectively. AGA: N-acetyl-L-glutamate. PP-ribose-P: 5-phosphoribosyl 1-pyrophosphate

charge of the adenylate system. The physiologic significance of the inhibition by other purine nucleotides is not clear. The activating effect of phosphoribosyl pyrophosphate is discussed later.

The same type of enzyme was recently found to exist also in *Ascaris* ovary and proved to have a similar sensitivity to inhibition by nucleotides and to activation by phosphoribosyl pyrophosphate (AOKI et al., 1975). GDP, dGDP, and other purine nucleotides are moderately inhibitory. In *Saccharomyces cerevisiae* and *Neurospora crassa*, the enzyme also catalyzes the first and committed step unique to the pyrimidine nucleotide biosynthesis de novo and is subject to inhibition by UTP (LACROUTE et al., 1965; DAVIS, 1967). There is apparently no documentation concerning effects of purine nucleotides.

Features of pyrimidine synthesis in eucaryotes and proeucaryotes should be mentioned prior to discussion of the events in bacteria (Fig. 2). Although carbamoylphosphate serves as the precursor for synthesis of both pyrimidine and arginine, the two pathways are spatially discrete and usually independent of each other in eucaryotes. There are two different types of carbamoyl-phosphate synthetase, and each is responsible for the supply of carbamoyl-phosphate for the respective pathways; for example, in mammals, ammonia- and acetylglutamate-dependent carbamoyl-phosphate synthetase (CPS I) is localized in mitochondria of liver cells serving as the first enzyme for the arginine and urea synthesis, whereas glutamine-dependent carbamoyl-phosphate synthetase (CPS II) is present in the cytosol of growing cells as well as of liver cells and provides carbamoyl-phosphate primarily for pyrimidine synthesis (for a review, TATIBANA and SHIGESADA, 1972b). In contrast, in *E. coli* and other bacteria, there is only one enzyme responsible for the synthesis of carbamoylphosphate, and its common cellular pool supplies carbamoyl-phosphate for both arginine and pyrimidine pathways (PIÉRARD and WIAME, 1964). Therefore, aspartate carbamoyltransferase is the first enzyme in a branched pathway leading to the synthesis of pyrimidine nucleotides and plays a principal role in the regulation of the synthesis (GERHART and PARDEE, 1962) discussed later. Along with this enzyme, carbamoyl-phosphate synthetase in *E. coli* is also subject to regulation in a more complex manner than is the pyrimidine-specific enzyme of eucaryotes. The *E. coli* enzyme is subject to feedback inhibition by UMP and is activated by IMP and ornithine (PIÉRARD et al., 1965; ANDERSON and MEISTER, 1966; PIÉRARD, 1966; ANDERSON and MARVIN, 1968). The presence of either effector (ornithine or IMP) decreases the ATP concentration required for half-maximal velocity, while the presence of the negative effector (UMP) has the opposite effect. The inhibition by UMP can be reversed by ornithine and is considered to be a mechanism which ensures the supply of carbamoyl-phosphate for the arginine synthesis, even when sufficient pyrimidine nucleotides are present, thereby leading to the inhibition of the synthetase (PIÉRARD, 1966). The physiologic significance of activation by IMP awaits further study.

Glutamine-dependent carbamoyl-phosphate synthetase from pea seedling is inhibited by UMP and UDP as well as by AMP, ADP, and GTP (O'NEAL and NAYLOR, 1968). Metabolic roles of the enzyme in pea seedling appear to be similar to those of the bacterial enzyme. TRAMELL and CAMPBELL (1970) found additional carbamoyl-phosphate synthetase (CPS III) in a land snail *Strophocheilus oblongus*; the enzyme uses glutamine as the preferred nitrogen donor and has an apparent dependence on acetylglutamate. The same type of enzyme was recently found in the liver of teleost fish (ANDERSON, 1976). The land snail enzyme is subject to inhibition by GTP, ITP, and AMP in descending order of potency. The teleost enzyme is inhibited by UTP, CTP, and GTP. The metabolic role of the newly found enzyme is not yet clear and, accordingly, the significance of the effects have not been evaluated.

II. Aspartate Carbamoyltransferase

Aspartate carbamoyltransferase (E.C.2.1.3.2), which catalyzes the first reaction unique to pyrimidine biosynthesis in E. coli, is inhibited by CTP, CDP, CMP, and cytidine in descending order of potency. Deoxycytidine derivatives are as effective as cytidine compounds, while uridine derivatives do not inhibit the native enzyme. ATP activates the enzyme, and both ATP and CTP compete for a single site on the regulatory subunit. GTP and dGTP are moderately inhibitory (GERHART and PARDEE, 1962; CHANGEUX et al., 1968). This pattern of regulation is not necessarily the case with the enzymes of other bacteria. Even though the pyrimidine biosynthetic pathway has a common sequence, and aspartate carbamoyltransferase is the first enzyme unique for the synthesis in all known bacteria, the control of activity of the enzyme differs from organism to organism. Such has been discussed by O'DONOVAN and NEUHART (1970).

Aspartate carbamoyltransferase of eucaryotes differs distinctly from that of E. coli in molecular and regulatory properties, reflecting its different function; as discussed above the enzyme is not the first but the second of the pyrimidine pathway (DAVIS, 1967; TATIBANA and ITO, 1967). The enzyme exists as a multienzyme complex with carbamoyl-phosphate synthetase in Neurospora (WILLIAMS et al., 1970) and Saccharomyces cerevisiae (LUE and KAPLAN, 1970), and further with dihydroorotase, the third enzyme of the pyrimidine pathway, in higher animals (SHOAF and JONES, 1971; KENT et al., 1975; MORI and TATIBANA, 1975b). The enzyme in Neurospora and Saccharomyces is inhibited by uridine compounds, and UTP is the most potent inhibitor. ATP does not activate the enzyme, in contrast to the case of the E. coli enzyme. The mammalian enzyme is rather insensitive to feedback inhibition (TATIBANA and ITO, 1967; INAGAKI and TATIBANA, 1970).

III. Orotate Phosphoribosyltransferase

Orotate phosphoribosyltransferase (E.C.2.4.2.10), which catalyzes the conversion of orotate to orotidylate in the presence of phosphoribosyl pyrophosphate, appears to play a regulatory role in the synthesis of uridylate in association with the next enzyme orotidylate decarboxylase. In mammals, the two enzymes exist as an enzyme complex (APPEL, 1968; BECKER et al., 1974; BROWN et al., 1975; REYES and GUGANIG, 1975; KAVIPURAPU and JONES, 1976). The transferase does not appear to be affected by natural nucleotides and related compounds except for the product orotidylate; UMEZU et al. (1971) observed no significant effect of uridine, cytidine, adenosine, and guanosine nucleotides on the transferase from bakers' yeast. The next step in the biosynthesis of uridylate is the irreversible decarboxylation of orotidylate to UMP.

IV. Orotidylate Decarboxylase

Orotidylate decarboxylase (E.C.4.1.1.23) is more sensitive than orotate phosphoribosyltransferase to regulation by nucleotides. The decarboxylase is inhibited by orotidylate and by certain analogues of orotate. The enzyme from brewers' yeast is inhibited by UMP ($K_i = 0.15$ mM), CMP, AMP, and GMP in a competitive manner with regard to orotidylate (CREASEY and HANDSCHUMACHER, 1961). UMEZU et al. (1971) reported inhibition of bakers' yeast enzyme by GMP, GDP, CMP, and CDP, but not by UMP. Thus, purine derivatives in yeast can control pyrimidine synthesis at this step.

The enzyme from rat liver is inhibited by UMP (BLAIR and POTTER, 1961), and brain enzyme purified 600-fold is inhibited by CMP, UMP, CDP, and CTP in the descending order shown (APPEL, 1968). AMP and GMP are moderately inhibitory to the latter enzyme.

It is notable that the reaction catalyzed by orotidylate decarboxylase is affected by several antimetabolites, including azauridine and allopurinol. Azauridine, an analogue of uridine that was developed as an antitumor agent, is converted to azauridine 5′-monophosphate by the catalysis of uridine kinase, and the nucleotide analogue then competitively inhibits the enzymatic decarboxylation of orotidylate to form UMP (PASTERNAK and HANDSCHUMACHER, 1959; HANDSCHUMACHER, 1960). Allopurinol [4,6-dihydroxypyrazolo(3,4-d)pyrimidine], analogue of hypoxanthine, is both a competitive inhibitor and a substrate of xanthine oxidase and is widely used as a hypouricemic agent. Several metabolites of this agent interfere with pyrimidine metabolism, and the site of action is also the decarboxylation reaction of orotidylate to form UMP. The details are discussed later.

V. Cytidine Triphosphate Synthetase

Cytidine triphosphate synthetase (E.C.6.3.4.2), which is responsible for the conversion of UTP to CTP, catalyzes the reaction:

$$\text{UTP} + \text{ATP} + \text{glutamine} \xrightarrow{\text{Mg}^{2+}} \text{CTP} + \text{ADP} + P_i + \text{glutamate}$$

This reaction is a critical step in nucleotide metabolism; there is no other known route for synthesis of cytidine nucleotides de novo, and CTP, the product of the reaction, is the starting substance for synthesis of other cytidine nucleotides. HURLBERT and KAMMEN (1960) were the first to demonstrate the synthesis of CTP in preparations from animal cells and further showed a requirement for guanosine phosphates. Studies on purified CTP synthetase from *E. colli* (LONG and PARDEE, 1967) showed that the presence of GTP is required as an allosteric effector. A K_a value for GTP was 0.08 mM, and the cellular level of GTP together with that of ATP can regulate the synthesis of CTP. The regulation of this enzyme is rather complex and unique, as UTP, the substrate of the enzyme, and CTP, the product, are both required in an approximately equal amount for the synthesis of RNA and DNA.

LONG and PARDEE (1967) showed that dependence of the reaction rate on the concentration of each substrate approximately follows the Michaelis equation when all other substrates are at near saturation. When other substrates are at low concentrations, the kinetics are strongly sigmoidal. The product CTP has been found to inhibit competitively with UTP and to activate the enzyme under other conditions, probably by replacing the allosteric activator GTP.

VI. Uridine-Cytidine Kinase

Uridine-cytidine kinase (E.C.2.7.1.48) catalyzes phosphorylation of uridine or cytidine to UMP or CMP, an important reaction in pyrimidine nucleotide synthesis by the salvage pathway. Deoxyribonucleosides are not phosphorylated by the enzyme from Ehrlich ascites cells (SKÖLD, 1960). ATP, dGTP, and dATP serve as the most effective phosphate donors for the kinase from rat hepatoma cells (ORENGO, 1969). UTP and CTP are potent inhibitors, and the inhibition by CTP is competitive with respect to ATP, but upon aging of the enzyme, the inhibitory effect of CTP is partially lost. On the basis of all the related data, it has been proposed that on the surface of the enzyme molecule there is a site for the regulatory ligand in addition to the sites for the phosphate donor and acceptor. Purine nucleotides do not appear to inhibit the enzyme.

D. Regulation of the Ribonucleotide System

The replication of DNA requires the presence of the four deoxyribonucleoside triphosphates, and syntheses of approximately equal amounts are required. The ribonucleotide reductase system is considered the supplier of building blocks for DNA synthesis in almost all cells (REICHARD, 1967).

The enzymic reactions are schematically represented as follows:

nucleoside diphosphate + thioredoxine-$(SH)_2$ $\xrightarrow{\text{ribonucleotide reductase}}$ deoxynucleoside diphosphate + thioredoxin-S_2

thioredoxin-S_2 + NADPH + H$^+$ $\xrightarrow{\text{thioredoxin reductase}}$ thioredoxin-$(SH)_2$ + NADP$^+$

The reaction and its regulation were studied in detail in the *E. coli* system (BROWN and REICHARD, 1969a; 1969b), but studies on mammalian systems have not been so extensive as those of the *E. coli* system. However, the results to date strongly indicate that the regulation of mammalian and bacterial systems is much the same (MOORE and REICHARD, 1964; MOORE and HURLBERT, 1966; REICHARD, 1972). Of considerable importance is the fact that one and the same enzyme catalyzes the reduction of a variety of ribonucleoside diphosphates but not of the corresponding mono- or triphosphates. The presence of allosteric effectors, nucleoside triphosphates, regulates both the overall activity and the substrate specificity of the enzyme. In the absence of effectors, the enzyme shows only limited activity. Addition of the positive effector ATP greatly enhances the reduction of the pyrimidine substrates CDP and UDP but not the reduction of the purine substrates. The reduction of GDP is stimulated by dTTP as effector, while the reduction of ADP requires the presence of dGTP. One may visualize here a sequential process that is initiated by the reduction of pyrimidine ribonucleotides, which leads to the formation of dTTP and triggers the reduction of purine ribonucleotides, GDP, and then ADP.

The reductase system is also subject to regulation by inhibition. dATP exerts the most profound inhibition on the reduction of all four substrates. In the sequential reduction of the nucleotides, dATP is the final product; thus, the general inhibition of the reaction by dATP can be considered the end-product inhibition. The inhibition by dATP is counteracted by ATP, and a second type of inhibition is exerted by the combination of dTTP and ATP. Under the proper conditions, the presence of these two nucleotides inhibits the reduction of the two pyrimidine ribonucleotides, thus directing the substrate specificity of the enzyme from pyrimidine to purine ribonucleotides. Purine and pyrimidine nucleotide reduction is, therefore, interrelated in this system.

Experiments were carried out with cultured mammalian cells in attempts to determine the correlation between the in vitro data and results obtained in vivo (REICHARD, 1972). By addition and withdrawal of hydroxyurea, a relatively specific inhibitor of the reductase, marked changes occurred in pool sizes of the four deoxyribonucleoside triphosphates, dCTP, dTTP, dGTP, and dATP. It was possible to correlate these results with the known behavior of the ribonucleotide reductase in vitro.

Lactobacillus leichmanii has a different reductase system, which catalyzes an analogous reaction, but is distinct from the *E. coli* system in that the reductase has an absolute requirement for a vitamin B_{12} cofactor and that it reduces ribonucleoside triphosphates but not diphosphates. The distribution of this system appears to be rather limited.

E. Disorders in Nucleotide Biosynthesis Induced by Exogenous Purines and Pyrimidines

I. Disorders in Purine Biosynthesis Induced by Orotate

STANDERFER and HANDLER (1955) found that when rats were fed a synthetic diet supplemented with orotic acid (1%) for 28 days, excessive neutral fat accumulated in their liver. Uracil and thymine, which are synthesized from orotic acid, were without effect. The fatty infiltration, unlike the development of fatty liver induced by a choline-deficient diet, is readily reversible and not accompanied by other serious pathologic disturbances. Such livers contain high levels of triglycerides (CREASEY et al., 1961) and cholesterol (RAJALAKSHMI et al., 1961). Furthermore, there is an inhibition of lipoprotein secretion (WINDMUELLER, 1964). HANDSCHUMACHER et al. (1960) could nullify the gross changes in lipid metabolism in rat liver by further supplementation of the diet with 0.25% adenine sulfate, thus suggesting that the alteration in nucleotide metabolism is responsible for development of the fatty liver. In fact, analysis of the acid-soluble nucleotides of the liver (VON EULER et al., 1963) indicated a four-fold increase of uridine nucleotides associated with a 50% decrease in adenosine nucleotides, including nicotinamide adenine dinucleotide phosphate and its reduced form. These changes, like the lipid accumulation, were largely nullified by further supplementation of 0.25% adenine sulfate to the diet. Based on in vitro studies with liver extracts, VON EULER et al. (1963) suggested that the increased synthesis of uridine nucleotides, with an ample supply of orotate, inhibited both the de novo and salvage pathways for purine nucleotide biosynthesis by competing with the common precursor, phosphoribosyl pyrophosphate.

Apparently inconsistent observations were reported by WINDMUELLER and SPAETH (1965), who found an enhanced synthesis of adenosine nucleotide in the liver of rats given orotic acid. Prior addition of 1% orotic acid to the purified basal diet for 2–5 days increased 3–15-fold the incorporation of radioactivity from [2-^{14}C]glycine or [^{14}C]formate into acid-soluble adenine and guanine as well as into nucleic acid purines. The kinetics of incorporation indicated an accelerated turnover of the acid-soluble pools of purine nucleotides. It was assumed that the acceleration of purine biosynthesis de novo induced by orotic acid resulted from a release of feedback inhibition imposed by hepatic purine nucleotides. Further studies by RAJA-LAKSHMI and HANDSCHUMACHER (1968) showed that the contradictory results reported by the two groups above only reflected two different phases of effects of orotic acid on purine metabolism in the liver. Orotic acid exerts a profound inhibitory effect on the biosynthesis of adenine from glycine both in vivo and in vitro. However, when the orotic acid-fed rats were fasted for 12 h prior to measuring the incorporation of glycine in vivo or preparing slices for studies in vitro, a twofold stimulation was demonstrated. The stimulatory effect was completely overcome by additional orotic acid in vivo and in vitro. Based on the results of experiments with liver slices or tissue extract, these workers suggested that the inhibition of purine synthesis is the result of depletion of the amount of phosphoribosyl pyrophosphate available for the reaction with glutamine, the first and committed step unique to the purine synthesis. Their interpretation was that the inhibitory effect of orotic acid continues while it is present in the liver, along with the inhibition of other reactions dependent upon phosphoribosyl pyrophosphate, and that the stimulation of purine synthesis then follows after the disappearance of orotic acid from the tissue. This may be a consequence of release from feedback control of the first enzyme of the purine pathway through a diminution of the pool of adenine nucleotides. The previously reported stimulation in purine synthesis caused by ingestion of orotic acid (WINDMUELLER and SPAETH, 1965) might reflect only the latter phase of the orotic acid effects.

KELLEY et al. (1970) provided evidence that orotic acid inhibits an early step of purine biosynthesis de novo in cultured human cells. Concentrations of orotic acid that inhibited purine synthesis also reduced intracellular levels of phosphoribosyl pyrophosphate. Orotic acid had no inhibitory effect in mutant cells (hypoxanthine-guanine phosphoribosyltransferase-defective) which hold high levels of phosphoribosyl pyrophosphate or in normal cells if depletion of phosphoribosyl pyrophosphate by orotic acid was prevented with azaorotate. These studies demonstrated that the inhibitory effect of orotic acid on purine synthesis in cultured human cells is due to a depletion of intracellular phosphoribosyl pyrophosphate. It should be noted that a series of diverse effects of orotic acid on purine metabolism in vivo appear to be limited to the liver, with no known effects on other tissues. This is apparently related to low permeability of many animal tissues other than liver and kidney to orotate, as reported by ORD and STOCKEN (1973).

II. Inhibition of Pyrimidine Nucleotide Synthesis by Adenine

Although adenine is readily used by mammalian cells grown in vitro, the compound is growth-inhibitory at concentrations of 1 mM or higher (HAKALA and TAYLOR, 1959; TOMIZAWA and ARONOW, 1960; McFALL and MAGASANIK, 1960). The toxic effect is not observed with similar concentrations of closely related compounds, such as adenosine, hypoxanthine, or inosine. Growth inhibition of cultured mouse fibroblasts strain L, caused by 1 mM adenine, is partially reversed by 0.1 mM uridine or cytidine (ARONOW, 1961). Uracil, cytosine, orotic acid, and orotidine were ineffective. Orotidylic acid was only partially effective, though not to the degree as observed with uridine or cytidine. Hypoxanthine, inosine, guanine, guanosine, ribose, and ribose 5-phosphate were completely ineffective. ARONOW (1961) noted an analogy of the growth-inhibitory effect by adenine and its specific reversal by pyrimidine nucleosides to orotic acid-induced fatty livers in rats and the restoring effect of adenine. He suggested that high concentrations of adenine directly inhibit certain enzymes involved in pyrimidine biosynthesis, repress the synthesis of these enzymes, or deplete a critical cofactor, for example, by competition with orotic acid for available phosphoribosyl pyrophosphate. In fact, in Ehrlich ascites tumor cells, adenine, and other purine bases could considerably reduce the intracellular level of phosphoribosyl pyrophosphate (HENDERSON and KHOO, 1965a).

The bacteriostatic effect of adenine was reported with *Aerobacter aerogenes* (BROOKE and MAGASANIK, 1954; MOYED, 1964) and *E. coli* (REMY and LOVE, 1968). HOSONO and KUNO (1974) studied the mechanism involved in the growth inhibition induced by adenine in *E. coli*. The syntheses of DNA, RNA, and protein were coordinately inhibited. As was observed with mammalian cells (ARONOW, 1961), the inhibition by adenine (2 mM) was reversed by the same concentration of uridine but not by adenosine, inosine, or guanosine. In the presence of adenine, the pool size of ATP increased twofold, while those of CTP and UTP were markedly reduced. These changes were reversed by uridine. The presence of adenine in the medium suppressed the incorporation of labeled uracil or orotic acid into nucleic acids but not of labeled uridine. Based on these results it was suggested that the growth inhibition provoked by adenine could be due primarily to inhibition of pyrimidine nucleotide biosynthesis de novo, probably at the step of orotic acid conversion of UMP. BAGNARA and FINCH (1974) intensively studied the effects of a variety of bases and nucleosides on the intracellular concentrations of nucleotides and phosphoribosyl pyrophosphate in *E. coli*. The primary purpose of the studies were to critically evaluate the interrelationship between the de novo and salvage pathways of purine and pyrimidine nucleotide biosyntheses. All purine precursors increased the levels of corresponding nucleotides, ATP or GTP, or both, concomitantly decreasing the levels of pyrimidine nucleotides, CTP and UTP. The purines at 0.1 mM or less, with the exception of guanosine, depleted the intracellular content of phosphoribosyl pyrophosphate to 10% or less of its normal value. Of the purine bases and nucleosides tested, adenine was the most potent in this effect. Their results suggest that the decreased availability of phosphoribosyl pyrophosphate, induced by the addition of preformed purine precursors such as adenine, is the cause for the immediate transient decreases in the level of pyrimidine nucleotides. It is notable that uracil was effective in *E. coli*, though weakly, in decreasing the levels of phosphoribosyl pyrophosphate and thus interferes with the purine nucleotide biosynthesis.

III. Interference of Adenosine and Other Purine Nucleosides with Pyrimidine Biosynthesis

Adenosine and several other purines including adenine have bacteriostatic effects on *Aerobacter aerogenes* (MOYED, 1964). Of the purine derivatives examined, adenosine was the most potent. The growth inhibition was reversed by either thiamine or by the pyrimidine portion of thiamine. As described above, BAGNARA and FINCH (1974) showed that various purine nucleosides decrease the levels of pyrimidine nucleotides and of phosphoribosyl pyrophosphate in E. coli.

KROOTH (1964) demonstrated the inhibitory action of adenosine on the growth of mutant human diploid fibroblasts obtained from persons with orotic aciduria. As a result of the extremely low levels of orotate phosphoribosyltransferase and orotidylate decarboxylase in the pathway of uridylate synthesis, the mutant cells were partially deprived of pyrimidine nucleotides. The growth of these strains was inhibited by adenosine, and the inhibition was overcome by uridine. The activity of orotidylate decarboxylase in mutant cells was reduced to about one-third in the presence of adenosine. It was suggested that the effect of adenosine on the cell was mediated by inhibition of enzyme synthesis.

ISHII and GREEN (1973) found that adenosine at concentrations as low as 5–50 μM was toxic to a number of established cell lines in culture. This effect was apparent only when the sera used in culture media were devoid of adenosine deaminase. The toxic effect can be prevented by uridine or other pyrimidine derivatives potentially convertible to uridine. In the presence of adenosine, the conversion of labeled aspartate to uridine nucleotides was reduced by 80–85%, and labeled orotate accumulated in both the cells and the culture medium. Xanthine, xanthosine, and guanosine at 1 mM, and guanine at 0.4 mM had no inhibitory effect on the growth of 3T6 cells. Adenine was toxic to 3T6 cells at 1 mM but not at lower concentrations. It is noteworthy that a mutant line (mouse fibroblast 3T6) deficient in adenosine kinase was 70-fold less sensitive to adenosine. The authors suggested that the toxic substance may be one of the adenosine nucleotides derived from adenosine by phosphorylation and that it inhibits the synthesis of uridylate at the stage of phosphoribosylation of orotate.

GREEN and CHAN (1973) presented direct evidence for depletion of the cellular pyrimidine nucleotide pool. Quantitative analyses of acid-soluble nucleotides of cultured 3T6 cells using high-pressure liquid chromatography showed that the presence of adenosine in the medium led to a 40–60% expansion of the pools of ADP and ATP, while UDP was reduced by 79% and UTP and CTP were reduced by more than 90%. They also found that two cultured cell lines of lymphoid origin were at least as sensitive to the cytotoxic effect of adenosine as the fibroblasts described earlier (ISHII and GREEN, 1973). Addition of uridine reversed the effects of adenosine on the lymphoid cells. The toxicity of adenosine depends on its direct conversion to AMP by adenosine kinase (ISHII and GREEN, 1973). The recently reported association between absence of adenosine deaminase and a human disease of the lymphoid system manifested by a greatly reduced number of lymphocytes and impaired immunity (GIBLETT et al., 1972; DISSING and KNUDSEN, 1972) was called to mind, and the authors suggested that the immune deficiency may be the result of the depletion of pyrimidine nucleotides induced by adenosine nucleotides in cells of the lymphoid system. However, there is the problem of why the lymphoid system should be particularly sensitive to the absence of adenosine deaminase. Cultured fibroblasts and lymphoid cell lines are equally sensitive to adenosine. Another factor to consider is the nature of adenosine nucleotide(s) itself, which apparently specifically inhibits the enzymes orotidylate phosphoribosyltransferase and orotidylate decarboxylase. There are no definitive data that an adenosine nucleotide can exert such a specific and potent inhibition on the two enzymes of the pyrimidine pathway that will lead to block of the pyrimidine nucleotide synthesis de novo and accumulation of orotate.

In short-term experiments in vitro with minces of chick oviduct and rat mammary gland, GÜLEN et al. (1974) found that adenosine or guanosine markedly inhibits the rate of $[^{14}C]$bicarbonate incorporation into orotic acid. Evidence presented indicates that the site of inhibition by purines of the de novo biosynthesis of pyrimidines is the initial reaction in the sequence, that catalyzed by glutamine-dependent carbamoyl phosphate synthetase.

PLANET and FOX (1976) reported investigations that are relevant to the above question regarding the mechanism of the adenosine effect. These researchers studied the effects of purine nucleosides on phosphoribosyl pyrophosphate synthesis in human erythrocytes in vitro and their work was based on previous observations that phosphoribosyl pyrophosphate synthesis was increased with nucleoside in mammalian cells when the concentration of inorganic phosphate concentration in medium exceeded 20 mM (HENDERSON and KHOO, 1965 b; HERSHKO et al., 1969) but was decreased with nucleoside in E. coli with 1.4 mM inorganic phosphate (BAGNARA and FINCH, 1974). In erythrocytes, when external inorganic phosphate was varied from 0–25 mM, adenosine, inosine, guanosine, or 6-mercaptopurine riboside (1.25 mM) produced a decrease in intracellular phosphoribosyl pyrophosphate. The nucleoside effect is attributable to decreased synthesis rather than to increased utilization. The authors noted that the nucleoside-related diminution of phosphoribosyl pyrophosphate was accompanied by a decrease of intracellular inorganic phosphate. Since the activity of phosphoribosyl pyrophosphate synthetase is known to be sensitive to small changes of inorganic phosphate (HERSHKO et al., 1969; WONG and MURRAY, 1969; SWITZER, 1969; FOX and KELLEY, 1971 b), it may be that decrease in the concentration of inorganic phosphate resulted in a reduction of phosphoribosyl pyrophosphate synthesis. Furthermore, decrease of the intracellular inorganic phosphate was produced both by those nucleosides that were eventually degraded by purine nucleoside phosphorylase (adenosine, inosine, and guanosine) and by nucleosides that were phosphorylated initially by adenosine kinase (methylmercaptopurine riboside and adenosine with erythro-9(2-hydroxyl-3-nonyl)-adenine). It was proposed that regulation of phosphoribosyl pyrophosphate formation by alteration of inorganic phosphate levels may account for a number of biological phenomena, such as cytotoxicity of adenosine toward cultured fibroblasts and lymphocytes (ISHII and GREEN, 1973; GREEN and CHAN, 1973). It should be noted, however, that the effect of adenosine on the intracellular concentration of inorganic phosphate is not specific. Other purine nucleosides, such as inosine, guanosine and methylmercaptopurine ribonucleoside, exert a similar effect, whereas cytotoxicity of adenosine to cultured cells is highly specific.

It is worthwhile considering alternate mechanisms other than depletion of inorganic phosphate that may be involved in the cytotoxicity of adenosine. The nucleoside is known to have some specific cellular effects that do not require metabolic conversion to other compounds. Such effects include the vasodilatory action on coronary arteries (BERNE, 1963; RUBIO et al., 1969) and activation of adenylate cyclase, leading to enhancement of cAMP levels in the brain (SATTIN and RALL, 1970; SHIMIZU and DALY, 1970; SCHULTZ and DALY, 1973). Adenosine and 3'-deoxyadenosine are also known to produce morphologic changes in cultured fibroblasts without alteration in intracellular cAMP levels (YIN and BERLIN, 1975). In view of these effects, the possibility has to be considered that adenosine as a bioactive substance not involving metabolic conversion may indirectly interfere with the synthesis or activity of certain enzymes of the pyrimidine biosynthetic pathway, thus leading to deprivation of pyrimidine nucleotides from the cells.

An interesting type of regulation of pyrimidine synthesis by purines was reported by ITO and UCHINO (1976). These workers demonstrated the inhibitory effects of guanine and guanosine as well as adenine on the induction of the two early enzymes of the pyrimidine pathway in phytohemagglutinin-stimulated human lymphocytes. When 1 mM guanine was added to the culture, the induction of the enzymes was inhibited, while that of uridine kinase was accelerated. [^{14}C]Bicarbonate incorporation into the acid-soluble uridine nucleotides via the de novo pathway was inhibited by guanine, and guanosine had a similar effect in this system.

IV. Effects of Allopurinol on Pyrimidine Biosynthesis De Novo

Allopurinol [4,6-dihydroxypyrazolo(3,4-d)pyrimidine] is an analogue of hypoxanthine. The compound is both a competitive inhibitor and a substrate of xanthine oxidase and is widely used as a hypouricemic agent. The administration to man of allopurinol or its major metabolic oxidation product, oxipurinol, consistently results in inhibition not only of uric acid synthesis but also of pyrimidine synthesis. FOX et al. (1970) found that when allopurinol was given to patients with hyperuricemia and also to normal subjects, increased amounts of orotidine (40–400 mg/day) were excreted in the urine. In experiments using the lysate of red blood cells, allopurinol exerted a significant inhibition on orotidylate decarboxylase activity in the presence of phosphoribosyl pyrophosphate but not in its absence. KELLEY and BEARDMORE (1970) also demonstrated the urinary excretion of orotidine and orotic acid using high-pressure anion-exchange chromatography. They clearly demonstrated that both allopurinol ribonucleotide and xanthosine 5'-monophosphate are potent competitive inhibitors for orotidylate decarboxylase in dialyzed human erythrocyte lysates. It was suggested that allopurinol in vivo is converted by a phosphoribosyltransferase to the ribonucleotide, which inhibits orotidylate decarboxylase and leads to accumulation of orotidine 5'-phosphate and then to excretion in the urine of its dephosphorylated product, orotidine. It was also likely that inhibition of xanthine oxidase by allopurinol leads to accumulation of xanthine, which is then converted to xanthosine 5'-monophosphate and inhibits orotidylate decarboxylase. In subsequent studies, indirect evidence suggested that several ribonucleotide derivatives of oxipurinol may also be potent inhibitors of orotidylate decarboxylase (FOX et al., 1971; BEARDMORE and KELLEY, 1971). An inhibitory effect of metabolites of allopurinol on pyrimidine synthesis has also been demonstrated in vivo in rats (BROWN et al., 1972) as well as in human fibroblasts in tissue culture (KELLEY et al., 1971). [^{3}H]Uridine incorporation was not inhibited by oxipurinol in cultured human lymphoblasts (BECKER et al., 1974).

The increased urinary excretion of orotidine and orotic acid following administration of allopurinol or oxipurinol is similar to that observed after administration of 6-azauridine, a pyrimidine analogue (FALLON et al., 1961). The latter compound is converted to its ribonucleotide, 6-azauridine-5′-monophosphate, and serves as a potent inhibitor of orotidylate decarboxylase (HANDSCHUMACHER, 1960).

FYFE et al. (1973) enzymatically synthesized and characterized 1- and 7-ribosyl 5′-phosphate of oxipurinol as well as 3-xanthosine 5′-phosphate and 1-ribosyl 5′-phosphate of allopurinol. When tested with orotidylate decarboxylase from yeast, the most effective inhibitor was found to be 1-ribosyloxipurinol 5′-phosphate, which has K_i values of 0.02 and 0.03 μM at high (12–48 μM) and low (0.5–2 μM) substrate concentrations, respectively. The corresponding N-7 derivative has corresponding K_i values of 0.7 and 0.06 μM. 1-Ribosylallopurinol 5′-phosphate, 3-xanthosine 5′-phosphate, and several naturally occurring nucleotides are less inhibitory. Nucleotide inhibitors stabilize the enzyme against loss of activity at 37° C. Inhibition constants determined with the enzyme from rat liver are similar to those found in yeast. The findings provided solid support for the view that it is the inhibition of orotidylate decarboxylase by the nucleotides of oxipurinol that is primarily responsible for the disorders in pyrimidine metabolism in subjects treated with allopurinol.

Another interesting effect of allopurinol was reported by Fox et al. (1970), who found that the administration of allopurinol was followed by a several-fold increase in the specific activity of orotate phosphoribosyltransferase in erythrocytes. An increase in the activity of orotidylate decarboxylase was also noted (Fox et al., 1971). The effect on these enzymes appeared to be similar to that of azauridine as reported by PINSKY and KROOTH (1967). These workers showed that in human fibroblasts cultured in the presence of added azauridine, a potent inhibitor of pyrimidine synthesis de novo as mentioned above, an increase in the levels of orotate phosphoribosyltransferase and orotidylate decarboxylase occurred and was attributed to an increase of enzyme protein. However, later studies demonstrated that the apparently analogous effects of allopurinol and azauridine are caused by different mechanisms. The increased activity of orotate phosphoribosyltransferase and orotidylate decarboxylase induced by allopurinol was attributed either to stabilization (Fox et al., 1971), activation of enzymes by allopurinol and its derivatives (BEARDMORE et al., 1972), or to both.

Further studies with cultured human lymphoblasts (BECKER et al., 1974) suggested that an inhibitor of orotidylate decarboxylase generated from oxipurinol upon incubation exerts the inhibitory action on the enzyme and also stabilized the enzyme complex containing orotate phosphoribosyltransferase and orotidylate decarboxylase. The complex obtained from the cells after incubation with oxipurinol behaves as a large molecular weight aggregate (108000), whereas the complex obtained from nontreated cells behaves as a smaller molecular weight form (41000). The enzymes from oxipurinol-treated cells showed an increased heat stability. GROBNER and KELLEY (1975) found that orotate phosphoribosyltransferase and orotidylate decarboxylase from human erythrocytes exist in a complex as three different molecular species with molecular weights of 55000, 80000, and 113000. The larger forms of the complex were more stable and paralleled the results seen with lymphoblasts (BECKER et al., 1974). In the presence of allopurinol ribonucleotide or oxipurinol-7-ribonucleotide but not the free bases, the largest, most stable species predominates. These observations reported by BECKER et al. (1974) and GROBNER and KELLEY (1975) support the possibility that the apparent increase in activity is due largely to stabilization of the complex during cell lysis and extraction rather than actual stabilization in vivo.

F. Role of Cellular Levels of Phosphoribosyl Pyrophosphate in Coordinate Control of Purine and Pyrimidine Nucleotide Biosynthesis

The intracellular concentration of phosphoribosyl pyrophosphate has been demonstrated to play a critical role in the regulation of purine metabolism (for a review, Fox and Kelley, 1971a). Some observations which support the view, e.g., orotate-induced inhibition of purine biosynthesis, are mentioned in the foregoing discussion. Phosphoribosyl pyrophosphate has been also shown to regulate pyrimidine nucleotide biosynthesis de novo; certain purine bases and nucleosides inhibit the pyrimidine synthesis by lowering the intracellular level of phosphoribosyl pyrophosphate in bacterial and animal cells, as has been discussed. Furthermore, nicotinamide, which also utilizes phosphoribosyl pyrophosphate for the synthesis of pyridine nucleotides, can affect purine and pyrimidine nucleotide biosyntheses. Ferris and Clark (1972) demonstrated that incorporation of [^{14}C]orotate into nucleic acids in regenerating rat liver was inhibited in a dose-dependent fashion by the previous injection of nicotinamide. It was suggested that a competition exists between the NAD synthesis, enhanced by administration of a large dose of nicotinamide, and purine and pyrimidine nucleotide synthesis for available phosphoribosyl pyrophosphate. In the experiments mentioned above, metabolism of pyrimidine is impaired only with unphysiologically high concentrations of adenine or nicotinamide, or with adenosine only in selected media devolid of adenosine deaminase activity. Notwithstanding, the observations are consistent with the physiologic importance of the intracellular level of phosphoribosyl pyrophosphate in the regulation of both purine and pyrimidine biosynthesis de novo as well as in coordination of the rates of two biosynthetic pathways.

An important function of phosphoribosyl pyrophosphate, which is critical in the regulation of pyrimidine biosynthesis de novo, was reported by Tatibana and Shigesada (1972a, 1972b). It was shown that a low concentration of phosphoribosyl pyrophosphate strongly stimulates the activity of glutamine-dependent carbamoylphosphate synthetase, the first committed step of the pyrimidine biosynthesis de novo, in hematopoietic mouse spleen. The effect is specific; ribose 5-phosphate, inorganic pyrophosphate, or a mixture of both cannot substitute for the compound. Evidence indicates the allosteric mechanism for the activating effect. In the presence of phosphoribosyl pyrophosphate, the K_m value of the synthetase for MgATP decreases without significant change in the maximal velocity. Thus, the extent of activation varies with the concentration of MgATP, a substrate; at a concentration of ATP as low as 1 mM, the extent was more than 10-fold. The apparent K_a for phosphoribosyl pyrophosphate is in the range of 4–9 μM. This range corresponds to the levels of phosphoribosyl pyrophosphate in various tissues (Fox and Kelley, 1971a; Hisata, 1975; Lalanne and Henderson, 1975). Activation by phosphoribosyl pyrophosphate antagonizes the inhibition of the synthetase by MgUTP (Tatibana and Shigesada, 1972b) or polyamine (Mori and Tatibana, 1975), and the inhibition is almost nullified at a high concentration of phosphoribosyl pyrophosphate (500 μM). The presence of these inhibitors considerably modifies the activating effect; the apparent K_a value for phosphoribosyl pyrophosphate increases in their presence, thus widening the range of its effective concentrations as an activator of the synthetase and also increases the apparent degree of amplification of the enzymatic activity by phospho-

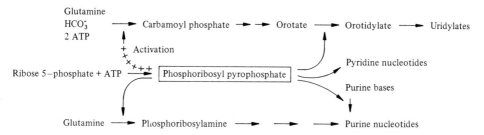

Fig. 3. Possible role of phosphoribosyl pyrophosphate in coordinate control of nucleotide biosyntheses

ribosyl pyrophosphate. The sensitivity to activation by phosphoribosyl pyrophosphate has been found with synthetases from mouse spleen (TATIBANA and SHIGESADA, 1972a), rat liver (MORI et al., 1975), Ehrlich ascites carcinoma (SHOAF and JONES, 1973), and rat ascites hepatoma (MORI and TATIBANA, 1975).

The control of glutamine-dependent carbamoyl phosphate synthetase by the level of phosphoribosyl pyrophosphate may play a significant role in coordination of the first step of pyrimidine synthesis with other critical steps in nucleotide syntheses that require phosphoribosyl pyrophosphate (TATIBANA and SHIGESADA, 1972a, 1972b) (Fig. 3). The two regulatory sites of pyrimidine biosynthesis, i.e., the production of carbamoyl phosphate and the conversion of orotate to orotidylate, are controlled by the level of phosphoribosyl pyrophosphate, so that the rates of both the early and later steps of uridylate synthesis de novo are more or less matched. In addition, the level of phosphoribosyl pyrophosphate can coordinate the first steps of both purine and pyrimidine syntheses de novo. The formation of 5-phosphoribosyl 1-amine from phosphoribosyl pyrophosphate and glutamine, the first committed reaction of the purine pathway, can be limited by supply of phosphoribosyl pyrophosphate (ROSENBLOOM et al., 1968; RAJALAKSHMI and HANDSCHUMACHER, 1968; FOX and KELLEY, 1971a), as has been discussed elsewhere in this volume. Thirdly, the initial step of the pyrimidine pathway might be related in some manner to salvage reactions of purine nucleotide biosynthesis catalyzed by adenine and hypoxanthine-guanine phosphoribosyltransferase, as well as to biosynthesis of pyridine nucleotides and other reactions involving phosphoribosyl pyrophosphate.

HISATA and TATIBANA have most recently obtained evidence that the control by phosphoribosyl pyrophosphate of the first enzyme of the pyrimidine pathway is operative in intact cells of hematopoietic mouse spleen in vivo and in vitro as well as Ehrlich ascites cells in vitro (manuscripts in preparation). Mouse spleen slices were incubated with varying concentrations (up to 1 mM) of adenine, 2,6-diaminopurine, hypoxanthine, or guanine, and incubation was continued upon addition of [^{14}C]bicarbonate as a tracer of pyrimidine synthesis. Tissues were analyzed for incorporation of ^{14}C into the acid-soluble uridine nucleotides and the intermediates of the orotic acid pathway as well as for the contents of phosphoribosyl pyrophosphate determined by the method of HISATA (1975). A considerable drop in the rate of uridylate synthesis was noted in tissues incubated with adenine or diaminopurine, but such was not the case with hypoxanthine or guanine. The level of phosphoribosyl pyrophosphate also showed a decrease in the tissues incubated with adenine or 2,6-diaminopurine but not with hypoxanthine or guanine. The different effects of two groups of purines are ascribable to the fact that adenine or diaminopurine and hypoxanthine or guanine are converted to nucleotides by distinct phosphoribosyltransferases, whose K_m values for phosphoribosyl pyrophosphate are different in animal cells (Fox and KELLEY, 1971a; HENDERSON and PATERSON, 1973). When the rate of ^{14}C incorporation into the pyrimidine pathway was plotted versus the level of phosphoribosyl pyrophosphate, a close correlation was evident. There was no significant change in the ATP level after incubation with adenine. In an attempt to determine the site of inhibition, a further analysis was made for the ^{14}C contents of the intermediates of the pathway, carbamoylaspartate, dihydroorotate, orotate, and orotidylate as well as of the end product, uridylates. Adenine suppressed the ^{14}C incorporation into both the early and later intermediates to an almost equal extent, and ^{14}C did not accumulate in orotate. These observations clearly indicate that under the experimental conditions, the primary site of control by the lowered level of phosphoribosyl pyrophosphate is the step of carbamoyl phosphate synthesis rather than the step of orotate conversion to orotidylate. Similar results were obtained in Ehrlich ascites cells in vitro.

The reaction of orotate with phosphoribosyl pyrophosphate to form orotidylate, catalyzed by orotate phosphoribosyltransferase, is generally considered as the site of regulation by phosphoribosyl pyrophosphate in the pyrimidine biosynthetic pathway. GREEN and CHAN (1973) and HOSONO and KUNO (1974) assumed that inhibition of orotidylate formation is primarily responsible for the suppression of pyrimidine synthesis de novo where depletion of phosphoribosyl pyrophosphate is conceivable. Considerations should be given, in such studies, to the possible involvement of the newly revealed function of phosphoribosyl pyrophosphate in control of the first committed reaction of pyrimidine biosynthesis.

The discovery of the regulatory role of the intracellular level of phosphoribosyl pyrophosphate has called attention to potential importance of regulation of its biosynthesis. This has been proved by a number of studies with regard to control of purine biosynthesis (for example, Fox and KELLEY, 1971a, 1971b; SPERLING et al., 1973; BECKER et al., 1973; CHAMBERS et al., 1974). The importance of the regulation also has to be considered with regard to coordinate control of purine and pyrimidine nucleotide syntheses. Since control of phosphoribosyl pyrophosphate synthetase is discussed by other authors in this volume, recent progress in tissue level studies on regulation of the synthesis of phosphoribosyl pyrophosphate will be discussed here in relationship to coordinated nucleotide biosyntheses.

CLIFFORD et al. (1972) reported the changes in purine nucleotide metabolism in rat liver as affected by diurnal variations in food ingestion and correlated the changes with those in liver polysome abundance and RNA content. Purine synthesis de novo, as measured by [^{14}C]glycine incorporation into free adenine and guanine nucleotides, was considerably stimulated to a great extent by ingestion of a protein-filled diet and conversely underwent a decrease following a 12-h period of fasting. Corresponding changes in the level of phosphoribosyl pyrophosphate were, however, not observed. On the other hand, LALANNE and HENDERSON (1975) reported a twofold diurnal variation in the level of phosphoribosyl pyrophosphate in mouse liver and investigated the effects of a variety of drugs and hormones on levels of this intermediate in vivo. Of the compounds tested, glucagon, insulin, epinephrine, ethyl-aminothiadiazole, and 2-deoxyglucose elevated the concentration of phosphoribosyl pyrophosphate 2-10-fold. HISATA and TATIBANA (manuscript in preparation; TATI-BANA, 1976) also observed similar changes in the level of phosphoribosyl pyrophosphate using the assay method of HISATA (1974) in freeze-clamped mouse liver. The level increased promptly from the basal level (about 6 nmol/g liver) to a value as high as about 20 nmol/g liver by ingestion of a 60% casein diet. No such increase was seen with ingestion of a protein-free diet. It is noteworthy that these changes in the hepatic level of phosphoribosyl pyrophosphate were closely related with those in the rates of purine and pyrimidine syntheses as measured by [^{14}C]glycine and [^{14}C]bi-carbonate incorporation into the respective acid-soluble nucleotides. HISATA and TATIBANA further studied a possible alteration in the levels of some factors that could affect phosphoribosyl pyrophosphate synthesis, such as adenylate energy charge (ATKINSON and FALL, 1967), ribose 5-phosphate, inorganic phosphate (PLANET and FOX, 1976), and cyclic nucleotides (CHAMBERS et al., 1974), and the activity of phos-phoribosyl pyrophosphate synthetase. The levels of those factors in the liver of mice fed a 60% casein diet did not significantly differ from those of animals fed a 0% casein diet (TATIBANA, 1976). Recent studies (HISATA and TATIBANA, manuscript in preparation) with isolated rat hepatocytes showed that glucagon increases the intra-cellular level of phosphoribosyl pyrophosphate and that a low concentration of colchicine inhibited the glucagon-induced increase. Molecular mechanisms involved in the elevation of phosphoribosyl pyrophosphate concentrations are yet to be clari-fied.

The possibility that the regulation of purine and pyrimidine syntheses by the level of phosphoribosyl pyrophosphate is an important part of the mechanisms for coor-dination of the syntheses of nucleotides with that of RNA in the liver has to be considered. A protein-containing diet leads to stimulation of RNA synthesis and polysome formation (CLIFFORD et al., 1972), to elevation of the concentration of phosphoribosyl pyrophosphate (LALANNE and HENDERSON, 1975; TATIBANA, 1976), as well as to stimulation in the syntheses of nucleotides (CLIFFORD et al., 1972; TATIBANA, 1976). The stimulation of RNA synthesis requires increased synthesis of purine and pyrimidine nucleotides as building blocks. A signal which directs the acceleration of nucleotide synthesis is the lowering of free nucleotide level, which releases the committed step of nucleotide synthesis from the feedback inhibition. This regulation may be called "control in series."

Control in series

Signal→RNA synthesis↑→Nucleotide synthesis↑

Control in parallel

Signal⟨ → RNA synthesis↑
       → Nucleotide synthesis↑

Another signal which directs increased synthesis of nucleotides is the enhanced level of phosphoribosyl pyrophosphate, which occurs by its increased synthesis; the signal transfer is apparently not mediated by RNA synthesis. In this mechanism, nucleotide synthesis and RNA synthesis are subject to "control in parallel," which probably would ensure a rapid supply of nucleotides as building blocks of RNA synthesis. Data supporting these speculations are awaited with great interest.

Observations on induction of phosphoribosyl pyrophosphate synthetase have been reported by CHAMBERS et al. (1974), who showed a 2–10-fold increase in phosphoribosyl pyrophosphate synthetase activity early in the process of concanavalin A activation of mouse spleen lymphocytes. The increase first appeared 8 h after addition of concanavalin A, and concomitant protein synthesis is a requirement. Induction of the synthetase occurs in parallel with increase in purine synthesis and precedes DNA synthesis. The induced activity of phosphoribosyl pyrophosphate synthetase is further stimulated 1.5–6-fold by the presence of cGMP (0.5 mM) in the enzyme assay, while the synthetase activity of untreated resting lymphocytes is not sensitive to the cyclic nucleotide. Addition of dibutyryl cAMP to concanavalin A-stimulated lymphocytes inhibits the appearance of cGMP-sensitive synthetase as well as DNA synthesis. GREEN and MARTIN (1974) found that phosphoribosyl pyrophosphate synthetase purified from HTC cells is activated 2–4-fold in the presence of a low concentration of cGMP (10 nM). These observations imply the presence of two different phosphoribosyl pyrophosphate synthetases: one present in nondividing cells and one induced and specifically adapted for the new cellular demand.

G. Possible Interrelationship Between Catabolism of Purine and Pyrimidine Nucleotides

Catabolism of purine nucleotides are extensively reviewed by other authors in this volume. In humans, purine nucleotides are degraded primarily to uric acid and excreted in the urine. In this conversion four different kinds of enzymatic reactions—dephosphorylation, deamination, cleavage of glycosidic bonds, and oxidation—are required. The catabolism of pyrimidine nucleotides also involves dephosphorylation, deamination, and glycosidic bond cleavage. Further metabolism of the pyrimidine bases is generally subject to reduction rather than to oxidation, in contrast to purine catabolism.

The reductive pathway of pyrimidine-base catabolism, which can lead to complete degradation of pyrimidines to carbon dioxide and ammonia, was worked out some years ago and has been reviewed by SCHULMAN (1961) and HENDERSON and PATERSON (1973). To our knowledge there has been no report concerning interference of purines, except for participation of pyridine nucleotides as the coenzymes, with the reductive pathway of pyrimidine catabolism. Catabolic processes of purine and pyrimidine nucleotides are presumably interrelated only at the steps of dephosphorylation and glycosidic bond cleavage. These will be briefly discussed.

I. Dephosphorylation of Purine and Pyrimidine Mononucleotides

Nucleoside monophosphates are converted to nucleosides by the catalysis of a variety of enzymes. Relatively nonspecific acid and alkaline phosphatases dephosphorylate nucleoside monophosphates, regardless of the base or of the position of the phosphate (2′, 3′, or 5′). Specific 5′-nucleotidases, which act selectively on nucleoside 5′-monophosphates and are known to exist in diverse mammalian tissues (BODAN-SKY and SCHWARTZ, 1968), do not generally discriminate between purine and pyrimidine 5′-ribonucleotides. Although precise physiologic roles of these enzymes remain unknown, their participation in nucleotide degradation is assumed. In such cases, purine and pyrimidine nucleotides can compete for the catalytic site of the enzymes and serve as competitive inhibitors.

More specific interference between catabolism of purines and pyrimidines is possible on 5′-nucleotidases. These enzymes are inhibited to some degree by their nucleoside products and also by nucleoside polyphosphates. Like 5′-nucleotidase from potato (KLEIN, 1957), the activity of rat liver microsomal 5′-nucleotidase, with 0.3 mM 5′-AMP as substrate was inhibited to the following extent by nucleosides (SEGAL and BRENNER, 1960): 0.025 M adenosine, 53%; 0.025M inosine, 54%; 0.05 M cytidine, 41%; 0.05 M uridine, 70%. Similar inhibition by nucleosides was noted for calf intestinal 5′-nucleotidase (CENTER and BEHAL, 1966). 5′-Nucleotidase from rat cardiac muscle is strongly inhibited by ATP > UTP > CTP > GTP (BAER et al., 1966) and also by ADP (SULLIVAN and ALPERS, 1971). The enzyme from sheep brain is strongly inhibited by low concentrations of nucleoside triphosphates, such as ATP, UTP, and CTP (IPATA, 1968). Nucleoside diphosphates are inhibitory but to a lesser extent. GTP and GDP are not effective. Two kinds of 5′-nucleotidases have been demonstrated in the liver of various animal species, the membrane-bound enzyme (for example, SONG and BODANSKY, 1967; WIDNELL and UNKELESS, 1968) and the enzyme present in soluble fraction (ITOH et al., 1967, 1968; FRITSON, 1969). The two enzymes differ in relative activities toward various 5′-mononucleotides and metal requirement. The soluble enzymes from various species are most active toward 5′-IMP. ITOH and TSUSHIMA (1972) fed a high protein diet to chickens and observed an increase in the activity of the soluble 5′-nucleotidase in the liver. They suggested the involvement of this enzyme in uricogenesis in the chicken. Both 5′-nucleotidases of liver, particulate and soluble, are only weakly, if at all, inhibited by nucleosides and nucleotides.

A unique and important 5′-nucleotidase has been identified in the soluble fraction of normal human erythrocytes (PAGLIA and VALENTINE, 1975). The enzyme dephosphorylates pyrimidine 5′-ribosemonophosphates but is not effective with purine nucleotides or with the 2′-, 3′-, or cyclic isomers of pyrimidine nucleotides. Apparent K_m values are 0.33 mM for UMP, 0.15 mM for CMP, and 1.0 mM for TMP. The enzyme is strongly inhibited by AMP, by adenosine, guanosine, and inosine and other nucleosides as well as by adenine and guanine. The discovery was made during a study of the pathogenesis of an unusual hereditary syndrome, which includes hemolytic anemia accompanied by markedly elevated erythrocyte pyrimidine nucleotides (VALENTINE et al., 1974). Thus, it appears that the pyrimidine-specific 5′-nucleotidase plays an important role in degradation of pyrimidine nucleotides, which are amply produced by degradation of nucleic acids in the process of erythrocyte maturation. With the help of this enzyme, the mature cells may acquire a balanced composition of purine and pyrimidine nucleotides (pyrimidine nucleotides are virtually absent in mature human erythrocytes). There is apparently no available evidence for the presence of this enzyme or similar purine- or pyrimidine-specific nucleotidases in other tissues.

II. Cleavage of Glycosidic Bond

Glycolysic bond cleavage is accomplished either phosphorolytically or hydrolytically and at either the nucleotide or nucleoside level. In most biological systems including tissues of higher animals, the major reaction is the phosphorolytic cleavage of nucleosides. The phosphorylase reaction is reversible and serves in the synthesis of nucleoside as well as its degradation. *Purine nucleoside phosphorylase* is ineffective toward pyrimidine nucleosides. *Uridine phosphorylase* catalyzes ribo- and deoxyribonucleosides of uracil and thymine, while *thymidine phosphorylase* acts on deoxyuridine and deoxythymidine. Thus, purines and pyrimidines do not interfere with the respective metabolism by these enzymes. However, since these phosphorolytic reactions are reversible with the equilibria lying in the direction of nucleoside formation, the synthesis or degradation of one nucleoside may change the amount of ribose phosphate, thus affecting the direction of nucleoside metabolism on the other nucleoside phosphorylase. Such an interference between purine and pyrimidine metabolism was reported by GOTTO et al. (1969), who showed that the incorporation of [^{14}C]uracil and [^{14}C]fluorouracil into the nucleic acids of Ehrlich ascites cells in vitro was strongly stimulated by the addition of inosine. Deoxyinosine enhanced the incorporation of 5-bromo[^{14}C]uracil into DNA. These data, together with the additional evidence, led to the suggestion that inosine and deoxyinosine exerted the stimulating effects by providing ribose 1-phosphate and deoxyribose 1-phosphate, rate-limiting substrates for the incorporation of uracil (or fluorouracil) and 5-bromouracil into RNA and DNA, respectively.

H. Possible Interference Between Purine and Pyrimidine Transport

Transfer of purines and pyrimidines between cells and tissues may have a considerable physiologic importance in their metabolism in the whole body, although to our knowledge definite and quantitative evaluations of the significance of the process have not been documented. Mechanisms for the entry of nucleosides among various forms of purine and pyrimidine into cells have been the subject of a number of investigations in recent years, thus reflecting the physiologic importance of this class of compounds. If the nucleoside transport across the cell membrane involves a special mechanism and the mechanism is of such broad specificity that is active for both purine and pyrimidine nucleosides, a competition between those nucleosides for the entry into or efflux from cells would evolve. Such a competition may interfere with the subsequent metabolism of nucleosides, provided that their entry into or efflux from the cells can be rate-limiting for their overall metabolism.

OLIVER and PATERSON (1971) studied transport of nucleosides by human erythrocytes by measuring disappearance of [^{14}C]uridine and [^{14}C]thymidine from incubation media or by following efflux of labeled uridine or thymidine from preloaded cells induced by an inward flow of various purine and pyrimidine ribo- and deoxynucleosides. Uridine and thymidine are not metabolized by human erythrocytes. The nucleoside transport is nonconcentrative, shows a saturation kinetics, and is competitively inhibited by formycin B, an analogue of inosine that does not undergo phosphorolytic cleavage. Based on these observations, these authors concluded that the transport of nucleosides across the plasma membrane of human erythrocytes is accomplished by a nonconcentrative facilitated diffusion mechanism of broad specificity. TAUBE and BERLIN (1972) showed that both purine and pyrimidine nucleosides are transported by a single system in rabbit polymorphonuclear leukocytes. Evidence presented includes observations that the system showed saturation kinetics, that nucleosides are competitive with each other, and that K_m values for a spectrum of nucleosides are identical with the K_i values as inhibitor. The most critical structural requirements for binding include the pyrimidine base moiety and 3'-OH configuration on the pentose.

In cells having a single nucleoside transport system of a broad specificity such as is seen in human erythrocytes and rabbit polymorphonuclear leucocytes, one may expect interference of purine and pyrimidine nucleoside transport and metabolism. However, it appears that not all eucaryotic cells possess the same transport mechanisms for nucleosides. Although the above reports as well as others (SCHOLTISSEK, 1968; KESSEL and SHURIN, 1968; STECK et al., 1969) suggest a nucleoside transport mechanism of rather broad specificity, other data indicate that more specific systems exist. It has been suggested that the thymidine transport mechanism in hamster cells may be distinct from that of uridine transport (BRESLOW and GOLDSBY, 1969; HARE, 1970). Studies using membrane vesicles from mouse fibroblast cells indicated that the uridine transport system in these vesicles is distinct from that of purine nucleosides (LI and HOCHSTADT, 1976). QUINLAN and HOCHSTADT (1976) demonstrated a group translocation mechanism specific for transport of the ribose moiety of inosine by vesicles of plasma membrane from SV-40 transformed 3 T 3 cells. Membrane-bound purine nucleoside phosphorylase is presumably involved in this process. This is the first unequivocal demonstration of the presence of a group translocation mechanism in animal cells and refers to an uptake process in which the exogenous transport substrate is enzymatically modified in the process of its passage across the membrane. The transport of adenine by membrane vesicles from *E. coli* is mediated by a translocation mechanism where adenine is converted to adenosine monophosphate by membrane-bound adenine phosphoribosyltransferase (HOCHSTADT-OZER and STADTMAN, 1971).

I. Conclusion

Purines and pyrimidines are present in nearly equal amounts in most types of cells and the turnover may be equally rapid. This in turn suggests close relationship between purine and pyrimidine metabolism. Enzymes of purine biosynthetic pathways are not significantly affected by pyrimidines, while certain enzymes of pyrimidine biosynthetic pathways are sensitive to regulation by purines. Roles of this regulation in coordinate control of the synthesis of pyrimidines and purines are conceivable but remain to be established with certainty.

Some purines, including allopurinol, adenine, and adenosine, interfere with pyrimidine metabolism, and orotate, a pyrimidine, does inhibit purine biosynthesis, particulary when organisms are treated with a relatively large amount of the agent. In many such cases, impairment of phosphoribosyl pyrophosphate metabolism is involved. The cellular level of phosphoribosyl pyrophosphate, a common precursor for syntheses of all nucleotides, regulates purine and pyrimidine nucleotide biosyntheses in a coordinate manner as a rate-limiting substrate or a specific activator of committed enzymes of both biosynthetic pathways. Considerable attention has been recently focused on molecular mechanisms for control of phosphoribosyl pyrophosphate synthesis and such observations have been described herein.

Possible reciprocal regulation of purines and pyrimidines in catabolism as well as membrane transport is briefly discussed.

Acknowledgement. The author wishes to thank M. Ohara, Kyoto University, for her invaluable help in preparing this manuscript.

References

Anderson, P. M.: A glutamine- and N-acetyl-L-glutamate-dependent carbamyl phosphate synthetase activity in the teleost *Micropterus salmoides*. Comp. Biochem. Physiol. **54 B**, 261—263 (1976)

Anderson, P. M., Marvin, S. V.: Effect of ornithine, IMP, and UMP on carbamyl phosphate synthetase from *Escherichia coli*. Biochem. biophys. Res. Commun. **32**, 928—934 (1968)

Anderson, P. M., Meister, A.: Control of *Escherichia coli* carbamyl phosphate synthetase by purine and pyrimidine nucleotides. Biochemistry **5**, 3164—3169 (1966)

Aoki, T., Oya, H., Mori, M., Tatibana, M.: Glutamine-dependent carbamoyl phosphate synthetase in *Ascaris* ovary and its regulatory properties. Proc. Jap. Acad. **51**, 733—736 (1975)

Appel, S. H.: Purification and kinetic properties of brain orotidine 5'-phosphate decarboxylase. J. biol. Chem. **243**, 3924—3929 (1968)

Aronow, L.: Reversal of adenine toxicity by pyrimidine nucleosides. Biochim. biophys. Acta (Amst.) **47**, 184—185 (1961)

Atkinson, D. E., Fall, L.: Adenosine triphosphate conservation in biosynthetic regulation. *Escherichia coli* phosphoribosylpyrophosphate synthase. J. biol. Chem. **242**, 3241—3242 (1967)

Atkinson, D. E., Walton, G. M.: Adenosine triphosphate conservation in metabolic regulation. Rat liver citrate cleavage enzyme. J. biol. Chem. **242**, 3239—3241 (1967)

Baer, H. P., Drummond, G. I., Duncan, E. L.: Formation and deamination of adenosine by cardiac muscle enzymes. Molec. Pharmacol. **2**, 67—76 (1966)

Bagnara, A. S., Finch, L. R.: The effects of bases and nucleosides on the intracellular contents of nucleotides and 5-phosphoribosyl 1-pyrophosphate in *Escherichia coli*. Europ. J. Biochem. **41**, 421—430 (1974)

Beardmore, T. D., Cashman, J. S., Kelley, W. N.: Mechanism of allopurinol-mediated increase in enzyme activity in man. J. clin. Invest. **51**, 1823—1832 (1972)

Beardmore, T. D., Kelley, W. N.: Mechanism of allopurinol-mediated inhibition of pyrimidine biosynthesis. J. Lab. clin. Med. **78**, 696—704 (1971)

Becker, M. A., Argubright, K. F., Fox, R. M., Seegmiller, J. E.: Oxipurinol-associated inhibition of pyrimidine synthesis in human lymphoblasts. Molec. Pharmacol. **10**, 657—668 (1974)

Becker, M. A., Kostel, P. J., Meyer, L. J., Seegmiller, J. E.: Human phosphoribosylpyrophosphate synthetase: increased enzyme specific activity in a family with gout and excessive purine synthesis. Proc. nat. Acad. Sci. (Wash.) **70**, 2749—2752 (1973)

Berne, R. M.: Cardiac nucleotides in hypoxia: possible role in regulation of coronary blood flow. Amer. J. Physiol. **204**, 317—322 (1963)

Blair, D. G. R., Potter, V. R.: Inhibition of orotidylic acid decarboxylase by uridine 5'-phosphate. J. biol. Chem. **236**, 2503—2506 (1961)

Blakley, R. L., Vitols, E.: The control of nucleotide biosynthesis. Ann. Rev. Biochem. **37**, 201—224 (1968)

Bodansky, O., Schwartz, M. K.: 5'-Nucleotidase. Advanc. clin. Chem. **11**, 277—328 (1968)

Breslow, R. E., Goldsby, R. A.: Isolation and characterization of thymidine transport mutants of chinese hamster cells. Exp. Cell Res. **55**, 339—346 (1969)

Brooke, M. S., Magasanik, B.: The metabolism of purines in *Aerobacter* aerogenes: a study of purineless mutants. J. Bacteriol. **68**, 727—733 (1954)

Brown, G. K., Fox, R. M., O'Sullivan, W. J.: Alteration of quaternary structural behaviour of an hepatic orotate phosphoribosyltransferase-orotidine 5'-phosphate decarboxylase complex in rats following allopurinol therapy. Biochem. Pharmacol. **21**, 2469—2477 (1972)

Brown, G. K., Fox, R. M., O'Sullivan, W. J.: Interconversion of different molecular weight forms of human erythrocyte orotidylate decarboxylase. J. biol. Chem. **250**, 7352—7358 (1975)

Brown, N. C., Reichard, P.: Ribonucleoside diphosphate reductase. Formation of active and inactive complexes of proteins B 1 and B 2. J. molec. Biol. **46**, 25—38 (1969a)

Brown, N. C., Reichard, P.: Role of effector binding in allosteric control of ribonucleoside diphosphate reductase. J. molec. Biol. **46**, 39—55 (1969b)

Caskey, C. T., Ashton, D. M., Wyngaarden, J. B.: The enzymology of feedback inhibition of glutamine phosphoribosylpyrophosphate amidotransferase by purine ribonucleotides. J. biol. Chem. **239**, 2570—2579 (1964)

Center, M. S., Behal, F. J.: Calf intestinal 5'-nucleotidase. Arch. Biochem. biophys. **114**, 414—421 (1966)

Chambers, D. A., Martin, Jr., D. W., Weinstein, Y.: The effect of cyclic nucleotides on purine biosynthesis and the induction of PRPP synthetase during lymphocyte activation. Cell **3**, 375—380 (1974)

Changeux, J.-P., Gerhart, J. C., Schachman, H. K.: Allosteric interactions in aspartate transcarbamylase. I. Binding of specific ligands to the native enzyme and its isolated subunits. Biochemistry **7**, 531—538 (1968)

Clifford, A. J., Riumallo, J. A., Baliga, B. S., Munro, H. N., Brown, P. R.: Liver nucleotide metabolism in relation to amino acid supply. Biochim. biophys. Acta (Amst.) **277**, 443—458 (1972)

Creasey, W. A., Handschumacher, R. E.: Purification and properties of orotidylate decarboxylases from yeast and rat liver. J. biol. Chem. **236**, 2058—2063 (1961)

Creasey, W. A., Hankin, L., Handschumacher, R. E.: Fatty livers induced by orotic acid. I. Accumulation and metabolism of lipids. J. biol. Chem. **236**, 2064—2070 (1961)

Davis, R. H.: Channeling in *Neurospora* metabolism. In: Vogel, H. J., Lampen, J. O., Bryson, V. (Eds.): Organizational Biosynthesis, pp. 303—322. New York: Academic Press 1967

Dissing, J., Knudsen, B.: Adenosine-deaminase deficiency and combined immunodeficiency syndrome. Lancet **1972 II**, 1316

Euler, L. H., von, Rubin, R. J., Handschumacher, R. E.: Fatty livers induced by orotic acid. II. Changes in nucleotide metabolism. J. biol. Chem. **238**, 2464—2469 (1963)

Fallon, H. J., Frei, E., III, Block, J., Seegmiller, J. E.: The uricosuria and orotic aciduria induced by 6-azauridine. J. clin. Invest. **40**, 1906—1914 (1961)

Ferris, G. M., Clark, J. B.: The control of nucleic acid and nicotinamide nucleotide synthesis in regenerating rat liver. Biochem. J. **128**, 869—877 (1972)

Fox, I. H., Kelley, W. N.: Phosphoribosylpyrophosphate in man: biochemical and clinical significance. Ann. intern. Med. **74**, 424—433 (1971a)

Fox, I. H., Kelley, W. N.: Human phosphoribosylpyrophosphate synthetase. Distribution, purification, and properties. J. biol. Chem. **246**, 5739—5748 (1971b)

Fox, R. M., Royse-Smith, D., O'Sullivan, W. J.: Orotidinuria induced by allopurinol. Science **168**, 861—862 (1970)

Fox, R. M., Wood, M. H., O'Sullivan, W. J.: Studies on the coordinate activity and lability of orotidylate phosphoribosyltransferase and decarboxylase in human erythrocytes, and the effects of allopurinol administration. J. clin. Invest. **50**, 1050—1060 (1971)

Fritson, P.: Nucleotidase activities in the soluble fraction of rat liver homogenate. Partial purification and properties of a 5'-nucleotidase with pH optimum 6.3. Biochim. biophys. Acta (Amst.) **178**, 534—541 (1969)

Fyfe, J. A., Miller, R. L., Krenitsky, T. A.: Kinetic properties and inhibition of orotidine 5'-phosphate decarboxylase. Effects of some allopurinol metabolites on the enzyme. J. biol. Chem. **248**, 3801—3809 (1973)

Gerhart, J. C., Pardee, A. B.: The enzymology of control by feedback inhibition. J. biol. Chem. **237**, 891—896 (1962)

Giblett, E. R., Anderson, J. E., Cohen, F., Pollara, B., Meuwissen, H. J.: Adenosine-deaminase deficiency in two patients with severely impaired cellular immunity. Lancet **1972 II**, 1067—1069

Gotto, A. M., Belkhode, M. L., Touster, O.: Stimulatory effects of inosine and deoxyinosine on the incorporation of uracil-2-^{14}C, 5-fluorouracil-2-^{14}C, and 5-bromouracil-2-^{14}C into nucleic acids by Ehrlich ascites tumor cells in vitro. Cancer Res. **29**, 807—811 (1969)

Green, H., Chan, T.-S.: Pyrimidine starvation induced by adenosine in fibroblasts and lymphoid cells: role of adenosine deaminase. Science **182**, 836—837 (1973)

Green, C. D., Martin, D. W., Jr.: A direct, stimulating effect of cyclic GMP on purified phosphoribosyl pyrophosphate synthetase and its antagonism by cyclic AMP. Cell **2**, 241—245 (1974)

Grobner, W., Kelley, W. N.: Effect of allopurinol and its metabolic derivatives on the configuration of human orotate phosphoribosyltransferase and orotidine 5'-phosphate decarboxylase. Biochem. Pharmacol. **24**, 379—384 (1975)

Gülen, S., Smith, P. C., Tremblay, G. C.: Evidence for the control of pyrimidine biosynthesis in tissue minces by purines. Biochem. biophys. Res. Commun. **56**, 934—939 (1974)

Hager, S. E., Jones, M. E.: Initial steps in pyrimidine synthesis in Ehrlich ascites carcinoma in vitro. II. The synthesis of carbamyl phosphate by a soluble, glutamine-dependent carbamyl phosphate synthetase. J. biol. Chem. **242**, 5667—5673 (1967a)

Hager, S. E., Jones, M. E.: A glutamine-dependent enzyme for the synthesis of carbamyl phosphate for pyrimidine biosynthesis in fetal rat liver. J. biol. Chem. **242**, 5674—5680 (1967b)

Hakala, M. T., Taylor, E.: The ability of purine and thymine derivatives and of glycine to support the growth of mammalian cells in culture. J. biol. Chem. **234**, 126—128 (1959)

Handschumacher, R. E.: Orotidylic acid decarboxylase: inhibition studies with azauridine 5'-phosphate. J. biol. Chem. **235**, 2917—2919 (1960)

Handschumacher, R. E., Creasey, W. A., Jaffe, J. J., Pasternak, C. A., Hankin, L.: Biochemical and nutritional studies on the induction of fatty livers by dietary orotic acid. Proc. nat. Acad. Sci. (Wash.) **46**, 178—186 (1960)

Hare, J. D.: Quantitative aspects of thymidine uptake into the acid-soluble pool of normal and polyoma-transformed hamster cells. Cancer Res. **30**, 684—691 (1970)

Henderson, J. F., Khoo, M. K. Y.: Availability of 5-phosphoribosyl 1-pyrophosphate for ribonucleotide synthesis in Ehrlich ascites tumor cells in vitro. J. biol. Chem. **240**, 2358—2362 (1965a).

Henderson, J. F., Khoo, M. K. Y.: Synthesis of 5-phosphoribosyl 1-pyrophosphate from ribonucleosides in Ehrlich ascites tumor cells in vitro. J. biol. Chem. **240**, 2363—2366 (1965b)

Henderson, J. F., Paterson, A. R. P.: Nucleotide Metabolism. An Introduction. New York: Academic Press 1973

Hershko, A., Razin, A., Mager, J.: Regulation of the synthesis of 5-phosphoribosyl-1-pyrophosphate in intact red blood cells and in cell-free preparations. Biochim. biophys. Acta (Amst.) **184**, 64—76 (1969)

Hill, D. L., Bennett, L. L., Jr.: Purification and properties of 5-phosphoribosyl pyrophosphate amidotransferase from adenocarcinoma 755 cells. Biochemistry **8**, 122—130 (1969)

Hisata, T.: An accurate method for estimating 5-phosphoribosyl 1-pyrophosphate in animal tissues with the use of acid extraction. Anal. Biochem. **68**, 448—457 (1975)

Hochstadt-Ozer, J., Stadtman, E. R.: The regulation of purine utilization in bacteria. II. Adenine phosphoribosyltransferase in isolated membrane preparations and its role in transport of adenine across the membrane. J. biol. Chem. **246**, 5304—5311 (1971)

Holmes, E. W., McDonald, J. A., McCord, J. M., Wyngaarden, J. R., Kelley, W. N.: Human glutamine phosphoribosylpyrophosphate amidotransferase. Kinetic and regulatory properties. J. biol. Chem. **248**, 144—150 (1973)

Holmes, E. W., Pehlke, D. M., Kelley, W. N.: Human IMP dehydrogenase. Kinetics and regulatory properties. Biochim. biophys. Acta (Amst.) **364**, 209—217 (1974)

Hosono, R., Kuno, S.: Mechanism of inhibition of bacterial growth by adenine. J. Biochem. (Tokyo) **75**, 215—220 (1974)

Hurlbert, R. B., Kammen, H. O.: Formation of cytidine nucleotides from uridine nucleotides by soluble mammalian enzymes: requirements for glutamine and guanosine nucleotides. J. biol. Chem. **235**, 443—449 (1960)

Inagaki, A., Tatibana, M.: Control of pyrimidine biosynthesis in mammalian tissues. III. Multiple forms of aspartate transcarbamoylase of mouse spleen. Biochim. biophys. Acta (Amst.) **220**, 491—502 (1970)

Ishii, K., Green, H.: Lethality of adenosine for cultured mammalian cells by interference with pyrimidine biosynthesis. J. Cell Sci. **13**, 429—439 (1973)

Ito,K., Nakanishi,S., Terada,M., Tatibana,M.: Control of pyrimidine biosynthesis in mammalian tissues. II. Glutamine-utilizing carbamoyl phosphate synthetase of various experimental tumors: distribution, purification and characterization. Biochim. biophys. Acta (Amst.) **220**, 477—490 (1970)

Ito, K., Uchino,H.: Control of pyrimidine biosynthesis in human lymphocytes. Inhibitory effect of guanine and guanosine on induction of enzymes for pyrimidine biosynthesis de novo in phytohemagglutinin-stimulated lymphocytes. J. biol. Chem. **251**, 1427—1430 (1976)

Itoh,R., Mitsui,A., Tsushima,K.: 5'-Nucleotidase of chicken liver. Biochim. biophys. Acta (Amst.) **146**, 151—159 (1967)

Itoh,R., Mitsui,A., Tsushima,K.: Properties of 5'-nucleotidase from hepatic tissue of higher animals. J. Biochem. (Tokyo) **63**, 165—169 (1968)

Itho,R., Tsushima,K.: Changes in 5'-nucleotidase activity in chick liver during development and dietary treatment. Biochim. biophys. Acta (Amst.) **273**, 229—235 (1972)

Ipata,P.L.: Sheep brain 5'-nucleotidase. Some enzymic properties and allosteric inhibition by nucleoside triphosphates. Biochemistry **7**, 507—515 (1968)

Jones,M.E.: Regulation of pyrimidine and arginine biosynthesis in mammals. Advanc. Enzyme Regul. **9**, 19—49 (1971)

Kavipurapu,P.R., Jones,M.E.: Purification, size, and properties of the complex of orotate phosphoribosyltransferase: orotidylate decarboxylase from mouse Ehrlich ascites carcinoma. J. biol. Chem. **251**, 5589—5599 (1976)

Kelley,W.N.: Purine and pyrimidine metabolism of cells in culture. In: Rothblat,G.H., Cristofalo,V.J. (Eds.): Growth, Nutrition, and Metabolism of Cells in Culture, Vol. 1, pp. 211—256. New York: Academic Press 1972

Kelley,W.N., Beardmore,T.D.: Allopurinol: alteration in pyrimidine metabolism in man. Science **169**, 388—390 (1970)

Kelley,W.N., Beardmore,T.D., Fox,I.H., Meade,J.C.: Effect of allopurinol and oxipurinol on pyrimidine synthesis in cultured human fibroblasts. Biochem. Pharmacol. **20**, 1471—1478 (1971)

Kelley,W.N., Fox,I.H., Wyngaarden,J.B.: Regulation of purine biosynthesis in cultured human cells. I. Effects of orotic acid. Biochim. biophys. Acta (Amst.) **215**, 512—516 (1970)

Kent,R.J., Lin,R.-L., Sallach,H.J., Cohen,P.P.: Reversible dissociation of a carbamoyl phosphate synthase-aspartate transcarbamoylase-dihydroorotase complex from ovarian eggs of *Rana catesbeiana*: Effect of uridine triphosphate and other modifiers. Proc. nat. Acad. Sci. (Wash.) **72**, 1712—1716 (1975)

Kessel,D., Shurin,S.B.: Transport of two non-metabolized nucleosides, deoxycytidine and cytosine arabinoside, in a sub-line of the L1210 murine leukemia. Biochim. biophys. Acta (Amst.) **163**, 179—187 (1968)

Klein,W.: Über Kartoffel-Nucleotidase. I. Reinigung und Isolierung des Fermentes. Z. physiol. Chem. **307**, 247—253 (1957)

Krooth,R.S.: Properties of diploid cell strains developed from patients with an inherited abnormality of uridine biosynthesis. Cold Spr. Harb. Symp. quant. Biol. **29**, 189—212 (1964)

Lacroute,F., Piérard,A., Grenson,M., Wiame,J.M.: The biosynthesis of carbamyl phosphate in *Saccaromyces cerevisiae*. J. gen. Microbiol. **40**, 127—142 (1965)

Lalanne,M., Henderson,J.F.: Effects of hormones and drugs on phosphoribosyl pyrophosphate concentrations in mouse liver. Canad. J. Biochem. **53**, 394—399 (1975)

Levine,R.L., Hoogenraad,N.J., Kretchmer,N.: Regulation of activity of carbamoyl phosphate synthetase from mouse spleen. Biochemistry **10**, 3694—3699 (1971)

Li,C.-C., Hochstadt,J.: Transport mechanisms in isolated plasma membranes. Nucleoside processing by membrane vesicles from mouse fibroblast cells grown in defined medium. J. biol. Chem. **251**, 1175—1180 (1976)

Long,C.W., Pardee,A.B.: Cytidine triphosphate synthetase of *Escherichia coli* B. I. Purification and kinetics. J. biol. Chem. **242**, 4715—4721 (1967)

Lue,P.F., Kaplan,J.G.: Metabolic compartmentation at the molecular level: the function of a multienzyme aggregate in the pyrimidine pathway of yeast. Biochim. biophys. Acta (Amst.) **220**, 365—372 (1970)

McFall, E., Magasanik, B.: The control of purine biosynthesis in cultured mammalian cells. J. biol. Chem. **235**, 2103—2108 (1960)

Moore, E. C., Hurlbert, R. B.: Regulation of mammalian deoxyribonucleotide biosynthesis by nucleotides as activators and inhibitors. J. biol. Chem. **241**, 4802—4809 (1966)

Moore, E. C., Reichard, P.: Enzymatic synthesis of deoxyribonucleotides. VI. The cytidine diphosphate reductase system from Novikoff hepatoma. J. biol. Chem. **239**, 3453—3456 (1964)

Mori, M., Ishida, H., Tatibana, M.: Aggregation states and catalytic properties of the multienzyme complex catalyzing the initial steps of pyrimidine biosynthesis in rat liver. Biochemistry **14**, 2622—2630 (1975)

Mori, M., Tatibana, M.: Glutamine-dependent carbamoyl phosphate synthetase: polyamines inhibit the activity and modify the activating effect of 5-phosphoribosyl 1-pyrophosphate. Biochem. biophys. Res. Commun. **67**, 287—293 (1975a)

Mori, M., Tatibana, M.: Purification of homogeneous glutamine-dependent carbamyl phosphate synthetase from ascites hepatoma cells as a complex with aspartate transcarbamylase and dihydroorotase. J. Biochem. (Tokyo) **78**, 239—242 (1975b)

Moyed, H. S.: Inhibition of the biosynthesis of the pyrimidine portion of thiamine by adenosine. J. Bacteriol. **88**, 1024—1029 (1964)

Muirhead, K. M., Bishop, S. H.: Purification of adenylosuccinate synthetase from rabbit skeletal muscle. J. biol. Chem. **249**, 459—464 (1974)

Murray, A. W.: Some properties of adenosine kinase from Ehrlich ascites-tumour cells. Biochem. J. **106**, 549—555 (1968)

Nierlich, D. P., Magasanik, B.: Regulation of purine ribonucleotide synthesis by end product inhibition. The effect of adenine and guanine ribonucleotides on the 5'-phosphoribosylpyrophosphate amidotransferase of *Aerobacter aerogenes*. J. biol. Chem. **240**, 358—365 (1965)

O'Donovan, G. A., Neuhard, J.: Pyrimidine metabolism in microorganisms. Bacteriol. Rev. **34**, 278—343 (1970)

Oliver, J. M., Paterson, A. R. P.: Nucleoside transport. I. A mediated process in human erythrocytes. Canad. J. Biochem. **49**, 262—270 (1971)

O'Neal, D., Naylor, A. W.: Purine and pyrimidine nucleotide inhibition of carbamyl phosphate synthetase from pea seedlings. Biochem. biophys. Res. Commun. **31**, 322—327 (1968)

Ord, M. G., Stocken, L. A.: Uptake of orotate and thymidine by normal and regenerating rat livers. Biochem. J. **132**, 47—54 (1973)

Orengo, A.: Regulation of enzymic activity by metabolites. I. Uridine-cytidine kinase of Novikoff ascites rat tumor. J. biol. Chem. **244**, 2204—2209 (1969)

Paglia, D. E., Valentine, W. N.: Characteristics of a pyrimidine-specific 5'-nucleotidase in human erythrocytes. J. biol. Chem. **250**, 7973—7979 (1975)

Pasternak, C. A., Handschumacher, R. E.: The biochemical activity of 6-azauridine: interference with pyrimidine metabolism in transplantalable mouse tumors. J. biol. Chem. **234**, 2992—2997 (1959)

Pausch, J., Wilkening, J., Nowack, J., Decker, K.: Control of pyrimidine biosynthesis in the perfused liver. Feedback inhibition of glutamine-dependent carbamoyl phosphate synthetase. Europ. J. Biochem. **53**, 349—356 (1975)

Piérard, A.: Control of the activity of *Escherichia coli* carbamoyl phosphate synthetase by antagonistic allosteric effectors. Science **154**, 1572—1573 (1966)

Piérard, A., Glansdorff, N., Mergeay, M., Wiame, J. M.: Control of the biosynthesis of carbamoyl phosphate in *Escherichia coli*. J. molec. Biol. **14**, 23—36 (1965)

Piérard, A., Wiame, J. M.: Regulation and mutation affecting a glutamine dependent formation of carbamyl phosphate in *Escherichia coli*. Biochem. biophys. Res. Commun. **15**, 76—81 (1964)

Pinsky, L., Krooth, R. S.: Studies on the control of pyrimidine biosynthesis in human diploid cell strains, I. Effect of 6-azauridine on cellular phenotype. Proc. nat. Acad. Sci. (Wash.) **57**, 925—932 (1967)

Planet, G., Fox, I. H.: Inhibition of phosphoribosylpyrophosphate synthesis by purine nucleosides in human erythrocytes. J. biol. Chem. **251**, 5839—5844 (1976)

Quinlan, D. C., Hochstadt, J.: Group translocation of the ribose moiety of inosine by vesicles of plasma membrane from 3T3 cells transformed by Simian virus 40. J. biol. Chem. **251**, 344—354 (1976)

Rajalakshmi, S., Handschumacher, R. E.: Control of purine biosynthesis de novo by orotic acid in vivo and in vitro. Biochim. biophys. Acta (Amst.) **155**, 317—325 (1968)

Rajalakshmi, S., Sarma, D. S. R., Sarma, P. S.: Studies on "orotic acid fatty liver". Biochem. J. **80**, 375—378 (1961)

Reichard, P.: The Biosynthesis of Deoxyribose. Ciba Lectures in Microbial Biochemistry. New York: John Wiley & Sons 1967

Reichard, P.: Control of deoxyribonucleotide synthesis in vitro and in vivo. Advanc. Enzyme Regul. **10**, 3—16 (1972)

Remy, C. N., Love, S. H.: Induction of adenosine deaminase in *Escherichia coli*. J. Bacteriol. **96**, 76—85 (1968)

Reyes, P., Guganig, M. E.: Studies on a pyrimidine phosphoribosyltransferase from murine leukemia P1534J. Partial purification, substrate specificity, and evidence for its existence as a bifunctional complex with orotidine 5'-phosphate decarboxylase. J. biol. Chem. **250**, 5097—5108 (1975)

Rosenbloom, F. M., Henderson, J. F., Caldwell, I. C., Kelley, W. N., Seegmiller, J. E.: Biochemical bases of accelerated purine biosynthesis de novo in human fibroblasts lacking hypoxanthine-guanine phosphoribosyltransferase. J. biol. Chem. **243**, 1166—1173 (1968)

Rubio, R., Berne, R. M., Katori, M.: Release of adenosine in reactive hyperemia of the dog heart. Amer. J. Physiol. **216**, 56—62 (1969)

Rudolph, F. B., Fromm, H. J.: Initial rate studies of adenylosuccinate synthetase with product and competitive inhibitors. J. biol. Chem. **244**, 3832—3839 (1969)

Sattin, A., Rall, T. W.: The effect of adenosine and adenine nucleotides on the cyclic adenosine 3', 5'-phosphate content of guinea pig cerebral cortex slices. Molec. Pharmacol. **6**, 13—23 (1970)

Scholtissek, C.: Studies on the uptake of nucleic acid precursors into cells in tissue culture. Biochim. biophys. Acta (Amst.) **158**, 435—447 (1968)

Schulman, M. P.: Purines and pyrimidines. In: Greenberg, D. M. (Ed.): Metabolic Pathways, Vol. II, pp. 389—457. New York: Academic Press 1961

Schultz, J., Daly, J. W.: Cyclic adenosine 3', 5'-monophosphate in guinea pig cerebral cortical slices. III. Formation, degradation, and reformation of cyclic adenosine 3', 5'-monophosphate during sequential stimulations by biogenic amines and adenosine. J. biol. Chem. **248**, 860—866 (1973)

Seegmiller, J. E., Grayzel, A. I., Laster, L., Liddle, L.: Uric acid production in gout. J. clin. Invest. **40**, 1304—1314 (1961)

Segal, H. L., Brenner, B. M.: 5'-Nucleotidase of rat liver microsomes. J. biol. Chem. **235**, 471—474 (1960)

Shiio, I., Ishii, K.: Regulation of purine ribonucleotide synthesis by end product inhibition. II. Effect of purine nucleotides on phosphoribosylpyrophosphate amidotransferase of *Bacillus subtilis*. J. Biochem. (Tokyo) **66**, 175—181 (1969)

Shimizu, H., Daly, J.: Formation of cyclic adenosine 3', 5'-monophosphate from adenosine in brain slices. Biochim. biophys. Acta (Amst.) **222**, 465—473 (1970)

Shoaf, W. T., Jones, M. E.: Initial steps in pyrimidine synthesis in Ehrlich ascites carcinoma. Biochem. biophys. Res. Commun. **45**, 796—802 (1971)

Shoaf, W. T., Jones, M. E.: Uridylic acid synthesis in Ehrlich ascites carcinoma. Properties, subcellular distribution, and nature of enzyme complexes of the six biosynthetic enzymes. Biochemistry **12**, 4039—4051 (1973)

Sköld, O.: Uridine kinase from Ehrlich ascites tumor: purification and properties. J. biol. Chem. **235**, 3273—3279 (1960)

Smith, P. C., Knott, C. E., Tremblay, G. C.: Detection of the feedback control of pyrimidine biosynthesis in slices of several rat tissues. Biochem. biophys. Res. Commun. **55**, 1141—1146 (1973)

Song, C. S., Bodansky, O.: Subcellular localization and properties of 5'-nucleotidase in the rat liver. J. biol. Chem. **242**, 694—699 (1967)

Sperling, O., Persky-Brosh, S., Boer, P., Vries de, A.: Human erythrocyte phosphoribosylpyrophosphate synthetase mutationally altered in regulatory properties. Biochem. Med. **7**, 389—395 (1973)

Standerfer, S. B., Handler, P.: Fatty liver induced by orotic acid feeding. Proc. Soc. exp. Biol. Med. (N.Y.) **90**, 270—271 (1955)

Steck, T. L., Nakata, Y., Bader, J. P.: The uptake of nucleosides by cells in culture. I. Inhibition by heterologous nucleosides. Biochim. biophys. Acta (Amst.) **190**, 237—249 (1969)

Sullivan, J. M., Alpers, J. B.: In vitro regulation of rat heart 5′-nucleotidase by adenine nucleotides and magnesium. J. biol. Chem. **246**, 3057—3063 (1971)

Switzer, R. L.: Regulation and mechanism of phosphoribosylpyrophosphate synthetase. I. Purification and properties of the enzyme from *Salmonella typhimurium*. J. biol. Chem. **244**, 2854—2863 (1969)

Tatibana, M.: Coordinate control of nucleotide biosynthetic pathways. J. Biochem. (Tokyo) **79**, 41 p—42 p (1976)

Tatibana, M., Ito, K.: Carbamyl phosphate synthetase of the hematopoietic mouse spleen and the control of pyrimidine biosynthesis. Biochem. biophys. Res. Commun. **26**, 221—227 (1967)

Tatibana, M., Ito, K.: Control of pyrimidine biosynthesis in mammalian tissues. I. Partial purification and characterization of glutamine-utilizing carbamyl phosphate synthetase of mouse spleen and its tissue distribution. J. biol. Chem. **244**, 5403—5413 (1969)

Tatibana, M., Shigesada, K.: Activation by 5-phosphoribosyl 1-pyrophosphate of glutamine-dependent carbamyl phosphate synthetase from mouse spleen. Biochem. biophys. Res. Commun. **46**, 491—497 (1972 a)

Tatibana, M., Shigesada, K.: Two carbamyl phosphate synthetases of mammals: specific roles in control of pyrimidine and urea biosynthesis. Advanc. Enzyme Regul. **10**, 249—271 (1972 b)

Tatibana, M., Shigesada, K.: Control of pyrimidine biosynthesis in mammalian tissues. V. Regulation of glutamine-dependent carbamyl phosphate synthetase: activation by 5-phosphoribosyl 1-pyrophosphate and inhibition by uridine triphosphate. J. Biochem. (Tokyo) **72**, 549—560 (1972 c)

Taube, R. A., Berlin, R. D.: Membrane transport of nucleosides in rabbit polymorphonuclear leukocytes. Biochim. biophys. Acta (Amst.) **255**, 6—18 (1972)

Tomizawa, S., Aronow, L.: Studies on drug resistance in mammalian cells. II. 6-Mercaptopurine resistance in mouse fibroblasts. J. pharmacol. exp. Ther. **128**, 107—114 (1960)

Tramell, P. R., Campbell, J. W.: Carbamyl phosphate synthesis in a land snail, *Strophocheilus oblongus*. J. biol. Chem. **245**, 6634—6641 (1970)

Umezu, K., Amaya, T., Yoshimoto, A., Tomita, K.: Purification and properties of orotidine-5′-phosphate pyrophosphorylase and orotidine-5′-phosphate decarboxylase from bakers' yeast. J. Biochem. (Tokyo) **70**, 249—262 (1971)

Valentine, W. N., Fink, K., Paglia, D. E., Harris, S. R., Adams, W. S.: Hereditary hemolytic anemia with human erythrocyte pyrimidine 5′-nucleotidase deficiency. J. clin. Invest. **54**, 866—879 (1974)

Weissman, S. M., Eisen, A. Z., Fallon, H., Lewis, M., Karon, M.: The metabolism of ring-labeled orotic acid in man. J. clin. Invest. **41**, 1546—1552 (1962)

Widnell, C. C., Unkeless, J. C.: Partial purification of a lipoprotein with 5′-nucleotidase activity from membranes of rat liver cells. Proc. nat. Acad. Sci. (Wash.) **61**, 1050—1057 (1968)

Williams, L. G., Bernhardt, S., Davis, R. H.: Copurification of pyrimidine-specific carbamyl phosphate synthetase and aspartate transcarbamylase of *Neurospora crassa*. Biochemistry **9**, 4329—4335 (1970)

Windmueller, H. G.: An orotic acid-induced, adenine-reversed inhibition of hepatic lipoprotein secretion in the rat. J. biol. Chem. **239**, 530—537 (1964)

Windmueller, H. G., Spaeth, A. E.: Stimulation of hepatic purine biosynthesis by orotic acid. J. biol. Chem. **240**, 4398—4405 (1965)

Wong, P. C. L., Murray, A. W.: 5-Phosphoribosyl pyrophosphate synthetase from Ehrlich ascites tumor cells. Biochemistry **8**, 1608—1614 (1969)

Wyngaarden, J. B., Ashton, D. M.: The regulation of activity of phosphoribosylpyrophosphate amidotransferase by purine ribonucleotides: a potential feedback control of purine biosynthesis. J. biol. Chem. **234**, 1492—1496 (1959)

Yin, H. H., Berlin, R. D.: The relation of endogenous adenosine cyclic 3′:5′-monophosphate to the antagonistic effects of adenosine and colchicine on cell shape. J. Cell Physiol. **85**, 627—634 (1975)

CHAPTER 7

Abnormalities of PRPP Metabolism Leading to an Overproduction of Uric Acid*

M. A. BECKER

A. Introduction

Abundant evidence has been presented in recent years indicating an important role for the intracellular concentration of 5-phosphoribosyl 1-pyrophosphate (PRPP)[1] in the regulation of the rate of purine nucleotide synthesis de novo. Extensive investigations of the effects of pharmacologic and genetic alterations in PRPP metabolism on human purine synthesis have been major sources of this evidence. In the present chapter, the metabolism of PRPP will be reviewed and particular emphasis will be given to determinants of PRPP synthesis and to genetically determined biochemical aberrations in which increased availability of PRPP leads to excessive purine nucleotide synthesis and thus uric acid overproduction in man.

B. Metabolism of PRPP

PRPP is an activated sugar phosphate that serves both as an intermediate in the synthesis of purine, pyrimidine, and pyridine nucleotides (KORNBERG et al., 1955) and as an allosteric regulator of the rate-limiting reaction in purine synthesis de novo (HOLMES et al., 1973a). Intracellular concentration of this compound is determined by the balance between the rate of PRPP production and the summed rates of the various reactions of PRPP utilization. Synthesis of PRPP involves transfer of the terminal pyrophosphate group of ATP to the C-1 carbon of ribose-5-P (KORNBERG et al., 1955) in a reaction catalyzed by the enzyme PRPP synthetase (E.C.2.7.6.1) (Fig. 1). The rate of intracellular PRPP production is subject to complex regulatory control effected in major part through diverse influences on the activity of PRPP synthetase which are discussed below.

I. Utilization of PRPP

PRPP is a substrate in several enzyme reactions by means of which its phosphoribosyl moiety is transferred to a nitrogenous base receptor on one or more of the naturally occurring or synthetic compounds listed in Table 1. These phosphoribo-

* The author acknowledges support from the Veterans Administration Research Service and from Grant AM-18197 from the National Institutes of Health.
[1] The abbreviations used in this chapter are: PRPP, 5-phosphoribosyl 1-pyrophosphate; ribose-5-P, ribose-5-phosphate; HGPRT, hypoxanthine-guanine phosphoribosyltransferase; APRT, adenine phosphoribosyltransferase; Pi, inorganic phosphate; G6PD, glucose-6-phosphate dehydrogenase; HEPES, 4-(2-hydroxyethyl)-1-piperazine ethanesulfonic acid; OPRT, orotate phosphoribosyltransferase.

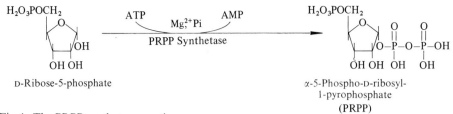

D-Ribose-5-phosphate → α-5-Phospho-D-ribosyl-1-pyrophosphate (PRPP)

Fig. 1. The PRPP synthetase reaction

Table 1. Phosphoribosyltransferase reactions using PRPP in mammalian tissues

Enzyme	Cosubstrates		Products
	Natural	Synthetic	
Amidophospho-ribosyltransferase (EC 2.4.2.14)	Glutamine Ammonia		Phosphorribosylamine Phosphoribosylamine
HGPRT (EC2.4.2.8)	Hypoxanthine Guanine Xanthine		IMP GMP XMP
		8-Azaguanine 6-Thioguanine 6-Mercapto-purine Allopurinol Oxipurinol	8-Aza-GMP 6-Thio-GMP 6-Mercaptopurine ribonucleotide Allopurinol-1-ribonucleotide Oxipurinol-1-ribonucleotide
APRT (EC 2.4.2.7)	Adenine Aminoimidazole-carboxamide		AMP Aminoimidazolecarboxamide ribotide
		2- or 8-azaadenine 2,6-Diamino-purine	2- or 8-aza-AMP 2,6-Diaminopurine ribonucleotide
OPRT (EC 2.4.2.10)	Orotate Uracil Cytosine Xanthine Uric acid		OMP UMP CMP N-3-(5′-phosphoribosyl)xanthine N-3-(5′-phosphoribosyl)uric acid
		Oxipurinol	Oxipurinol-7-ribonucleotide
Imidazoleacetate Phosphoribo-syltransferase (EC 6.3.4.a)	Imidazoleacetate		5′-Phosphoribosylimidazoleacetate
Nicotinate phosphoribo-syltransferase (EC 2.4.2.11)	Nicotinate		5′-Phosphoribosylnicotinate
Nicotinamide phosphoribosyl-transferase (EC 2.4.2.12)	Nicotinamide		5′-Phosphoribosylnicotinamide
Quinolinate phosphoribo-syltransferase (EC 2.4.2a)	Quinolinate		5′-Phosphoribosylquinolinate

syltransferase reactions constitute the major routes of PRPP utilization, although hydrolysis of PRPP by nonspecific phosphatases also occurs (FOX and MARCHANT, 1974). In the face of considerable competition for PRPP, the extent to which utilization of this compound is directed toward purine synthesis de novo is dictated by the concentration of PRPP, the relative and absolute affinities of the individual catabolizing enzymes for the compound, and the availability of co-substrates. The marked increases in intracellular PRPP concentrations, which accompany increased rates of purine synthesis de novo in cells severely deficient in HGPRT (ROSENBLOOM et al., 1968; WOOD et al., 1973a, b), imply that at least certain cells normally have high rates of PRPP utilization in this pathway of purine base salvage which are redirected toward purine synthesis de novo in this enzyme deficiency state. In contrast, the normal PRPP concentrations and rates of purine synthesis in cells deficient in APRT (HERSHFIELD et al., 1976) and OPRT suggest lower rates of PRPP utilization for nucleotide synthesis by these pathways in the normal cell. Despite the role of PRPP as a direct donor of the phosphoribosyl moiety of pyrimidine and pyridine nucleotides as well as purine nucleotides, major interest in PRPP as a regulatory intermediate has centered on purine nucleotide synthesis in which the alternative biosynthetic pathways share a common requirement for this compound.

In the pathway of purine nucleotide synthesis de novo, a series of 10 enzymatic reactions (see Chapter 1) is required for the incorporation of small molecule precursors of uric acid into a purine ring that is synthesized on a ribose phosphate backbone donated by PRPP in the initial reaction. This reaction, which involves the irreversible formation of 5-phosphoribosyl-1-amine, glutamate, and inorganic pyrophosphate from PRPP, glutamine, and water (HARTMAN and BUCHANAN, 1958) is catalyzed by amidophosphoribosyltransferase, an enzyme with regulatory properties that agree well with the proposed rate-determining role of this reaction in the pathway (WYNGAARDEN and ASHTON, 1959; CASKEY et al., 1964; HILL and BENNETT, 1969; WOOD and SEEGMILLER, 1973c; HOLMES et al., 1973a, b). The activity of human amidophosphoribosyltransferase is inhibited by purine nucleotides (WOOD and SEEGMILLER, 1973c; HOLMES, 1973a). This inhibition is antagonized by PRPP, a substrate whose usual intracellular concentrations are well below the Michaelis constant of the enzyme for this compound. The enzyme's substrate kinetics are converted from hyperbolic to sigmoidal in the presence of purine nucleotides (HOLMES et al., 1973a). Thus, PRPP is at once a potential rate-limiting substrate and an allosteric activator of amidophosphoribosyltransferase.

These regulatory effects on enzyme activity have their structural correlates in the actions of PRPP and purine nucleotides on the quaternary structure of amidophosphoribosyltransferase (see Chapter 2). A molecular model (HOLMES et al., 1973b) consistent with the large body of evidence (reviewed by BECKER and SEEGMILLER, 1974) suggesting antagonistic roles for the concentrations of PRPP and purine nucleotides in determining the rate of purine synthesis de novo has thus been provided.

In the alternate pathway of purine nucleotide synthesis, APRT and HGPRT catalyze single-step conversions of the purine bases adenine and hypoxanthine or guanine, respectively, to their mononucleotides by reaction with PRPP. Among factors likely to govern the reciprocol relationship between the rates of salvage and de novo pathways of purine synthesis, competition for the common substrate PRPP and inhibition by the purine nucleotide products common to the pathways would appear most important. The purine re-utilization pathway, which requires 1 mol of ATP (for PRPP synthesis)/mol of nucleotide product, represents a more economical source of purine nucleotides in terms of cellular energy expenditure than does its more complex counterpart, which requires 6 mol of ATP for the assembly of 1 mol of IMP. Seen in this light, preferential utilization of PRPP for purine salvage, which can be inferred from studies in human cells (WOOD et al., 1973 a) showing the purine phosphoribosyltransferases to have higher affinities and amidophosphoribosyltransferase to have lower affinity for PRPP, would seem highly appropriate.

II. Intracellular PRPP Concentration

Measurement of intracellular PRPP concentration has proved useful in establishing the biochemical correlates of genetic abnormalities of purine metabolism and in assessing the mechanisms of action of certain drugs and chemicals on the rate of purine synthesis. Although radiochemical methods have generally replaced spectrophotometric procedures (KORNBERG et al., 1955) for the assay of PRPP, all of the available assay procedures continue to utilize the reaction of PRPP with a purine or pyrimidine base in the presence of an excess of the appropriate endogenously or exogenously supplied phosphoribosyltransferase enzyme. Commonly employed isotopic procedures include: measurement of AMP formation from labeled adenine in the presence of APRT (HENDERSON and KHOO, 1965a); measurement of IMP formation from labeled hypoxanthine in the presence of HGPRT (HERSHKO et al., 1969); and measurement of $[^{14}CO_2]$ evolution from carboxyl-labeled orotate in the presence of both OPRT and orotidylic acid decarboxylase (KORNBERG et al., 1955).

Intracellular PRPP content has been determined under a variety of conditions in several mammalian cell types, including erythrocytes (GREENE and SEEGMILLER, 1969; FOX et al., 1970; SPERLING et al., 1972a; GORDON et al., 1974), leukocytes (BROSH et al., 1976), lymphocytes (WOOD et al., 1973c), liver (CLIFFORD et al., 1972; LALANNE and HENDERSON, 1974), cultured fibroblasts (ROSENBLOOM et al., 1968; ZOREF et al., 1975; BECKER, 1976a), lymphoblasts (WOOD et al., 1973a; NUKI et al., 1974), and neuroblastoma (WOOD et al., 1973b). Representative results are shown in Table 2. A twofold diurnal variation in PRPP concentration has been described in mouse liver (LALANNE and HENDERSON, 1975).

III. Determinants of PRPP Synthesis

1. PRPP Synthetase

PRPP synthetase catalyzes synthesis of PRPP from ATP (as a magnesium-ATP complex) and ribose-5-P in a reaction dependent upon P_i and Mg^{2+} (Fig. 1). The reaction appears to follow an ordered Bi Bi mechanism with ribose-5-P, the first substrate bound by the human enzyme and PRPP the last product released (FOX and KELLEY, 1972). For PRPP synthetase from S. typhimurium, the order of substrate binding is reversed, although the reaction mechanism is of a similar type (SWITZER, 1971).

The role of the reaction product PRPP as a determinant of the rate of purine synthesis de novo (see below) and the marked disparity between the catalytic capacity of this enzyme and the actual rate of intracellular PRPP formation (HERSHKO et

Table 2. Intracellular PRPP content in mammalian cells

Species	Cell type	PRPP content	Approximate PRPP concentration (μM)
Human	Erythrocyte	1.5–7.0 nmol/ml packed cells	2–7
	Fibroblast[b]	0.23–0.55 nmol/10⁶ cells	
		0.05–0.28 nmol/mg protein	4–15
	Lymphocyte	8–13 pmol/10⁶ cells	—
	Leukocyte	2.0–5.5 nmol/ml packed cells	—
	Lymphoblast[b]	10–15 pmol/10⁶ cells	—
Rat	Liver	—	8–11
Mouse	Liver	50–100 nmol/g wet weight	14.5–29
	Neuroblastoma[b]	76 pmol/10⁶ cells	

[a] Values are representative of those stated in references given in text; measurements were made under a variety of conditions of preparation and used several different assay procedures.
[b] Cultured cells.

al., 1969) make intracellular control of PRPP synthetase activity seem likely. In fact, studies of PRPP production by intact cells (HERSHKO et al., 1969; BAGNARA et al., 1974), as well as detailed kinetic analyses of preparations of the enzyme purified from microbial (SWITZER, 1969, 1971; SWITZER and SOGIN, 1973) and mammalian (FOX and KELLEY, 1972; BECKER et al., 1975; ROTH et al., 1974; ROTH and DEUEL, 1974; WONG and MURRAY, 1969) sources, show that PRPP synthetase activity is influenced by a wide array of compounds, including inhibitors, activators, and products as well as substrates.

2. Substrates

Among naturally occurring nucleoside triphosphates, only ATP and dATP (which serve equally well) are substrates for mammalian PRPP synthetases (WONG and MURRAY, 1969; FOX and KELLEY, 1971a; ROTH et al., 1974); Michaelis constants (K_m) of PRPP synthetase for MgATP range from $1.4 \times 10^{-5} M$ for the purified human erythrocyte enzyme (FOX and KELLEY, 1972) to $2.2 \times 10^{-4} M$ for the purified rat liver enzyme (ROTH et al., 1974). PRPP synthetase also shows a high degree of specificity for ribose-5-P as the pyrophosphate acceptor, although ribulose-5-phosphate may be a substrate for the human erythrocyte enzyme. Apparent K_m values for ribose-5-P range from $3.3 \times 10^{-5} M$ to $2.9 \times 10^{-4} M$ (Fox and KELLEY, 1972; ROTH et al., 1974).

In the presence of an excess of Mg^{2+}, the initial velocity of PRPP synthetase reactions shows hyperbolic responses to increasing concentrations of both MgATP and ribose-5-P (WONG and MURRAY, 1969; FOX and KELLEY, 1972; ROTH et al., 1974; BECKER et al., 1975). A sigmoidal relationship between MgATP concentration and initial velocity was observed, however, when rat liver PRPP synthetase was studied with ATP in excess of Mg^{2+} or at equimolar concentrations of each (ROTH et al., 1974). The significance of this finding with respect to the activity of the enzyme in the cell is uncertain, but the importance of Mg^{2+} as well as MgATP as a determinant

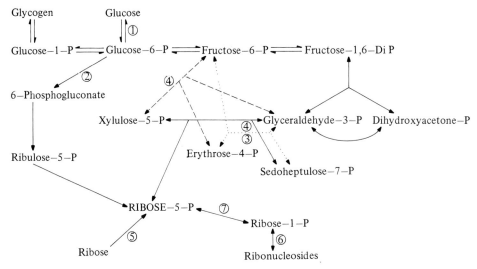

Fig. 2. Pathways of ribose-5-P biosynthesis. The enzyme activities catalyzing the numbered reactions are: 1) glucose-6-phosphatase; 2) glucose-6-phosphate dehydrogenase; 3) transaldolase; 4) transketolase; 5) ribokinase; 6) nucleoside phosphorylase; 7) phosphoribomutase

of catalytic activity is highlighted. Michaelis constants of mammalian PRPP synthetases for MgATP are substantially lower than intracellular ATP concentrations, implying the likelihood of saturation of the enzyme with this substrate under normal circumstances. However, alterations in the distribution of free and bound Mg^{2+}, the presence of significant concentrations of the competitive inhibitor ADP, and perhaps effects on the conformation of the enzyme resulting from the binding of ligands at distant sites are all factors that may alter the interaction of MgATP with the enzyme and thus affect the enzyme reaction in the cell.

Sources of intracellular ribose-5-P (Fig. 2) include: the oxidative and nonoxidative pentose phosphate pathways; the phosphorolysis of purine and pyrimidine nucleosides with production of ribose-1-phosphate, followed by conversion of this compound to ribose-5-P in the phosphoribomutase reaction; and (potentially) the direct conversion of ribose to ribose-5-P in a reaction with ATP catalyzed by ribokinase. Of these, the conversion of sugar phosphates by means of the pentose phosphate pathways constitutes the major source of ribose-5-P production. The oxidative pentose phosphate pathway is a sequence of reactions initiated by conversion of glucose-6-phosphate to 6-phosphogluconate in a reaction catalyzed by G6PD and accompanied by generation of NADPH. The rate of operation of this pathway is dependent in part upon the regulation of G6PD activity by the ratio of [NADPH]/[NADP] (KREBS and EGGLESTON, 1974). In such tissues as liver, adrenal cortex, adipose tissue, and leukocytes, the oxidative pathway is very active and contributes in major proportion to the utilization of glucose and the production of ribose-5-P. In the nonoxidative pentose phosphate pathway, conversion of fructose-6-phosphate and glyceraldehyde-3-phosphate to ribose-5-P occurs in a series of reactions including transaldolase and transketolase reactions which involve erythrose-4-phosphate, sedoheptulose-7-phosphate, and xylulose-5-phosphate as intermediates. This anaerobic pathway contributes in varying degrees in different tissues to the generation of ribose-5-P either in conjunction with the oxidative pathway or, as in the case of striated muscle, exclusive of it.

Although only a small proportion of the ribose-5-P generated by the pentose phosphate pathway is ordinarily converted to PRPP (KATZ and ROGNSTAD, 1967), intracellular steady-state concentrations of ribose-5-P appear to be below or near the Michaelis constant of PRPP synthetase for this compound (BECKER, 1976b). In the face of these findings, assignment to ribose-5-P of a primary role in governing the rate of intracellular PRPP production remains a controversial matter. Nevertheless, support for such a role is provided by a number of studies that report or imply stimulation of PRPP synthesis under circumstances in which ribose-5-P availability is increased either through acceleration of the oxidative pentose phosphate pathway or through increased rates of nucleoside phosphorolysis. Thus, glucose, fructose, and galactose stimulate the phosphogluconate oxidation pathway in bacteria (LOVE and GOTS, 1955) and in mammalian cells in culture (HARRINGTON, 1958; HENDERSON and KHOO, 1965a), an effect accompanied by increased PRPP production and purine synthetic rates; methylene blue, an artificial election acceptor that stimulates the oxidative pathway by accelerating NADPH oxidation (BRIN and YONEMOTO, 1958), increases ribose-5-P and PRPP synthesis in human erythrocytes (HERSHKO et al., 1969) and fibroblasts (KELLEY et al., 1970a; BECKER, 1976b) as well as Ehrlich ascites tumor cells (HENDERSON and KHOO, 1965a); thyroid stimulating hormone (LINDSAY et al., 1969) and adrenocorticotropic hormone (McKERNS, 1969), which stimulate G6PD in bovine thyroid slices and adrenal homogenates respectively, also increase nucleotide synthesis and conversion of orotate to uridylate, presumably through increased PRPP production; and, finally, nucleosides such as inosine increase ribose-5-P and PRPP concentrations in Ehrlich ascites tumor cells (HENDERSON and KHOO, 1965b) and human fibroblasts (BECKER, 1976b) by direct donation of the ribose moiety of the nucleoside to PRPP through ribose-phosphate intermediates.

In contrast to these observations, other studies have reported that increases in PRPP synthesis in response to measured or presumed increases in ribose-5-P concentrations are dependent on the P_i concentration of the incubation medium and fail to occur at physiologic extracellular P_i concentrations. As a result of these studies in human erythrocytes (HERSHKO et al., 1969), and peripheral blood leukocytes (BROSH et al., 1976), and in rat liver slices (BOER et al., 1976), P_i has been postulated (HERSHKO et al., 1969) to exert primary control over PRPP synthetase catalytic activity with rate-limiting control by ribose-5-P being manifested only at optimal P_i concentrations. Resolution of the role of ribose-5-P in the control or PRPP synthetase will be of great interest, since as will be described later, increased ribose-5-P availability as the basis of increased PRPP generation and concomitant excessive purine nucleotide synthesis is an attractive mechanism to explain the uric acid overproduction of certain individuals.

3. Inhibitors

Inhibitors of mammalian PP-ribose-P synthetases include: purine pyrimidine and pyridine nucleotides (FOX and KELLEY, 1972; ROTH and DEUEL, 1974; WONG and

MURRAY, 1969); 2,3-diphosphoglycerate (FOX and KELLEY, 1972; BECKER et al., 1975); and the reaction products PRPP and AMP (FOX and KELLEY, 1972). The kinetics of inhibition of the PRPP synthetase reaction by these compounds indicate at least three separable sites of interaction between the enzyme and its various inhibitors (FOX and KELLEY, 1972). ADP, which is the most potent inhibitor of the enzyme, is a competitive inhibitor of PRPP synthetase with respect to the substrate MgATP (FOX and KELLEY, 1972; ROTH and DEUEL, 1974; WONG and MURRAY, 1969). For the human erythrocyte enzyme, the inhibition constant (K_i) for ADP (0.01 mM) is below the prevailing intracellular ADP concentration, suggesting a potential physiologic role for the competitive interaction of adenylates in controlling enzyme activity. On the basis of similar observations in $E.\ coli$, ATKINSON and FALL (1967) have postulated that PRPP synthetase activity is regulated in part by cellular "energy charge," and studies of the enzyme from Ehrlich ascites tumor cells (WONG and MURRAY, 1969), rat liver (ROTH and DEUEL, 1974), and human erythrocytes (FOX and KELLEY, 1972) are consistent with this concept. In the presence of ADP, inhibition of PRPP synthetase activity is accompanied by a change from a hyperbolic to a sigmoidal function of the curve relating P_i concentration to reaction velocity (HERSHKO et al., 1969). This relationship suggests the possibility of an allosteric interaction involving the enzyme, P_i, and ADP.

Both 2,3-diphosphoglycerate and the reaction product PRPP inhibit erythrocyte PRPP synthetase by a mechanism that is competitive with respect to ribose-5-P (FOX and KELLEY, 1972), thus revealing a second site of potential regulation of enzyme activity. Since for the human enzyme the inhibition constant (K_i) for PRPP is substantially higher than the intracellular concentration of this compound, inhibition by PRPP of its own synthesis is unlikely to be important under normal circumstances. On the other hand, the K_i for 2,3-diphosphoglycerate, 5.3 mM (FOX and KELLEY, 1972) is comparable to the concentration of this compound in the erythrocyte, indicating that competition between ribose-5-P and 2,3-diphosphoglycerate may play a role in the control of PRPP synthetase activity. Such a formulation might also predict that PRPP synthesis in the erythrocyte is dependent on changes in state of hemoglobin oxygenation that are accompanied by changes in intracellular concentrations of free 2,3-diphosphoglycerate, free magnesium, and (to a lesser degree) MgATP (BUNN et al., 1971), all important effectors of PRPP synthetase activity.

Inhibitors of human PRPP synthetase exclusive of ADP, PRPP, and 2,3-diphosphoglycerate exhibit a mechanism of inhibition that is noncompetitive with respect to both substrates (FOX and KELLEY, 1972). These compounds include the reaction product AMP as well as pyridine nucleotides and certain mono-, di-, and triphosphates of purine and pyrimidine nucleosides. The relatively high inhibitory constants for these inhibitors, the failure of combinations of these compounds to inhibit PRPP synthetase synergistically, and the increasing enzyme inhibition observed with unphysiologically high inhibitor concentrations have led to the postulation of the mechanism of "heterogeneous metabolic pool inhibition" (STADTMAN, 1970) directed at a third site on the enzyme to explain these observations (FOX and KELLEY, 1972). While a similar type of inhibition has been described for PRPP synthetase from $S.\ typhimurium$ (SWITZER, 1971), studies of rat liver PRPP synthetase (ROTH and DEUEL, 1974b) have shown the enzyme to be inhibited by a much more restricted range of compounds. In fact, under conditions in which rat liver PRPP synthetase is "stabilized" by the presence of EDTA and albumin, neither "heterogeneous metabolic pool inhibition" nor inhibition by 2,3-diphosphoglycerate was observed.

4. Activators

Although activation of mammalian PRPP synthetases by Mg^{2+}, P_i, and cyclic GMP has been described, the mechanisms of activation by these compounds are, in general, less well appreciated than is the case for the enzyme inhibitors. Divalent cation is an absolute requirement for PRPP synthetase activity, and Mg^{2+} is the most effective divalent cation in fulfilling this requirement (Fox and KELLEY, 1971a; WONG and MURRAY, 1969). Since the effects of Mg^{2+} on PRPP synthetase are rather complicated, however, this compound might be regarded as an activator as well as a cofactor. Initial velocity studies with Mg^{2+} showed that this cation binds sequentially to both human (Fox and KELLEY, 1972) and bacterial (SWITZER, 1971) PRPP synthetases independently of the formation of the MgATP substrate complex. The site of this sequential binding of magnesium to the enzyme is unknown, but, as will be described below, the effects of Mg^{2+} on PRPP synthetase quaternary structure are consistent with a potential activating role for this metal ion.

The presence of P_i is also an essential requirement for expression of PRPP synthetase activity (HERSHKO et al., 1969; Fox and KELLEY, 1971a; ROTH et al., 1974; WONG and MURRAY, 1969). Replacement of P_i by dialysis of enzyme preparations against buffers containing Tris-HCl or HEPES results in no major loss of enzyme activity as long as the enzyme is subsequently assayed in the presence of P_i (ROTH et al., 1974). Stimulation of enzyme activity is dramatic, extends over a wide range of P_i concentrations and is maximal at concentrations (varying from 10–100 mM, depending on the source of the enzyme) well above those generally regarded as physiologic (approximately 0.5–1.5 mM). The P_i activation curves of purified mammalian PRPP synthetases are hyperbolic. Addition of ADP to the human erythrocyte enzyme results, however, in a change in the P_i activation curve to a sigmoid function (HERSHKO et al., 1969). Although the mechanism of activation of PRPP synthetase by P_i is presently unknown, studies of PRPP generation in intact erythrocytes suggest a primary role for P_i in governing the intracellular catalytic activity of the enzyme and thus the rate of PRPP synthesis (HERSHKO et al., 1969).

Stimulation of the activity of rat hepatoma tissue culture (HTC) cell PRPP synthetase by cyclic GMP is accompanied by an increase in the apparent affinity of the enzyme for the substrate ATP (GREEN and MARTIN, 1974). This interesting phenomenon has not been observed in the purified human erythrocyte enzyme.

The foregoing discussion of inhibitors and activators of PRPP synthetase has suggested a variety of mechanisms for the regulation of the activity of this enzyme. Definitive proof of the operation in vivo of all these mechanisms has not yet been provided. However, mutant forms of human (SPERLING et al., 1973; ZOREF et al., 1975) and rat hepatoma cell (GREEN and MARTIN 1973, 1974) PRPP synthetase have been identified, in which diminished responsiveness of the aberrant enzymes to one or more inhibitor or activator is associated with increased enzyme activity, increased PRPP production, and excessive rates of purine nucleotide synthesis. Thus it seems that regulation of PRPP synthetase activity by small molecule effectors is functionally significant in the intact cell.

5. Structure and Activity of PRPP Synthetase

The relationship between the structure and activity of human erythrocyte PRPP synthetase has been studied (Fox and KELLEY, 1971a; BECKER et al., 1977) and provides a plausible molecular model for control of enzyme activity by certain of the effectors discussed above. Analyses of preparations of this enzyme, purified to electrophoretic and ultracentrifugal homogeneity, show that PRPP synthetase is composed of a single polypeptide subunit of molecular weight 33 200 (BECKER et al., 1977) that undergoes reversible enzyme concentration-dependent and ligand-mediated self-association to a number of polymeric states (Fox and KELLEY, 1971a; BECKER et al., 1977). Aggregated forms of PRPP synthetase containing 2, 4, 8, 16, and 32 subunits have been identified by gel filtration and sucrose density gradient ultracentrifugation studies carried out in the presence of various effectors.

Association of subunits to aggregates containing 16 and 32 subunits results from incubation of the enzyme with any one or combination of the following effectors in the presence of P_i: MgATP, Mg^{2+}, purine nucleotide inhibitors of enzyme activity and reaction products. In the presence of any given effector combination, increasing enzyme concentration favors more extensive subunit self-association. Neither P_i nor ribose-5-P alone or in combination alters the state of subunit association, but 2,3-diphosphoglycerate dissociates the enzyme to forms as small as the monomer and antagonizes subunit aggregation in response to MgATP or Mg^{2+} (BECKER et al., 1977).

The reversible effects of these compounds on the quaternary structure of PRPP synthetase take on potential regulatory significance in light of the establishment of a definite relationship between enzyme activity and state of subunit association. The largest aggregated forms of the enzyme, composed of 16 and 32 subunits are fully active, while the monomeric and smaller aggregated forms of PRPP synthetase containing 2, 4, and 8 subunits show minimal or no enzymatic activity (less than 4% of the activity of the larger forms per mole of subunit) (MEYER and BECKER, 1977). These findings confirm the suggestion, based on considerations of enzyme stability and on intracellular ATP and Mg^{2+} concentrations, that the activity of PRPP synthetase in cells resides in the largest aggregates (Fox and KELLEY, 1971a).

Some interesting possibilities concerning the structural basis of regulation of PRPP synthetase activity are suggested by these findings. For instance, the inhibitory effects of 2,3-diphosphoglycerate on enzyme activity might be mediated by dissociation of the enzyme into smaller inactive forms in response either to increases in concentration of this effector or to decreases in ribose-5-P availability. On the other hand, the inhibitory effects of purine nucleotides appear to result from direct inactivation of the larger enzyme aggregates rather than from interference with the process of aggregation itself. Thus, rather than altering enzyme quaternary structure, these compounds are likely to exert their inhibitory effects either through direct competition for substrate binding sites (ADP) or through changes in enzyme conformation at the level of secondary or tertiary protein structure (noncompetitive nucleotide inhibitors). The kinetically separable sites of enzyme-inhibitor interaction discussed earlier (Fox and KELLEY, 1972) may have their disparate structural correlates in these proposed effects. While the subunit aggregating effect of Mg^{2+} might be related to its role in enzyme activation, a structural basis for the stimulation of enzyme activity by

P_i has not been revealed. Potentiation by P_i of subunit association in response to MgATP or Mg^{2+} is of far lesser magnitude than the stimulation of enzyme activity by comparable concentrations of P_i (BECKER et al., 1977).

6. Control of the Amount of PRPP Synthetase

In *S. typhimurium*, synthesis of PRPP synthetase is repressed by uridine nucleotides (OSLZOWY and SWITZER, 1972). Neither purine nucleotides nor other pyrimidine nucleotides exhibit this effect. No conclusive information is available concerning the effects of specific metabolites on the rates of synthesis and degradation of mammalian PRPP synthetases. Nevertheless, in human fibroblasts in culture, specific enzyme activities of PRPP synthetase show a roughly inverse relationship with cell density. When cultures reach a confluent state, relatively constant specific enzyme activities from one half to one fourth those of nonconfluent cultures are found (MARTIN and MALER, 1976; BECKER, unpublished). By means of immunochemical inactivation studies using specific antiserum to the enzyme, these variations in specific enzyme activity have been shown to reflect corresponding variations in the amount of PRPP synthetase protein.

A second example suggesting control of the amount of PRPP synthetase in mammalian cells has been found in the case of deficiency of a specific erythrocyte pyrimidine nucleotidase that results in a hemolytic anemia characterized by high concentrations of erythrocyte pyrimidine nucleotides (VALENTINE et al., 1972, 1974). In erythrocytes from affected individuals, activity of PRPP synthetase is approximately 30% of that found in normal erythrocytes of comparable age. This mild deficiency of PRPP synthetase activity appears, from antibody inactivation studies, to result from a corresponding decrease in PRPP synthetase protein (BECKER, unpublished). Whether it is the rate of PRPP synthetase production or its rate of degradation that is altered in the above cases is not yet known.

Recently, increased activity of PRPP synthetase has been reported in mutagenized rat hepatoma cells (GRAF et al., 1976) and in human fibroblasts (MARTIN and MALER, 1976) deficient in HGPRT activity. Increased amounts of structurally normal PRPP synthetase appear to account for these findings. As a result MARTIN and associates have proposed that the HGPRT locus regulates the rate of production of PRPP synthetase in addition to serving as the structural gene for HGPRT.

Increased PRPP synthetase activity has not been found in HGPRT-deficient erythrocytes (BECKER et al., 1973a) or, for that matter, in HGPRT-deficient fibroblasts (BECKER, 1976a) lymphoblasts (WOOD et al., 1973a) or neuroblastoma (WOOD et al., 1973b) by other investigators who have, in addition, found no evidence for increased PRPP production in these cells (ROSENBLOOM et al., 1968; BECKER, 1976a). The reason for these discrepancies are unclear. Resolution of this problem is of importance, since increased PRPP synthetase activity could account, at least in part, for the elevated PRPP concentrations in HGPRT-deficient cells that have previously been ascribed to diminished PRPP utilization (see below).

C. PRPP Availability and the Rate of Purine Synthesis De Novo

A wide array of investigations support the concept of PRPP availability as a determinant of the rate of purine synthesis de novo in man. For convenience in this discussion, these studies can be broadly classified into three groups: 1) studies of amido-phosphoribosyltransferase and the interaction of effectors on this allosterically regulated enzyme: 2) studies of the actions of certain pharmacologic and chemical agents on PRPP concentrations and purine synthetic rates; 3) studies of PRPP metabolism in individuals with excessive uric acid production and in their cells in tissue culture.

I. Studies of Amidophosphoribosyltransferase and Its Effectors

As mentioned previously, in vitro studies of human amidophosphoribosyltransferase (HOLMES et al., 1973a, b) have provided a structural model for the antagonism of PRPP and purine nucleotides in influencing the rate of purine synthesis de novo. The sigmoidal response of amidophosphoribosyltransferase to increasing concentrations of PRPP in the presence of purine nucleotide inhibitors indicates that within a range of concentrations of PRPP subsaturating for the enzyme, PRPP acts as an allosteric activator. Thus, if intracellular PRPP concentrations are within the lower range of the substrate-velocity curve for this effector, small increments in PRPP concentration should result in disproportionately greater stimulation of enzyme activity and, as a consequence, of purine nucleotide synthetic rate. In two studies, the concentrations of PRPP at which the velocity of the human amidophosphoribosyltransferase reaction was half maximal were found to be 0.25 and 0.48 mM (WOOD and SEEGMILLER, 1973; HOLMES et al., 1973a), concentrations well above the prevailing intracellular PRPP concentrations determined in normal human erythrocytes, fibroblasts, and lymphoblasts, and rodent neuroblastoma and liver (Table 2). On the other hand, as will be detailed below, PRPP concentrations are increased in cells from individuals with either excessive PRPP synthetase activity or HGPRT deficiency, and the excessive purine synthetic rates observed in these cells appear to be explainable in terms of the consequent activation of amidophosphoribosyltransferase.

II. Effects of Pharmacologic Agents on PRPP Concentration and Purine Synthetic Rate

A variety of pharmacologic and chemical agents that either utilize or increase the generation of PRPP produce corresponding alterations in the rate of purine synthesis in man. Administration of allopurinol (FOX et al., 1970; YÜ and GUTMAN, 1964), adenine (SCHULMAN et al., 1971; SEEGMILLER et al., 1968), orotic acid (KELLEY et al., 1970c), or imidazoleacetic acid (BECKER and SEEGMILLER, unpublished) to volunteers results in diminished erythrocyte PRPP concentrations and is accompanied by decreases in purine synthetic rates as measured either by daily urinary purine excretion or by the rate of labeled glycine incorporation into urinary uric acid. In addition, incubation of cultured human fibroblasts with adenine (FOX and KELLEY, 1971b), orotic acid (KELLEY et al., 1970b), or nicotinic acid (BOYLE et al., 1972) results in diminution in both PRPP concentrations and rates of purine synthesis de novo. Conversely, administration of the experimental antitumor agent 2-ethylamino-1,3,4-thiadiazole to human subjects results in a marked stimulation of the rate of labeled glycine incorporation into purine compounds, including uric acid (SEEGMILLER et al., 1963); increased hepatic PRPP concentration, which has been demonstrated in mice receiving this drug (LALANNE and HENDERSON, 1975) provides a likely basis for this stimulation, although the mechanism responsible for the elevated PRPP level is unknown. Finally, as discussed earlier, incubation of cultured fibroblasts with methylene blue results in increased PRPP concentrations, which is accompanied by increased rates of purine synthesis de novo (KELLEY et al., 1970a; BECKER, 1976b).

D. Studies of PRPP Metabolism in Uric Acid Overproducers Without Recognized Enzyme Defects

Study of cells of individuals with gout and excessive uric acid production due to enzyme defects such as HGPRT deficiency or excessive PRPP synthetase activity has confirmed that increased PRPP availability is one type of aberration in the normal regulatory mechanism that can result in excessive purine synthesis. Nevertheless, only a minority of patients with purine overproduction have presently identifiable enzyme abnormalities (BECKER and SEEGMILLER, 1974); in the great majority of patients with primary gout and purine overproduction, a causal relationship between increased PRPP availability and excessive purine nucleotide synthesis is much less clear. Prior to a discussion of the well-defined or proposed specific enzyme defects resulting in abnormal PRPP metabolism, therefore, the more limited evidence for increased PRPP availability in primary gout warrants mention.

Direct evidence for abnormal PRPP metabolism in at least some patients with gout and excessive uric acid excretion was first presented by JONES et al. (1962), who administered [^{14}C] glucose and imidazoleacetic acid to seven normal individuals and nine patients with gout. Increased rates of *PRPP turnover*, indicated by higher specific activities and rates of incorporation of label into the ribose moiety of imidazoleacetic acid ribonucleoside, were shown by only the three patients with gout and urinary excretion greater than 600 mg uric acid/day. Subsequent studies from Israel reported increased *PRPP generation* in the erythrocytes of some patients with primary gout (HERSHKO et al., 1968) and excessive uric acid excretion (SPERLING et al., 1971). In these studies, however, considerable overlap in the incorporation of labeled purine bases into erythrocyte nucleotides was observed between gouty overproducers and normal controls; in fact, the mean values for PRPP generation assessed in this manner were strongly influenced by a small number of extremely high values. In addition, increased PRPP generation in the erythrocytes of patients with primary gout has not been a usual finding in studies reported from the United States (MEYSKENS and WILLIAMS, 1971; FOX and KELLEY, 1971b). Still other studies have shown increased *PRPP concentrations* in cultured fibroblasts from certain patients with uric acid overproduction (HENDERSON et al., 1968). The later identification of partial HGPRT deficiency (KELLEY et al., 1967) or excessive PRPP synthetase activity (SPERLING et al., 1972b; BECKER, 1973b, 1976a) among certain of the patients described in these studies explains some of the above findings.

It appears clear, however, that abnormalities in PRPP concentration and generation do occur in the cells of at least some uric acid overproducers in whom HGPRT and PRPP synthetase activities are grossly normal. In a recent study (BECKER, 1976a) in which PRPP concentration and generation and ribose-5-P concentration were determined in fibroblasts derived from seven such individuals, PRPP concentration was increased in all strains, and PRPP generation was increased in five of the seven.

Table 3. Proposed classification of abnormalities associated with excessive purine production

Subgroup	PP-ribose P		Ribose-5-phosphate concentration	Example of associated enzyme abnormality
	Concentration	Generation		
1	Increased	Increased	Increased	Glucose-6-phosphatase deficiency[a]
2	Increased	Increased	Normal or decreased	Increased PP-ribose-P synthetase activity
3	Increased	Normal	Normal	Hypoxanthine-guanine phosphoribosyltransferase deficiency
4	Normal or decreased	Increased	Normal	Feedback resistant PP-ribose-P aminotransferase[a]

[a] Association of enzyme abnormality with pattern of PP-ribose-P and ribose-5-P determinations proposed but not yet demonstrated. Reproduced from Becker (1976a) by permission of The Journal of Clinical Investigation.

In studies directed by the results of these three measurements (Table 3), two of these individuals were found to have an enzyme with altered kinetic characteristics (one in HGPRT, another in PRPP synthetase) to explain their abnormal PRPP metabolism; in three others with normal ribose-5-P concentrations, patterns of PRPP generation resembled those found in cells from individuals with these enzyme defects. The fibroblasts from the two additional patients showed increased ribose-5-P concentrations. The possibility that purine overproduction in the latter two individuals was a consequence of increased ribose-5-P availability, leading to increased PRPP generation and concentration was suggested. The basis of the increased ribose-5-P concentration in these cells is as yet unknown, but the possibility of a defect in the pentose phosphate pathways is under investigation.

Another point made in this study was the apparent superiority of fibroblast PRPP determinations compared with those made in erythrocytes in distinguishing normal and overproducer populations. Although the overall correlation between erythrocyte and fibroblast PRPP determinations was excellent ($r = 0.92$), erythrocyte PRPP values were within 2 SD of the normal mean in two of the six patients in whom the determination was made, while fibroblast PRPP values in all seven patients were more than 2 SD above the normal fibroblast mean value. The poorer resolution between normal and abnormal populations afforded by erythrocyte PRPP determinations may in part explain the reported low frequency of increased erythrocyte PRPP concentrations among patients with primary gout and uric acid overproduction (Fox and Kelley, 1971b; Greene and Seegmiller, 1969; Becker, 1973a). It may also explain the occasional reports of male patients with purine overproduction, partial deficiency of HGPRT, and normal erythrocyte PRPP concentration (Greene and Seegmiller, 1969; Sperling et al., 1972a).

In summary, abnormalities in PRPP turnover, generation, and concentration have been described among patients with primary gout and uric acid overproduction. The frequency of these abnormalities and the extent to which they contribute to the disordered rates of purine synthesis are not yet as clearly understood as in the case of certain specific enzyme abnormalities that lead to altered PRPP metabolism and to which attention will now be directed.

Table 4. Proposed enzyme abnormalities in man in which alterations in PRPP metabolism result in excessive purine production

Mechanism	Enzyme abnormality	Mode of inheritance
Increased PRPP production	Excessive PRPP synthetase activity	Possibly X-linked recessive
	Glucose-6-phosphatase deficiency (type-1 glycogen storage disease)	Autosomal recessive
	Increased glutathione reductase activity	Autosomal dominant
Decreased PRPP utilization	Severe HGPRT deficiency (Lesch-Nyhan syndrome)	X-linked recessive
	Partial HGPRT deficiency	X-linked recessive
	Purine nucleoside phosphorylase deficiency	Autosomal recessive

E. PRPP Metabolism in Enzyme Defects Associated with Uric Acid Overproduction

Increased availability of PRPP for purine synthesis de novo could presumably result from either increased PRPP production or diminished PRPP use in alternative reactions. Among the inborn metabolic errors associated with excessive uric acid production, both mechanisms appear to be represented: increased production in excessive PRPP synthetase activity, and decreased use in HGPRT deficiency. In addition to these extensively studied enzyme abnormalities, altered PRPP generation or use has been suggested (although not established) as a contributing factor in the development of gout in individuals with several other enzyme defects. Table 4 lists, according to the likely mechanism, those enzyme abnormalities in which deranged PRPP metabolism has been proposed or established as the basis for purine overproduction.

I. Increased PRPP Production

An increased rate of PRPP generation has been proposed as the mechanism leading to uric acid overproduction in three enzyme abnormalities associated with gout. This mechanism has been conclusively demonstrated only in the case of excessive PRPP synthetase activity. There is conflicting evidence (discussed previously) concerning the role of ribose-5-P concentration in the control of intracellular PRPP synthesis. Nevertheless, demonstration of increased ribose-5-P concentration in the fibroblasts of two patients with increased rates of PRPP and purine synthesis (BECKER, 1976a) reinforces the view that any disorder leading to increased ribose-5-P availability could potentially result in increased PRPP generation and purine overproduction. Indeed, increased activity of the oxidative pentose phosphate pathway with consequent excessive ribose-5-P and thus PRPP generation has been hypothesized to underlie uric acid overproduction in glucose-6-phosphatase deficiency (ALEPA et al., 1967; KELLEY et al., 1968a). A similar scheme for the association of gout with a variant form of glutathione reductase that has increased enzyme activity has been proposed (LONG, 1970), although in this enzyme abnormality evidence for purine overproduction has not been presented.

1. Excessive PRPP Synthetase Activity

Detailed studies of three families in which affected members have structurally altered and overactive PRPP synthetases in conjunction with marked purine overproduction have clearly established the relationship between excessive PRPP production and the rate of purine synthesis de novo. Increased PRPP synthetase activity was first described by SPERLING and associates (1972 b) in erythrocyte lysates from one of two brothers with gouty arthritis, uric acid urolithiasis, dramatic uric acid overexcretion (2200–2400 mg/day), and excessive erythrocyte PRPP concentration and rate of synthesis (SPERLING et al., 1972 c). PRPP synthetase from the affected patient demonstrated increased activity only at P_i concentrations below 2 mM (Fig. 3 A), and subsequent kinetic studies showed a normal maximal velocity and normal affinities for P_i, ATP, and ribose-5-P in partially purified preparations of the enzyme (SPERLING et al., 1973). The structural basis for the abnormally active enzyme was revealed, however, by experiments in which the sensitivity of the mutant enzyme to inhibition by purine nucleotides and 2,3-diphosphoglycerate was shown to be significantly reduced (SPERLING et al., 1973).

Fibroblasts cultured from this patient were subsequently shown to have increased PRPP concentration, and generation and a PRPP synthetase specific enzyme activity more stikingly increased at 1.6 mM than at 50 mM P_i (ZOREF et al., 1975). In addition, these cells demonstrated a 3-fold increased incorporation of [^{14}C] formate into intracellular nucleotides and a 15-fold increased rate of labeled purine excretion into the incubation medium. The decreased sensitivity of the PRPP synthetase of this patient to feedback inhibition of enzyme activity by purine nucleotides was also confirmed in the fibroblasts. These findings are consistent with the following sequence of abnormalities suggested by SPERLING and associates (ZOREF et al., 1975) to relate the excessively active enzyme in this family to their uric acid overproduction: feedback-resistance of PRPP synthetase; superactivity of the enzyme under physiologic conditions; increased PRPP generation and concentration; and increased rate of purine synthesis de novo.

A second and different structural alteration in PRPP synthetase has been described in two brothers with gout and uric acid overproduction (BECKER et al., 1973 a, b, c). In these individuals, in whom the rate of [^{14}C] glycine incorporation into urinary uric acid was 3–5-fold greater than normal, erythrocyte and fibroblast PRPP synthetase activities exceeded normal mean values by 2.5–3-fold at all concentrations of P_i (Fig. 3 B). Increased PRPP concentrations and rates of PRPP generation in these cell types and increased purine synthetic rates in the fibroblasts were demonstrated and attested to the functional significance of the excessive enzyme activity in the intact cell.

PRPP synthetase from affected members of this family was electrophoretically distinct from the normal enzyme with an isoelectric point of 4.85, compared to 5.10 for the normal enzyme (BECKER et al., 1975). While the homogeneously purified mutant enzyme showed normal affinity constants for the substrates and Mg^{2+} and inhibitory constants for ADP, GDP, AMP, and 2,3-diphosphoglycerate, the maximal velocity (Vmax) of the enzyme was elevated 2.2-fold. On the basis of antibody inactivation, quantitative precipitin, and immunodiffusion studies using rabbit antiserum developed to purified normal PRPP synthetase, the increased activity of the mutant

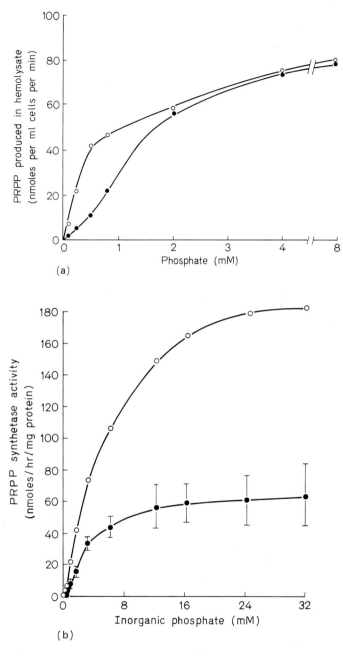

Fig. 3a and b. Effect of Pi concentration on the activity of PRPP synthetase in hemolysates from normal individuals and from affected members of two families with excessive PRPP synthetase activity. (a) ●———●, normal hemolysate; ○———○, hemolysate from the patient described by SPERLING et al. (1972b) (Reproduced by permission of Biochemical Medicine). (b) ●———●, mean values in dialyzed hemolysates from 15 normal subjects; ○———○, dialyzed hemolysate from one of the affected patients described by BECKER et al. (1973b) (Reproduced by permission of The American Journal of Medicine)

enzyme was shown to result from increased catalytic activity per enzyme molecule. Thus, in contrast to the feedback-resistant PRPP synthetase previously described, increased enzyme activity in this family appeared to result from increased enzyme specific activity per molecule due either to primary mutation in the structural gene for PRPP synthetase or to a post-transcriptional alteration in enzyme structure.

Still a third distinctive structural variant of PRPP synthetase associated with excessive intracellular PRPP concentration and generation as well as purine overproduction has been described (BECKER, 1976a). The enzyme from the erythrocytes and cultured fibroblasts of the two affected brothers in this family was normally active at saturating substrate concentrations. PRPP synthetase from these sources, however, showed 3–4-fold higher affinity for ribose-5-P than did the enzyme from normal individuals. Thus, it appears likely that at prevailing intracellular ribose-5-P concentrations, this genetically altered PRPP synthetase catalyzes synthesis of PRPP at a significantly increased rate. The ribose-5-P concentration in fibroblasts from one of these individuals, was, in fact, significantly diminished in comparison to the values in fibroblasts from normal individuals and from patients with the second form of abnormal PRPP synthetase described above (BECKER, 1976a). Partially purified erythrocyte PRPP synthetase with increased affinity for ribose-5-P showed diminished electrophoretic mobility providing further evidence for a structural defect in the protein.

To date, screening of erythrocyte lysates by routine measurement of PRPP synthetase activity has been carried out in several hundred additional individuals with uric acid overproduction and has revealed only a single additional individual with excessive enzyme activity (MÜLLER and FRANK, 1974). In this patient, in contrast to those mentioned above, increased purine production was accompanied by benign symmetric lipomatosis. Increased PRPP synthetase activity has not been found in other patients with this latter disorder.

The obvious differences in the enzyme defects described above exemplify the heterogeneity in mutational events giving rise to similar enzyme abnormalities (in this case, excessive PRPP synthetase activity) and suggest that additional mutations at the PRPP synthetase structural locus may well account for purine overproduction in other patients with primary gout. The subtle nature of two of the three described abnormalities in this enzyme, however, may explain the low yield in identifying abnormalities in PRPP synthetase by routine screening of enzyme activities. As discussed above, early experience with an alternative approach (BECKER, 1976a) using the measurement of PRPP generation and concentration and ribose-5-P concentration in fibroblast cultures from uric acid overproducers without gross enzyme defects, has proved encouraging in permitting categorization of such individuals (Table 3) for more intensive investigation of the enzymes most likely to be affected.

The mode of inheritance of excessive PRPP synthetase activity is uncertain. In the family described by SPERLING and associates (1972b, c) the mother of the propositus was clinically normal and showed entirely normal findings in her erythrocytes but was found to excrete excessive quantities of uric acid in the daily urine. Fibroblasts cultured from this woman (ZOREF et al., 1975) showed increased PRPP synthetase activity at 1.6 mM P_i, diminished response of the enzyme to purine nucleotide inhibitors, increased PRPP concentration and generation, and an increased rate of purine synthesis de novo. In all of these determinations (except inhibitor responsiveness), values for the mother's cells were intermediate, greater than those for normal control cells but less than those for cells from her affected son.

Attempts at demonstration of two populations of fibroblasts in cultures from this woman, using a modification of a previously described selective medium (GREEN and MARTIN, 1973) in which cells with increased PRPP synthetase activity survive while normal cells do not, were unsuccessful (ZOREF et al., 1975). This failure, however, may have been due to the phenomenon of metabolic cooperation by means of which cells with normal enzyme activity are supplied with an unknown factor, allowing survival in the selective medium (ZOREF et al., ˙1976a). Taking care to prevent metabolic cooperation, SPERLING and associates have recently reported evidence for two populations of cells in this woman's fibroblast culture indicating X-linkage of the structural gene for PRPP synthetase (ZOREF et al., 1976b). The pedigree of the involved family, showing the propositus' father and four sons to be entirely normal clinically and biochemically and the mother to have abnormalities that are attenuated is consistent with this suggestion.

In the family with a PRPP synthetase of increased enzyme activity per molecule, a daughter of one of the affected brothers shows mild hyperuricemia and excessive uric acid excretion (BECKER, 1973a). Erythrocyte enzyme activity is entirely within the range of her affected father and uncle; this finding suggests that if the genetic locus for PRPP synthetase is on the X-chromosome, either nonrandom X-chromosome inactivation or subsequent selection against erythrocyte precursors with normal enzyme activity is occurring. (Similar alternatives exist to explain the normal erythrocyte findings in the mother of the propositus described by SPERLING et al. (1972c), although nonrandom inactivation or selection in that case apparently operates against the abnormal enzyme).

Fibroblasts from this girl show findings similar to those of the affected males (BECKER, 1976a), although enzyme activity in her cells is slightly but consistently lower than theirs. Autosomal dominant inheritance has been proposed for the abnormality in PRPP synthetase in this family (BECKER et al., 1973a); the data, however, are not inconsistent with X-linked inheritance, especially since: 1) no evidence for a normal as well as a mutant form of the enzyme has been adduced in purified enzyme preparations from the affected males (BECKER et al., 1975); 2) Nonrandom X-chromosome inactivation or selection against mutant or normal cell populations after random inactivation is known to occur, as in the case of the erythrocytes of obligate heterozygote carriers of severe HGPRT deficiency (NYHAN et al., 1970).

An infant with hypouricemia, seizures, and mental retardation in whom erythrocyte PRPP synthetase activity was about 10% of normal has been reported from Japan (WADA et al., 1974). Both parents of this child were clinically normal but were shown to have intermediate values for the enzyme, suggesting autosomal recessive inheritance of the defect. This deficiency of PRPP synthetase, however, has not been shown to involve enzyme structure, and, in fact, enzyme activity was apparently restored to normal values following treatment of the child's seizures with ACTH (Y. WADA, Personal communication).

2. Glucose-6-phosphatase Deficiency

Among the multiple biochemical abnormalities found in patients with glucose-6-phosphatase deficiency (type I glycogen storage or Von Gierke's disease) is severe hyperuricemia frequently resulting in gout. At least two mechanisms for the development of hyperuricemia in these individuals have been established. First, the increased serum lactate and ketone body concentrations resulting from hypoglycemia interfere with renal secretion of uric acid (Yü et al., 1957; GOLDFINGER et al., 1965). Second, in these patients, an increased rate of uric acid synthesis de novo has been demonstrated by [^{14}C] glycine incorporation into urinary uric acid (ALEPA et al., 1967; KELLEY et al., 1968a; JACOVCIC and SORENSON, 1967). While increased hepatic PRPP production resulting from excessive activity of the oxidative pathway of glucose-6-phosphate catabolism has been hypothesized as the driving force to increased purine synthesis, studies of hepatic PRPP synthesis and concentration in patients with this autosomal recessive disorder have yet to be reported. Normal PRPP concentrations have been found in erythrocytes from these patients (GREENE and SEEGMILLER, 1969), but this is not surprising since glucose-6-phosphatase activity is normally restricted to liver, kidneys, and gastrointestinal tract.

3. Increased Glutathione Reductase Activity

Glutathione reductase catalyzes reduction of glutathione by NADPH and H$^+$ with generation of NADP. Increased glutathione reductase activity has been hypothesized (LONG, 1970) to stimulate the rate of the oxidative pentose phosphate pathway through providing increased NADP for the early reactions in this sequence (Fig. 2). Consequent increased ribose-5-P and PRPP generation might, then, account for the reported association of hyperuricemia and gout with an electrophoretically faster migrating form of the erythrocyte enzyme, which has 28% higher than normal acitivity (LONG, 1967). Measurements of PRPP generation and concentration in individuals with this variant of glutathione reductase have not been reported, nor has the associated gout been demonstrated to result from excessive uric acid production. In addition, activation of glutathione reductase in certain disease states and by vitamin compounds such as riboflavin and nicotinamide have raised concern about the accuracy of previous measurements of glutathione reductase activity (BEUTLER, 1969). Finally, doubt has been expressed concerning a rate-determining role for NADP in the phosphogluconate oxidative pathway (PANIKER et al., 1970).

II. Decreased PRPP Use

PRPP is a substrate in a wide array of phosphoribosyltransferase reactions, including amidophosphoribosyltransferase; increased PRPP availability for purine synthesis de novo might potentially result from deficiency in any other enzyme normally using this compound. In fact, the affinities of the various phosphoribosyltransferases for PRPP, the availability of cosubstrates, and the concentration of PRPP resulting from the particular enzyme defect (a function of the normal rate of use of PRPP in that pathway), are among the factors governing purine synthetic rate in phosphoribosyltransferase deficiency states. In all tissues examined to date, deficiencies of HGPRT, both severe (SEEGMILLER et al., 1967) and partial (KELLEY et al., 1967), are accompanied by increased PRPP concentrations and excessive rates of purine synthesis de novo. The weight of evidence suggests underuse (ROSENBLOOM et al., 1968) rather than increased production of PRPP as the basis of increased concentration in HGPRT-deficient cells; the increased PRPP concentration, in turn, appears to be the most acceptable explanation for the increased rate of purine synthesis de novo in the absence of evidence of diminished purine nucleotide inhibitor concentrations (Ro-SENBLOOM et al., 1968; NUKI et al., 1976; BECKER, 1976b). Intrinsic to such a formulation for the purine overproduction that occurs with HGPRT deficiency but not with deficiencies of other phosphoribosyltransferases is a high rate of normal use of PRPP in the HGPRT reaction; this remains to be proved directly, and, indeed, without such proof alternative mechanisms to explain purine overproduction in HGPRT deficiency remain possible.

1. HGPRT Deficiency

A spectrum of HGPRT deficiency ranging from nearly total absence of enzyme activity (SEEGMILLER et al., 1967) to milder deficiencies (KELLEY et al., 1969) associated with easily identifiable residual activity has been described. Within the two major subcategories of severe and partial HGPRT deficiencies, which generally (but not invariably) correlate well with the clinical manifestations of the Lesch-Nyhan syndrome (LESCH and NYHAN, 1964) and a later-onset syndrome of gout and uric acid urolithiasis, respectively, a great deal of genetic heterogeneity has been demonstrated. Thus, while the characteristics of residual HGPRT of affected members within a single family are constant, a great deal of variation in substrate or inhibitor binding, thermal responsiveness (KELLEY and MEADE, 1971), growth characteristics in selective media, electrophoretic migration (FOX and LACROIX, 1976), and identifiable cross-reactive material (UPCHURCH et al., 1975; GHANGAS and MILMAN, 1975) is encountered among the enzymes from different affected families. Although in many cases evidence for a defect in the X-linked structural gene for HGPRT has been provided by the above studies, some HGPRT deficiencies may result from mutations in other genetic loci controlling either synthesis or degradation of the enzyme. These observations, which are discussed in Chapter 3, concern us here insofar as increased PRPP concentration is the only well-established and constant abnormal biochemical correlate of the purine overproduction common to all forms of HGPRT deficiency.

There are at least two mechanisms readily available to explain enhanced purine synthesis de novo in HGPRT deficiency. Diminished reuse of hypoxanthine or guanine by the purine salvage pathway, which is dependent on HGPRT activity, could result in IMP and GMP deficiencies. Since these and other purine nucleotides act as feedback inhibitors of both amidophosphoribosyltransferase (HOLMES et al., 1973a) and PRPP synthetase (BAGNARA et al., 1974), nucleotide deficiency could result in increased purine synthesis de novo by engendering a dual imbalance in the normal regulation of amidophosphoribosyltransferase activity through both diminished feedback control and excessive PRPP production. Comparative measurements of purine nucleotide pool sizes in normal and HGPRT-deficient fibroblasts (ROSEN-BLOOM et al., 1968; BECKER, 1976b) and lymphoblasts (NUKI et al., 1976) have failed to confirm purine nucleotide deficiency in the mutant cells. The low concentrations of GMP and particularly IMP in these cell types, however, temper the interpretation of these findings. In addition, no direct comparison of purine nucleotide pool sizes in normal and mutant liver or neural tissue has been reported. Thus, it is still possible, although perhaps unlikely, that decreased nucleotide concentrations contribute to the pathogenesis of excessive purine synthesis in HGPRT deficiency.

A second and presently more satisfactory mechanism to explain increased purine synthesis de novo in cells deficient in HGPRT relates to the accompanying increase in PRPP concentrations. In one study of heterozygote carriers of partial HGPRT deficiency, an inverse relationship between the erythrocyte PRPP concentration and residual HGPRT activity was found (GORDON et al., 1974); in another study of males with partial HGPRT deficiency, purine overexcretion was correlated with degree of enzyme deficiency (KELLEY et al., 1969). As a substrate and allosteric activator of amidophosphoribosyltransferase, PRPP in greater than normal concentrations would be expected to stimulate this enzyme and thus accelerate purine synthetic rates. The primacy of this mechanism in the purine overproduction of HGPRT deficiency is supported by several observations: the constancy of increased PRPP concentration in HGPRT-deficient cells; the diminution toward normal of the rates of purine syntheses of mutant fibroblasts partially depleted of PRPP by treatment with orotic acid (KELLEY et al., 1970b) or nicotinic acid (BOYLE et al., 1972); and the association of purine overproduction with increased PRPP availability in cells with excessive PRPP synthetase activity (SPERLING et al., 1972b; BECKER et al., 1973a).

Increased concentrations of PRPP in HGPRT-deficient cells appear to result from underuse of this compound in purine base salvage. No increase has been found in PRPP generation in fibroblasts derived from individuals with severe and partial enzyme deficiencies (ROSENBLOOM et al., 1968; BECKER, 1976a). Although increased PRPP synthetase activity has been reported in HGPRT-deficient human fibroblasts (MARTIN and MALER, 1976) and rat hepatoma cells (GRAF et al., 1976), the findings in fibroblasts contrast with similar determinations in other laboratories. In addition, the high PRPP concentrations of HGPRT-deficient erythrocytes cannot be accounted for by increased PRPP synthetase activity, since activities of the latter enzyme are normal in these cells (BECKER et al., 1973a). Nevertheless, pending corroboration of the increased PRPP synthetase activity in mutant fibroblasts, the possibility exists of both excessive PRPP generation and decreased PRPP use operating to different degrees in different HGPRT-deficient cells as determinants of PRPP concentration.

2. APRT Deficiency

Partial deficiency of erythrocyte APRT is not rare, occurring in about 1% of individuals tested (FOX et al., 1976; SRIVASTAVA et al., 1972). The association of partial APRT deficiency with gout described in a number of reports, however, probably reflects a sampling bias since patients with gout constitute the major population tested to date (FOX et al., 1976). The occurrence of partial APRT deficiency in the absence of hyperuricemia and gout (KELLEY et al., 1968b), discordance between APRT deficiency and hyperuricemia in the family members of some propositi with both traits (FOX et al., 1973; DELBARRE et al., 1974), and the inconstant evidence for increased PRPP concentration and purine overproduction in affected individuals (FOX et al., 1973; EMMERSON et al., 1975; FOX et al., 1976) are all consistent with the view that partial deficiency of this enzyme is not pathogenetically a direct cause of gout.

Two aspects of partial deficiency of APRT are of particular interest. First, despite pedigree studies suggesting that affected individuals have a heterozygous deficiency for an autosomal trait (HENDERSON et al., 1969), deficiencies of erythrocyte APRT result in considerably less than 50% normal residual enzyme activity. Inactivation of a dimeric enzyme by a mutant subunit could account for this more severe degree of deficiency than is expected in the heterozygous state (HENDERSON et al., 1969). Indeed, human erythrocyte APRT appears to be composed of subunits of molecular weight 11000 arranged in dimeric, trimeric, and hexameric forms (THOMAS et al., 1973). Second, fibroblasts cultured from individuals with partial deficiency of the erythrocyte enzyme do not show deficient APRT activity, while leukocytes from some but not all of these patients do (Fox et al., 1976). Thus, a genetic basis for at least some of these partial deficiency states awaits further delineation.

Severe APRT deficiency has been found in two children in different families who showed relative hyperuricemia and excretion of crystals and urinary calculi composed of 2,8-dihydroxyadenine (CARTIER and HAMET, 1974; VAN ACKER et al., 1976). This autosomal recessive inherited enzyme deficiency state is associated with excessive adenine but apparently normal uric acid excretion. Information regarding PRPP metabolism in these patients is incomplete, but in cultured human lymphoblasts selected for severe APRT deficiency, neither increased PRPP concentration nor excessive purine synthesis de novo was found (HERSHFIELD et al., 1976). At present, then, it would appear that APRT deficiency does not lead to a degree of PRPP underuse sufficient to increase intracellular concentrations of this compound and thus accelerate purine synthesis.

3. Purine Nucleoside Phosphorylase Deficiency

Purine nucleoside phosphorylase (E.C.2.4.2.1) catalyzes the conversion of inosine and guanosine to the purine bases hypoxanthine and guanine, respectively, with production of equimolar amounts of ribose-1-phosphate. Deficiency of this enzyme has recently been described in association with immunologic deficiency predominantly involving T-cell-mediated functions (GIBLETT et al., 1975; HAMET et al., 1976; WADMAN et al., 1976). In one such patient, purine overproduction in the form of excessive urinary excretion of purine nucleoside phosphorylase substrates (mainly inosine) has been demonstrated (COHEN et al., 1976). Of particular interest in this patient is the reported increase in erythrocyte PRPP concentration in the face of normal fibroblast PRPP concentration, PRPP synthetase activity, and rate of purine synthesis de novo, despite demonstration of the enzyme defect in these cultured cells.

Since the genetic defect in this individual involves the enzyme immediately proximal to HGPRT in the purine salvage cycle (i.e., IMP→inosine→hypoxanthine→IMP), relative sparing of PRPP would be expected in affected tissues because of an inability to provide hypoxanthine or guanine for the HGPRT reaction. In erythrocytes, increased PRPP concentration is compatible with such a PRPP-sparing effect, and, indeed, the purine overproduction of this patient may reflect the operation of this mechanism in the major sites of purine synthesis de novo. The dissociation between the findings in the patient's fibroblasts and erythrocytes with respect to PRPP concentration and between the cultured cells and the whole patient with respect to rates of purine synthesis suggest that in HGPRT-deficient fibroblasts significant PRPP-sparing does not occur. By extension, then, the increased PRPP concentration in HGPRT-deficient fibroblasts is hypothesized (COHEN et al., 1976) to result from increased PRPP synthetase activity in these cells rather than from PRPP underuse. These interesting findings thus have obvious implications for the above discussion of altered PRPP metabolism in HGPRT deficiency and point to the importance of the study of additional patients with nucleoside phosphorylase deficiency.

References

Acker, K. J. Van, Simmonds, A. H., Cameron, J. S.: Complete deficiency of adenine phosphoribosyltransferase (APRT): Report of a family. Z. klin. Chem. klin. Biochem. **14**, 277 (1976)

Alepa, F. P., Howell, R. R., Klinenberg, J. R., Seegmiller, J. E.: Relationships between glycogen storage disease and tophaceous gout. Amer. J. Med. **42**, 58—66 (1967)

Atkinson, D. E., Fall, L.: Adenosine triphosphate conservation in biosynthetic regulation. *Escherichia coli* phosphoribosylpyrophosphate synthetase. J. biol. Chem. **242**, 3241—3242 (1967)

Bagnara, A. S., Letter, A. A., Henderson, J. F.: Multiple mechanisms of regulation of purine biosynthesis de novo in intact tumor cells. Biochim. biophys. Acta (Amst.) **374**, 259—270 (1974)

Becker, M. A.: Patterns of phosphoribosylpyrophosphate and ribose-5-phosphate concentration and generation in fibroblasts from patients with gout and purine overproduction. J. clin. Invest. **57**, 308—318 (1976a)

Becker, M. A.: Regulation of purine nucleotide synthesis: effects of inosine on normal and hypoxanthine-guanine phosphoribosyltransferase-deficient fibroblasts. Biochim. biophys. Acta (Amst.) **435**, 132—144 (1976b)

Becker, M. A., Meyer, L. J., Huisman, W. H., Lazar, C., Adams, W. B.: Human erythrocyte phosphoribosylpyrophosphate synthetase: subunit analysis and states of subunit association. J. biol. Chem. (in press) (1977)

Becker, M. A., Meyer, L. J., Seegmiller, J. E.: Gout with purine overproduction due to increased phosphoribosylpyrophosphate synthetase activity. Amer. J. Med. **55**, 232—242 (1973a)

Becker, M. A., Meyer, L. J., Wood, A. W., Seegmiller, J. E.: Purine overproduction in man associated with increased phosphoribosylpyrophosphate synthetase activity. Science **179**, 1123—1126 (1973b)

Becker, M. A., Kostel, P. J., Meyer, L. J., Seegmiller, J. E.: Human phosphoribosylpyrophosphate synthetase: increased enzyme specific activity in a family with gout and excessive purine synthesis. Proc. nat. Acad. Sci. (Wash.) **70**, 2749—2752 (1973c)

Becker, M. A., Kostel, P. J., Meyer, L. J.: Human phosphoribosylpyrophosphate synthetase: Comparison of purified normal and mutant enzymes. J. biol. Chem. **250**, 6822—6830 (1975)

Becker, M. A., Seegmiller, J. E.: Genetic aspects of gout. Ann. Rev. Med. **25**, 15—28 (1974)

Beutler, E.: Effect of flavin compounds on glutathione reductase activity: in vivo and in vitro studies. J. clin. Invest. **48**, 1957—1966 (1969)

Boer, P., Lipstein, B., Vries, A. de, Sperling, O.: The effect of ribose-5-phosphate and 5-phosphoribosyl-1-pyrophosphate availability on de novo synthesis of purine nucleotides in rat liver slices. Biochim. biophys. Acta (Amst.) **432**, 10—17 (1976)

Boyle, J. A., Raivio, K. O., Becker, M. A., Seegmiller, J. E.: Effects of nicotinic acid on human fibroblast purine biosynthesis. Biochim. biophys. Acta (Amst.) **269**, 179—183 (1972)

Brin, M., Yonemoto, R. H.: Stimulation of the glucose oxidative pathway in human erythrocytes by methylene blue. J. biol. Chem. **230**, 307—317 (1958)

Brosh, S., Boer, P., Kupfer, B., Vries, A. de, Sperling, O.: De novo synthesis of purine nucleotides in human peripheral blood leukocytes. J. clin. Invest. **58**, 289—297 (1976)

Bunn, H. F., Ransil, B. J., Chao, A.: The interaction between erythrocyte organic phosphates, magnesium ion and hemoglobin. J. biol. Chem. **246**, 5273—5279 (1971)

Cartier, P., Hamet, M.: Une nouvelle maladie métabolique: Le déficit complet en adénine-phosphoribosyltransferase avec lithiase de 2,8-dihydronyadénine. CR. Acad. Sci. (Paris) **279**, 883—886 (1974)

Caskey, C. T., Ashton, D. M., Wyngaarden, J. B.: The enzymology of feedback inhibition of glutamine phosphoribosylpyrophosphate amidotransferase by purine ribonucleotides. J. biol. Chem. **239**, 2570—2579 (1964)

Clifford, A. J., Riumallo, J. A., Baliga, B. S., Munro, H. N., Brown, P. R.: Liver nucleotide metabolism in relation to amino acid supply. Biochim. biophys. Acta (Amst.) **277**, 443—458 (1972)

Cohen, A., Doyle, D., Martin Jr., D. W., Ammann, A. J.: Abnormal purine metabolism and purine overproduction in a patient deficient in purine nucleoside phosphorylase. New Engl. J. Med. **295**, 1449—1454 (1976)

Delbarre, F., Auscher, C., Amor, B., Gery, A. de: Gout with adenine phosphoribosyltransferase deficiency. Advanc. exp. Med. Biol. [A] **41**, 333—342 (1974)

Emmerson, B. T., Gordon, R. B., Thompson, L.: Adenine phosphoribosyltransferase deficiency: its inheritance and occurrence in a female with gout and renal disease. Aust. N.Z. J. Med. **5**, 440—446 (1975)

Fox, I. H., Kelley, W. N.: Human phosphoribosylpyrophosphate synthetase: distribution, purification and properties. J. biol. Chem. **246**, 5739—5748 (1971a)

Fox, I. H., Kelley, W. N.: Phosphoribosylpyrophosphate in man: biochemical and clinical significance. Ann. intern. Med. **74**, 424—433 (1971b)

Fox, I. H., Kelley, W. N.: Human phosphoribosylpyrophosphate synthetase: kinetic mechanism and end product inhibition. J. biol. Chem. **247**, 2126—2131 (1972)

Fox, I. H., Lacroix, S.: Electrophoretic variation in partial deficiencies of hypoxanthine-guanine phosphoribosyltransferase (HGPRT). Z. klin. Chem. klin. Biochem. **14**, 288 (1976)

Fox, I. H., Lacroix, S., Moore, M.: Adenine phosphoribosyltransferase (APRT) deficiency: evidence for genetic heterogeneity. Clin. Res. **24**, 294 A (1976)

Fox, I. H., Marchant, P.: Phosphoribosyl pyrophosphate degradation in human tissues. Canad. J. Biochem. **52**, 1162—1166 (1974)

Fox, I. H., Meade, J. C., Kelley, W. N.: Adenine phosphoribosyltransferase deficiency in man: report of a second family. Amer. J. Med. **55**, 614—620 (1973)

Fox, I. H., Wyngaarden, J. B., Kelley, W. N.: Depletion of erythrocyte phosphoribosylpyrophosphate in man. A newly observed effect of allopurinol. New Engl. J. Med. **283**, 1177—1182 (1970)

Ghangas, G. S., Milman, G.: Radioimmune determination of hypoxanthine phosphoribosyltransferase cross-reacting material in erythrocytes of Lesch-Nyhan patients. Proc. nat. Acad. Sci. (Wash.) **72**, 4147—4150 (1975)

Giblett, E. R., Ammann, A. J., Wara, D. W.: Nucleoside phosphorylase deficiency in a child with severely defective T-cell immunity and normal B-cell immunity. Lancet **1975 I**, 1010—1013

Goldfinger, S., Klinenberg, J. R., Seegmiller, J. E.: Renal retention of uric acid induced by infusion of betahydroxybutyrate and acetoacetate. New Engl. J. Med. **272**, 351—355 (1965)

Gordon, R. B., Thompson, L., Emmerson, B. T.: Erythrocyte phosphoribosylpyrophosphate concentrations in heterozygotes for hypoxanthine-guanine phosphoribosyltransferase deficiency. Metabolism **23**, 921—927 (1974)

Graf Jr., L. H., McRoberts, J. A., Harrison, T. M., Martin Jr., D. W.: Increased PRPP synthetase activity in cultured rat hepatoma cells containing mutations in the hypoxanthine-guanine phosphoribosyltransferase gene. J. Cell Physiol. **88**, 331—342 (1976)

Green, C. D., Martin Jr., D. W.: Characterization of a feedback-resistant phosphoribosylpyrophosphate synthetase from cultured, mutogenized hepatoma cells that overproduce purines. Proc. nat. Acad. Sci. (Wash.) **70**, 3698—3702 (1973)

Green, C. D., Martin Jr., D. W.: A direct stimulating effect of cyclic GMP on purified phosphoribosylpyrophosphate synthetase and its antagonism by cyclic AMP. Cell **2**, 241—245 (1974)

Greene, M. L., Seegmiller, J. E.: Elevated erythrocyte phosphoribosylpyrophosphate in X-linked uric acidemia: importance of PRPP concentration in the regulation of human purine biosynthesis. J. clin. Invest. **48**, 32 a (1969)

Hamet, M., Griscelli, C., Cartier, P., Ballet, J. J., Bruyn, C. H. M. M. de, Hösli, P.: A second case of inosine phosphorylase deficiency with severe T-cell abnormalities. Program Abstr., 2nd Int. Symp. on Purine Metab. in Man, Vienna, 1976

Harrington, H.: Effect of glucose and various nucleosides of purine synthesis by Ehrlich ascites tumor cells in vitro. J. biol. Chem. **233**, 1190—1193 (1958)

Hartman, S. C., Buchanan, J. M.: Biosynthesis of the purines. XXI. 5-Phosphoribosylpyrophosphate amidotransferase. J. biol. Chem. **233**, 451—455 (1958)

Henderson, J. F., Khoo, M. K. Y.: Synthesis of 5-phosphoribosyl-1-pyrophosphate from glucose in Ehrlich ascites tumor cells in vitro. J. biol. Chem. **240**, 2349—2357 (1965a)

Henderson, J. F., Khoo, M. K. Y.: Synthesis of 5-phosphoribosyl-1-pyrophosphate from ribonucleosides in Ehrlich ascites tumor cells in vitro. J. biol. Chem. **240**, 2363—2366 (1965b)

Henderson, J. F., Rosenbloom, F. M., Kelley, W. N., Seegmiller, J. E.: Variations in purine metabolism of cultured fibroblasts from patients with gout. J. clin. Invest. **47**, 1511—1516 (1968)

Henderson, J. F., Kelley, W. N., Rosenbloom, F. M., Seegmiller, J. E.: Inheritance of purine phosphoribosyltransferase in man. Amer. J. hum. Genet. **21**, 61—70 (1969)

Hershfield, M., Spector, E., Seegmiller, J. E.: Purine synthesis and excretion in human lymphoblasts mutants deficient in adenosine kinase (AK) and adenine phosphoribosyltransferase (APRT). Z. klin. Chem. klin. Biochem. **14**, 297 (1976)

Hershko, A., Hershko, C., Mager, J.: Increased formation of 5-phosphoribosyl-1-pyrophosphate in red blood cells of some gouty patients. Israel J. Med. Sci. **4**, 939—944 (1968)

Hershko, A., Razin, A., Mager, J.: Regulation of the synthesis of 5-phosphoribosyl-1-pyrophosphate in intact red blood cells and in cell-free preparations. Biochim. biophys. Acta (Amst.) **184**, 64—76 (1969)

Hill, D. L., Bennett, Jr., L. L.: Purification and properties of 5-phosphoribosyl pyrophosphate amidotransferase from adenocarcinoma 755 cells. Biochemistry **8**, 122—130 (1969)

Holmes, E. W., McDonald, J. A., McCord, J. M., Wyngaarden, J. B., Kelley, W. N.: Human glutamine phosphoribosylpyrophosphate amidotransferase: kinetic and regulatory properties. J. biol. Chem. **248**, 144—150 (1973a)

Holmes, E. W., Wyngaarden, J. B., Kelley, W. N.: Human glutamine phosphoribosylpyrophosphate amidotransferase: two molecular forms interconvertible by purine ribonucleotides and phosphoribosylpyrophosphate. J. biol. Chem. **248**, 6035—6040 (1973b)

Jacovcic, S., Sorenson, L. B.: Studies of uric acid metabolism in glycogen storage disease associated with gouty arthritis. Arthr. and Rheum. **10**, 129—134 (1967)

Jones, O. W., Ashton, D. M., Wyngaarden, J. B.: Accelerated turnover of phosphoribosylpyrophosphate, a purine nucleotide precursor, in certain gouty subjects. J. clin. Invest. **41**, 1805—1815 (1962)

Katz, J., Rognstad, R.: The labeling of pentose phosphate from glucose-^{14}C and estimation of the rates of transaldolase, transketolase: the contribution of the pentose cycle, and ribose phosphate synthesis. Biochemistry **6**, 2227—2247 (1967)

Kelley, W. N., Fox, I. H., Wyngaarden, J. B.: Essential role of phosphoribosylpyrophosphate (PRPP) in regulation of purine biosynthesis in cultured human fibroblasts. Clin. Res. **18**, 457 (1970a)

Kelley, W. N., Fox, I. H., Wyngaarden, J. B.: Regulation of purine biosynthesis in cultured human cells. I. Effects of orotic acid. Biochim. biophys. Acta (Amst.) **215**, 512—516 (1970b)

Kelley, W. N., Greene, M. L., Fox, I. H., Rosenbloom, F. M., Levy, R. I., Seegmiller, J. E.: Effects of orotic acid on purine and lipoprotein metabolism in man. Metabolism **19**, 1025—1035 (1970c)

Kelley, W. N., Greene, M. L., Rosenbloom, F. M., Henderson, J. F., Seegmiller, J. E.: Hypoxanthine-guanine phosphoribosyltransferase deficiency in gout. Ann. intern. Med. **70**, 155—206 (1969)

Kelley, W. N., Levy, R. I., Rosenbloom, F. M., Henderson, J. F., Seegmiller, J. E.: Adenine phosphoribosyltransferase deficiency: a previously undescribed genetic defect in man. J. clin. Invest. **47**, 2281—2289 (1968b)

Kelley, W. N., Meade, J. C.: Studies on hypoxanthine-guanine phosphoribosyltransferase in fibroblasts from patients with Lesch-Nyhan syndrome: evidence for genetic heterogeneity. J. biol. Chem. **246**, 2953—2958 (1971)

Kelley, W. N., Rosenbloom, F. M., Henderson, J. F., Seegmiller, J. E.: A specific enzyme defect in gout associated with overproduction of uric acid. Proc. Natl. Acad. Sci. U.S.A. **57**, 1735—1739 (1967)

Kelley, W. N., Rosenbloom, F. M., Seegmiller, J. E., Howell, R. R.: Excessive production of uric acid in type I glycogen storage disease. J. Pediat. **72**, 488—496 (1968a)

Kornberg, A., Lieberman, I., Simms, E. S.: Enzymatic synthesis and properties of 5-phosphoribosylpyrophosphate. J. biol. Chem. **215**, 389—402 (1955)

Krebs, H. A., Eggleston, L. V.: The regulation of the pentose phosphate cycle in rat liver. Advanc. Enzyme Regul. **12**, 421—434 (1974)

Lalanne, M., Henderson, J. F.: Determination of 5-phosphoribosyl-1-pyrophosphate in mouse liver. Analyt. Biochem. **62**, 121—133 (1974)

Lalanne, M., Henderson, J. F.: Effects of hormones and drugs on phosphoribosyl pyrophosphate concentrations in mouse liver. Canad. J. Biochem. **53**, 394—399 (1975)

Lesch, M., Nyhan, W. L.: A familial disorder of uric acid metabolism and central nervous system function. Amer. J. Med. **36**, 561—570 (1964)

Lindsay, R. H., Cash, A. G., Hill, J. B.: TSH stimulation of orotic acid conversion to pyrimidine nucleotides and RNA in bovine thyroid. Endocrinology **84**, 534—543 (1969)

Long, W. K.: Glutatione reductase in red blood cells: Variant associated with gout. Science **155**, 712—713 (1967)

Long, W. K.: Association between glutathione reductase variants and plasma uric acid concentration in a Negro population. Amer. J. hum. Genet. **22**, 14a—15a (1970)

Love, S. H., Gots, J. S.: Purine metabolism in bacteria. III. Accumulation of a new pentose-containing arylamine by a purine-requiring mutant. J. biol. Chem. **212**, 647—654 (1955)

Martin Jr., D. W., Maler, B. A.: Phosphoribosylpyrophosphate synthetase is elevated in fibroblasts from patient with the Lesch-Nyhan syndrome. Science **193**, 408—411 (1976)

McKerns, K. W.: Adrenocorticotropin-induced generation of 5'-phosphoribosylpyrophosphate and its relation to nucleotide synthesis in the adrenal cortex. Biochim. biophys. Acta (Amst.) **192**, 318—325 (1969)

Meyer, L. J., Becker, M. A.: Human erythrocyte phosphoribosylpyrophosphate synthetase: Dependence of activity on state of subunit association. J. biol. Chem. (1977) (in press)

Meyskens, F. L., Williams, H. E.: Concentration and synthesis of phosphoribosylpyrophosphate in erythrocytes from normal, hyperuricemic and gouty subjects. Metabolism **20**, 737—742 (1971)

Müller, M. M., Frank, O.: Lipid and purine metabolism in benign symmetric lipomatosis. Advanc. exp. Med. Biol. [A] **41**, 509—516 (1974)

Nuki, G., Lever, J., Seegmiller, J. E.: Biochemical characteristics of 8-azaguanine resistant human lymphoblast mutants selected in vitro. Advanc. exp. Med. Biol. [A] **41**, 255—268 (1974)

Nuki, G., Astrin, K., Brenton, D., Cruikshank, M., Lever, J., Seegmiller, J. E.: Purine and pyrimidine nucleotide concentrations in cells with decreased hypoxanthine-guanine phosphoribosyltransferase (HGPRT) activity. Z. klin. Chem. klin. Biochem. **14**, 311 (1976)

Nyhan, W. L., Bakay, B., Connor, J. B., Marks, J. F., Keele, D. K.: Hemizygous expression of glucose-6-phosphate dehydrogenase in erythrocytes of heterozygotes for the Lesch-Nyhan syndrome. Proc. nat. Acad. Sci. (Wash.) **65**, 214—218 (1970)

Oslzowy, J., Switzer, R. L.: Specific repression of phosphoribosylpyrophosphate synthetase by uridine compounds in *Salmonella typhimurium*. J. Bacteriol. **110**, 450—451 (1972)

Paniker, N. V., Srivastava, S. K., Beutler, E.: Glutathione metabolism of the red cells: effect of glutathione reductase deficiency on the stimulation of hexose monophosphate shunt under oxidative stress. Biochim. biophys. Acta (Amst.) **215**, 456—460 (1970)

Rosenbloom, F. M., Henderson, J. F., Caldwell, I. C., Kelley, W. N., Seegmiller, J. E.: Biochemical bases of accelerated purine biosynthesis de novo in human fibroblasts lacking hypoxanthineguanine phosphoribosyltransferase. J. biol. Chem. **243**, 1166—1173 (1968)

Roth, D. G., Shelton, E., Deuel, T. F.: Purification and properties of phosphoribosylpyrophosphate synthetase from rat liver. J. biol. Chem. **249**, 291—296 (1974)

Roth, D. G., Deuel, T. F.: Stability and regulation of phosphoribosyl pyrophosphate synthetase from rat liver. J. biol. Chem. **249**, 297—301 (1974)

Schulman, J. D., Greene, M. L., Fujimoto, W. Y., Seegmiller, J. E.: Adenine therapy for the Lesch-Nyhan syndrome. Pediat. Res. **5**, 77—82 (1971)

Seegmiller, J. E., Grayzel, A. I., Liddle, L., Wyngaarden, J. B.: The effect of 2-ethylamino-1,3,4-thiadiazole on the incorporation of glycine into urinary purines and uric acid in man. Metabolism **12**, 507—515 (1963)

Seegmiller, J. E., Rosenbloom, F. M., Kelley, W. N.: Enzyme defect associated with a sex linked human neurological disorder and excessive purine synthesis. Science **155**, 1682—1684 (1967)

Seegmiller, J. E., Klinenberg, J. R., Miller, J., Watts, R. W. E.: Suppression of glycine-^{15}N incorporation into urinary uric acid by adenine-8-^{13}C in normal and gouty subjects. J. clin. Invest. **47**, 1193—1203 (1968)

Sperling, O., Ophir, R., Vries, A. de: Purine base incorporation into erythrocyte nucleotides and erythrocyte phosphoribosyltransferase activity in primary gout. Rev. Europ. Etud. clin. Biol. **16**, 147—151 (1971)

Sperling, O., Eilam, G., Persky-Brosh, S., Vries, A. de: Simple method for determination of 5-phosphoribosyl-1-pyrophosphate in red blood cells. J. Lab. clin. Med. **79**, 1021—1026 (1972a)

Sperling, O., Boer, P., Persky-Brosh, S., Kanarek, E., Vries, A. de: Altered kinetic property of erythrocyte phosphoribosylpyrophosphate synthetase in excessive purine production. Rev. Europ. Etud. clin. Biol. **17**, 703—706 (1972b)

Sperling, O., Eilam, G., Persky-Brosh, S., Vries, A. de: Accelerated 5-phosphoribosyl-1-pyrophosphate synthesis. A familial abnormality associated with excessive uric acid production and gout. Biochem. Med. **6**, 310—316 (1972c)

Sperling, O., Persky-Brosh, S., Boer, P., Vries, A. de: Human erythrocyte phosphoribosylpyrophosphate synthetase mutationally altered in regulatory properties. Biochem. Med. **7**, 389—395 (1973)

Srivastava, S. K., Villacorte, D., Beutler, E.: Correlation between adenylate metabolizing enzymes and adenine nucleotide levels of erythrocytes during blood storage in various media. Transfusion (Philad.) **12**, 190—197 (1972)

Stadtman, E. R.: Mechanisms of enzyme regulation in metabolism. In: Boyer, P. D. (Ed.): The Enzymes, Vol. 1, 3rd ed., p. 454. New York: Academic Press 1970

Switzer, R. L.: Regulation and mechanism of phosphoribosylpyrophosphate synthetase. I. Purification and properties of the enzyme from *Salmonella typhimurium*. J. biol. Chem. **244**, 2854—2863 (1969)

Switzer, R. L.: Regulation and mechanism of phosphoribosylpyrophosphate synthetase. III. Kinetic studies of the reaction mechanism. J. biol. Chem. **246**, 2447—2458 (1971)

Switzer, R. L., Sogin, D. C.: Regulation and mechanism of phosphoribosylpyrophosphate synthetase. V. Inhibition by end products and regulation by adenosine diphosphate. J. biol. Chem. **248**, 1063—1073 (1973)

Thomas, C. B., Arnold, W. J., Kelley, W. N.: Human adenine phosphoribosyltransferase. Purification, subunit structure and substrate specificity. J. biol. Chem. **248**, 2529—2535 (1973)

Upchurch, K. S., Levya, A., Arnold, W. J., Holmes, E. W., Kelley, W. N.: Hypoxanthine-guanine phosphoribosyltransferase deficiency. Association of reduced catalytic activity with reduced levels of immunologically detectable enzyme protein. Proc. nat. Acad. Sci. (Wash.) **72**, 4142—4146 (1975)

Valentine, W. N., Anderson, H. M., Paglia, D. E., Jaffe, E. R., Konrad, P. N., Harris, S. R.: Studies on human erythrocyte nucleotide metabolism. II. Nonspherocytic hemolytic anemia, high red cell ATP, and ribosephosphate pyrophosphokinase (RPK, E.C.2.7.6.1) deficiency. Blood **39**, 674—684 (1972)

Valentine, W. N., Fink, K., Paglia, D. E., Harris, S. R., Adams, W. S.: Hereditary hemolytic anemia with human erythrocyte pyrimidine 5'nucleotidase deficiency. J. clin. Invest. **54**, 866—879 (1974)

Wada, Y., Nishimura, Y., Tanabu, M., Yoshimura, Y., Iinuma, K., Yoshida, T., Arakawa, T.: Hypouricemic, mentally retarded infant with a defect of 5-phosphoribosyl-1-pyrophosphate synthetase of erythrocytes. Tohoku J. exp. Med. **113**, 149—157 (1974)

Wadman, S. K., Bree, P. K. de, Gennip, A. H. Van, Stoop, J. W., Zegers, B. J. M., Staal, G. E. J., Siegenbeek Van Heukelom, L. H.: Urinary purines in a patient with a severely defective T-cell immunity and a purine nucleoside phosphorylase deficiency in the erythrocytes and lymphocytes. Z. klin. Chem. klin. Biochem. **14**, 326 (1976)

Wood, A. W., Becker, M. A., Seegmiller, J. E.: Purine nucleotide synthesis in lymphoblasts cultured from normal subjects and a patient with Lesch-Nyhan syndrome. Biochem. Genet. **9**, 261—274 (1973a)

Wood, A. W., Becker, M. A., Minna, J. D., Seegmiller, J. E.: Purine metabolism in normal and thioguanine-resistant neuroblastoma. Proc. nat. Acad. Sci. (Wash.) **70**, 3880—3883 (1973b)

Wood, A. W., Seegmiller, J. E.: Properties of 5-phosphoribosyl-1-pyrophosphate amidotransferase from human lymphoblasts. J. biol. Chem. **248**, 138—143 (1973)

Wood, A. W., Astrin, K. H., McCrea, M. E., Becker, M. A.: Purine metabolism in human lymphocytes during phytohemagglutinin (PHA)-induced blastogenesis. Fed. Proc. **32**, 652a (1973c)

Wong, P. C. L., Murray, A. W.: 5-Phosphoribosyl pyrophosphate synthetase from Ehrlich ascites tumor cells. Biochemistry **8**, 1608—1614 (1969)

Wyngaarden, J. B., Ashton, D. M.: The regulation of activity of phosphoribosylpyrophosphate amidotransferase by purine ribonucleotides: a potential feedback control of purine biosynthesis. J. biol. Chem. **234**, 1492—1496 (1959)

Yü, T. F., Gutman, A. B.: Effect of allopurinol (4-hydroxypyrazolo(3,4-d)pyrimidine) on serum and urinary uric acid in primary and secondary gout. Amer. J. Med. **37**, 885—898 (1964)

Yü, T. F., Sirota, J. H., Berger, L., Halpern, M., Gutman, A. B.: Effect of sodium lactate infusion on urate clearance in man. Proc. nat. Acad. Sci. (Wash.) **96**, 809—813 (1957)

Zoref, E., Vries, A. de, Sperling, O.: Mutant feedback-resistant phosphoribosylpyrophosphate synthetase associated with purine overproduction and gout. J. clin. Invest. **56**, 1093—1099 (1975)

Zoref, E., Vries, A. de, Sperling, O.: Metabolic cooperation between human fibroblasts with normal and with superactive phosphoribosylpyrophosphate synthetase. Nature (Lond.) **260**, 786—788 (1976a)

Zoref, E., Vries, A. de, Sperling, O.: Evidence for X-linkage of phosphoribosylpyrophosphate (PRPP) synthetase. Z. klin. Chem. klin. Biochem. **14**, 328 (1976b)

CHAPTER 8

Urate Excretion in Nonmammalian Vertebrates

W. H. DANTZLER

A. Introduction

Urates[1] are the major renal excretory products of nitrogen metabolism for many nonmammalian tetrapod vertebrates. This chapter concerns this excretory process. No attempt is made to discuss the overall metabolism or biochemistry of nitrogen-containing compounds in these animals. The latter subject has been extensively reviewed by others (CAMPBELL, 1970; CAMPBELL and GOLDSTEIN, 1972). Instead, the present discussion concerns the occurrence of renal urate excretion as a major process among nonmammalian vertebrates, the nature and mechanism of the excretory process, and the relationship of urate excretion to such problems as the conservation of water and the excretion of ions.

B. Occurrence of Urates as the Primary Excretory Products of Nitrogen Metabolism

The principal end products of nitrogen metabolism excreted in the urine of nonmammalian tetrapods are urates, urea, and ammonia. The percentage of urinary nitrogen appearing in each of these forms is shown for some birds, reptiles, and amphibians in Table 1. Urates have low solubilities in water (from 0.384 mmol/l for uric acid to 12.06 mmol/l for monopotassium urate) and, therefore, can be excreted with very little water. For this reason, their occurrence as the primary excretory products of nitrogen metabolism has often been considered to be connected with life in an arid habitat and the need to conserve water. Although the importance of urates in water conservation is probably not solely a function of their low solubility (see below), and many other adaptations account for the survival of nonmammalian vertebrates in arid environments, some relationship between the relative magnitude of urate excretion and the aridity of the environment can be seen in Table 1.

All birds primarily excrete urates regardless of habitat (Table 1). However, significant amounts of ammonia are also present in the urine (Table 1), and the fraction of excretory nitrogen appearing as ammonia is greater for aquatic than for terrestrial birds. Moreover, ammonia excretion in aquatic birds increases with increasing urine flow (STEWART et al., 1969). In domestic fowl, the partition of urinary nitrogen among urates, urea, and ammonia is unaffected by the amount or source of the dietary proteins (TASAKI and OKUMURA, 1964; TEEKILL et al., 1968; MCNABB and MCNABB, 1975).

---

[1] The term "urate" in this paper is used to refer to all forms that contain the urate anion (uric acid, uric acid dihydrate, and monobasic urate salts).

Among the reptiles, urate is the major excretory end product of nitrogen metabolism in the Crocodilia, Squamata, Rhyncocephalia, and many of the Testudinea (Table 1). However, large quantities of ammonia are consistently excreted by the semiaquatic crocodiles, and MINNICH (1972) has even found significant amounts of ammonium excreted with precipitated urates in cloacal samples from a number of terrestrial snakes and lizards (see below).

Among the Testudinea, urates occur as the primary form of excretory nitrogen only in species living in arid terrestrial environments (Table 1). However, some investigations have suggested that change in hydration can alter the percentage of excretory nitrogen in the forms of urate and urea. Thus, studies of *Testudo leithii* and *T. sulcata* by KHALIL and HAGGAG (1955) and of *Chelodina longicollis* by ROGERS (1966) indicated that with dehydration the percentage of nitrogen excreted as urates increased and that excreted as urea decreased. These investigators, however, studied spontaneous excretions (KHALIL and HAGGAG, 1955) or bladder samples (ROGERS, 1966). Urates can be stored in the bladder of terrestrial tortoises and may be voided spontaneously (DANTZLER and SCHMIDT-NIELSEN, 1966). Moreover, water and urea may be absorbed from the bladders of both terrestrial tortoises and semiaquatic

Table 1. Approximate percentage of total urinary nitrogen in the form of urates, urea, and ammonia in some nonmammalian vertebrates

	Percent of total urinary nitrogen appearing as:			References
	Urates	Urea	Ammonia	
Birds				
Terrestrial				
Gallus domesticus				
(chicken)	55–72	2–11	11–21	MCNABB and MCNABB, 1975
Aquatic				
Anas platyrhynchos				
(duck)	54	1.5	29	STEWART et al., 1949
Reptiles				
Testudinea				
Wholly aquatic	5	20–25	20–25	
Semiaquatic	5	40–60	6–15	
Wholly terrestrial				MOYLE, 1969
Mesic environment	7	30	6	BAZE and HORNE, 1970
Xeric environment	50–60	10–20	5	
Gopherus agassizii				
(desert tortoise)	20–50	15–50	3–8	DANTZLER and SCHMIDT-NIELSEN, 1966
Pseudemys scripta				
(freshwater turtle)	1–24	45–95	4–44	DANTZLER and SCHMIDT-NIELSEN, 1966
Crocodilia	70	0–5	25	KHALIL and HAGGAG, 1958
Squamata				
Sauria	90	0–8	Insignificant— ?highly significant	KHALIL, 1951; DESSAUER, 1952; PERSCHMANN, 1956; MINNICH, 1972

Table 1 (continued)

	Percent of total urinary nitrogen appearing as:			References
	Urates	Urea	Ammonia	
Ophidia	98	0–2	Insignificant— ?highly significant	KHALIL, 1948a, b; MINNICH, 1972
Rhyncocephalia				
Sphenodon punctatum	65–80	10–28	3–4	HILL and DAWBIN, 1969
Amphibians				
Anurans				
Mesic-xeric terrestrial				
Chiromantis xerampelina[a] (African tree frog)	60–75	20–35	1–8	LOVERIDGE, 1970
Chiromantis petersi[b] (African tree frog)	70–97	1	2	HILLMAN (personal communication)
Phyllomedusa sauvagei[b] (South American tree frog)	80–90	3–11	5	
Phyllomedusa pailona[b] (South American tree frog)	50–80	9–40	7–9	
Phyllomedusa iherengi[b] (South American tree frog)	50–80	14–37	4–7	
Phyllomedusa hypochondrialis[b] (South American tree frog)	20–80	18–75	2–4	SHOEMAKER and McCLANAHAN, 1975
Pachymedusa dacnicolor[b] (Mexican tree frog)	2–7	90	5	
Mesic terrestrial—semiaquatic				
Hyla pulchella[b] (South American tree frog)	0	94	6	
Rana catesbiana (bullfrog)	0	84	12	MUNRO, 1953
Aquatic environment				
Xenopus laevis[c] (South African aquatic toad)		20–28	72–80	MUNRO, 1953 McBEAN and GOLDSTEIN, 1967

[a] Values are percents of dried urine.
[b] Values are percents of urinary nitrogen appearing as urates, urea, and ammonia.
[c] Values are for animals in freshwater.

turtles (DANTZLER and SCHMIDT-NIELSEN, 1966; BENTLEY, 1976). Therefore, studies of spontaneous excretions or bladder samples will not give an accurate indication of a change in the renal excretion of urates and urea with changes in hydration. It is necessary to collect ureteral urine. Data for two individual species of Testudinea are shown in Table 1, because these are the only ones in which the partition of total urinary nitrogen was obtained with ureteral urine. When such urine from desert tortoises *(Gopherus agassizii)* was analyzed, the proportions of urates and urea showed no consistent change with hydration or dehydration (DANTZLER, 1964).

Although terrestrial and semiaquatic anuran amphibians are generally considered to be ureotelic, recent studies (LOVERIDGE, 1970; SHOEMAKER, 1972; SHOEMAKER and McCLANAHAN, 1975) have shown that there are a number of species which can excrete predominantly urate. Two of these (*Chiromantis xerampelina* and *C. petersi*) are African tree frogs and the others are four species of South American tree frogs of the genus *Phyllomedusa* (*P. sauvagei, P. pailona, P. iherengi,* and *P. hypochondrialis*) (Table 1). All of these are capable of living in relatively xeric environments. However, other closely related arboreal frogs can inhabit xeric regions without the ability to excrete significant amounts of urate (e.g., *Pachymedusa dacnicolor;* Table 1). One of the urate-excreting species *(Phyllomedusa sauvagei)* and probably two others (*Chiromantis xerampelina* and *C. petersi*) excrete predominantly urate under all circumstances (LOVERIDGE, 1970; SHOEMAKER and McCLANAHAN, 1975; HILLMAN, personal communication). The other urate-excreting species (*P. pailona, P. iherengi,* and *P. hypochondrialis*) excrete 80% of their urinary nitrogen in the form of urate only during dehydration. At this time, however, urine output and total nitrogen excretion are low, and much waste nitrogen actually accumulates in the body fluids in the form of urea. When urate excretion in these species is calculated as a percentage of the total waste nitrogen produced or as a percentage of the nitrogen excreted during hydration, it amounts to about 50% for *P. pailona* and *P. iherengi* and about 20% for *P. hypochondrialis* (SHOEMAKER and McCLANAHAN, 1975). The predominantly ureotelic or ammonotelic nature of some mesic terrestrial or semiaquatic and aquatic anuran species is also shown in Table 1 for comparison.

C. The Process of Renal Excretion of Urates

I. Filtration at the Glomerulus

In an early micropuncture study, BORDLEY and RICHARDS (1933) found that urate was freely filtered through the glomerulus of snakes (*Thamnophis sirtalis, Storeria occipitomaculata,* and *S. dekayi*) and frogs *(Rana pipiens)*. Studies of this type have not been repeated, although the method for determining the urate concentration used by BORDLEY and RICHARDS (1933) was less sensitive and less specific than those now available. In fact, since the frogs studied are not uricotelic and have a low plasma urate concentration, they had to be injected with urate to raise the plasma concentration to levels that could be measured with the method available (BORDLEY and RICHARDS, 1933). However, recent equilibrium dialysis studies have shown no binding of urate to serum proteins from frogs or snakes (unnamed species) (SIMKIN, 1972). These findings support the idea that urate is freely filtered in frogs and snakes, and it is generally assumed that this is the case for all reptiles and amphibians. Although this may well be true, additional direct studies in vivo on other reptiles as well as those anuran amphibians found to be uricotelic appear warranted.

No direct in vivo studies on the filtration of urate through the avian glomerulus have been attempted to date. However, in the equilibrium dialysis studies mentioned above (SIMKIN, 1972), significant binding (about 18%) of urate to proteins in chicken serum was observed at $4°$ C with hypoosmotic buffers. On the other hand, ultrafiltration studies at room temperature have shown that 71% (LEVINE et al., 1947), 94% (MARTINDALE, 1976), or 100% (MAYRS, 1924; SHANNON, 1938) of the plasma urate in chickens is ultrafilterable. Whether any significant protein binding occurs in vivo and influences filtration at the glomerulus has yet to be determined. Therefore, it is not possible to state at present whether or not urate is completely freely filtered at the avian glomerulus.

II. Transport by the Renal Tubules

1. Direction of Net Urate Transport

The studies of renal tubular transport of urate in vivo in nonmammalian vertebrates have involved standard clearance techniques or modifications of these. Since the cloaca or bladder may modify, or even transport, the urates (see below), ureteral urine should be collected directly in order to determine the role of renal tubular transport in the process of urate excretion. Unless otherwise specified, the clearance data presented in this chapter have been limited to those obtained in studies involving direct collections of ureteral urine.

MAYRS (1924) and GIBBS (1929) first suggested that urate might be secreted by the renal tubules of birds on the basis of the observation that its concentration in the urine of chickens was much higher than that in the plasma. SHANNON (1938) clearly demonstrated net tubular secretion in these animals by showing that the urate clearance greatly exceeded the simultaneous inulin clearance. Although some cloacal contamination may have occurred in SHANNON's studies and the method for determining urate was not as specific as later ones, the basic findings have been confirmed in subsequent studies on chickens (NECHAY and NECHAY, 1959; BERGER et al., 1960), ducks (STEWART et al., 1969), and mourning doves (SHOEMAKER, 1967, 1972). No evidence of tubular reabsorption has been found, even when secretion is markedly inhibited with drugs (NECHAY and NECHAY, 1959; BERGER et al., 1960).

Complete ultrafilterability of urate was assumed in the above studies. However, if some urate is bound to plasma proteins, the fraction of excreted urate that is secreted by the renal tubules would be even larger. Even with the assumption that urate is freely filtered, these clearance studies on chickens, ducks, and mourning doves indicate that 85–95% of the urate in the ureteral urine comes from tubular secretion (SHANNON, 1938; STEWART et al., 1969; SHOEMAKER, 1967, 1972).

In vivo measurements of net tubular urate secretion in birds may be complicated by urate synthesis in the renal tubule cells. Significant xanthine dehydrogenase activity has been measured in vitro in the kidneys as well as the livers of chickens (MORGAN, 1926; LANDON and CARTER, 1960). From the amounts of urate precursors present in chick kidneys, CHOU (1972) even suggested that more than 40% of the total urate production could occur in the kidneys. Recently, QUEBBEMANN (1973), using the SPERBER (1948) technique for supplying substrates directly to the renal tubule cells of one kidney via the renal portal system, demonstrated that urate could be formed from xanthine in the tubule cells of chickens in vivo and secreted directly into the tubular urine. This process could be blocked by the administration of allopurinol, a known inhibitor of xanthine oxidase in mammals and, presumably, of xanthine dehydrogenase in chickens.

The importance of renal urate synthesis in terms of total urate excretion in chickens was investigated by MARTINDALE (1976) who found that it apparently contributed less than 3% of the total urate clearance in animals that had been fasted 18 h. This has been confirmed by CHIN and QUEBBEMANN (personal communication). Therefore, previous evaluations of transepithelial tubular secretion by clearance methods in fasted chickens are probably reasonably reliable.

However, CHIN and QUEBBEMANN (personal communication) also found that renal synthesis accounted for about 20% of excreted urate in normally fed chickens and that, if hypoxanthine was administered to these animals via the systemic circulation, as much as half of the excreted urate could be of renal origin. The administration of hypoxanthine to fasted animals also increased the rate of renal synthesis of urate. Therefore, in normally fed chickens or in chickens administered precursors for urate synthesis, renal synthesis of urate will contribute significantly to clearance measurements of apparent transepithelial tubular secretion.

In other species of birds, renal synthesis of urate may be even more important. For example, in pigeons, there appears to be little xanthine dehydrogenase activity in the liver, and final conversion of hypoxanthine to urate occurs in the kidney and pancreas (EDSON et al., 1936). Although tubular secretion has not been evaluated in these birds, it is likely that tubular synthesis would contribute markedly to the apparent transepithelial tubular secretion.

Since tubular synthesis of urate has not been examined in ducks or mourning doves, it is possible that it contributes to the tubular secretion described above. However, the fraction of excreted urate that apparently comes from tubular secretion in these birds when they are fasted is the same as in chickens (SHANNON, 1938; STEWART et al., 1969; SHOEMAKER, 1967, 1972). Moreover, the clearance of urate in fasted ducks and mourning doves is the same as the simultaneous clearance for para-aminohippurate (PAH), an exogenous substance which is secreted by the renal tubules (STEWARD et al., 1969; SHOEMAKER, 1967, 1972). This observation suggests that the apparent tubular secretion of urate in ducks and mourning doves primarily represents transepithelial transport. Nevertheless, in assessing the magnitude of transepithelial tubular secretion of urate in avian species, the contribution of renal tubular synthesis, if any, to the apparent tubular secretion should be determined.

In those reptiles on which clearance data have been obtained (*Pseudemys scripta*, *Gopherus agassizii*, *Natrix* spp.) (DANTZLER and SCHMIDT-NIELSEN, 1966; DANTZLER, 1967b, 1968, 1970a), net tubular secretion of urate occurs, since the urate clearance always exceeds the inulin clearance. Moreover, a stop-flow study of renal function in unanesthetized water snakes (*Natrix* spp.) revealed no evidence of net tubular reabsorption of urate (DANTZLER, 1967b). These studies were performed on fed animals at 28° C. The possibility of renal urate synthesis has not been investigated in reptiles.

In one uricotelic amphibian species (*Phyllomedusa sauvagei*), preliminary clearance studies on fed animals kept out of water at 30° C indicate that 90–95% of the urate excreted in the urine is secreted by the renal tubules (SHOEMAKER, personal communication). Although some of these measurements were made on bladder collections, they probably are a reasonable indication of the magnitude of the tubular secretion, unless there is significant reabsorption or secretion of urate or reabsorption of the volume marker in the bladder. No studies on the possible role of renal tubular synthesis in urate secretion have been performed in these amphibians.

2. Sites of Tubular Transport

Among the nonmammalian vertebrates, the segment or segments of the renal tubules in which urate secretion takes place have been identified only in reptiles, and among them, only in snakes of the genus *Thamnophis*. Studies with isolated segments of snake tubules perfused in vitro in a manner similar to that first described by BURG et al. (1966) indicate that urate can be transported from bathing medium to lumen against a concentration gradient throughout the proximal tubule but not in the distal tubule (DANTZLER, 1973, 1976). When tubules were perfused with no urate in the initial perfusate and 2×10^{-5} mol/l urate in the bathing medium, the mean ratio of the concentration of urate in the collected tubule fluid to that in the bath (TF/B ratio) was about 2.0 throughout the proximal tubule but only about 0.1 in the distal tubule (Table 2). Moreover, net transepithelial transport in the distal tubule was less than one-tenth that in the proximal tubule (Table 2).

Although the site of tubular secretion of urate in the avian kidney has not yet been determined, it is of particular interest because of the heterogeneous nephron population. The avian kidney contains a mixture of nephrons resembling those of reptiles and those of mammals. Most nephrons resemble reptilian nephrons with simple proximal and distal tubules without loops of HENLE. These nephrons empty at right angles into collecting ducts. The other nephrons have loops of HENLE which, together with vasa recta and parallel collecting ducts, form medullary cones. These structures appear to function as countercurrent multipliers, as in the mammalian kidney, to allow the production of a concentrated urine (SKADHAUGE and SCHMIDT-NIELSEN, 1967). In each medullary cone the collecting ducts fuse to form increasingly larger ducts, until they leave the cone as a single ureteral branch (see BRAUN and DANTZLER, 1972 for illustration). It would be of great interest to determine if urate were secreted by one of these types of nephrons only. Since the reptilian-type nephrons are very short and simple, empty at right angles into the collecting ducts, and do not contribute directly to the concentrating mechanism, large quantities of urate should be able to move through them and into the collecting ducts without interfer-

Table 2. Urate and PAH transport

	Urate transport	
	TF/B	Net urate transport moles mm^{-1} min$^{-1} \times 10^{-15}$
Proximal tubule	2.12 ± 0.21 (23)	54.86 ± 7.91 (23)
Distal tubule	0.13 ± 0.06 (6)	4.57 ± 2.27 (6)
	PAH transport	
	TF/B	Net PAH transport moles mm^{-1} min$^{-1} \times 10^{-15}$
Proximal-proximal tubule	0.85 ± 0.19 (7)	45.3 ± 9.92 (7)
Distal-proximal tubule	6.02 ± 0.61 (23)	249.9 ± 35.60 (23)

Values are means $\pm$ SE. Figures in parentheses indicate number of tubules. These data have been published previously (DANTZLER, 1973, 1974a, 1976).

ing with the concentrating mechanism. On the other hand, large quantities of urate secreted by the mammalian-type nephrons might precipitate in the loops of HENLE and significantly interfere with the concentrating mechanism.

Cortical slices from chicken kidneys do accumulate urate in vitro (PLATTS and MUDGE, 1961; DANTZLER, 1969). If this uptake across the peritubular sides of the cells can be considered an adequate indication of urate secretion, then the reptilian-type nephrons must secrete urate, because they make up about 80% of the nephron tissue in the cortex (BRAUN and DANTZLER, 1972). However, whether the mammalian-type nephrons contribute significantly to urate secretion cannot be determined from these data. Slices of medullary cones do not accumulate urate in vitro, suggesting that the loops of HENLE of the mammalian-type nephrons and the larger collecting ducts do not contribute to urate secretion (DANTZLER, 1969).

3. Process of Tubular Transport

Most of the data now available on the steps in the tubular transport process for urate in nonmammalian vertebrates have come from work with isolated, perfused snake renal tubules. However, some information also has come from kidney slice or clearance studies on other reptiles or birds.

The urate concentration was measured in the cell water of isolated, perfused snake proximal tubules during net transport from bathing medium to lumen (DANTZLER, 1973). This concentration was consistently greater than that in the bath or the collected tubule fluid (Fig. 1). Since no significant amount of urate accumulated in the cell water during studies of efflux from lumen to bath (DANTZLER, 1973), there was no evidence for significant binding of urate within the cells. Therefore, the data on the urate concentration in the cell water, lumen, and bath during net transepithelial transport (Fig. 1) are consistent with active transport of urate into the cells across the peritubular membrane and passive movement down a concentration gradient into the lumen. This model for net transepithelial transport of urate from bath to lumen is also shown in Figure 1.

The apparent permeability of the luminal membrane of these isolated tubules to urate was determined from the net transepithelial transport and the concentration difference between the cells and the lumen (DANTZLER, 1973). The apparent permeability of the peritubular membrane to urate was determined from the efflux of urate from tubules with oil-filled lumens (DANTZLER, 1974b, 1976). The permeability of the peritubular membrane was $3.10 \pm 0.61 \times 10^{-5}$ cm s^{-1} (mean $\pm$ SE for five tubules), while that of the luminal membrane was only $0.75 \pm 0.26 \times 10^{-5}$ cm s^{-1} (mean $\pm$ SE for nine tubules) (Fig. 1). A luminal membrane permeability much lower than the peritubular membrane permeability suggests an ineffective system if urate transported into the cells across the peritubular membrane is to diffuse into the lumen and not back into the bath. Therefore, the transport system may be more complicated than the model shown in Figure 1.

In this regard, transport into the cells across the peritubular membrane may depend partially on perfusion through the tubule. When nonperfused tubules were incubated with urate under the same conditions as the perfused tubules, they maintained only one-third the cellular urate concentration of the latter (DANTZLER, 1973). This failure of the nonperfused tubules to maintain a high urate concentration

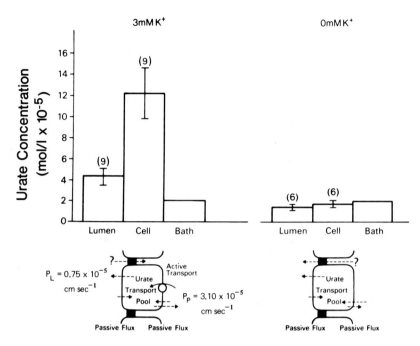

Fig. 1. Models for transepithelial urate transport by isolated, perfused snake (*Thamnophis* spp.) renal proximal tubules in the presence and absence of potassium in the bathing medium. Model on left represents control (3 mmol/l, potassium) situation. That on right represents experimental (potassium-free) situation. Circle and solid arrow represent active transport. Broken arrows indicate passive fluxes. Bars in upper part of figure indicate mean urate concentrations in bath, tubule fluid, and cell water at end of perfusion period. Vertical lines indicate SE. Numbers in parentheses indicate number of tubules. Apparent urate permeabilities for luminal membrane (P_L) and peritubular membrane (P_P) are shown for control model. Redrawn with modifications from DANTZLER (1973) and RANDLE and DANTZLER (1973)

difference between cell water and bath may be explained by the high peritubular membrane permeability. However, the much higher cellular concentration maintained in the perfused tubules would indicate some stimulation of the active transport step during perfusion. Although the nature of such regulation is not yet clear, it might be important in vivo in reducing accumulation of urate by the cells of nephrons that are not filtering. The nephrons of reptiles and amphibians and the reptilian-type nephrons of birds do not all filter continuously (FORSTER, 1942; SCHMIDT-NIELSEN and FORSTER, 1954; SAWYER, 1951; DANTZLER and SCHMIDT-NIELSEN, 1966; DANTZLER, 1967a; BRAUN and DANTZLER, 1972).

Net transepithelial transport from bath to tubule lumen in these isolated, perfused tubules also varied directly with the flow rate through the tubule (DANTZLER, 1973). This would be expected to occur if the transepithelial permeability for urate were great enough to permit significant back-diffusion. The amount of urate lost from the lumen of the tubule by this process would depend on the concentration in the luminal fluid and, thus, on the flow rate through the tubule. At high perfusion rates, when the urate concentration in the lumen was low, the back-diffusion would

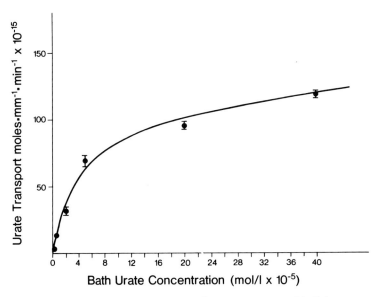

Fig. 2. Effect of changes in bath urate concentration on net transepithelial urate secretion by isolated, perfused snake (*Thamnophis* spp.) renal proximal tubules. Values are from four tubules. Vertical lines indicate SD. Perfusion rate was constant ($2\,nl\,min^{-1}$) in all periods. Curve was fitted by eye. Redrawn from DANTZLER (1973)

be reduced, and the net secretion of urate correspondingly increased. The opposite would occur at low perfusion rates when the luminal concentration of urate was high. This would appear to be another important mechanism, in addition to reduction of uptake on the peritubular side, for preventing continued accumulation of urate in nephrons that are not filtering.

As predicted, significant efflux, varying inversely with flow rate, was found to occur from lumen to bath (DANTZLER, 1973). The transepithelial permeability determined directly from this efflux ($2.42 \pm 1.09 \times 10^{-5}\,cm\,s^{-1}$; mean $\pm$ SE for seven tubules) was four times that ($0.60 \times 10^{-5}\,cm\,s^{-1}$) calculated from the independently measured luminal and peritubular membrane permeabilities given above (DANTZLER, 1976). This observation suggests that a large fraction of urate can move passively between the cells and that this is the region in which most of the back leak occurs. This paracellular pathway is indicated by a dashed arrow and a question mark in Figure 1.

Saturation of the transepithelial transport process for urate was also examined in these isolated, perfused tubules (DANTZLER, 1973). When the concentration in the bathing medium was varied over a 200-fold range at a constant rate of perfusion through the tubule, the transport system tended to saturate (Fig. 2). Complete saturation was not achieved with the maximum concentration used (0.40 mmol/l), but it appeared that this saturation would not occur at a bath concentration below 1.0 mmol/l. The failure of the transport process to saturate completely at lower bath concentrations appears appropriate, because other studies on snakes (DANTZLER, 1968, 1970a) indicate that the plasma urate concentration may average 0.4–

0.5 mmol/l. The apparent K_m for urate calculated from a reciprocal plot of the data in Figure 2 is about 0.6 mmol/l. No measurements of the maximum rate of tubular transport for urate have been made in these animals in vivo.

Among birds, SHANNON (1938), using clearance techniques, found that a maximum rate for tubular transport of urate was attained in chickens at a plasma concentration of about 1.2 mmol/l. Using the SPERBER (1948) technique, ZMUDA and QUEBBEMANN (1975) studied the tubular secretion of preformed urate and urate synthesized within the renal tubule cells in normal and gouty chickens of the same strain. In the gouty animals, which had been shown previously to have reduced overall tubular secretion of urate (AUSTIC and COLE, 1972), the secretion of preformed urate was impaired, but that of urate formed in the tubule cells from guanine was not. On the basis of these findings, ZMUDA and QUEBBEMANN (1975) postulated that a major transport step for the secretion of preformed urate is located at the peritubular membrane and that this mechanism is defective in gouty chickens. This concept also agrees with data showing significant uptake of urate by chicken kidney slices in vitro (PLATTS and MUDGE, 1961; DANTZLER, 1969; AUSTIC and COLE, 1976) and with the model for tubular urate transport derived from the study of isolated, perfused snake renal tubules (Fig. 1).

The effects of certain inorganic ions on the tubular transport of urate were studied with avian and reptilian kidney slices and isolated, perfused snake renal tubules in order to determine whether there is any dependency of this transport process on the transport of inorganic ions (DANTZLER, 1969, 1970b, 1971; RANDLE and DANTZLER, 1973; AUSTIC and COLE, 1976). The preparation and incubation of kidney slices from garter snakes (*Thamnophis* spp.), desert spiny lizards (*Sceloporus magister*), and chickens in potassium-free medium reduced the uptake of urate (DANTZLER, 1969, 1970b, 1971). Although the depletion of tissue potassium was comparable in kidney slices from chickens and both reptilian species, the reduction in urate uptake was most marked with chicken kidney slices. It was less marked with *Thamnophis* slices and least marked with *Sceloporus* slices. Moreover, incubation in high potassium (40 mmol/l medium), which led to similar increases in potassium concentration in slices from these three species, resulted in a marked increase in urate uptake by *Sceloporus* slices, much less increase by chicken slices, and no increase by *Thamnophis* slices. The physiologic meaning of these differences, if any, is not clear. Since *Sceloporus*, like the garter snake, is carnivorous, the marked stimulatory effect of potassium on urate uptake by slices from its kidneys is probably unrelated to any normal need to eliminate large amounts of urate as potassium urate, in contrast to the situation that may prevail in herbivorous forms (see below).

AUSTIC and COLE (1976) found that more potassium was required in the bathing medium to initiate urate accumulation by kidney slices from chickens with hyperuricemia and gout than by kidney slices from normal chickens of the same strain. However, slices from the gouty animals, which showed less uptake even under control conditions than slices from the normal animals, also required less potassium than slices from the normal animals to attain a maximum level of uptake. The potassium requirement for urate accumulation by slices from the normal chickens was similar to that observed previously (DANTZLER, 1969).

Since the slice technique does not permit evaluation of transepithelial transport or localization of sites of transport, the effects of inorganic ions on urate transport were evaluated with isolated, perfused snake (*Thamnophis* spp.) proximal tubules (RANDLE and DANTZLER, 1973). Removal of potassium from the bathing medium at a constant perfusion rate led to a significant depression of the net transfer of urate from bath to lumen within 20 min and to a maximum depression to about 25% of control within 60 min. With potassium absent from the bathing medium, net urate secretion remained depressed at all perfusion rates. Furthermore, in the absence of potassium, the urate concentration in the cell water at the time of maximum depression of urate transport (1.8×10^{-5} mol/l) was lower than that in the bath (2×10^{-5} mol/l) but greater than that in the lumen (1.5×10^{-5} mol/l) (Fig. 1). These findings, which contrast markedly with those in control tubules (Fig. 1), suggest that the active transport across the peritubular membrane is eliminated in the absence of potassium and that urate moves from bath to lumen by a purely passive process. This model for urate transport in the absence of potassium is shown in Figure 1. At the same time, the apparent unidirectional transepithelial permeability from bath to lumen ($1.95 \pm 0.39 \times 10^{-5}$ cm s^{-1}; mean $\pm$ SE for 11 tubules), calculated assuming completely passive movement, was not different from that determined from passive efflux from lumen to bath (see above). Evidently, the removal of potassium from the bathing medium does not significantly alter the transepithelial permeability for urate. This observation strengthens the concept that potassium influences the active step in the transport process. Moreover, the similarity of the two measurements of the transepithelial permeability suggests that some urate moves between the cells in the absence of potassium. This is indicated by the dashed arrow and question mark in the model in Figure 1.

When potassium was restored to the bath, even after the tubules had been perfused in potassium-free medium for more than 2 h, the net transfer of urate from bath to lumen increased significantly in 40 min and was restored to control levels in 60 min. The effects of potassium removal are thus readily reversible. However, in other tubules, when the medium potassium concentration was raised from the control level (3 mmol/l) to 40 mmol/l, a slight but probably significant depression of net urate secretion occurred. The importance of this slight effect is not clear. No depression of urate uptake by snake or chicken kidney slices with 40 mmol/l potassium in the bathing medium was observed in previous studies (DANTZLER, 1969).

The effects of sodium, as well as those of potassium, on urate transport were studied with isolated, perfused snake renal tubules (RANDLE and DANTZLER, 1973). Replacing all the sodium in the bathing medium and perfusion fluid with choline had no effect on net transepithelial transport of urate over periods as long as 4 h. However, sodium appears to be important for urate transport by avian kidneys. Reducing the sodium concentration in the bathing medium to 50 mmol/l or less significantly inhibited urate uptake by chicken kidney slices (DANTZLER, 1969; AUSTIC and COLE, 1976).

The cellular concentrations of potassium and sodium varied with the changes in the media concentrations (DANTZLER, 1969; RANDLE and DANTZLER, 1973). However, it is not possible to determine whether the changes in urate transport by isolated snake renal tubules or urate uptake by snake and chicken kidney slices resulted solely from changes in these concentrations, changes in the rates of transport of these inorganic ions, or a combination of these. Studies of the effects of cardiac glycosides, such as ouabain, on urate uptake by snake and chicken kidney slices or urate transport by isolated snake renal tubules have failed to clarify this situation (DANTZLER, 1969; RANDLE and DANTZLER, 1973). Ouabain, even in a concentration of 10^{-3} mol/l, has no effect on urate transport by snake renal tubules or urate uptake by snake kidney slices (DANTZLER, 1969; RANDLE and DANTZLER, 1973). However, this is probably due to the insensitivity of Na-K-ATPase in this tissue to ouabain, since other data (DANTZLER, 1969, 1972) indicate that both the tissue potassium concentration and the heavy microsomal ATPase activity are only affected by ouabain concentrations of 10^{-2} mol/l. A concentration of 10^{-2} mol/l ouabain did have some effect on urate uptake by snake kidney slices (DANTZLER, 1969), but the meaning of this effect is not clear. In the case of avian kidney slices, even 10^{-5} mol/l ouabain inhibits urate uptake (DANTZLER, 1969). Presumably, ouabain inhibits the Na-K-ATPase in this case. It is possible that this enzyme is involved in supplying energy directly to the urate transport system. However, the effects of ouabain on urate transport may be related to the depression of potassium uptake.

Although acetate had been found to stimulate the uptake of urate and other organic acids by mammalian kidney slices (CROSS and TAGGART, 1950; PLATTS and MUDGE, 1961), no stimulatory effect was found with slices from kidneys of chickens, mesophilic snakes (*Thamnophis* spp., *Natrix* spp.), or xerophilic lizards *(Sceloporus magister)* (DANTZLER, 1969, 1970a, 1971), or with isolated, perfused renal tubules from snakes (*Thamnophis* spp.) (DANTZLER, unpublished observations). Similarly, no stimulation of urate uptake by snake (*Natrix* spp.) kidney slices was observed with lactate or pyruvate, but some slight inhibition of uptake was observed with malate, fumarate, and succinate (DANTZLER, 1970a).

Acid-base balance may also affect tubular urate transport and may be related to the effects of inorganic ions on such transport. Tubular secretion of urate in unanesthetized water snakes (*Natrix* spp.) increased during an acute alkalosis (produced by i.v. infusion of sodium bicarbonate) but did not change during an acute acidosis (produced by i.v. infusion of hydrochloric acid) (DANTZLER, 1968). The increase in urate secretion during alkalosis seemed correlated with an increase in arterial blood pH and not with urine pH, for urate secretion was unaffected by the administration of sufficient acetazolamide to produce an alkaline urine without a change in blood pH. Since much of the uric acid may be in the form of the sodium or potassium salt (see below), an increase in tubular secretion during metabolic alkalosis could be important in eliminating base in the same fashion as an increase in the excretion of sodium bicarbonate.

ULLRICH (1976) suggested recently that organic acid transport by renal tubules, including urate transport, may not proceed by a primary active transport system driven by ATP. He suggests that the transport may proceed by a co- or countertransport system involving sodium and potassium. Since hydrogen ion secretion is sodium-dependent and ouabain-sensitive, the hydrogen ion-hydroxyl ion transport process may provide the link to the transport of organic acids. He notes that in kidney cells a gradient exists for passive hydrogen ion flux into the cells and hydroxyl ion flux out of the cells. Since the hydroxyl ion flux into the interstitium would be much greater than urate uptake, only a small part would have to be coupled in a countertransport system to account for urate uptake.

In avian renal tissue, where urate uptake by slices is moderately sensitive to sodium, such a system at least seems plausible. However, much more needs to be known about the steps in transport at the luminal and peritubular membranes, the electrical properties of the membranes, and the response of the membranes to changes in the pH gradient before it can be determined with certainty that such a system is correct. In the case of reptilian renal tubules, where more details on the steps in the urate transport system are available, the lack of effects of sodium make this particular countertransport system far less plausible. Moreover, this stimulatory effect of alkalosis (or, more precisely, an increased peritubular pH) is difficult to reconcile with hydroxyl ion-urate countertransport. It is possible that alkalosis stimulates transport of potassium into the proximal tubule cells at the peritubular membrane (as it probably does in the distal tubule cells) (GIEBISCH, 975) and that urate transport is coupled in some way to this transport. However, this relationship certainly has not been proven. The urate transport seems just as likely to be a primary active process with the potassium effects unrelated to co-transport.

4. Specificity of Tubular Transport

It has generally been assumed that in nonmammalian vertebrates urate shares a common secretory system in the renal tubules with other organic anions, such as para-aminohippurate (PAH). Recently, however, a number of studies have suggested that this may not always be the case (DANTZLER, 1970a, 1976; ZMUDA and QUEBBEMANN, 1975). Among birds, the most suggestive evidence for a separate transport system for urate comes from the study of gouty chickens by ZMUDA and QUEBBEMANN (1975). They found that although tubular urate secretion was impaired (apparently from impairment of transport into the cells at the peritubular side; see above), PAH secretion was not. However, AUSTIC and COLE (1974) found about 60% inhibition of PAH secretion in the same strain of gouty chickens. The plasma PAH concentrations were low in the former study but approached the level for maximum tubular transport in the latter. Earlier studies had also shown that high plasma PAH concentrations could reduce tubular transport of urate in normal chickens (BERGER et al., 1960).

Others have suggested that two pathways may be available for the tubular secretion of organic anions and that only one of these is the major pathway for urate (WEINER and TINKER, 1972). ZMUDA and QUEBBEMANN (1975) suggested that, if PAH is transported by both pathways, but only the urate pathway is defective in gouty chickens, then the secretion of PAH may appear normal when the amount infused is low and impaired when the amount infused is high. Although this is certainly possible, it is obvious that the differences between the urate and PAH transport systems in the avian kidney are not yet clearly defined.

The clearest evidence for a specific transport system for urate that is separate from that for PAH and other organic anions is found among the ophidian reptiles. Ligation of the renal portal vein during clearance studies on water snakes (*Natrix* spp.) completely eliminated tubular secretion of PAH but reduced tubular secretion of urate only when such secretion was very high (DANTZLER, 1970a). These data suggested that, although the sites for urate and PAH secretion might overlap, the sites for urate secretion involved a greater portion of each renal tubule than those for PAH secretion. It also appeared that the renal portal system supplied only those regions where PAH secretion occurred. This difference in the location of the sites for urate and PAH secretion was confirmed in the studies on isolated, perfused snake renal tubules (DANTZLER, 1973, 1974a). Whereas urate was transported from bath to lumen against a concentration gradient throughout the proximal tubule (see above), PAH was transported from bath to lumen against a concentration gradient only in the distal portion of the proximal tubule (Table 2). Moreover, net transepithelial transport of PAH was about five times as great in the distal portion of the proximal tuble as in the proximal portion (Table 2).

High plasma concentration of PAH (3 mmol/l or 50 mg/100 ml) infused in vivo had no effect on tubular urate secretion (DANTZLER, 1970a). Also, PAH in a concentration 3000 times that of urate failed to reduce urate uptake by snake kidney slices (DANTZLER, 1970a). Similarly, a concentration of urate 20 times that of PAH did not affect PAH transport by isolated, perfused renal tubules or uptake by snake kidney slices (DANTZLER, 1970a, 1974a). These data indicate that urate and PAH do not compete for the same transport mechanism.

Other differences between urate and PAH transport have also been defined in studies on isolated, perfused snake renal tubules. During transepithelial transport of PAH from bath to lumen against a concentration gradient, the concentration in the cell water was greater than in the bath or tubule lumen (DANTZLER, 1974a). As in the case of urate transport, these data are compatible with active transport into the cells on the peritubular membrane and passive movement down a concentration gradient into the lumen. In contrast to urate, however, the apparent permeability of the luminal membrane to PAH ($3.50 \pm 0.91 \times 10^{-5}$ cm s^{-1}; mean $\pm$ SE for 15 tubules) was about seven times that of the peritubular membrane ($0.50 \pm 0.07 \times 10^{-5}$ cm s^{-1}; mean $\pm$ SE for five tubules) (DANTZLER, 1974a, 1974b). These findings are quite compatible with the model for PAH transport, indicating active accumulation at the peritubular membrane and passive movement into the lumen. Moreover, net transepithelial transport of PAH did not vary with perfusion rate the way that for urate did (DANTZLER, 1974a, 1976). This suggested that the backflux of PAH from lumen to bath was not great. Indeed, this was the case. In addition, the transepithelial permeability for PAH determined from the efflux from lumen to bath ($0.67 \pm 0.17 \times 10^{-5}$ cm s^{-1}; mean $\pm$ SE for nine tubules) was about the same as the calculated from the independently determined luminal and peritubular membrane permeabilities (0.44×10^{-5} cm s^{-1}) (DANTZLER, 1976). This suggests that, unlike urate, the PAH backflux that does occur is primarily transcellular.

The PAH transport system in the isolated perfused renal tubules saturated at a bath concentration of about 0.06 mmol/l, a concentration far below that for urate (DANTZLER, 1974a). Moreover, the apparent K_m for PAH transport calculated from these saturation data was about 0.01 mmol/l. Since the K_m for urate transport is about 0.6 mmol/l, it appears that the affinity for PAH transport is more than 50 times that for urate transport.

Alterations in the potassium and sodium concentrations affected PAH transport by isolated, perfused snake renal tubules differently from urate transport. Removing potassium from the bathing medium depressed PAH transport as it did urate transport, but the active transport step into the cells on the peritubular membrane was not completely eliminated (DANTZLER, 1974b). Furthermore, no change occurred in the apparent permeabilities for the luminal and peritubular membranes. A more significant difference, however, occurred in the effect of high potassium concentration (10 mmol/l and 40 mmol/l) on transepithelial transport. In contrast to urate, such an increase in ·potassium concentration from the control level rapidly but reversibly depressed transepithelial PAH transport (DANTZLER and BENTLEY, 1975). Under these circumstances, the apparent permeabilities of the luminal and peritubular membranes were markedly reduced, and these reductions alone appear to have accounted for the decrease in transepithelial transport.

Also, in contrast to urate transport, transepithelial PAH transport was sensitive to the sodium concentration in the bathing medium. When the sodium in the bathing medium was replaced with choline, net PAH transport was dramatically but reversibly depressed (DANTZLER and BENTLEY, 1976). Under these circumstances, the active step for PAH transport appeared to be markedly inhibited but not eliminated. Moreover, the permeability of the peritubular membrane was double the control level, suggesting that an increased back leak from the cells into the bath as well as a depressed active transport step accounted for the depressed transepithelial transport. The sensitivity of the PAH transport system to sodium as well as potassium suggests that the transport step at the peritubular membrane may involve a countertransport step of the type suggested by ULLRICH (1976) and discussed above. However, in view of the striking effects of the alteration in concentration of inorganic ions on the membrane permeabilities, a primary transport step also seems quite plausible. In any case, the evidence favors a urate transport step separate from that for PAH in the renal tubules of ophidian reptiles.

No detailed studies of the specificity of the renal tubular transport system have been made in uricotelic amphibians. However, urate is capable of blocking the uptake of phenol red by pieces of developing kidney from ureotelic frogs *(Rana pipiens)* (JAFFEE, 1954). A similar interaction between urate and the transport system for other organic acids may also occur in uricotelic anurans.

D. Chemical Forms of Urates in Urine

I. Forms in Liquid Phase of Urine

The solubility of the acid form of urate is very low in water (0.384 mmol/l), but it is very unlikely that a significant amount of urate actually exists in this form in the liquid phase of the urine. The pK_a for the monobasic urate salt is about 5.7 (GUDZENT, 1908), and that for the dibasic salt is about 10.2 (ATSMON et al., 1963). Since the pH of the ureteral urine of most nonmammalian tetrapods varies from about 5 to 9 but is normally only slightly acid (e.g., turtles, DANTZLER and SCHMIDT-NIELSEN, 1966; snakes, DANTZLER, 1968; MINNICH, 1972; carnivorous lizards, MINNICH, 1972; birds, WOLBACH, 1955) or even alkaline (e.g., crocodilians, COULSON and HERNANDEZ, 1964; herbivorous lizards, MINNICH, 1972; birds, WOLBACH, 1955), most of the urate in solution must exist as the monobasic salt. The cations associated with urate will probably be mainly sodium and potassium, the predominant one depending upon whether the animal is carnivorous or herbivorous. In crocodilians, of course, where large amounts of ammonia are excreted in an alkaline urine, ammonium urate may be the important salt.

Although the solubilities of the monobasic urate salts in water are not great (6.76 mmol/l for sodium urate; 12.06 mmol/l for potassium urate) (GUDZENT, 1908), they are much greater than that of the acid form. In turtles, the concentrations of urate, sodium, potassium, and ammonia in the liquid phase of the ureteral urine are low enough so that the urate salts can exist in a true solution (DANTZLER and SCHMIDT-NIELSEN, 1966). However, this is not always the case for other reptiles and birds. For example, the concentrations of urate, sodium, and potassium in the liquid phase of the ureteral urine of lizards *(Dipsosaurus dorsalis)* (MINNICH, 1976b), snakes (*Natrix* spp.) (DANTZLER, 1968, and unpublished observations), pigeons *(Columbia livia)* (McNABB and POULSON, 1970), and domestic fowl *(Gallus demosticus)* (McNABB et al., 1973b; McNABB, 1974) are above those at which the urate salts can exist in solution. As these authors note, such findings indicate that some of the urate in the liquid phase of the urine is in a colloidal state. The property of urates to form lyophobic colloids in aqueous solutions has been known for many years (SCHADE and BODEN, 1913; BECHHOLD and ZIEGLER, 1914; YOUNG and MUSGRAVE, 1932; PORTER, 1963b).

As MINNICH (1976b) points out, the small size of the colloidal particles prevents the formation of large precipitated masses as long as the colloid is stable. In the reptiles and birds mentioned above, however, the concentrations of urates in the liquid phase of the urine often exceed the stability limits for lyophobic colloidal urate in aqueous solutions (PORTER, 1963b; MINNICH, 1976b; McNABB et al., 1973b; McNABB, 1974). These findings suggest that the lyophobic urate colloidal particles are converted to a lyophilic state by absorption to lyophilic macromolecules (PORTER, 1963b). These lyophilic colloids can exist in the liquid phase of the urine in concentrations above the stability limits for lyophobic colloids.

Mucoid materials, consisting of muco- and glycoproteins and acid mucopolysaccharides, that may serve as appropriate lyophilic macromolecules have been identified by histochemic techniques in the kidneys of a number of species of birds (LONGLEY et al., 1963; McNABB et al., 1973a). These are present in the greatest amounts in the ureters and collecting ducts where urate concentrations would be highest, but their abundance does not increase with increasing urate excretion (McNABB et al., 1973a). Preliminary attempts to isolate and identify these mucoid materials suggest that many of them may come from the plasma (McNABB and McNABB, 1975). MINNICH (1976b, and personal communication) has obtained preliminary evidence for a urate-binding protein that may serve a similar function in the ureteral urine of a lizard *(Dipsosaurus dorsalis)*.

Therefore, it appears that the liquid phase of the urine in many reptiles and birds contains lyophilic colloids as well as lyophobic colloids and urate salts in solution. The apparent formation of lyophilic colloids through the interaction of urate particles with lyophilic macromolecules permits much more urate to remain in the liquid phase than would otherwise be the case. This may be important in protecting the urinary system by reducing the amount of urate precipitation. It should also be noted that, during renal failure in birds, plasma urate levels that are normally too low to present problems in solubility rise to very high levels without precipitation (LEVINE et al., 1947). It appears that much of this urate may also be transported in the form of ultrafiltrable colloids (LEVINE et al., 1947). Studies on the form of urate in the liquid phase of amphibian urine have yet to be made.

II. Forms in Urine Precipitates

Urates are also present in the urine in precipitates. These are found not only in the cloaca or bladder, where it appears that much urate from the liquid phase is precipitated, but also in the ureters and collecting ducts of both the avian kidney (GIBBS, 1928; HART and ESSEX, 1942; MCNABB and POULSON, 1970) and the reptilian kidney (MINNICH and PIEHL, 1972; DANTZLER, unpublished observations). Precipitated urate in the ureteral urine of a number of lizards and snakes is exclusively in the form of smooth-walled spheres (2–10 μ in diameter) (MINNICH and PIEHL, 1972). Similar spheres have also been found in the urine of birds (FOLK, 1969a, b; LONSDALE and SUTOR, 1971). The cause of this spherical shape is not known (LONSDALE and SUTOR, 1971). However, MINNICH (1976b) suggests that the lyophilic urinary macromolecules mentioned above may be important. He suggests that the formation of spherical precipitates occurs by the "salting out" of lyophilic colloidal urates. This process may be initiated by the presence of additional electrolytes secreted by the renal tubules. However, as MINNICH (1976b) notes, the trapping of a considerable amount of the water of hydration by the lyophilic macromolecules during precipitation could cause crystals to grow in a disordered state. The disordered layer structure of the spherical precipitates in bird urine has been defined by the X-ray diffraction studies of LONSDALE and SUTOR (1971).

These spheres may be important in enabling precipitated urates to move through the collecting ducts and ureters without clogging or stone formation. The spheres may not form large precipitated masses or hard stones very readily because of their smooth surfaces and the presence of the urinary macromolecules (MINNICH, 1976b). The like charge and high degree of solvation of the latter may cause the spheres to repel one another (MINNICH, 1976b). The lyophilic urinary macromolecules may also lubricate the urinary tract for the spherical precipitates, although such a role for these substances has not been demonstrated (MINNICH and Piehl, 1972; MCNABB et al., 1973a; MCNABB and MCNABB, 1975; MINNICH, 1976b). MINNICH (1976b) also suggests that these spheres may deform, much like an erythrocyte, during their passage through narrow tubular structures, such as the renal tubules and ureters.

The exact chemical nature of these urate precipitates and their relationship to inorganic ions in the urine of birds and reptiles are the subjects of continuing investigation and some controversy. The precipitates in avian urine, whether studied from cloacal droppings or ureteral urine, initially appear to be spheres with a disordered layer structure (LONSDALE and SUTOR, 1971; MCNAAB and MCNABB, 1975). However, precipitates in the cloacal urine of reptiles contain ordered crystalline precipitates of urates as well as spheres (MINNICH and PIEHL, 1972). Since only spheres appear in the ureteral urine of reptiles, MINNICH (1976b) suggests that the unstable disordered structure of the spheres is transformed into an ordered crystalline state during storage in the cloaca or bladder. LONSDALE and SUTOR (1971), using X-ray diffraction and ashing techniques, found primarily uric acid dihydrate and almost no urate salts in the precipitated fraction of bird urine. Nevertheless, the precipitates in bird urine contain large amounts of sodium and potassium (MCNABB et al., 1973b; MCNABB, 1974; BRAUN, personal communication). The molar ratios of sodium plus potassium to urate in these precipitates vary from 0.7 to 3.4, depending upon the diet and drinking regimen (MᴄNᴀʙʙ et al., 1973b). This observation appears to confirm the results of Lᴏɴsᴅᴀʟᴇ and Sᴜᴛᴏʀ (1971), since ratios greater than 1.0 should not occur if only monobasic urate salts were present, and the pH of avian urine is never sufficiently high for appreciable amounts of the dibasic salts to exist. Moreover, the ratios found by MᴄNᴀʙʙ et al. (1973b) are actually underestimates, since they do not include the contribution of ammonium, calcium, and magnesium (MᴄNᴀʙʙ, 1974; MᴄNᴀʙʙ and MᴄNᴀʙʙ, personal communication).

The MᴄNᴀʙʙs (MᴄNᴀʙʙ et al., 1973b; MᴄNᴀʙʙ, 1974) have explained these findings by proposing that charge configurations hold sodium and potassium in the spaces that exist between the layers of uric acid dihydrate described by Lᴏɴsᴅᴀʟᴇ and Sᴜᴛᴏʀ (1971). The latter investigators did describe layers of unspecified water-soluble material between the layers of uric acid dihydrate. The MᴄNᴀʙʙs' (MᴄNᴀʙʙ and MᴄNᴀʙʙ, 1975) also feel that this trapping of sodium and potassium between layers of uric acid dihydrate could explain the observation that urine samples containing much precipitated urate favor the precipitation of both sodium and potassium but not ammonium (MᴄNᴀʙʙ, 1974). This order of precipitation is not in accord with the expected preferential precipitation of sodium urate when lyophobic colloids flocculate (Pᴏʀᴛᴇʀ, 1963b) or with the low solubility of ammonium urate (Pᴏʀᴛᴇʀ, 1963a). However, the negative charges on the urate colloids may hold the smaller cations between the layers of uric acid dihydrate, while the larger, polar molecules like ammonium may be excluded from this structure (MᴄNᴀʙʙ and MᴄNᴀʙʙ, 1975). This could also explain the inclusion of large amounts of calcium and magnesium in the urate precipitates of avian urine (MᴄNᴀʙʙ and MᴄNᴀʙʙ personal communication).

The MᴄNᴀʙʙs' hypothesis, although reasonable, is not proven. It is also possible that the large amounts of cations in the precipitates in avian urine exist as soluble salts with some anion other than urate. Little chloride has been found in the precipitates (MᴄNᴀʙʙ and MᴄNᴀʙʙ, personal communication), but other anions could be present. Also, if lyophilic colloids are present in the liquid phase of the urine, their flocculation may lead to an order of cation precipitation different from that expected for lyophobic colloids.

Although it seems unlikely that the X-ray diffraction studies of Lᴏɴsᴅᴀʟᴇ and Sᴜᴛᴏʀ (1971) are in error, it is possible that hydrated urate salts could have given a pattern similar to that of uric acid dihydrate. However, recent thermogravimetric and differential thermal analyses of precipitates from avian urine do not show any evidence of monobasic urate salts (MᴄNᴀʙʙ and MᴄNᴀʙʙ, personal communication). Thus, it seems probable that most of the insoluble precipitate in avian urine is uric acid dihydrate and that many, if not all, of the cations present are held by physical forces.

The situation may be different in the urine of reptiles. Mɪɴɴɪᴄʜ (1972) determined the cations bound (i.e., not readily soluble in water) in the dried urinary pellets of 43 species of lizards, 17 species of snakes, and the desert tortoise, *Gopherus agassizii*. He found that most of the cations were not readily soluble in water. Of these, potassium was the most abundant in precipitates from lizards (except *Varanus* spp.), boid snakes, and the desert tortoise. As might be expected, it was particularly abundant in precipitates from herbivorous lizards and the herbivorous desert tortoise. Sodium and ammonium occurred in smaller amounts. In the precipitates from most snakes (except the boas) and the monitor lizards (*Varanus* spp.), ammonium was more abundant than sodium or potassium. The molar ratio of the cations (sodium, potassium, and ammonium) to urate averaged about 0.8, and the total cationic content was close to that predicted from the pH of the liquid phase of the urine. This molar ratio and the low solubility of the cations are compatible with the existence of monobasic urate salts in the precipitates (MINNICH, 1972). MINNICH (personal communication) feels that this is generally the case for reptilian urinary precipitates.

Recently, however, NAGY (1975) found large amounts of precipitates with molar ratios of potassium to urate greater than 3.0 in the urine of chuckwallas *(Sauromalus obesus)*. Since the potassium could not be readily extracted from the precipitate with water, he did not feel that it could be electrostatically or physically trapped between layers of uric acid dihydrate. Although it is not possible to explain the high molar ratio of potassium to urate at present, other anions such as phosphates, with which the potassium could be combined, or proteins, to which it could be absorbed, may be involved in these precipitates. NAGY (1975) did not actually measure urate in the precipitates but assumed that all the nitrogen in the precipitates was in the form of urate. Of course, if some were not in the form of urate, the molar ratios would be even higher. However, if much nitrogen were in the form of proteins to which potassium was absorbed or if other anions were present in the precipitates, the observed ratios would be higher than the true ones.

The uricotelic amphibians excrete urate precipitates containing significant amounts of water insoluble cations (SHOEMAKER and MCCLANAHAN, 1975; HILLMAN, personal communication). When these animals are deprived of free water, 40%–80% of the excreted ammonia is included with the urate precipitates as insoluble ammonium. More potassium than sodium is excreted with the urate precipitates (SHOEMAKER and MCCLANAHAN, 1975; HILLMAN, personal communication); moreover, a larger percentage of excreted potassium than sodium is in the bound form. The largest amounts of insoluble cations excreted with urates are found in the urine of the most completely uricotelic species (*Phyllomedusa sauvagei* and *Chiromantis petersi*). About 20–30% of the excreted sodium and about 50% of the excreted potassium are in the insoluble form in the urine of these species. Molar ratios of excreted cations to urate are not available for these uricotelic anurans, and it is difficult to estimate whether or not the precipitates are predominantly monobasic urate salts.

No attempts have yet been made to analyze the chemical form of the precipitates in reptilian or amphibian urine by physical techniques. Clearly, much more work must be done to determine the true chemical form. However, the presence of high concentrations of potassium in the urate precipitates of reptilian urine and of sodium and potassium in the urate precipitates of avian urine may reflect the importance of these ions in the tubular transport processes discussed above. Moreover, the cations in the urate precipitates, whatever their chemical form, can be excreted without contributing to the osmotic pressure of the urine. Thus, the limited concentrating ability of the avian kidney and the absence of any concentrating ability in the reptilian and amphibian kidneys do not necessarily indicate the true capacity of these kidneys for excreting ions.

III. Modification of Form and Ionic Content of Urates by Transport Processes in Bladder or Cloaca

Although urate precipitates have been found in the ureteral urine of many birds and reptiles, further precipitation occurs in the bladder or cloaca. Precipitated urates are found in the coprodeum and distal large intestine of birds (SKADHAUGE, 1973), distal large intestine and cloaca of snakes (DANTZLER, 1968; MINNICH, 1972; MINNICH and PIEHL, 1972), in the cloaca of lizards (MINNICH, 1970, 1972; MINNICH and PIEHL, 1972) and crocodilians (KHALIL and HAGGAG, 1958; COULSON and HERNAN-DEZ, 1964), in the bladder of a number of turtles (DANTZLER and SCHMIDT-NIELSEN, 1966; BAZE and HORNE, 1970; MINNICH, 1976a), apparently in the bladder or cloaca of the tuatara (HILL and DAWBIN, 1969), and in the bladder of uricotelic amphibians (SHOEMAKER and McCLANAHAN, 1975). In very few cases, however, is there clear information on the degree to which urate precipitation occurs in the cloaca or bladder compared with the ureters.

Precipitation of urates could be produced by the absorption of water in the cloaca or bladder. As noted above, urate precipitates are present in the ureteral urine of birds. However, these normally move retrograde from the ureters into the coprodeum and distal large intestine (SKADHAUGE, 1973). Solute-linked as well as osmotically driven water absorption occurs in this region, its magnitude depending upon the degree of hydration (SKADHAUGE, 1973), and this could result in further precipitation of urates. Water absorption may also account for precipitation of urates in the bladder or cloaca of numerous reptiles. For example, in the desert tortoise (*Gopherus agassizii*) ureteral urine contains no precipitated urate, but the bladder urine of dehydrated tortoises always contains large amounts of urate precipitates (DANTZLER and SCHMIDT-NIELSEN, 1966; MINNICH, 1976b). The ureteral urine in these animals is always hypoosmotic to the plasma, but it becomes isoosmotic with the plasma as water is absorbed during storage in the bladder. This water absorption is probably important in the precipitation process.

Although urate precipitates can be present in the ureteral urine of lizards and snakes (see above), much water is present also (MINNICH, 1976b; DANTZLER, 1968). However, the cloacal urine spontaneously voided by dehydrated lizards is a hard mass of urate with little water (MINNICH, 1976a, b). Similarly, the spontaneous excretions of snakes contain mostly a soft mass of precipitate with apparently less water than the ureteral urine (DANTZLER, unpublished observations). These observations suggest that absorption of water by the cloaca helps to precipitate urates. Water absorption, solute-linked or osmotically driven, has been described for the cloaca of a number of lizards (*Dipsosaurus dorsalis, Varanus gouldii, Amphibolerus ornatus*, and *A. inermis*), for the cloaca and large intestine of several snakes (genera *Xenoden, Phylodiia*, and *Crotalus*) (JUNQUEIRA et al., 1966; MURRISH and SCHMIDT-NIELSEN, 1970; BRAYSHER and GREEN, 1970; BENTLEY and BRADSHAW, 1972; MINNICH, 1976b), and for the cloaca of crocodilians (*Crocodylus acutus*) (SCHMIDT-NIELSEN and SKADHAUGE, 1967). It also seems likely that absorption of water in the bladders of uricotelic anurans would stimulate urate precipitation, but this has not been studied.

Precipitation of urates could also be initiated by acidification of the urine in the bladder or cloaca. This acidification would convert the urate salts to the less soluble uric acid, permitting further absorption of sodium. Acidification would also promote precipitation of urates, because the flocculation limits for lyophobic colloidal urates decrease with decreasing pH (PORTER, 1963b).

If major acidification occurs in the cloaca of snakes, it appears reasonable that tubular urate secretion did not change during acidosis (see above; DANTZLER, 1968). Cloacal acidification would permit the continued excretion of nitrogenous waste during acidosis while sodium was being conserved and acid eliminated. However, if acidification could occur only through obligatory absorption of sodium in exchange for hydrogen ions, an extrarenal route might be required for the excretion of excess absorbed sodium (SCHMIDT-NIELSEN et al., 1963). Acidification of the urine does occur within the bladders of turtles, and this may result from either absorption of bicarbonate (SCHILB and BRODSKY, 1966) or secretion of hydrogen ions (STEINMETZ, 1967). Cloacal acidification of the urine has also been demonstrated in some lizards (*V. gouldii* and *D. dorsalis*) (GREEN, 1969; MINNICH, 1970).

Secretion of cations, such as potassium, by the bladder or cloaca could also cause colloidal urate to precipitate. Such potassium secretion has been demonstrated only in the cloaca of chickens (SKADHAUGE, 1973) and the lizards *V. gouldii* (BRAYSHER and GREEN, 1970) and *D. dorsalis* (MINNICH, 1976b).

Additional secretion of urate by the bladder or cloaca could lead to increased precipitation of urate by increasing the amount of urate that must be held in solution or colloidal suspension. If sufficient secretion occurred and the concentrations of other buffers were low, some decrease in the pH of the cloacal fluid could occur. So far, secretion of urate by the cloaca has been demonstrated only in the lizard, *D. dorsalis* (MINNICH, 1976b, in press). This is a very interesting finding, but it is not yet clear whether this contributes significantly to the magnitude of urate secretion. Moreover, it has not yet been determined whether this represents transepithelial transport or synthesis of urate by the cloacal epithelium.

E. Concluding Remarks

Urate is the primary excretory product of nitrogen metabolism in birds, most reptiles, and some amphibians. It is secreted by the renal tubules by a transport process that may be distinct from that for other organic anions. It passes along the urinary tract in forms which may involve soluble salts, colloidal suspensions, and precipitates. These forms may be modified in the cloaca or bladder. The final excretion of urates as well as their transport by the renal tubules may be intimately involved with requirements for the excretion of cations and even with acid-base balance. These factors may be more significant for the animals than the simple conservation of water through the low solubility of urates. The basic steps in the transport processes and the chemical forms of the urates are only beginning to be adequately described. In view of the complexity of the processes, the apparent differences among species, and the relatively few basic studies that have been made, much more work needs to be done before urate excretion in nonmammalian vertebrates is well understood.

Acknowledgments. The personal research reported here was supported by National Science Foundation Research Grant PCM 76-18679.

References

Atsmon, A., DeVries, A., Frank, M.: Uric Acid Lithiasis. New York: Elsevier 1963

Austic, R. E., Cole, R. K.: Impaired renal clearance of uric acid in chickens having hyperuricemia and articular gout. Amer. J. Physiol. **223**, 525—530 (1972)

Austic, R. E., Cole, R. K.: Specificity of the renal transport impairment in chickens having hyperuricemia and articular gout. Proc. Soc. exp. Biol. (N.Y.) **146**, 931—935 (1974)

Austic, R. E., Cole, R. K.: Hereditary variation in uric acid transport by avian kidney slices. Amer. J. Physiol. **231**, 1147—1151 (1976)

Baze, W. B., Horne, F. R.: Ureogenesis in chelonia. Comp. Biochem. Physiol. **34**, 91—100 (1970)

Bechhold, H., Ziegler, J.: Vorstudien über Gicht. III. Biochem. Z. **64**, 471—489 (1914)

Bentley, P. J.: Osmoregulation in reptiles. In: Gans, C. (Ed.): Biology of the Reptilia, Vol. V. London: Academic Press 1976

Bentley, P. J., Bradshaw, S. D.: Electric potential difference across the cloaca and colon of the Australian lizards *Amphibolarus ornatus* and *A. inermis*. Comp. Biochem. Physiol. [A] **42**, 465—472 (1972)

Berger, L., Yü, T. F., Gutman, A. B.: Effect of drugs that alter uric acid excretion in man on uric acid clearance in the chicken. Amer. J. Physiol. **198**, 575—580 (1960)

Bordley, J. III., Richards, A. N.: Quantitative studies of the composition of glomerular urine. VIII. The concentration of uric acid in glomerular urine of snakes and frogs, determined by an ultramicroadaptation of Folin's method. J. biol. Chem. **101**, 193—221 (1933)

Braun, E. J., Dantzler, W. H.: Function of mammalian-type and reptilian-type nephrons in kidney of desert quail. Amer. J. Physiol. **222**, 617—629 (1972)

Braysher, M., Green, B.: Absorption of water and electrolytesfrom the cloaca of an Australian lizard, *Varanus gouldii* (Gray). Comp. Biochem. Physiol. **35**, 607—614 (1970)

Burg, M., Grantham, J., Abramow, M., Orloff, J.: Preparation and study of fragments of single rabbit tubules. Amer. J. Physiol. **210**, 1293—1298 (1966)

Campbell, J. W. (Ed.): Comparative Biochemistry of Nitrogen Metabolism, Vol. 2: The Vertebrates. New York: Academic Press 1970

Campbell, J. W., Goldstein, L. (Eds.): Nitrogen Metabolism and the Environment. London-New York: Academic Press 1972

Chou, S. T.: Relative importance of liver and kidney in synthesis of uric acid in chickens. Canad. J. physiol. Pharmacol. **50**, 936—939 (1972)

Coulson, R. A., Hernandez, T.: Biochemistry of the Alligator. Baton Rouge: Louisiana State University Press 1964

Cross, R. J., Taggart, J. V.: Renal tubular transport: accumulation of p-aminophippurate by rabbit kidney slices. Amer. J. Physiol. **161**, 181—190 (1950)

Dantzler, W. H.: The Role of the Kidneys and Bladder in the Handling of Water and Solutes in the Fresh-water turtle *(Pseudemys scripta)* and the Desert Tortoise *(Gopherus agassizii)*. Ph.D. Thesis, Duke University, Durham 1964

Dantzler, W. H.: Glomerular and tubular effects of arginine vasotocin in water snakes *(Natrix sipedon)*. Amer. J. Physiol. **212**, 83—91 (1967a)

Dantzler, W. H.: Stop-flow study of renal function in conscious water snakes *(Natrix sipedon)*. Comp. Biochem. Physiol. **22**, 131—140 (1967b)

Dantzler, W. H.: Effect of metabolic alkalosis and acidosis on tubular urate secretion in water snakes. Amer. J. Physiol. **215**, 747—751 (1968)

Dantzler, W. H.: Effects of K, Na, and ouabain on urate and PAH uptake by snake and chicken kidney slices. Amer. J. Physiol. **217**, 1510—1519 (1969)

Dantzler, W. H.: Comparison of renal tubular transport of urate and PAH in water snakes: evidence for differences in mechanisms and sites of transport. Comp. Biochem. Physiol. **34**, 609—623 (1970a)

Dantzler, W. H.: Kidney function in desert vertebrates. In: Benson, G. K., Phillips, J. G. (Eds.): Memoirs of the Society for Endocrinology. Hormones and the Environment, Vol. 18, pp. 157—190. London-Cambridge: University Press 1970b

Dantzler, W. H.: Relation of potassium to urate accumulation by kidney slices from desert spiny lizards *(Sceloporus magister)*. Comp. Biochem. Physiol. **40**, 467—477 (1971)

Dantzler, W. H.: Effects of incubations in low potassium and low sodium media on Na-K-ATPase activity in snake and chicken kidney slices. Comp. Biochem. Physiol. **41**, 79—88 (1972)

Dantzler, W. H.: Characteristics of urate transport by isolated perfused snake proximal renal tubules. Am. J. Physiol. **224**, 445—453 (1973)

Dantzler, W. H.: PAH transport by snake proximal renal tubules: differences from urate transport. Amer. J. Physiol. **226**, 634—641 (1974a)

Dantzler, W. H.: K$^+$ effects on PAH transport and membrane permeabilities in isolated snake renal tubules. Amer. J. Physiol. **227**, 1361—1370 (1974b)

Dantzler, W. H.: Comparison of uric acid and PAH transport by isolated perfused snake renal tubules. In: Silbernagl, S., Lang, F., Greger, R. (Eds.): Amino Acid Transport and Uric Acid Transport. Stuttgart: Georg Thieme Verlag 1976

Dantzler, W. H., Bentley, S. K.: High K$^+$ effects on PAH transport and permeabilities in isolated snake renal tubules. Amer. J. Physiol. **229**, 191—199 (1975)

Dantzler, W. H., Bentley, S. K.: Low Na$^+$ effects on PAH transport and permeabilities in isolated snake renal tubules. Amer. J. Physiol. **230**, 256—262 (1976)

Dantzler, W. H., Schmidt-Nielsen, B.: Excretion in fresh-water turtle *(Pseudemys scripta)* and desert tortoise *(Gopherus agassizii)*. Amer. J. Physiol. **210**, 198—210 (1966)

Dessauer, H. C.: Biochemical studies on the lizard. *Anolis carolinensis.* Proc. Soc. exp. Biol. (N.Y.) **80**, 742—744 (1952)

Edson, N. L., Krebs, H. A., Model, A.: The synthesis of uric acid in the avian organism: hypoxanthine as an intermediary metabolite. Biochem. J. **30**, 1380—1385 (1936)

Folk, R. L.: Spherical urine in birds: Petrography. Science **166**, 1516—1519 (1969a)

Folk, R. L.: Petrography of avian urine. Tex. J. Sci. **21**, 117—129 (1969b)

Forster, R. P.: The nature of the glucose reabsorptive process in the frog renal tubule. Evidence for intermittency of glomerular function in the intact animal. J. Cell. Comp. Physiol. **20**, 55—69 (1942)

Gibbs, O. S.: The function of the fowl's ureters. Amer. J. Physiol. **87**, 594—601 (1928)

Gibbs, O. S.: The secretion of uric acid by the fowl. Amer. J. Physiol. **88**, 87—100 (1929)

Giebisch, G.: Some reflections on the mechanism of renal tubular potassium transport. Yale J. biol. Med. **48**, 315—336 (1975)

Green, B.: Water and electrolyte balance of the sand goanna *Varanus gouldii* (Gray). Ph.D. Thesis, Univ. Adelaide, S. Aust. 1969

Gudzent, F.: Physikalisch-chemische Untersuchungen über das Verhalten der harnsauren Salze in Lösungen. Z. physiol. Chem. **56**, 150—179 (1908)

Hart, W. M., Essex, H. E.: Water metabolism of the chicken with special reference to the role of the cloaca. Amer. J. Physiol. **136**, 657—668 (1942)

Hill, L., Dawbin, W. H.: Nitrogen excretion in the tuatara, *Sphenodon punctatus.* Comp. Biochem. Physiol. **31**, 453—468 (1969)

Jaffee, O. C.: Phenol red transport in the pronephros and mesonephros of the developing frog (Rana pipiens). J. Cell Comp. Physiol. **44**, 347—361 (1954)

Junqueira, L. C. U., Malnic, G., Monge, C.: Reabsorptive function of the ophidian cloaca and large intestine. Physiol. Zool. **39**, 151—159 (1966)

Khalil, F.: Excretion in reptiles. II. Nitrogen constituents of urinary concretions of the oviparous snake *Zamensis diadema.* J. biol. Chem. **172**, 101—103 (1948a)

Khalil, F.: Excretion in reptiles. III. Nitrogen constituents of urinary concretions of the viviparous snake *Eryx thebaicus.* J. biol. Chem. **172**, 105—106 (1948b)

Khalil, F.: Excretion in reptiles. IV. Nitrogenous constituents in excreta of lizards. J. biol. Chem. **189**, 443—445 (1951)

Khalil, F., Haggag, G.: Ureotelism and uricotelism in tortoises. J. exp. Zool. **130**, 423—432 (1955)

Khalil, F., Haggag, G.: Nitrogenous excretion in crocodiles. J. exp. Biol. **35**, 552—555 (1958)

Landon, E. J., Carter, C. E.: The preparation properties and inhibition of hypoxanthine dehydrogenase of avian kidney. J. biol. Chem. **235**, 819—824 (1960)

Levine, R., Wolfson, W. Q., Lenel, R.: Concentration and transport of true urate in the plasma of the azotemic chicken. Amer. J. Physiol. **151**, 186—191 (1947)

Longley, J. B., Burtner, H. J., Monis, B.: Mucous substances in excretory organs: a comparative study. Ann. N.Y. Acad. Sci. **106**, 493—501 (1963)

Lonsdale, K., Sutor, D. J.: Uric acid dihydrate in bird urine. Science **172**, 958—959 (1971)

Loveridge, J. P.: Observations on nitrogenous excretion and water relations of *Chiromantis xerampelina* (Amphibia, Anura). Arnoldia (Rhodesia) **5**, 1—6 (1970)

McBean, R. L., Goldstein, L.: Ornithine-urea cycle activity in Xenopus laevis: adaptation to saline. Science **157**, 931—932 (1967)

McNabb, R. A.: Urate and cation interactions in the liquid and precipitated fractions of avian urine, and speculations on their physico-chemical state. Comp. Biochem. Physiol. [A] **48**, 45—54 (1974)

McNabb, F. M. A., Poulson, T. L.: Uric acid excretion in pigeons, *Columba livia*. Comp. Biochem. Physiol. **33**, 933—939 (1970)

McNabb, F. M. A., McNabb, R. A., Steeves, H. R. III.: Renal mucoid materials in pigeons fed high and low protein diets. Auk **90**, 14—18 (1973 a)

McNabb, F. M. A., McNabb, R. A.: Proportions of ammonia, urea, urate, and total nitrogen in avian urine and quantitative methods for their analysis on a single urine sample. Poultry Sci. **54**, 1498—1505 (1975)

McNabb, R. A., McNabb, F. M. A., Hinton, A. P.: The excretion of urate and cationic electrolytes by the kidney of the male domestic fowl. J. Comp. Physiol. **82**, 47—57 (1973 b)

McNabb, R. A., McNabb, F. M. A.: Minireview: Urate excretion by the avian kidney. Comp. Biochem. Physiol. [A] **51**, 253—258 (1975)

Martindale, L.: Renal urate synthesis in the fowl *(Gallus domesticus)*. Comp. Biochem. Physiol. [A] **53**, 389—391 (1976)

Mayrs, E. B.: Secretion as a factor in elimination by the bird kidney. J. Physiol. (Lond.) **58**, 276—287 (1924)

Minnich, J. E.: Water and electrolyte balance of the desert iguana, *Dipsosaurus dorsalis*, in its natural habitat. Comp. Biochem. Physiol. **35**, 921—933 (1970)

Minnich, J. E.: Excretion of urate salts by reptiles. Comp. Biochem. Physiol. **41**, 535—549 (1972)

Minnich, J. E.: Water procurement and conservation by desert reptiles in their natural environment. Israel J. Med. Sci. **12**, 740—758 (1976 a)

Minnich, J. E.: Adaptations in the reptilian excretory system for excreting insoluble urates. Israel J. Med. Sci. **12**, 854—861 (1976 b)

Minnich, J. E., Piehl, P. A.: Spherical precipitates in the urine of reptiles. Comp. Biochem. Physiol. [A] **41**, 551—554 (1972)

Morgan, E. J.: Distribution of xanthine oxidase. I. Biochem. J. **20**, 1282—1291 (1926)

Moyle, V.: Nitrogenous excretion in chelonian reptiles. Biochem. J. **44**, 581—584 (1949)

Munro, A. F.: The ammonia and urea excretion of different species of amphibia during their development and metamorphosis. Biochem. J. **54**, 29—36 (1953)

Murrish, D. E., Schmidt-Nielsen, K.: Water transport in the cloaca of lizards: active or passive? Science **170**, 324—326 (1970)

Nagy, K. A.: Nitrogen requirement and its relation to dietary water and potassium content in the lizard *Sauromalus obesus*. J. Comp. Physiol. **104**, 49—58 (1975)

Nechay, B. R., Nechay, L.: Effects of probenecid, sodium salicylate, 2,4-dinitrophenol and pyrazinamide on renal secretion of uric acid in chickens. J. Pharmacol. exp. Ther. **126**, 291—295 (1959)

Perschmann, C.: Über die Bedeutung der Nierenpfortader insbesondere für die Ausscheidung von Harnstoff und Harnsäure bei *Testudo Hermanni* Gml. und *Lacerta viridis* Laur. sowie über die Funktion der Harnblase bei *Lacerta viridis* Laur. Zool. Beitr. **2**, 447—480 (1956)

Platts, M. M., Mudge, G. H.: Accumulation of uric acid by slices of kidney cortex. Amer. J. Physiol. **200**, 387—391 (1961)

Porter, P.: Physico-chemical factors involved in urate calculus formation. I. Solubility. Res. Vet. Sci. **4**, 580—591 (1963 a)

Porter, P.: Physico-chemical factors involved in urate calculus formation. II. Colloidal flocculation. Res. Vet. Sci. **4**, 592—602 (1963 b)

Quebbemann, A. J.: Renal synthesis of uric acid. Amer. J. Physiol. **224**, 1398—1402 (1973)

Randle, H. W., Dantzler, W. H.: Effects of K^+ and Na^+ on urate transport by isolated perfused snake renal tubules. Amer. J. Physiol. **255**, 1206—1214 (1973)

Rogers, L. J.: The nitrogen excretion of *Chelodina longicollis* under conditions of hydration and dehydration. Comp. Biochem. Physiol. **18**, 249—260 (1966)

Sawyer, W. H.: Effect of posterior pituitary extracts on urine formation and glomerular circulation in the frog. Amer. J. Physiol. **164**, 457—464 (1951)

Schade, H., Boden, E.: Über die Anamolie der Harnsäurelöslichkeit (Kolloides Harnsäure). Z. physiol. Chem. **83**, 347—380 (1913)

Schilb, T. P., Brodsky, W. A.: Acidification of mucosal fluid by transport of bicarbonate ion in turtle bladders. Amer. J. Physiol. **210**, 997—1008 (1966)

Schmidt-Nielsen, B., Forster, R. P.: The effect of dehydration and low temperature on renal function in the bullfrog. J. Cell. Comp. Physiol. **44**, 233—246 (1954)

Schmidt-Nielsen, B., Skadhauge, E.: Function of the excretory system of the crocodile (*Crocodylus acutus*). Amer. J. Physiol. **212**, 973—980 (1967)

Schmidt-Nielsen, K., Borut, A., Lee, P., Crawford, Jr., E.: Nasal salt excretion and the possible function of the cloaca in water conservation. Science **142**, 1300—1301 (1963)

Shannon, J. A.: The excretion of uric acid by the chicken. J. Cell. Comp. Physiol. **11**, 135—148 (1938)

Shoemaker, V. H.: Renal function in the mourning dove. Amer. Zool. **7**, 736 (1967)

Shoemaker, V. H.: Osmoregulation and excretion in birds. In: Farner, D. S., King, J. R. (Eds.): Avian Biology, Vol. II, pp. 527—574. New York: Academic Press 1972

Shoemaker, V. H., McClanahan, Jr., L. L.: Evaporative water loss, nitrogen excretion and osmoregulation in phyllomedusine frogs. J. comp. Physiol. **100**, 331—345 (1975)

Simkin, P. A.: Uric acid binding to serum proteins: differences among species. Proc. Soc. Exp. Biol. (N.Y.) **139**, 604—606 (1972)

Skadhauge, E.: Renal and cloacal salt and water transport in the fowl (*Gallus demosticus*). Dan. Med. Bull. **20** (Suppl. I), 1—82 (1973)

Skadhauge, E., Schmidt-Nielsen, B.: The renal medullary electrolyte and urea gradient in roosters and turkeys. Amer. J. Physiol. **212**, 1313—1318 (1967)

Sperber, I.: The excretion of some glucuronic acid derivatives and phenol sulfuric esters in the chicken. Ann. roy. Agr. Coll. (Sweden) **15**, 317—349 (1948)

Steinmetz, P. R.: Characteristics of hydrogen ion transport in urinary bladder of water turtle. J. clin. Invest. **46**, 1531—1540 (1967)

Stewart, D. J., Holmes, W. N., Fletcher, G.: The renal excretion of nitrogenous compounds by the duck (*Anas platyrhynchos*) maintained on freshwater and on hypertonic saline. J. exp. Biol. **50**, 527—539 (1969)

Tasaki, I., Okumura, J.: Effect of protein level of diet on nitrogen excretion in fowls. J. Nutr. **83**, 34—38 (1964)

Teekill, R. A., Richardson, C. E., Watts, A. B.: Dietary protein effects on urinary nitrogen components of the hen. Poultry Sci. **47**, 1260—1266 (1968)

Ullrich, K. J.: Renal tubular mechanisms of organic solute transport. Kidney Int. **9**, 134—148 (1976)

Weiner, I. M., Tinker, J. P.: Pharmacology of pyrazinamide: metabolic and renal function studies related to the mechanism of drug-induced urate retention. J. Pharmacol. exp. Ther. **180**, 411—434 (1972)

Wolbach, R. A.: Renal regulation of acid-base balance in the chicken. Amer. J. Physiol. **181**, 149—156 (1955)

Young, E. G., Musgrave, F. F.: The formation and decomposition of urate gels. Biochem. J. **26**, 941—953 (1932)

Zmuda, M. J., Quebbemann, A. J.: Localization of renal tubular uric acid transport defect in gouty chickens. Amer. J. Physiol. **229**, 820—825 (1975)

Urinary Excretion of Uric Acid in Nonhuman Mammalian Species

F. ROCH-RAMEL and G. PETERS

A. Introduction

Ideas on the renal elimination of uric acid from the beginning of the 19th century up to the 1930's have been extensively reviewed by GUTMAN and YÜ (1972). Most investigators primarily interested in renal physiology made the mode of renal excretion of uric acid fit their preferred concepts of the formation of urine. Thus, uric acid had to be secreted into tubular fluid for BOWMAN (1842), who thought that urinary solutes were secreted by the tubules into water filtered at the glomeruli. For LUDWIG (1844), uric acid, like all other plasma solutes, had to be filtered by the glomeruli to be subsequently concentrated in tubular fluid by "passive" abstraction of water. For CUSHNY (1917), uric acid had to be filtered by the glomeruli and subsequently partly reabsorbed by an active transport mechanism supposed to transport a fluid of constant composition resembling Locke's solution (but probably containing more uric acid) from the tubules to the peritubular capillaries. The renal handling of uric acid as such became interesting to physicians when A. B. GARROD (1859), on the basis of presumably invalid measurement of urinary uric acid, suggested that human gout could be due to a primary failure of renal uric acid excretion. It is easier to imagine a functional incapacity of a secretory process than a disturbance in the filtration-reabsorption mechanism, resulting in retention. Thus, most investigators who followed this lead carried out experiments in birds, the uric acid of which is transported into the urine by net tubular secretion (see GUTMAN and YÜ, 1972). Extrapolation from birds to mammals, however, cannot easily be justified because the large amounts of uric acid produced in the metabolism of the uricotelic phyla (birds and reptiles) may be expected to be excreted by other mechanisms than in the ureotelic phyla (amphibia and mammals) in which uric acid is an intermediary metabolite, or sometimes the end product, of purine metabolism (KEILIN, 1958).

The present review is exclusively concerned with the fate of uric acid (urate) in the kidneys of nonhuman mammals. After many controversies during the last 40 years (GUTMAN and YÜ, 1972), the fundamental nature of uric acid translocation within the mammalian kidney may be considered firmly established (FORSTER, 1967; GUTMAN and YÜ, 1972). Urate ions (uric acid is practically completely dissociated at pH 7.4) are filtered through the glomerular membrane and are subsequently reabsorbed from tubular fluid, but are also secreted from peritubular blood into tubular fluid. The main differences in the pattern of urinary urate excretion between different mammalian species are due to variation in the relative rates of tubular secretion and reabsorption.

Among mammals, only man and the great apes (chimpanzee, *Pongo pygmaeus* or "orang-utan" and gorilla) depend on the renal excretion of urate for health and survival. Only in these species is uric acid the end product of purine metabolism; it reaches plasma concentrations near the limit of its (rather low) solubility (FANELLI et al., 1970a; CHRISTEN et al., 1970a, 1970b).

In all lower mammalian species investigated, uricase present in body tissues, mainly in the liver, catalyzes the degradation of most of the uric acid formed into allantoin, which is excreted by the kidneys (FLORKIN and DUCHATEAU, 1943). In these species, the concentration of uric acid in the blood is 5–20 times lower than in man, resulting in a very small filtered load. The excretion of uric acid as such is biologically unimportant to the subanthropoid mammals. We shall demonstrate that, in spite of this fact, the kidneys of the lower mammals possesss the same transport mechanisms as those of man and anthropoids, but use them at a quantitatively different level. Studies on lower mammalian species provided information on the sites of secretion and reabsorption, and on mechanisms of drug action that appear applicable to man.

The term "secretion" will be used here to denote an inflow of urate from peritubular blood into tubular fluid, and the term "reabsorption" to denote an outflow of urate from tubular fluid to peritubular blood: the use of neither term implies any judgment on the mechanism of translocation, which may be diffusional or carrier mediated, and may or may not imply energy consumption. The term "net secretion" will be taken to indicate predominance of secretion over reabsorption in a given segment of the nephron or in the whole kidney. Similarly "net reabsorption" will be used to denote predominance of the reabsorptive over the secretory flow.

Any decrease in the fractional excretion of urate $(C_{urate}/C_{inulin} = FE_{urate})$ may result from either a depression of urate secretion or an enhancement of urate reabsorption; conversely, any increase of the fractional excretion of urate may be due to either diminished reabsorption or increased secretion. Unless the authors of published contributions arrive at other conclusions, we shall, throughout this review interpret published data by assuming that any drug-induced decrease of FE_{urate} is due to an inhibition of the secretory movement, and any increase of FE_{urate} to a depression of the reabsorptive flow. It should also be stressed that the apparent absence of a uricosuric or an antiuricosuric effect of a drug may be due either to simultaneous enhancement and depression of transtubular urate transports in both directions or to the absence of an effect on transtubular urate movements.

The following abbreviations will be used in this review: C_{urate} = urinary clearance of urate; C_{in} = urinary clearance of inulin = glomerular filtration rate (GFR); C = urinary clearance of a substance denoted by a subscript; FE = fractional excretion of a substance denoted by a subscript; FE_{urate} = fractional excretion of urate = C_{urate}/C_{in}; P_{urate} = concentration of urate in plasma. Concentrations of urate will be expressed either as mg-% = mg uric acid/100 ml urine, plasma or tissue water, or as mM = mmol/liter urine, plasma or tissue water.

B. Methods of Investigation

Evaluation of proposed mechanisms of urate excretion requires knowledge of the methods of investigation used and of their limitations, which have recently been reviewed by TORRETTI and WEINER (1976).

I. Clearance Methods

In most recent studies on the influence of drugs or of physiologic changes on urinary urate excretion, C_{in} was used as a measure of GFR. Unfortunately, in some studies in the dog or the rabbit, the clearance of exogenous creatinine and, sometimes even of endogeneous creatinine was taken as a measure of GFR. Creatinine is known to be secreted and presumably also reabsorbed by renal tubules of dogs and of other mammals, and the secretion of creatinine is known to be inhibited by drugs interfering with transport of uric acid, such as probenecid, salicylate, or p-aminohippurate (PAH) (WESSON, 1969). Therefore a simultaneous depression of both urate and creatinine secretion by a drug may obscure changes of urate transport.

In the rabbit, creatinine has been found not to be subject to transtubular transport (WESSON, 1969; NOLAN and FOULKES, 1971). Other investigators, however, found that in the rabbit the urinary clearance of creatinine is depressed by probenecid (MØLLER, 1966b) and that urate reabsorption is depressed by creatinine (BEECHWOOD et al., 1964). Experimental studies based on measurement of GFR as $C_{creatinine}$ are, therefore, difficult to interpret.

II. Stop-flow Analysis

The stop-flow method has been applied to the study of urate excretion in dogs (YÜ et al., 1960; MUDGE et al., 1968b) rabbits (MØLLER, 1965a; BEECHWOOD et al., 1964) and Cebus monkeys (FANELLI et al., 1970b). Such studies should lead to correct conclusions about sites of net secretion and of net reabsorption if carried out carefully, with prior (rather than simultaneous) determination of the PAH peak, indicating a proximal site of movement (in order to avoid the possible interference of PAH with urate transports), and in the presence of a clear-cut sodium and chloride dip that identifies distal samples.

When urate is injected into the renal artery during the period of stopped urine flow ("modified stop-flow" experiments) the secretory urate flow can be detected even in species in which reabsorption predominates over secretion (ZINS and WEINER, 1968). This method, however, shows secretion occurring along a concentration gradient.

III. The Double-Isotope-Precession Method

When pelvic urine and renal venous blood are continuously sampled after a bolus injection of ^{14}C-urate and ^{3}H-inulin, temporal precession of ^{14}C over ^{3}H in urine indicates secretion, while an increase of the $^{14}C/^{3}H$ ratio in renal venous blood beyond that present in the injectate demonstrates urate reabsorption (SILVERMAN et al., 1970). This method has been used to analyse drug effects on renal urate excretion (NOLAN and FOULKES, 1971).

IV. Micropuncture Methods

1. Microinjection Technique

Microinjection of ^{14}C-urate and ^{3}H-inulin into various sites of proximal or distal convoluted tubules has been performed only in rats (KRAMP et al., 1971; WEINMAN et al., 1975). Fluid overloading of a tubule, which is difficult to avoid because of the low specific radioactivity of ^{14}C-2-urate may create artifactual changes.

As proposed by KRAMP and LENOIR (1975b), secretory movements of urate can be studied by continuous sampling of the urine from one kidney after microinjection of the labeled compound mixture into a peritubular capillary. In a simplified variant of the latter technique, capillary microinjection of a ^{14}C-urate-^{3}H-inulin mixture is replaced by placing a droplet of the mixture on the decapsulated surface of the kidney (KRAMP and LENOIR, 1975; ROCH-RAMEL and WEINER, 1975).

2. Microperfusion of Tubular Segments In Vivo

Tubular reabsorption of urate has been studied in the rat by microperfusing tubular segments, with the technique described by DEETJEN and SILBERNAGL (1972). In such experiments, tubular segments were perfused with ^{14}C-2-urate dissolved in either isotonic saline (ROCH-RAMEL et al., 1976a), or, when movements of urate were to be evaluated independently of water movements, in solutions containing raffinose or mannitol (LANG et al., 1972; ROCH-RAMEL et al., 1976a; WEINMAN et al., 1976a). The process of reabsorption measured under these conditions differs from physiologic reabsorption in that it always occurs along a favorable concentration gradient.

Urate secretion has also been investigated by microperfusion, by measuring the movements of unlabeled urate into tubular perfusate in the absence or the presence of a concentration gradient (LANG et al., 1972, 1973; ROCH-RAMEL et al., 1976a).

3. Microperfusion of Isolated Tubular Segments from Rabbits In Vitro

This technique, developed originally by BURG (1972), has only been used for rabbit kidneys.

4. Free-flow Micropuncture

The renal fate of uric acid in rats has been investigated with the free-flow micropuncture technique (ABRAMSON and LEVITT, 1975; GREGER et al., 1971; ROCH-RAMEL et al., 1976a), in dogs (ROCH-RAMEL et al., 1976c), in rabbits (ROCH-RAMEL et al., 1976b), and in Cebus monkeys (ROCH-RAMEL and WEINER, 1973, 1975). Free-flow micropuncture experiments lead to conclusions about the net addition or net withdrawal of urate from tubular fluid at different sites of superficial nephrons. Since not all segments of superficial nephrons are accessible to micropuncture, and since a different handling of urate by juxtamedullary convoluted tubules can never be excluded it may be difficult to interpret differences between fractions of urate that have escaped tubular reabsorption or have been added to tubular fluid at various sites of superficial nephrons and the FE_{urate} (ROCH-RAMEL et al., 1970).

5. Uptake of Uric Acid by Renal Tissue

In species that show an overall net secretion of urate, renal cortical slices concentrate urate, presumably by transport across their peritubular membranes (CROSS and TAGGART, 1950). In intact animals of several species, drugs known to interfere with urate transport (in either direction) inhibit this uptake (PLATTS and MUDGE, 1961).

Similarly, urate is concentrated in the cells of suspensions of rabbit renal tubules prepared by treating renal cortical tissue with collagenase (method first described by BURG and ORLOFF, 1962).

V. Analytic Methods Used for Measuring Urate Concentrations in Body Fluids

In lower mammals the plasma concentration of urate generally is equal to or even much lower than 1 mg-% (MUDGE et al., 1973). Measurement of plasma concentrations, therefore, is difficult unless large blood samples are obtained. Therefore, studies have frequently been carried out in animals loaded with urate. The analytic method used in clearance studies, in which fairly large volumes of urine and plasma were available, has generally been the highly specific uricase-UV absorption method described by POULSEN and PRAETORIUS (1954), which may be considered a standard for evaluating any other method. The phosphotungstic acid method of FOLIN and DENIS (1912) used in all older studies has been shown to be nonspecific (YÜ and GUTMAN, 1957) because reducing substances other than uric acid present in urine react with phosphotungstate.

In free-flow micropuncture studies quantities of urate as low as 10^{-10} g (6×10^{-13} mol) must be measured in samples of tubular fluid. The Poulsen-Praetorius method is not sensitive enough for such measurements. Ultramicroanalytic methods for this purpose have been developed by adapting the nonspecific colorimetric method of Folin to ultramicrodimensions (GREGER et al., 1971), by reducing an enzymatic and fluorometric procedure described by BLOCH and LATA (1970) to ultradimensions (ROCH-RAMEL and WEINER, 1973) and, finally, by infusing ^{14}C-urate and separating it from ^{14}C-allantoin by chromatography of samples of tubular fluid, plasma and urine (ABRAMSON et al., 1974). All three types of ultramicroanalytic methods have been used in free-flow micropuncture experiments in rats.

VI. Overall Renal Function and Plasma Concentrations of Uric Acid in Various Mammalian Species

As stated in the introduction, the combination of different rates of metabolic degradation, renal and intestinal excretion, and uric acid production results in widely different physiologic plasma concentrations in different species of mammals. These concentrations, as well as the prevalent values of fractional excretion present in the different species are summarized in Table 1. Present-day knowledge on the renal fate of urate in those species that have been investigated most extensively will be discussed in the subsequent sections.

C. Rabbit

The rabbit was the preferred experimental animal of early investigators interested in uric acid for its own sake. It has sometimes also been used in attempts to obtain more general insights into mechanisms of the formation of the urine. In the latter context, HEIDENHAIN and NEISSER (1874) felt that they had demonstrated tubular secretion of an important urinary constituent when they saw "aggregates" of crystalline and

Table 1. Plasma concentration and fractional excretion of uric acid in different species of mammals

	P_{urate}		FE_{urate}	References
	mg-%	(μM/Liter)		
Rat	0.5–0.7	(30–40)	0.2–0.3	DE ROUGEMONT et al., 1976
	3.0–3.2[a]	(180–190)	0.5–0.6	DE ROUGEMONT et al., 1976
Guinea pig	0.2–0.9	(30–55)	0.6	LEMIEUX et al., 1973a
			2.0–4.0	from MUDGE et al., 1973
Rabbit	0.2–0.5	(10–30)	0.2–0.95	from MUDGE et al., 1973
	3.3–3.5	(190–210)	1.5–1.6[a]	ROCH-RAMEL et al., 1976b
Dalmatian dog	0.6–0.8	(35–50)		from MUDGE et al., 1973
	2.8–3.0[a]	(170–180)	1.3–1.5[a]	ROCH-RAMEL et al., 1976c
				LEMIEUX and PLANTE, 1968
Non-Dalmatian dog	0.2–0.4	(10–20)	0.2–0.4	from MUDGE et al., 1973
	2.8–3.0[a]	(170–180)	0.4–0.5[a]	ROCH-RAMEL et al., 1976c
				LEMIEUX and PLANTE, 1968
Cat	?		0.6–1.0	from MUDGE et al., 1973
Goat	0.3–1.0	(20–60)	?	from MUDGE et al., 1973
	?		1.3–3.8	from MUDGE et al., 1973
Calf	0.6	(35)		from MUDGE et al., 1973
	?		1.2	from MUDGE et al., 1973
Pig	<0.1	(<5)		SIMMONDS et al., 1976
	0.1–0.4[a]	(5–20)	1.0–3.0[a]	SIMMONDS et al., 1976
Rhesus monkey (*Macaca mulatta*)	<0.5	(<30)	2.0–3.5	FANELLI et al., 1970a
Cebus monkey (*Cebus albifrons*)	1.5–6	(100–350)	0.04–0.15	FANELLI et al., 1970a
Chimpanzee (*Pan troglodytes*)	2.0–5.0	(120–300)	0.03–0.15	FANELLI et al., 1970a
Man	3.0–7.0	(180–420)	0.07–0.13	from MUDGE et al., 1973

Figures italicized are for normal levels of uric acid and the fractional excretion at these levels.
[a] Animals overloaded by i.v. infusion of uric acid.

amorphous urate in tubular lumina of rabbits after injecting urate into the aorta: the uric acid found in the tubules was further identified by recrystallization and/or the murexide reaction (oxidation to alloxan and treatment with ammonia, yielding ammonium purpurate) (confirmed by EBSTEIN and NICOLAIER, 1896; and by ECKERT, 1913). Heidenhain's interpretation was challenged by CUSHNY (1917), who stated that the precipitation of urate in tubular fluid could also be explained by the concentration of filtered urate as a consequence of water reabsorption. This interpretation was supported by microscopic observations by SCHULTZ (1931), who, after single i.v. injections of large doses of lithium urate in rabbits, found urate crystals and crystal aggregates between the glomerular tufts and in Bowman's capsule, but interpreted his data as an expression of secretion of urate by glomerular capillaries.

    CUSHNY (1917) was aware of the fact that the urinary clearance of uric acid (mainly in the dog) is rather small. His interpretation of the appearance of crystals in tubular fluid was based on the assumption that uric acid is a "nonthreshold" substance, i.e., is not reabsorbed from tubular fluid. Thus he proposed that plasma uric acid could not be completely filterable through glomerular capillaries due to its "colloidal state" in the plasma. There is, however, no evidence of the existence of "colloidal solutions" of uric acid in the sense given to this term in the early twentieth century. When present at high concentrations, which are frequently reached in the urine of all species and under pathologic conditions in human plasma, uric acid forms supersaturated solutions. There is no reason to assume that supersaturation influences particle size or interferes with ultrafiltrability. The ultrafiltrability of plasma urate could be limited by protein binding. However, more recent evidence suggests that this is not so.

Plasma urate levels in rabbits are low as a consequence of uricase activity located mainly in the liver. Subtotal (90%) hepatectomy results in large increases of P_{urate} and of the urinary urate excretion (McMASTER and DRURY, 1929). In spite of the presence of uricase, 2–3 i.v. injections of 160 to 250 mg/kg (1.0–1.5 mmol/kg) of urate (injected with 1.4–2 mmol/kg Li_2CO_3), given at 24 h intervals, induced acute anuria, uremia, and death within 12 h after the last injection (MARZANI, 1964a, 1964b). Similar results were obtained by BODA et al. (1966).

I. Ultrafilterability of Urate

BEECHWOOD et al. (1964) and MØLLER (1965a) using the ultrafiltration procedure of TORIBARA et al. (1957) found that more than 95% of the urate present in rabbit plasma was ultrafilterable through the cellophane membrane. This conclusion was confirmed by SHEIKH and MØLLER (1968), who studied protein binding of uric acid by three different methods: equilibrium dialysis (HUGHES and KLOTZ, 1956), ultrafiltration through a cellophane membrane under a CO_2 atmosphere (TORIBARA et al., 1957), and gel filtration (ALVSAKER, 1965). Comparing human and rabbit serum at 4° C and 20° C resp., the latter being enriched to a urate concentration of 5 mg-% (0.3 mM), they found that 26% of the urate present in man and 16% in the rabbit were bound to plasma proteins at 4° C, but that protein binding did not exceed 5% in either species at 20° C. SIMKIN (1972a), using the equilibrium-dialysis method, however, did not find any binding at 4° C. The possibility that the apparent absence of protein binding found at plasma levels of 5 mg-% (0.3 mM) in rabbit could be due to a saturation of the binding sites at relatively low urate concentrations, is ruled out by experiments of BEECHWOOD et al. (1964) who found no evidence for protein binding in the plasma of rabbits that were not loaded with urate, i.e., at plasma concentrations of 0.2–0.4 mg/100 ml (0.012–0.024 mM).

II. Fractional Excretion of Urate

At physiologic urate concentrations in plasma (0.1–0.5 mg/100 ml = 0.006–0.03 mM) the fractional excretion of urate (C_{urate}/GFR) in the rabbit varies from 10–80% and tends to increase with increasing plasma concentrations (MØLLER, 1962, 1966a; POULSEN and PRAETORIUS, 1954). When the plasma urate concentration is raised to levels of 1–4 mg/100 ml (0.06–0.24 mM) by infusion, the fractional excretion usually rises above 100% and may reach values as high as 200% (POULSEN and PRAETORIUS,

1954; MØLLER, 1966a). In this respect, however, there are large non-sex-related differences between individual rabbits, even when studied in the same laboratory (BEECHWOOD et al., 1964). It is, therefore, not surprising that different investigators working in different laboratories apparently reached contradictory results. Thus, at the plasma urate concentration of 3 mg/100 ml (0.18 mM) POULSEN and PRAETORIUS (1954), as well as MØLLER (1966a), found fractional excretion above unity, i.e., net secretion, while BEECHWOOD et al. (1964) found a fractional excretion around 80% and, thus, net reabsorption. Both MØLLER (1966a) and BEECHWOOD et al. (1964) used inulin for measuring GFR. POULSEN and PRAETORIUS (1954) used creatinine, which might have interfered with transtubular urate transports (see below), but reached results that agree with those of MØLLER (1966a).

The change from tubular net reabsorption to net secretion with increasing plasma concentrations of urate presumably indicates an increasing prevalence of secretory vs. reabsorptive transtubular transport. In the absence of data on the two unidirectional fluxes in the rabbit kidney in vivo, it cannot be determined whether, at high plasma levels, secretion prevails over reabsorption by a primary enhancement of the secretory process or by a primary depression of the reabsorptive process. The fact that in urate-loaded rabbits net secretion is depressed by salicylate and is actually converted into net reabsorption by probenecid (POULSEN, 1955) demonstrates that reabsorption occurs simultaneously with secretion and may, furthermore, argue for an enhanced rate of the unidirectional secretory flux as the primary determinant of net secretion. If the plasma-urate concentration is raised to extremely high levels (34–60 mg/100 ml = 2–4 mM), the secretory flux is saturated (MØLLER, 1966a).

The conversion of net reabsorption into net secretion with increasing plasma concentrations of urate, also demonstrated in other mammalian species (see below), suggests that there may be a control mechanism for stabilizing the concentration of urate in the circulating blood. Nothing is known at the present time about the nature or the purpose of such a hypothetical regulatory system.

The secretory transport of urate across tubular walls usually occurs against a chemical (and presumably also against an electrochemical) gradient, and may be assumed to be a carrier mediated process. The reabsorptive flux from tubular fluid to peritubular plasma may also be assumed to be carrier mediated. It has been shown by MØLLER (1962) in rabbits infused with lactate at a physiologic plasma concentration of urate, that net reabsorption may occur against a concentration gradient: under these conditions the concentration of urate was lower in the urine than in plasma.

Changes in the rate of urine flow in urate-loaded rabbits affect the fractional excretion of urate to a minor extent: any increase of urine flow by five- to tenfold resulted maximally in a 10% increase of the fractional excretion (BEECHWOOD et al., 1964; MØLLER, 1966a; MUDGE et al., 1968b). At physiologic plasma concentrations of urate, however, MØLLER (1962) found a pronounced increase of the fractional excretion of urate, resulting in a conversion of net reabsorption into net secretion at high rates of urine flow. In these experiments, diuresis was induced by infusing a 0.9% NaCl solution containing either mannitol or sulfate at a rate of 2–7 ml/min, along with creatinine (0.4 g/l) as a glomerular marker. The rapid infusion of this solution not only induced diuresis, but also increased the tubular load of creatinine from 8 to 28 mg/min. Smaller amounts of creatinine than represented by this difference have been shown to interfere with urate reabsorption in stop-flow experiments in rabbits

(BEECHWOOD et al., 1964). The uricosuria ascribed to osmotic diuresis by MØLLER (1962) may in fact have been due to an effect of the creatinine.

By stop-flow experiments, the secretory mechanism of transtubular urate transport has been localized to the proximal tubule: the peak of secretion was located at the same site as that of PAH (BEECHWOOD et al., 1964; MØLLER, 1965a, 1965b). A proximal secretory peak of urate concentration in stop-flow experiments was also observed in animals in a state of net reabsorption of urate. This peak could be turned into a reabsorptive dip by injecting probenecid (BEECHWOOD et al., 1964). The existence and suppression of the peak demonstrate the simultaneous occurrence of secretion and reabsorption.

No changes in urate concentration were observed in "distal samples" in stop-flow experiments: no net transtubular movements of urate appear to occur at this site (BEECHWOOD et al., 1964).

III. Micropuncture Studies and Microperfusion of Isolated Tubular Segments

Free-flow micropuncture data have been obtained only for convoluted proximal tubules on the surface of the kidney (ROCH-RAMEL et al., 1976b). In urate-loaded rabbits (plasma concentration 3–4 mg/100 ml = 0.2 mM) excreting 160% of the filtered load in their urine, only 80% of the filtered load was recovered in proximal tubular micropuncture samples. Thus net reabsorption occurred in proximal convoluted tubules, and the overall net secretion must be assumed to be due to net secretion, either in the straight parts of proximal tubules or in lower segments of the nephron.

Studies in vitro on different isolated segments of the rabbit nephron (CHONKO et al., 1975, 1976) showed that the only segment capable of secreting urate against a chemical gradient is the pars recta, which also appears to be the site of the most rapid secretion of PAH (TUNE et al., 1969).

IV. Uptake of Urate into Renal Cortical Tissue In Vitro

Cortical slices from rabbits have been shown to concentrate urate up to 2–3 times the level of concentration in the bathing fluid (BERNDT and BEECHWOOD, 1965; PLATTS and MUDGE, 1961). In suspensions of separated cortical tubules, the concentration factor for 2-C^{14}-urate reached the value of 3–4 (SHEIKH and MØLLER, 1971). Thus, cells of renal cortex concentrate 2-C^{14}-uric acid as well as nonlabeled uric acid. This finding excludes the possibility that the high concentration of intracellular urate in slices is due only to intracellular synthesis, as suggested by JONES and DESPOPOULOS (1974). Uptake into cortical slices has not been confirmed by DESPOPOULOS (1959) or JONES and DESPOPOULOS (1974). These workers do not provide data on the fractional excretion of urate and may, therefore, have used a strain of rabbits that does not secrete uric acid. Uptake of urate into slices depends on the presence of oxygen and is enhanced by high concentrations of potassium (40 mM) in the bath, but is not affected to any notable extent by varying the pH of the incubation medium (7.1–7.9). Rubidium and cesium in high concentrations also increase urate uptake (BERNDT and

BEECHWOOD, 1965), and it is not depressed by reduction of the sodium concentration of the bathing medium to 65 mM.

The uptake of urate into renal cortical tissue critically depends on its concentration in the bathing medium: at or below 0.1 mM in the medium, the concentration in suspended tubules was actually lower than in the medium, but at 0.75 mM it was higher (SHEIKH and MØLLER, 1971). In slices the maximal concentration was reached at 0.5 mM urate in the medium; it most likely decreased as a consequence of saturation of the concentrating mechanism at concentrations above 1.0 mM (PLATTS and MUDGE, 1961). Lower levels of urate in tubules suspended in a bathing medium at 0.1 mM (SHEIKH and MØLLER, 1971) may reflect the presence of an active extrusion mechanism (MØLLER and SHEIKH, 1976). Such an extrusion mechanism at the peritubular surface of tubular cells could be part of the system for tubular urate reabsorption. This view is supported by the fact that PAH, which is only slightly reabsorbed from mammalian tubules (CHO and CAFRUNY, 1970), does not show this phenomenon (CROSS and TAGGART, 1950).

The effects of endogenous substrates such as lactate, pyruvate, and Krebs-cycle metabolites are shown in Table 2. Some of them stimulate, while others decrease urate uptake. Some of the changes observed may be explained by an increase in metabolic energy supply. These substrates, however, are also organic anions, which may compete with uric acid for tubular secretion or even reabsorption. Similar dual effects are exerted by endogenous metabolites on PAH uptake by rabbit renal slices (HEWITT et al., 1976).

The efflux of urate from loaded slices has been studied by BERNDT et al. (1965) and was found to be quite dissimilar to the efflux of PAH (TAGGART et al., 1953). Urate efflux was unaffected by sodium acetate and was stimulated by sodium succinate and by the absence of potassium from the medium.

V. Drug Effects

The effects of many different drugs on various aspects of tubular urate transport in rabbits are summarized in Table 2.

The data are self-explanatory. In general, drugs that in man are known to be uricosuric, in rabbits either decrease the fractional excretion of urate or are inactive. Pyrazinoic acid, a well-known inhibitor of the secretion of uric acid in man, enhances the proximal tubular secretory peak of the rabbit in stop-flow experiments, presumably by depressing reabsorption, without, however, increasing FE_{urate}. The interactions with PAH indicate that both compounds may partially share a common pathway for secretion. In the rabbit, urate infusion depresses PAH secretion (MØLLER, 1967a, 1967b). Urate inhibits the uptake of PAH seen in slices (DESPOPOULOS, 1959). Thus urate and PAH, compete for the secretory transport mechanism, the affinity of urate being slightly smaller than that of PAH (MØLLER, 1967a, 1967b). It is particularly noteworthy that creatinine, at a dose of 18 mg/kg, like hydrochlorothiazide, pyrazinoic acid and ouabain, increases the stop-flow proximal secretory peak, presumably by depressing reabsorption, but does not actually induce uricosuria (BEECHWOOD et al., 1964). Creatinine is neither a cation nor an anion but is secreted by the tubules of the chicken and of some mammalian species by a carrier-mediated system sensitive to both inhibitors of the organic cation and the inorganic

Table 2. Effects of drugs and metabolites on renal urate excretion in rabbits

Drug	Dose mg/kg	Effects				Effects on uptake into slices or separated tubules		
		FE_{urate}		Proximal[b] secretory peak in stop flow	Concentration in renal cortex (in vivo)	Concentration M	Slices	Tubules (in vitro)
		At low P_{urate}	At high P_{urate}					
Pyrazionic acid	30–100		—	2) ↗		10^{-3}	↗10)	
Probenecid	30–50	small↗ 1) 2) 3)	↗ 3) 11) 12)	Reversed to →reabsorption 2) 4)	↗11)	10^{-6}–10^{-4}	↗↘9) 10)	→6) 7)[a] 8)[a]
Salicylate	50–200	— 1) 2), —5)	1) 2), ↗11) 12), —5)	—2)	↗11)	10^{-4}–10^{-3}	→9) 10)	
Benziodarone	1–8					10^{-5}–10^{-4}	↗10)	
Phenylbutazone						10^{-4}	↗10)	
Sulfinpyrazone						10^{-5}–10^{-4}	↗10)	
Cinchophene						10^{-4}–10^{-3}	↗10)	
2-Phenyl-3-OH-cinchoninic acid								↗14)
Barbituric acid						$> 10^{-3}$	↗10)	
p-Diethyl-sulfamyl-benzoic acid						10^{-4}–10^{-3}		↗14)
Benzoic acid						$> 10^{-3}$		
p-Aminohippurate	20–100		↗11) 12)	↗12)	↗11)	$> 10^{-3}$	↗↗10)	↗6)
Hippurate						10^{-4}–10^{-3}	↗↗10)	↗6)
Diodone	25–150		↗11) 12), —2)	↗12)		10^{-4}–10^{-3}	↗10)	↗14)
Chlorothiazide	10–30		—2)	↗2)		10^{-4}–10^{-3}	↗10)	↗14)
Ethacrynic acid						10^{-4}–10^{-3}		↗14)
Acetazolamide						10^{-3}		↗14)
Tienilic acid	50	—16)	—16)					
Ouabain	0.04		↗9)	↗9)		10^{-5}–10^{-4}	↗↗9)	→7)[a] 8)[a]
2,4-Dinitrophenol	10		↗11) 12)		↗11)	10^{-5}–10^{-4}	↗10)	↗6)
Fumarate	100–150		↗11) 12)		↗11)	10^{-2}	↗10)	
Succinate	100–150		↗11) 12)		↗11)	10^{-2}	↗↗10)	
α-Ketoglutarate			↗2)	↗2)		10^{-2}	↗↗10)	
Pyruvate	200–500	↗15)[c]				10^{-2}	—10)	↗13)
Lactate		↗2)	↗2)			10^{-2}	—10)	
Acetate		—				10^{-3}	↗↗10)	
Creatinine	18	—	↗2)	↗2)		$> 10^{-3}$	↗10)	—13)

↗ Increase. ↘ Decrease. — No change.

[a] Isolated perfused pars recta. [b] ↗ Possibly due to a decrease in reabsorption. [c] GFR measured as creatine clearance.

1) POULSEN (1955); 2) BEECHWOOD et al. (1964); 3) MØLLER (1966b); 4) MØLLER (1965a); 5) LEMIEUX et al. (1973b); 6) SHEIKH and MØLLER (1971); 7) CHONKO et al. (1975); 8) CHONKO et al. (1976); 9) BERNDT and BEECHWOOD (1965); 10) PLATTS and MUDGE (1961); 11) MØLLER (1967a); 12) MØLLER (1967b); 13) KIPPEN and KLINENBERG (1976b); 14) KIPPEN and KLINENBERG (1976a); 15) MØLLER (1962); 16) LEMIEUX et al. (1976).

anion transport systems (WESSON, 1969). However, no net secretion of creatinine has been observed in the rabbit (WESSON, 1969; NOLAN and FOULKES, 1971).

It should be stressed that the apparent absence of a drug effect on the fractional excretion of urate may show an equal inhibition of transport in the secretory and in the reabsorptive direction. Any change in the fractional excretion of urate reflects a change of prevalence between reabsorption and secretion; unfortunately, it is generally impossible to state which of the two transports is primarily altered.

VI. Conclusion

In the rabbit, the physiologic plasma-urate level is very low. Plasma urate is probably completely filterable through glomerular capillaries at the physiologic plasma level and certainly is nearly completely filterable at higher plasma levels. In the proximal convoluted tubule, urate is both reabsorbed and secreted; the rates of the uni-directional fluxes are unknown. The result of the transport across the walls of proximal convoluted tubules appears to be net reabsorption of smaller or larger magnitude, as long as the plasma concentration remains below 30 times the physiologic level. For the whole kidney, net reabsorption prevails at physiologic and slightly increased plasma concentrations of urate, but reverts to net secretion at high plasma concentrations or urate. Overall net secretion is most probably due to net secretion by the straight portion of the proximal tubules. No transtubular movements of urate appear to occur across the walls of distal convoluted tubules or of collecting ducts. Most drugs that are uricosuric in man, in the rabbit inhibit the secretory flux more than the reabsorptive flux, and thereby exert an antiuricosuric effect. Thiazide diuretics and pyrazinoic acid may predominantly inhibit the reabsorptive urate flux, but this effect can only be demonstrated under stop-flow conditions. The only drug that has a definite uricosuric effect in the rabbit is ouabain.

The secretory pathway for urate across proximal tubules of the rabbit may be partly identical with the mechanism for the secretion of organic anions, e.g., PAH. An active transport mechanism located in the peritubular membrane may play a role in the reabsorption of urate.

D. Dog

I. Comparison of Dalmatian and Non-Dalmatian Dogs

Differences in uric acid metabolism between different races and strains of dogs have never been systematically investigated. The chance discovery of a larger and a more rapid excretion in the urine of the dalmatian coach hound than in other dogs made by BENEDICT (1915) resulted in many studies in which the dalmatian was compared to other races summarily called "mongrel dogs." Dalmatians excrete 10 times more urate within 24 h than mongrel dogs under normal conditions. Were this difference a primarily renal phenomenon, one would expect the plasma concentration of uric acid to be low in dalmatians. In fact, it is 2–4 times higher than in mongrel dogs, and this hyperuricemia is accompanied by a relatively low concentration of allantoin (and a low urinary excretion of this compound) (YÜ et al., 1971). Increased urinary excretion of urate in the dalmatian does not reflect an accelerated turnover of purine bases since the sum of urate plus allantoin excreted is the same in dalmatian and in mongrel dogs (Yü et al., 1971). The hyperuricemia of dalmatians (DUNCAN et al., 1961; FRIEDMAN and BYERS, 1948a; Yü et al., 1960; Yü et al., 1971) appears to be due to a slow rate of conversion into allantoin (BENEDICT, 1915; FOLIN et al., 1924; FRIEDMAN and BYERS, 1948a; DUNCAN et al., 1961; Yü et al., 1971). The uricase activity of dalmatian liver, however, has consistently been found to equal that found in other dogs (WELLS, 1918; KLEMPERER et al., 1938; ANDREINI et al., 1966); uricase has also been demonstrated to be present in liver peroxisomes (AFZELIUS, 1965; Yü et al., 1971). There is no reason to assume that extrahepatic uricase activity in the dalmatian could be lower than in the mongrel dog. In the latter, some conversion of urate into allantoin occurs even after total hepatectomy (BOLLMAN and MANN, 1933). The decreased rate of urate oxidation in the dalmatian coach hound is presently thought to be due to the presence of an impediment to urate inflow into uricase-containing liver cells (KLEMPERER et al., 1938). Similarly, a transport system for urate into red blood cells, present in mongrel dogs (HARVEY and CHRISTENSEN, 1964) and in man (OVERGAARD-HANSEN and LASSEN, 1959; LUCAS-HERON and FONTENAILLE, 1976), appears to be absent in dalmatians.

The slow rate of hepatic conversion of urate into allantoin in dalmatian coach hounds adequately explains the hyperuricemia: there is no need to assume an altered rate of disposal by other means. The concentration of urate in CSF was found to be as low as in mongrel dogs (BYERS and FRIEDMAN, 1949), an observation that presumably reflects an equally rapid rate of transport of urate from CSF to blood in both types of dogs. The rate of excretion of uric acid into the gut of dalmatian coach hounds does not appear to have been investigated: in normal dogs this rate may be high, since the clearance of urate into 100 g small intestine perfused with water has been found to be equal to the urinary clearance (KNAPOWSKI et al., 1963).

The increased rate of urinary excretion of urate in dalmatians cannot be due to a primary increase of the plasma concentration because (1) the kidney of dalmatians has been shown to excrete urate at a more rapid rate than the kidney of mongrels at plasma concentrations made equal by different rates of urate infusion (ROCH-RAMEL et al., 1976c) and (2) in mongrel dogs, inhibition of the conversion of urate into allantoin to a level similar to that observed in dalmatians does not result in a rise of the urinary urate clearance to a "dalmatian" level (Yü et al., 1971). Dalmatian coach hounds thus appear to differ from mongrel dogs both in a decreased rate of prerenal urate oxidation and by an increase of FE_{urate}.   Though the dog kidney is capable of oxidizing xanthine into urate (MORGAN, 1926), the rate of production is not higher in the dalmatian than in the mongrel kidney (QUEBBEMAN et al., 1975). Neither the mongrel nor the dalmatian kidney appears to have uricase activity (QUEBBEMAN et al., 1975). The difference in the renal fate of urate between dalmatians and other dogs is not due to a difference in ultrafiltrability of urate: urate does not appear to be bound to plasma proteins in either normals dogs (MUDGE et al., 1968b) or in dalmatians, even in equilibrium dialysis experiments at 4° C (SIMKIN, 1972a). The difference between FE_{urate} in dalmatians and in mongrel dogs is evidently of tubular origin and could represent either a genetically determined primary difference in tubular functions, or be due to the presence in dalmatians or in mongrel dogs of blood-borne uricosuric or antiuricosuric factors. Published data on reciprocal transplantation experiments do not allow a distinction to be made between the two possibilities. Thus, dalmatian dogs bearing one single transplanted mongrel dog's kidney have been shown to excrete as much urate, and mongrel dogs bearing one single transplanted dalmatian kidney as little urate as they did before transplantation (APPLEMAN et al., 1966). Unfortunately, renal functions were not studied in these experiments. As expected, reciprocal liver transplantations between dalmatians and non-dalmatians demonstrated that the amount of urate excreted per 24 h was determined by the type of liver present in the organism rather than by the other body tissues comprising the kidney (KUSTER et al., 1967; TOMPKINS et al., 1967; KUSTER et al., 1972). The presence of a dalmatian liver appeared to increase the urinary clearance of urate in the recipient (TOMKINS et al., 1967).

It was shown a long time ago that the urinary clearance of urate is higher than C_{urea} in dalmatians but lower in mongrel dogs (SCHAFFER et al., 1941) and is either equal to (FRIEDMAN and BYERS, 1948a) or higher than (WOLFSON et al., 1950; BEYER, 1954) the clearance of exogeneous creatinine in dalmatians, but lower in mongrel dogs. These observations were originally interpreted as indicating the presence of a tubular secretory mechanism for urate in dalmatians that was absent and replaced by a reabsorptive mechanism in other dogs. Both mechanisms were shown by stop-flow experiments to be located in the proximal tubule (KESSLER et al., 1959). At present there is ample evidence to indicate that both tubular secretion and reabsorption occur in both dalmatian and non-dalmatian dogs and that the difference between the two types of dogs depends on the relative rates of secretion and absorption. Thus, the occurrence of reabsorption simultaneously with secretion in dalmatians is demonstrated by the fact that treatment with probenecid or pyrazinamide depresses FE_{urate} to values as low as 0.7 (YÜ et al., 1960; BEYER et al., 1951). Under particular experimental conditions, FE_{urate} values lower than unity have been observed at normal plasma levels (YÜ et al., 1960) or even after urate loading (REEM and VANAMEE, 1964). On the other hand, the presence of a secretory mechanism for urate in mongrel dogs was suggested by the very old observations of microscopically demonstrated urate crystals in tubules (MINKOWSKI, 1898), and of a depression of urinary urate excretion by cyanide (GREMELS and BODO, 1926). Proof of tubular secretion was provided by the demonstration of net secretion ($FE_{urate} = 1.1$–1.3) in dogs loaded with urate and mannitol (LATHEM et al., 1960; YÜ et al., 1960). Similar to man (BERLINER et al., 1950), the Cebus monkey (FANELLI et al., 1970b), and the rat (BOUDRY, 1971a), mongrel dogs increase their FE_{urate} with increasing urate loads. Furthermore, after a simultaneous injection of ^{14}C-urate and ^{3}H-inulin into the renal artery of mongrel dogs, a smaller fraction of ^{14}C-urate than of ^{3}H-inulin was recovered from the renal vein (NOLAN and FOULKES, 1971); this observation indicates uptake of urate by the kidney, which may or may not have been followed by secretion into the tubules.

All investigators using stop-flow procedures arrived at the conclusion that secretion of urate in dalmatians and reabsorption both in dalmatians and in other dogs occur in proximal tubules (KESSLER et al., 1959; YÜ et al., 1960; MUDGE et al., 1968b; ZINS and WEINER, 1968). That secretion of urate in mongrel dogs also occurs in proximal tubules was definitely established by ZINS and WEINER (1968). They used inulin as a nonreabsorbed indicator, enhanced the secretory movement by infusing urate into the renal artery during stop flow, and observed a single large proximal secretory peak (confirmed by MUDGE et al., 1968b and by NOLAN and FOULKES, 1971). Previous observations of a single distal secretory peak for urate in mongrel dogs (YÜ et al., 1961; DAVIS et al., 1965), as well as a distal and a proximal secretory peak in a few dalmatian coach hounds were probably due to methodologic errors (ZINS and WEINER, 1968) resulting from the use of creatinine as an indicator of water reabsorption. Creatinine is unreliable in this respect (SWANSON and HAKIM, 1962; O'CONNEL et al., 1962).

In free-flow micropuncture experiments in both mongrel and dalmatian dogs infused with urate, at rates calculated to yield similar plasma concentrations (ROCH-RAMEL et al., 1976c), net reabsorption of about 50% of filtered urate was shown to occur in the proximal convoluted tubules of mongrel dogs. That this represented the sum of proximal secretory and reabsorptive flows was demonstrated by an increase of net fractional urate reabsorption produced by pyrazinoic acid, a known inhibitor of urate secretion. In dalmatian coach hounds, on the other hand (ROCH-RAMEL et al., 1976c), net reabsorption of urate occurred in some, but net secretion in other proximal convoluted tubules, so that the mean net movement in this tubular segment was zero. Net secretion in the dalmatian was shown to occur between the late proximal convolutions and the early distal convolutions, presumably analogous to the net secretion in rabbit (see above), in the straight portion of the proximal tubule. The large C_{urate} in dalmatian dogs thus appears to be due to a decreased prevalence of reabsorption over secretion in proximal convoluted tubules and a net secretory transport (absent in mongrel dogs) in the straight portion of the proximal tubules.

No net movements of urate through distal tubules or collecting ducts appeared to occur in these micropuncture experiments. Large corticomedullary gradients of tissue-water urate concentration were, however, observed in nondiuretic mongrel dogs infused with large amounts of urate (EPSTEIN and PIGEON, 1964), but disappeared in mannitol or in water diuresis. As in monkeys (CANNON et al., 1968), the papillary tissue water urate concentration in the nondiuretic dogs often exceeded that found in pelvic urine. This observation may reflect the existence of precipitated urate, crystallized or amorphous, in the papilla.

An increase in the rate of urine flow in mongrel dogs results in a moderate (YÜ et al., 1960; LATHEM et al., 1960) or even extremely small (MUDGE et al., 1968b; PLANTE and LEMIEUX, 1968) increase of FE_{urate}; whatever back diffusion may occur from lower nephron segments is not influenced by variation of the urine pH from 5 to 8 (MUDGE et al., 1968b; LATHEM et al., 1960; PLANTE and LEMIEUX, 1968). Furthermore, rates and mechanisms of renal excretion of uric acid appear to be similar in male and female dogs (MUDGE et al., 1968b). Decreases of renal arterial blood pressure do not appear to depress FE_{urate} (BERGER et al., 1964). An increase in the plasma urate concentration in hemorrhagic hypotension (COWSERT et al., 1966; JONES et al., 1968; SIMEONE et al., 1975) appears to be due to an increase in uric acid production by degradation of adenine and guanine nucleotides, while uricase activity is unchanged.

FE_{urate} was not decreased in non-dalmatian or dalmatian dogs after a 12 day fasting period; in man, such a fasting period would decrease the FE_{urate} secondary to the accumulation of ketone bodies. In dog, however, no ketosis developed (LEMIEUX and PLANTE, 1968).

II. Effects of Drugs

Drug effects on the renal excretion of urate in mongrel dogs are summarized in Table 3, and in dalmatian coach hounds in Table 4. As the tables show, the observations on uricosuric or antiuricosuric effects of most drugs are incomplete. PAH in modified stop-flow experiments in mongrel dogs converted the proximal secretory flux of urate to reabsorption, and caused a small depression of the overall clearance of urate (ZINS and WEINER, 1968); this indicates that the same mechanism may be responsible for the secretory proximal transport of urate and of PAH. Superimposition of sodium cyanide on PAH, however, reconverted the proximal reabsorptive peak into a secretory peak (ZINS and WEINER, 1968). The proximal secretory transport of urate did not appear to be completely blocked by PAH. Metabolic inhibitors such as ouabain (ZINS and WEINER, 1968) or cyanide (GREMELS and BODO, 1926; ZINS and WEINER, 1968; JOHNSON and FOULKES, 1973) inhibit the tubular reabsorption of urate.

In addition to the tabulated data, it should be mentioned that intravenous injections of 3–7.5 g sorbitol, sucrose, fructose, or glycerol in mongrel dogs increased the rate of urate excretion (GRABFIELD and SWANSON, 1942): there is no proof that this apparent uricosuric effect was renal: the simultaneous increase of allantoin excretion observed suggests a metabolic effect. Glucose, xylose, maltose, galactose, mannitol, or dulcitol had no effect on urinary urate excretion under these conditions.

III. Conclusion

Urate is both reabsorbed and secreted in proximal convoluted tubules of mongrel dogs and dalmatian coach hounds. In the proximal convoluted tubules of mongrel dogs, reabsorption prevails over secretion, while no net urate movement occurs downstream from the end of the proximal convoluted tubules. In dalmatians, rates of secretion and reabsorption in proximal convoluted tubules are similar, and net secretion occurs in the straight portion of proximal tubules. These data do not support the idea that the increased excretion of urate in the dalmatian kidney might be due to the presence of an impediment to reabsorption analogous to the impediment to transport of urate into uricase-containing sites of the liver. Drugs that affect uric acid transport in one direction usually also affect the transport in the opposite direction. Secretory transport mechanisms may be more sensitive than the reabsorptive ones to some drugs. Organic anions secreted into proximal tubular fluid appear to compete mainly with the secretory transport of urate but not to block it completely.

E. Rat

I. Plasma Concentration and Ultrafilterability of Urate

The normal urate concentration in rat plasma is low: values reported by different investigators under slightly varying conditions range from 0.4 to 1.5 mg-% (20–90 μM). Plasma urate is scarcely bound to protein: equilibrium dialysis experiments indicated less than 5% protein-binding at 37° C (GREGER et al., 1971, 1974b; LANG, 1976). A

Table 3. Effects of drugs and metabolites on renal urate excretion in mongrel dogs

Drug	Dose mg/kg i.v.	Effects on FE_{urate} At low P_{urate}	At high P_{urate}	Reabsorption proximal dip (stop-flow)	Proximal secretory peak[d] (in modified stop-flow)	2-^{14}C-urate recovery in urine[e]
Probenecid[a]	25–80	↗1)[a] 2)[a] 3) 5)	↗1)[a] 2)[a] 3) 4)[a] 5)	↘3) 6) —5)	↘9)	—7)
	200					↗8)
Salicylate	50–200	↗5) 10)[c] 11)[b]			↘12)	
Sulfinpyrazone	10–15		↗3)			
Benziodarone	0.1/min	—13)[c]	—13)[c]			
Zoxazolamine	30–70		—14)			
Diodone (Iodopyracet)	200–250	↗11)[b]				
Oxipurinol	20–50	↗15)				
Pentobarbital	22	—5)		—5)		
Ouabain	0.05–0.08 (0.05 into renal artery)	—5)		—5)	↗12)	
2-4-Dinitrophenol	10	—5)		—5)		
Cyanide	0.05–0.11/min into renal artery				↗12)	↗8)
Etacrynic acid	2–80				↘9)	
Furosemide	>40				↘9)	
Chlorothiazide	50				↘12) 9)	
Chlormerodrin	7				—9)	
Meralluride	?	—11)[b]				
Mersalyl	>1.5	—22)				
Tienilic acid	50	↗16)	↗16) (net secretion)			
Pyrazinoic acid (or pyrazinamide)	20–120 500–600	↘5)	↘18) 19) ↗17)		↘17) 9)	
p-Aminohippurate	30 150–200		↘12)		↘9) 12)	↗8)
Lactate	100–1000 800–1700		—20) 21)		↘9)	
β-Hydroxybutyrate	?		—21)			
Ethanol	?		—21)			

↗ Increase. ↘ Decrease. — No change.
[a] For other sulfamylbenzoic acid derivates, see Beyer (1954)
[b] No measurement of GFR.
[c] Creatinine used as glomerular marker.
[d] ↗ is due to inhibition of reabsorption.
[e] Double isotope dilution, renal intra-arterial injection; ↗ is due to inhibition of reabsorption.

1) Beyer et al. (1951); 2) Beyer (1954); 3) Yü et al. (1960); 4) Lathem et al. (1960); 5) Mudge et al. (1968b); 6) Kessler et al. (1959); 7) Berger and Yü (1970); 8) Johnson and Foulkes (1973); 9) Nolan and Foulkes (1971); 10) Friedman and Byers (1948b); 11) Miller et al. (1951); 12) Zins and Weiner (1968); 13) Lemieux et al. (1973a); 14) Maroske and Weiner (1968); 15) Elion et al. (1968); 16) Lemieux et al. (1976); 17) Weiner and Tinker (1972); 18) Yü et al. (1961); 19) Roch-Ramel et al. (1976c); 20) Reem and Vanamee (1964); 21) Plante and Lemieux (1968); 22) Fanelli et al. (1973a).

Table 4. Effects of drugs and metabolites on renal urate excretion in Dalmatian coach hounds

Drug	Dose [mg/kg]	FE_{urate}	Comment
Probenecid	i.v. 25–80	↘1) 2) 3) 4) 5)	Net secretion reversed to net reabsorption
Salicylate	i.v. 50–200	—6)	Creatinine as glomerular marker
		—7)	No measurement of GFR
Benziodarone	i.v. 0.1/min	—8)	
Pyrazinoic acid	i.v. 30–70	↘9) 10)	Net secretion reversed to net reabsorption
Oxipurinol	i.v. 20–50	—11)	
Lactate	i.v. 100–1000	—12)	

↗ Increase.   ↘ Decrease.   — No change.

1) YÜ et al. (1960); 2) BEYER (1954), 3) BEYER et al. (1951); 4) KESSLER et al. (1959); 5) BERGER and YÜ (1970); 6) FRIEDMAN and BYERS (1948b); 7) MILLER et al. (1951); 8) LEMIEUX et al. (1973a); 9) YÜ et al. (1961); 10) ROCH-RAMEL et al. (1976c); 11) ELION et al. (1968); 12) REEM and VANAMEE (1964).

higher protein-bound fraction was found by this procedure at 4° C. The urate concentration found in glomerular fluid of Munich-Wistar rats was 5–10% lower than expected when Donnan factors and plasma-water content are taken into consideration (ROCH-RAMEL et al., 1976a). Thus, at least 90–95% of plasma urate is freely ultrafilterable in normal rats.

II. Fractional Excretion of Urate

The fractional excretion of urate in the rat, at physiologic plasma concentrations, varies from 20% to 40% (Table 1). Much higher values were reported by two groups of investigators using labeled urate infusions. Thus, KRAMP et al. (1971) using 2-^{14}C-urate found a fractional excretion of 60%, but in fact, the sum of urate plus allantoin was measured both in blood and in urine. Uricase activity in rats is very high, so that in animals constantly infused with ^{14}C-urate only 15–25% of the ^{14}C in plasma and only 5–10% of the ^{14}C in urine represent urate; the remainder is allantoin (ABRAMSON et al., 1974). The high FE_{urate} found by ABRAMSON and LEVITT (1975) is more difficult to explain. In their study 2-^{14}C-urate was infused and 2-^{14}C-urate separated from ^{14}C-allantoin by column chromatography. These investigators carefully controlled their radiochemical methods and concluded that chemical methods were not applicable to the rat; it is difficult to pinpoint any error. Using 6-^{14}C-urate, however, COOK et al. (1975) found perfect agreement between radiochemical and chemical results: both yielded FE_{urate} values of 30%.

As in mongrel dogs, FE_{urate} increases with increasing plasma concentrations both in anesthetized (KRAMP and LENOIR, 1975a; DE ROUGEMONT et al., 1976) and in un-anesthetized (BOUDRY, 1971a) rats. However, in Boudry's experiments (1971a), the steepness of the increase differed considerably between two strains of unanesthetized "Wistar" rats; surprisingly, at very low plasma levels, an increase of P_{urate} from 0.7 to 1.5 mg-% (40→90 µM) resulted in a decrease of FE_{urate} from 25 to 15%. This finding was interpreted as evidence for the presence of a secretory mechanism saturated at very low plasma concentrations (BOUDRY, 1971a). This interpretation, however, is incompatible with direct measurements of the secretory flux (see below). Although FE_{urate} increases with increasing plasma concentration, it very rarely exceeds 100% (net secretion); such values were observed in 4 out of 12 clearance periods of anesthetized rats infused with mannitol, by GREGER et al. (1971) and in 4 out 146 clearance periods, in unanesthetized rats, by BOUDRY (1971a). Net secretion was also observed by GREGER (1976) in some rats treated with oxonate. Again in contrast to other investigators, ABRAMSON and LEVITT (1975) found no increase of FE_{urate} with increasing plasma concentrations.

Variation of the rate of urine flow from 0.04–1.7 ml/kg body wt · min did not change the FE_{urate} (BOUDRY, 1971a; STEELE et al., 1974; COOK et al., 1975), whether the rate of urine flow was increased by saline or mannitol infusion or by water loading. In the diabetes-insipidus-like state induced by a 7-day treatment with 4–6 mg/kg · day LiCl, FE_{urate} was increased (MARTINEZ-MALDONADO et al., 1975; data given by STEELE et al., 1974). The increase was suspected of being due to an impairment of proximal reabsorption (MARTINEZ-MALDONADO et al., 1975). The large increases of FE_{urate} resulting from an increase of urine flow up to 1.8 ml/kg body wt · min observed in normal rats (GREGER et al., 1971) or in rats either hepatectomized or treated with oxonate (GREGER, 1976) may have been due to variations in the plasma concentration of urate due to the simultaneous infusion of mannitol and of urate (normal rats) or to variable inhibition of uricase activity in oxonate-treated and hepatectomized animals (GREGER, 1976).

It is noteworthy that at much lower rates of urine flow, when urine flow was increased from 0.02–0.05 ml/kg body wt · min as calculated from the U/P_{inulin} values given by GREGER et al. (1971), an increase of FE_{urate} from 20 to 40% was observed in rats at physiologic P_{urate}. This increase may be explained by an increased rate of fluid flow through Henle's loops, rather than through the collecting ducts (see below).

Changes in extracellular fluid volume strongly influence FE_{urate}. In rats expanded by infusion of isotonic saline (10% body wt), FE_{urate} reached 45–50%, whereas in rats with chronic volume depletion induced by furosemide and a low sodium diet, FE_{urate} fell to less than 10% (WEINMAN et al., 1975). An increase of FE_{urate} during acute volume expansion was also noted by ABRAMSON and LEVITT (1975). The relationship between sodium and urate reabsorption will be discussed below.

Changes of urine pH induced by bicarbonate or NH_4Cl had no effect on FE_{urate} in acute experiments on unanesthetized rats (BOUDRY, 1971a). In microperfusion experiments, increasing the pH of the perfusion fluid from 5 to 8 (an increase that could be expected to increase the ionized fraction of urate from 14% to nearly 100%) had no effect on the proximal reabsorption of urate (SONNENBERG et al., 1965; LANG, 1976). Though apparently small, the change of the gradient of the undissociated species between tubular fluid and plasma in such experiments may be expected to be large. The data suggest that undissociated uric acid is not preferentially reabsorbed. Clearance studies, thus, indicate that in the rat, urate reabsorption prevails over the concomitant secretion. High P_{urate} values favor secretion. Back diffusion from lower nephron segments does not appear to play an important role in reabsorption. The tubular transfer mechanisms for undissociated uric acid have not been shown to differ from those for urate ions.

III. Site and Nature of Transtubular Movements of Urate

For technical reasons, the rat is the species in which transport of urate across tubular walls has been studied most extensively by micropuncture and microperfusion methods (for a review, see LASSITER, 1975). The main difficulty in free-flow micropuncture experiments has been in the choice or the development of a suitable ultramicroanalytic method for urate. The three types of ultramicroanalytic methods used in micropuncture experiments and their limitations have been discussed above (Sect. 2. e).

The compound 2-^{14}C-urate can be used only in tubular microperfusion experiments for measuring the reabsorptive flux of urate and in capillary microperfusion experiments for measuring the secretory flux if recirculation of labeled urate can be excluded (LANG et al., 1974). The kidney of rats contains either extremely little (HASHIMOTO, 1974; GRAHAM and KARNOVSKY, 1965; TRUSZKOWSKI and GOLDMANOWNA, 1933) or no uricase activity (STRAUS, 1956; BERNHEIM and BERNHEIM, 1947; THOENES and LANGER, 1969); the radioactivity measured in such experiments, therefore, is entirely due to uric acid.

On the other hand, renal tissues of rats and other mammals have xanthine oxidase activity (FRIEDMAN and BYERS, 1953; BERNHEIM and BERNHEIM, 1947; RICHERT and WESTERFELD, 1951; BASS et al., 1950) and synthesize a certain amount of urate in vivo (ALEXANDER et al., 1966), apparently too little to produce a detectable increase of urate secretion. The secretory flux of urate measured in microperfusion experiments was not increased by the i.v. infusion of xanthine (LANG, 1976), and the fractional excretion of urate was not influenced by infusing either allopurinol or hypoxanthine when the plasma concentration of urate was kept constant (STEELE and UNDERWOOD, 1976).

1. Proximal Convoluted Tubules

At P_{urate} up to 200 µM (3–4 mg-%) urate was reabsorbed from proximal convoluted tubules (ROCH-RAMEL et al., 1976 a; DE ROUGEMONT et al., 1976). Only when P_{urate} was raised to 600 µM (10 mg-%) did net secretion of urate occur in the first half of the proximal convoluted tubules (DE ROUGEMONT et al., 1976). An apparent net secretion at much lower plasma concentrations described by other investigators (GREGER et al., 1971) may be considered an experimental artifact caused by the use of a nonspecific analytic method for tubular fluid (overestimation of urate concentration) and a specific method for plasma and urine (ROCH-RAMEL et al., 1976a). A small proximal net reabsorption of urate (comparable to that found by DE ROUGEMONT et al. (1976) at $P_{urate} = 200$ µM was also found in animals infused with 2-^{14}C-urate after elimination of the uricase activity by subtotal hepatectomy or treatment with oxonate (GREGER, 1976). Though the investigators do not indicate P_{urate} values in the latter experiments, they must be assumed to have been 3–4 times larger than the initial levels 1 h after inhibition of uricase activity (JOHNSON et al., 1969). The group of investigators using the column chromatographic-radiochemical procedure (ABRAMSON and LEVITT, 1975), found a 30% reabsorption of filtered urate from the early proximal, but a subsequent 20% secretion into the late proximal convoluted tubules. As the fractional excretion was 90% of filtered urate (see Table 5), which is in contradiction to all other data reported, these data cannot be interpreted.

Table 5. Physiologic cconcentration and fractional urinary excretion of urate in rats

References	P_{urate} in normal, unloaded rats		No. of rats	Fractional excretion %	Urine-flow rate µl/kg min	Analytic method
	mg-%	µM				
ABRAMSON and LEVITT, 1975	0.34 ±0.04	20± 2	7	0.90±0.02	~ 20	Column chromatography of 2-^{14}C-urate
BOUDRY, 1971a	1.1 ±0.1	65± 6	8	0.10±0.01	300	Enzymatic-UV
	1.5 ±0.1	89± 6	6	0.18±0.03		
COOK et al., 1975	1.53±0.36	91±21	5	0.29±0.09	—	6-^{14}C-urate
			5	0.21±0.07	—	Phosphotungstic acid
GREGER et al., 1971	1.5	90±10	13	0.38±0.05	< 50	Enzymatic-UV
KRAMP et al., 1971	—	—	8	0.76±0.09	< 20	2-^{14}C-urate
KRAMP and LENOIR, 1975a	0.75±0.09	45± 5	9	0.33±0.06	>200	Enzymatic-UV
DE ROUGEMONT et al., 1976	0.63±0.05	38± 3	13	0.32±0.02	120	Fluorometric
STEELE et al., 1974	0.4 ±0.006	24± 1	6	0.13±0.02	~100	Enzymatic-UV
WEINMAN et al., 1975	1.15±0.09	68± 5	9	0.12±0.06	< 50	Enzymatic-O_2 electrode

Net reabsorption (or secretion at very high plasma levels) of urate in proximal convoluted tubules represents the sum of a reabsorptive and a secretory flux. The reabsorptive flux has been measured by tubular microperfusion techniques using 2-^{14}C-urate and has been found to correspond to 15% of the amount of urate perfused per mm of tubular length (SONNENBERG et al., 1965; LANG et al., 1972; ROCH-RAMEL et al., 1976a). A larger reabsorptive flux (30% of the amount perfused per mm of tubular length) has been found by WEINMAN et al. (1976a), who started collecting perfused fluid immediately after initiating the tubular perfusion; the other investigators quoted waited 2 min before beginning the collection. In microinjection experiments (KRAMP et al., 1971; WEINMAN et al., 1975) only 15% of the amount injected into proximal tubular fluid was found to be reabsorbed along the whole proximal tubule. The apparent discrepancy between the results of microperfusion and microinjection experiments could be due to depression of urate reabsorption by increased tubular volume after microinjection, or to other technical factors.

Reabsorptive urate fluxes measured by both techniques may be underestimated because a fraction of the microperfused or microinjected urate could be secreted back into tubular fluid from the large "unstirred layer" situated between the contraluminal membrane of tubular cells and capillary blood (ROCH-RAMEL et al., 1976a).

The transport capacity of the reabsorptive flux is very large: increasing the urate concentration in perfused fluid up to 300 µM (LANG et al., 1972) or up to 830 µM (ROCH-RAMEL et al., 1976a) or even up to 1.5 mM (WEINMAN et al., 1976a) did not appear to result in saturation. A small decrease in fractional reabsorption was, however, observed by LANG (1976) at the rather high concentration of 1 mM. Saturation of reabsorption reported to have been observed in microinjection experiments (KRAMP et al., 1971) was in fact explained by the erroneous use of a logarithmic scale when plotting reabsorption against urate concentration in the microinjectate (ROCH-RAMEL et al., 1976a). Thus, saturation of reabsorption cannot be invoked for explaining the change from net proximal reabsorption to net secretion when P_{urate} is increased from 200 to 600 µM.

It has been proposed that a hypothetical saturable component of the reabsorptive flux of urate would depend on water reabsorption (GREGER et al., 1976). The proximal reabsorption of urate, however, does not depend on sodium (and water) reabsorption. The rate of urate reabsorption was the same when tubules were perfused with isotonic saline (i.e., in the presence of sodium and water reabsorption), or with a so-called equilibrium solution containing raffinose or mannitol and little sodium (in order to inhibit sodium and water reabsorption) (ROCH-RAMEL et al., 1976a). Furthermore, in free-flow micropuncture experiments, the injection of chlorothiazide induced a decrease of proximal sodium and water reabsorption but not of the proximal fractional reabsorption of urate (WEINMAN et al., 1976a). The fact that a few compounds studied more recently are both natriuretic and uricosuric cannot be said to demonstrate a dependence of urate on sodium or water reabsorption: it has been shown that one of these compounds (MK 196 = (6,7-dichloro-2-methyl-1-oxo-2-phenyl-5-indanyloxy acetic acid) in proximal tubules inhibits urate reabsorption and has no influence on sodium reabsorption, but does inhibit sodium reabsorption from lower segments of the nephron (WEINMAN et al., 1976a).

At low P_{urate} levels, proximal reabsorption doubtlessly occurs against a chemical (and an electrochemical) gradient (DE ROUGEMONT et al., 1976). The speculation that this apparently active transport could be due to a downhill transport of unionized uric acid from more acidic tubular fluid to more alkaline plasma (GREGER et al., 1976) meets with the objection that the permeability of proximal tubular walls to undissociated uric acid has not been shown to be greater than to urate ions (see above).

The proximal secretory flux of urate was found to be approximately equal to the reabsorptive flux when measured in microperfusion experiments in which the tubules were perfused with urate-free solutions and P_{urate} kept constant by i.v. infusion (ROCH-RAMEL et al., 1976a). The secretory flux may have been underestimated less than the reabsorptive flux since an "unstirred layer" possibly present on the luminal surface of the cells should be smaller than on the contraluminal surface. The secretory flux did not show any signs of saturation up to plasma urate concentrations above 300 µM (ROCH-RAMEL et al., 1976a). A much larger secretory flux reported by LANG et al. (1972, 1973) probably represents an experimental artifact due to an overestimation of the concentration of urate in recollected perfusate by recourse to the nonspecific phosphotungstate method. Tubular secretion of urate was also demonstrated by the capillary microinjection technique at injection rates from 2 pmol/s up to 20 pmol/s (KRAMP and LENOIR, 1975b). Flux rates cannot be calculated from such experiments.

There is no doubt that secretion occurs simultaneously with reabsorption in the same segment of proximal convoluted tubules. Renal cortical slices from rats, unlike those from rabbits, but like those from mongrel dogs, are unable to concentrate uric acid (PLATTS and MUDGE, 1961). This fact may indicate that the transport mechanism is not located in the contraluminal membrane of tubular cells.

2. Henle's Loops

As usual in micropuncture language, Henle's loop will be taken to include the straight portion of the proximal tubule, the descending and the ascending limbs of Henle's loops, and the very early part of the distal convoluted tubule.

In free-flow micropuncture experiments no significant, or at best a very small reabsorption of urate from Henle's loops was found in rats during slow saline diuresis (ROCH-RAMEL et al., 1976a) or in moderate mannitol diuresis (DE ROUGEMONT et al., 1976). A much larger rate of reabsorption from this segment was found by GREGER et al. (1971) in antidiuretic rats.

Reabsorption of urate (2-^{14}C-urate) was also measured in microperfusion experiments, and at a perfusion rate of 22 nl/min was found to average 9% of the amount perfused at a concentration of 83 μM, and 5.7% at a concentration of 830 μM (ROCH-RAMEL et al., 1976a). Higher rates of reabsorption were measured in similar microperfusion experiments by GREGER et al. (1974a), who also found that the rate of absorption varied from 43% at a perfusion rate of 10 nl/min to 14% at a perfusion rate of 40 nl/min. There is no explanation offered for the discrepancy between the results of the two laboratories.

The concentration of urate in the renal tissue increases from cortex to inner medulla (LANG, 1976). The cortical-medullary urate gradient does not need to be explained by urate movements across the walls of Henle's loops because it was not greater than the corticomedullary gradient of the concentrations of inulin, a solute that does not cross tubular walls, and because the concentration of urate in papillary tissue water did not exceed that in pelvic urine.

3. Distal Convoluted Tubules

No net transtubular movements of urate were found in this segment in free-flow micropuncture studies (ROCH-RAMEL et al., 1976a; DE ROUGEMONT et al., 1976). A very small reabsorption was described by other investigators (GREGER et al., 1974a). In microperfusion experiments (OELERT et al., 1969; LANG, 1976) and in microinjection experiments (KRAMP et al., 1971; KRAMP and LENOIR, 1975a; WEINMAN et al., 1975) the distal convoluted tubules were found to be practically impermeable to urate.

4. Collecting Ducts

In free-flow micropuncture experiments, the fractions of nonreabsorbed urate recovered from end-distal tubules and from pelvic urine were equal (ROCH-RAMEL et al., 1976a; DE ROUGEMEONT et al., 1976). An apparent difference found by GREGER et al. (1971) may be explained by the use of the nonspecific phosphotungstic acid method for end-distal samples and that of a specific method for pelvic urine. These observations suggest practical impermeability of collecting ducts to urate, and this was confirmed by microinjections of 2-^{14}C-urate into distal tubules (KRAMP et al., 1971), i.e., the label was completely recovered in pelvic urine. In another study by the same group (KRAMP and LENOIR, 1975a) a very small fraction (5%) of the injected labeled urate was found to be absorbed from the collecting ducts. The small amount of reabsorption appeared to be carrier-mediated since it could be blocked by an excess of unlabeled urate or by benziodarone (KRAMP and LENOIR, 1975a).

Thus, the bulk of the transports of urate across tubular walls appears to occur in the convoluted part and to a minor extent in the straight portion of the proximal tubules and/or in the loops of Henle, while lower nephron segments do not appear to contribute greatly to modulating the urinary urate excretion.

IV. Effects of Drugs

The effects of drugs are summarized in Table 6. The effects of drugs known to be uricosuric or antiuricosuric in man have effects in rat that are consistently small and difficult to demonstrate. The uricosuric drugs tend to increase FE_{urate} only at low values of P_{urate}. An effect of antiuricosuric drugs can only be demonstrated at high P_{urate}, i.e., at high baseline rates of fractional urate excretion (Table 6).

As a prototype of a substance transported by the proximal secretory mechanism for organic anions, p-aminohippurate (PAH) is of special interest. In rabbits (Sect. C V) and dogs (Sect. D II), though not in man, PAH inhibits the secretion of urate. In unanesthetized intact rats the infusion of PAH (25 mg/kg + 2–3 mg/kg · min) induced a 10–35% depression of FE_{urate} only in animals heavily loaded with urate (BOUDRY, 1971b). In microinjection experiments, however, the secretion of urate injected into peritubular capillaries was not inhibited by PAH (1.5–6.4 mM) added to the injected fluid, but pyrazinamide (1.6–3 mM) did inhibit urate secretion (KRAMP and LENOIR, 1975b). Similarly, PAH did not inhibit urate secretion in experiments based on a modification of the dilution technique of SILVERMAN (FOULKES, 1975). An apparent inhibitory effect of PAH on urate secretion observed in tubular microperfusion experiments with a solution containing unlabeled urate after intra-aortic injection of 2-^{14}C-urate (ROCH-RAMEL and BOUDRY, 1971) cannot be accepted as definite evidence because the baseline values proved difficult to reproduce. On the other hand, in tubular microinjection experiments, PAH appeared to inhibit the reabsorption of urate (KRAMP et al., 1971).

The observation that PAH interferes with the secretion of urate only at high P_{urate} levels in the rat may indicate that urate is secreted by two different mechanisms, one of them being the anion secretory mechanism that is also responsible for the secretion of PAH. In the rat, the anion secretory mechanism appears to participate in the secretion of urate only at high plasma levels, possibly because urate at low plasma levels is excluded from access to this mechanism by the presence of endogenous anions with a higher affinity.

It should be added that the influence of a large number of drugs on the excretion of urate in the rat has been studied by MARTIN (1948) in experiments in which GFR was not measured, and urinary urate concentration measured with a rather unreliable method. The data, therefore, are difficult to interpret. Acetanilide, o-aminobenzoate, acetylsalicylate, salicylate, phenacetin, and sulfanilate were found to increase the urinary excretion of urate, while m-aminobenzoate and benzoate depressed it.

Table 6. Drugs effects in rats

	Dose in mg/kg i.v., where not otherwise stated	Effects on FE_{urate}		Proximal reabsorptive flux	Proximal secretory flux
		Low P_{urate}	High P_{urate}		
Probenecid	200	↗1)	—1)		
	100	—1)		↘2) m.i.	
				—9) m.pe	
Salicylate	100	↗12)[a]			
Sulfinpyrazone	50	—1)	—1)		
Benziodarone	10	↗3)	—3)	↘3) m.i.	
Benzbromarone	10	↗3)	—3)	↘3) m.i.	
Hydrochlorothiazide	5	—1)	—1)		
Chlorothiazide	25	—4)		—4) m.pe	—4) m.pe (droplet)
Clopamide	16/24 h i.v. + i.p.	—14)			
Furosemide	5/24 h i.v.	↘14)			
Indanylacetic acid (MK 196)	0.8/min	↗5) 10)		↘5) m.i.	↘5) m.pe (droplet)
Pyrazinoic acid	100	↘13)		↘13) m. pu. ↘2) m.i.	↘13) m.pu ↘6) m.i. 1.3–3 mM in the fluid m.i. cap
Pyrazinamide	50		—1)		
	100	small ↘1)	↘1)		
p-Aminohippurate	25	—1)	↘1)		
	4/min			↘2) m.i.	—6) 1.5–6.4 mM in the fluid m.i. cap. —7) double isotope dilution 0.05 mM i.ao ↘8) m.pe
Glycine	50	—12) 15)[a,b]			
Oestrone	0.003		↗11)[a]		
Ethinylostradiol	0.03		↗11)[a]		

↗ Increase.   ↘ Decrease.   — No change.   — No change.

[a] Creatinine for glomerular marker.

[b] FE_{urate} calculated from $C_{creatinine}$ and C_{urate}, nonstatistically significant; conclusion in contradiction with that given by the author.

Abbreviations: m.i., microinjection technique; m.pe, microperfusion technique; m.pu, free-flow micropuncture: indirect inferences on fluxes; m.i. cap., microinjection into peritubular capillary blood; m.pe, tubular microperfusion m.pe (droplet), urale applied as droplet on surface of the kidney, i.ao, intraaortic.

1) Boundry (1971b); 2) Kramp et al. (1971); 3) Kramp and Lenoir (1975a); 4) Weinman et al. (1976a); 5) Weinman et al. (1976b); 6) Kramp and Lenoir (1975b); 7) Foulkes (1975); 8) Roch-Ramel and Boudry (1971) (see Section 5.d); 9) Lang (1976); 10) McKenzie et al. (1976); 11) Musil and Sandow (1976): rats treated with oxonic acid; 12) Friedman (1948); 13) Abramson and Levitt (1976) (see Section 5.b); 14) Imbs et al. (1975): rats with remnant kidney and azotemia; clopamide, though nonuricosuric, increased P_{urate} by 42% in 24 h; furosemide given at dose levels inducing same natriuresis as clopamide (preceding line), depressed uricosuria by 27%, and increased P_{urate} by 44%; 15) Friedman (1947).

V. Experimental Hyperuricemia

The high uricase activity present mainly in the liver of rodents and other mammals is responsible for the low P_{urate} concentrations found under normal conditions. In order to increase P_{urate} and/or to make the rat more similar to man for studying the metabolism of uric acid or the pathogenesis of gout, many investigators have attempted to eliminate the liver uricase activity in rats in order to induce acute or chronic hyperuricemia.

Uricase activity can be depressed either by inhibitory drugs, by destroying large parts of the liver, or by diminishing the blood flow through the liver. The parmacologic uricase inhibitors used in such experiments were either salts of oxonic acid, a symmetrical triazine (FRIDOVICH, 1965; JOHNSON et al., 1969), or analogs of hypoxanthine or xanthine (IWATA et al., 1973). Among the latter, 2,8-diaza-hypoxanthine has been reported (IWATA et al., 1973) to be a more potent inhibitor of uricase activity (bovine kidney or rat liver homogenates) than either 2-aza-hypo-xanthine or 8-aza-hypoxanthine, 8-aza-xanthine, or even oxonate, and to induce a longer-lasting and more pronounced hyperuricemia and decrease of plasma allantoin concentrations when injected into rats in acute experiments (IWATA et al., 1973).

Oxonates have been used to induce hyperuricemia lasting several hours, either as single injections (GREGER, 1976; BODA et al., 1973) or as single injections followed by i.v. infusion (DE ROUGEMONT et al., 1976). Acute oxonate hyperuricemia was considerably augmented by the induction of tourniquet shock (BODA et al., 1973), the mechanism of the augmentation being either renal failure or a decrease of hepatic blood flow or both. Tourniquet shock plus oxonate administration induced visible precipitation of uric acid both in tubules and in interstitial tissue (BODA et al., 1973).

Chronically feeding oxonate (2% in diet) for 3 weeks induced a nonsignificant, minor ($\sim 30\%$) rise of P_{urate} and an increase of the daily urate excretion to twice the control value (WAISMAN et al., 1974). Feeding potassium oxonate (5% in diet), supplemented by i.p. injections on the 4th and the 5th day, doubled P_{urate} (STAVRIC et al., 1976); simultaneous feeding of fructose in doses that by themselves cause an increase of P_{urate} by 30%, resulted in an increase of FE_{urate} to a level five times the control value. In order to obtain higher sustained levels of P_{urate}, several investigators added both oxonate (2–5%) and various urates (1–3%) to the diet for periods from 3–10 weeks (STAVRIC et al., 1969; MWASI et al., 1976; STAVRIC et al., 1973; BLUESTONE et al., 1975; WAISMAN et al., 1974). This type of chronic treatment consistently entails an increase of P_{urate} by 40—100% and a simultaneous 7–16-fold increase of the daily urinary excretion of urate. Since GFR has not been measured simultaneously with urinary urate excretion in any of these studies, it cannot be decided whether chronic hyperuricemia (or chronic treatment with oxonate) influences transtubular urate transport.

In all animals consistently fed with oxonate plus urate the urate concentration in renal tissue was considerably increased and microscopic examination revealed the presence of uric acid and urate crystals in medullary tubules (STAVRIC et al., 1969; MWASI et al., 1976; STAVRIC et al., 1973; WAISMAN et al., 1974) and also in medullary interstitial tissue. Interstitial urate deposits often actually looked like tophi; intratubular deposits often developed into stones (BLUESTONE et al., 1975). The histologic picture of the kidneys suggested the presence of progressive interstitial nephritis, secondary to tubular obstruction and precipitation of uric acid and urates in interstitial tissue. No primary glomerular changes were seen (Mwasi et al., 1976; Stavric et al., 1973) in acute renal failure induced by the rapid i.v. injection of uric acid plus lithium carbonate (300 mg/kg of uric acid within 5 min). There was, however, precipitation of uric acid and urates not only in tubules and in interstitial tissue but also to a large extent in the medullary vasa recta (Conger et al., 1976).

Hyperuricemia has been induced in acute experiments by partial destruction of the liver (Greger, 1976) either by clamping the celiac and the superior and inferior mesenteric arteries or by clamping only the hepatic artery and establishing a bypass between the portal and the right jugular vein. Damage to the liver induced by poisoning with carbon tetrachloride also induces chronic hyperuricuria and formation of urate calculi (Ungar, 1951). Subtotal hepatectomy induces an increase of P_{urate} and of urinary urate excretion in short-term experiments (Byers et al., 1947).

Circulatory exclusion of a fraction of the total liver tissue by surgical establishment of an end-to-side portacaval anastomosis ("Eck fistula") always resulted in a large increase of the daily urate excretion and a decrease in that of allantoin, and often induced the formation of renal calculi (Lauterburg et al., 1977).

VI. Conclusion

Proximal convoluted tubules are the main site of transtubular urate transport in rats. Reabsorption and secretion occur simultaneously at the same levels of these structures, and the two unidirectional fluxes are of approximately equal magnitude. Prevalence of one flux over the other depends on experimental conditions. Only a minor reabsorptive movement has been demonstrated to occur between late proximal and early distal convoluted tubules, presumably in the straight portion of the proximal tubules. There are no data about a possible secretory flux at this site. Uricosuric drugs, with the exception of one single recently developed uricosuric and diuretic compound, do not show clear-cut uricosuric effects in rats, presumably because of simultaneous interference with both reabsorption and secretion. PAH, in the rat, interferes with urate secretion to a much lesser extent than in dogs or rabbits, but does appear to exert a minor inhibitory effect on urate reabsorption.

F. Mouse

The mechanisms of renal excretion of urate have not been studied in mice. This species has, however, been used for screening diuretic and uricosuric compounds by measuring the rate of urate excretion during 2–4 h in metabolic cages (Thuillier et al., 1974). In male Swiss C.D. mice, a high dose of benziodarone (100 mg/kg p.o.) had a slight uricosuric effect, while the same dose of tienilic acid and two related drugs had more pronounced uricosuric and large diuretic effects. Furosemide and ethacrynic acid at markedly diuretic doses (20 mg/kg p.o.) did not enhance the urinary excretion of urate, as measured by a rather nonspecific analytic method.

G. Guinea Pig

The physiologic plasma concentration of urate is low (0.5–0.9 mg-% = 30–54 μM). Protein binding of urate has been found to be negligible at room temperature (Mudge et al., 1968a), but around 20% at 4° C (Simkin, 1972a). At the physiologic

Table 7. Effects of drugs and metabolites on renal urate excretion in guinea pigs

Drug	Dose mg/kg i.v.	Effects on FE_{urate} Low P_{urate}	Effects on FE_{urate} High P_{urate}	Proximal secretory peak in stop-flow	Effects on urate uptake into cortical slices concentration M
Probenecid	50		↘ reversed to net reabsorption	↘ reversed to reabsorption	10^{-6}–10^{-4} ↘
Pyrazinoic acid	25–50			↘	10^{-3}–10^{-2} ↘
Benziodarone	< 1–3	—1)			
Chlorothiazide	15–20			—	
Phenylbutazone					10^{-5}–10^{-4} ↘2)
Lactate	250–1000			—	
Acetate					10^{-3} ↗2)
Succinate					10^{-2} ↘
Ouabain	0.04–0.20			—	10^{-6}–10^{-5} ↘
2,4-Dinitrophenol					$5 \cdot 10^{-4}$ ↘

↗ Increase.   ↘ Decrease.   — No change.
Most data were taken from MUDGE et al. (1968a).
1) Data from LEMIEUX et al. (1973). 2) Data from PLATTS and MUDGE (1961).

Table 8. Renal excretion of pyrazinoate (PZA) in different species

Species	P_{PZA} mg/L	P_{PZA} (mM)	FE_{PZA}	Effects of PZA on urate transport	Reference
Guinea pig	?		3.6	decrease in proximal secretory peak	MUDGE et al. (1968a)
Rabbit	?		0.45	increase in proximal secretory peak	MUDGE et al. (1968a)
Dalmatian dog	110–120	(0.9–1.0)	0.1–0.15	decrease in FE_{urate}	ROCH-RAMEL et al. (1976c)
Non-Dalmatian dog	50–120	(0.4)	0.15	decrease in proximal	WEINER and TINKER (1972)
	400–450	(3.0–3.5)	0.3	secretory peak increase in FE_{urate}	
Pig	70	(0.6)	0.1	no change in FE_{urate}	SIMMONDS et al. (1976)
	430–570	(3.5–4.6)	0.8		
Cebus monkey	5–10	(0.04–0.08)	0.9–1.2	decrease in FE_{urate}	WEINER and TINKER (1972)
(C. albifrons)	150–200	(1.2–1.6)	0.8–1.1		
Chimpanzee	70	(0.56)	1.2–1.5	decrease in FE_{urate}	FANELLI and WEINER (1973)
(P. troglodytes)	700–800	(5.6–6.5)	1.4–1.6	increase in FE_{urate}	

plasma concentration FE_{urate} was ~60% (LEMIEUX et al., 1973a). When P_{urate} was increased to 1.5 mg-% (89 μM) by loading, FE_{urate} was 0.6; when the plasma concentration was increased to 3 mg-% (178 μM) a pronounced net secretion (FE_{urate} 2.0–4.0) was found to occur (MUDGE et al., 1968a). In stop-flow experiments a secretory peak was found in proximal urine samples, while the distal nephron appeared to be impermeable to urate (MUDGE et al., 1968a). Slices of renal cortical tissue have been found by one group of investigators (MUDGE et al., 1968a), to concentrate urate in vitro, but no concentration was found by another investigator

(BRAUN, 1961). The effects of drugs and metabolites on the urinary excretion of urate and the concentration of urate in renal slices that have been studied are summarized in Table 7.

The effects of probenecid were comparable to those seen in the dalmatian coach hound and in the rabbit. Pyrazinoic acid (PZA), which in the rabbit, as judged from stop-flow experiments, inhibited reabsorption and had no effect on FE_{urate}, in the guinea pig, reversed the proximal secretory peak and changed FE_{urate} from net secretion to net reabsorption (BEECHWOOD et al., 1964). The difference between the effects in the two species may or may not be related to the different mechanisms of urinary excretion of pyrazinoate. In rabbits, the fractional excretion of this compound was 0.45, and in guinea pigs it was secreted at a $FE_{PZA} = 3.6$. The data summarized in Table 8, however, do not suggest any clear correlation between the mode of the urinary excretion of pyrazinoate and its effect on FE_{urate}. Ouabain, which was highly uricosuric in the rabbit, had no such effect in the guinea pig.

H. Pig

Urate excretion in this species has been studied by one group of investigators (SIMMONDS et al., 1976). The normal plasma concentration of urate in pig is even lower than in other uricase-endowed mammals; it amounts to less than 0.1 mg-% ($<6\ \mu M$). Excretion studies, therefore, were only done in pigs infused with urate. Under these conditions the protein binding of urate amounted to 12%.

The fractional excretion of urate was 160% at P_{urate} values from 0.1–0.4 mg-% (6–24 μM). With an increase of P_{urate} to 1 mg-% (60 μM), net secretion was considerably enhanced, and FE_{urate} reached 330%; no further increase of FE_{urate} occurred with higher values of P_{urate}. At a P_{urate} of 6 mg-% (360 μM), GFR fell and other signs of reversible acute renal failure appeared (SIMMONDS et al., 1976). FE_{urate} in the pig proved to be independent of the rate of urine flow.

Probenecid (0.25 mg/kg · min) depressed FE_{urate} but did not convert net secretion into reabsorption. Neither pyrazinamide (1 mg/kg · min), nor pyrazinoic acid (3 mg/kg · min), had any effect on FE_{urate} in contrast to observations made in the dalmatian coach hound (ROCH-RAMEL et al., 1976c).

J. Nonhuman Primates

An extensive review of metabolism and renal transport of uric acid in nonhuman primates has been published by FANELLI and BEYER (1974). Among the nonhuman primates, two groups must be distinguished in respect to the metabolism of uric acid. Apes, like man, have lost all uricase activity and metabolize purines into uric acid excreted by the kidneys and by the gut. Monkeys, on the other hand, still have some uricase activity and metabolize a variable fraction of the uric acid to allantoin (NAKAJIMA and BOURNE, 1970). The uricase found in several tissues, mostly in the liver of monkeys, however, differs from that found in lower mammals in its lability and its rapid inactivation in vitro (CHRISTEN et al., 1970a, 1970b; LOGAN et al., 1976). No uricase activity was found in the renal tissue of the Rhesus *(Macaca mulatta)* (TISHER et al., 1968). In respect to the renal excretory mechanisms for urate, old-world monkeys differ from new-world monkeys.

I. Old-World Monkeys

In this family of animals, P_{urate} is usually below 1 mg-% (59 μM) and total body uricase activity is high (CHRISTEN et al., 1970a, 1970b; FANELLI et al., 1970a). FE_{urate} is above unity in most species. Net tubular secretion of urate has been found in all old-world monkeys with the exception of the bushbaby *(Galago crassicaudatus)* (FANELLI et al., 1970a). In female Rhesus monkeys *(M. mulatta)* in the antidiuretic state, infused with a highly concentrated urate solution, the urate concentration in renal tissue has been found to increase 1.3–9-fold from the cortex to the papillary tip, with intermediate concentrations in the outer and in the inner medulla. In turn, the urate concentrations found in the papillary tip were 1.5–5 times greater than in final urine (CANNON et al., 1968). The latter fact suggests the occurrence of some medullary countercurrent multiplication of urate concentrations in the rhesus. The cortico-medullary gradient of urate concentration, which was greater than in human kidneys obtained at autopsy, however, cannot be interpreted in the absence of measurements of tissue inulin concentrations. In rats (see above) the corticomedullary urate gradient was equal but not superior to the inulin gradient.

II. New-World Monkeys

In most species of new-world monkeys, P_{urate} is relatively high (1.5–6.0 mg-% = 90–360 μM). The high P_{urate} level found in one family of new-world monkeys (the Cebus monkeys) has been interpreted as evidence for the absence of uricase activity (SKEITH and HEALEY, 1968). In fact, uricase activity is present in all new-world monkeys, though it is lower than in the old-world monkeys (CHRISTEN et al., 1970a, 1970b). The turnover of uric acid has been shown to be much larger than in man (10 mg = 59 μmol/kg body wt/day) both in the woolly monkey (LOGAN et al., 1976) and in Cebus monkeys (SIMKIN, 1971); in the latter species it attained 72 mg = 428 μmol/kg body wt/day (NOLL and DUGAN, 1971). In most species of new-world monkeys, FE_{urate} is far below unity; thus these animals, such as the Cebus monkey, resemble man both in their high P_{urate} and in net tubular reabsorption. There are, however, a few exceptional species: in the red howler monkey *(Alouatta semiculus)* FE_{urate} reached 1.8; net tubular secretion of urate has also been found to occur in the moustached tamami *(Sagunus mystax)* and in the squirrel monkey *(Saimiri sciureus)*. In these three species P_{urate} has been found to be as low as in old-world monkeys (FANELLI et al., 1970a).

Mechanisms of the renal excretion of urate have been studied extensively by stop-flow and micropuncture experiments only in Cebus monkeys, a group of species that has attracted considerable attention because of its similarity to man (see above) and its high sensitivity to drugs known to interfere with urate transport in man (SKEITH and HEALEY, 1968). In contrast to Rhesus monkeys, in which ∼20% of the plasma urate was found to be bound to proteins, urate in the Cebus monkey is not bound to plasma proteins (SIMKIN, 1971; FANELLI et al., 1970b).

P_{urate} in normal Cebus monkeys varies from 1 to 3 mg-% (59–175 μM) and FE_{urate} from 5 to 10% (SKEITH and KEALEY, 1968; BLANCHARD et al., 1972; FANELLI et al., 1970b). FE_{urate} appeared to be lower in *Cebus capucinus* than in *C. albifrons* or in *C. apella*, and was equal in the two latter species (FANELLI et al., 1970b). No difference in

FE_{urate} between males and females was found in *C. capucinus* and in *C. apella* (FANELLI et al., 1970b). The value reported for FE_{urate} in female *C. albifrons* by BLANCHARD et al. (1972) was somewhat lower than that found in male animals of the same species by FANELLI et al. (1970b). The difference, however, may reflect different experimental conditions rather than a sex difference.

As in lower mammalian species, FE_{urate} in Cebus monkeys increases with increasing P_{urate} values up to a maximum of 35%, which is reached at P_{urate} levels of 20–30 mg-% (1.19–1.78 mM). For these high plasma levels an apparent maximal rate of reabsorptive transport (Tm of 1.7–2.2 mg/min) is reached (FANELLI et al., 1970b). This apparent Tm value is of course much smaller than the actual Tm for the reabsorptive flux because tubular secretion occurs at the same P_{urate} level as reabsorption (FANELLI et al., 1970b).

Changes of the rate of urine flow had as little influence on FE_{urate} in Cebus monkeys as in dogs, rats, and rabbits (BLANCHARD et al., 1972).

Classic and modified stop-flow experiments showed that net reabsorption occurs mainly in proximal convoluted tubules (FANELLI et al., 1970b; LEMIEUX et al., 1973b). While this conclusion has been confirmed in micropuncture experiments (ROCH-RAMEL and WEINER, 1973, 1975), a small distal secretory peak found in modified stop-flow experiments by LEMIEUX et al. (1973b) has not been substantiated in the micropuncture studies quoted.

These studies showed that, in moderate osmotic diuresis, most of the filtered urate in Cebus monkeys is reabsorbed along the proximal convoluted tubules. No net movement of urate occurred across Henle's loops or along the distal convoluted tubules. Some urate disappeared out of tubular fluid between late superficial distal convoluted tubules and pelvic urine. This disappearance could reflect reabsorption from the collecting ducts, or else a more complete reabsorption of urate from total juxtamedullary nephrons than from superficial nephrons (ROCH-RAMEL and WEINER, 1973). The net proximal tubular reabsorption of urate observed was the sum of a large reabsorptive and a smaller secretory flux since net proximal reabsorption increased under the influence of pyrazinoic acid (ROCH-RAMEL and WEINER, 1975).

1. Effects of Drugs and Metabolites

In the olive baboon, the normal net secretion of urate ($FE_{urate} \sim 2$) was converted to net reabsorption (FE_{urate} of 0.8) by pyrazinoic acid, as well as by infusion of PAH (FANELLI and BEYER, 1974). Thus a reabsorptive flux is present in monkeys that show net tubular secretion of urate. On the other hand, pyrazinoic acid did not significantly depress FE_{urate} in the woolly monkey (LOGAN et al., 1976).

Again, Cebus monkeys were more extensively studied than other species of monkeys; the Cebus monkeys are sensitive to all drugs known to be uricosuric in man, with the exception of zoxazolamine (FANELLI and WEINER, 1975). The monkeys are, however, less sensitive to these drugs than man. The effects of different drugs and metabolites on renal urate excretion are summarized in Table 9. As shown in the table, PAH depressed FE_{urate}; conversely, very large amounts of urate depressed the fractional excretion of PAH (FANELLI et al., 1970b). Inasfar as both anions used the same secretory transport system, the affinity of the latter for PAH appeared to be greater than for urate. Fructose had no renal uricosuric effect in Cebus monkeys, but

Table 9. Effects of drugs and metabolites on renal urate excretion in Cebus monkeys

Drug	Dose mg/kg	FE_{urate}	Comment
Probenecid	p.o. > 12.5–100	↗1)	At high as well as low P_{urate}
	i.v. 1.2– 50	↗1) 2)	
	i.v. > 1/min	↗4)	
2-Nitroprobenecid			
2-Chloroprobenecid	0.2–2/min	↗4)	Proximal inhibitory effect of
2-Hydroxyprobenecid			2-nitroprobenecid 10) 11)
Carinamide	p.o. 50	—1)	
	i.v. 50	—1)	
Salicylate	0.5–3/min	↘3)	Animals infused with mannitol
	0.5–3/min	↗3)	Animals infused with bicarbonate
m-Hydroxybenzoic acid	1–2/min	↘5)	Totally suppresses urinary urate excretion
			No uricosuric effect even at high dose level
Phenylbutazone	i.v. 25	↗1)	
Sulfinpyrazone	p.o. 15–30	↗1)	
	i.v. 25–50	↗1) 2)	
Benziodarone	p.o. 15	↗1) 7) 8)	
Zoxazolamine	p.o. 15	—1)	
	i.v. 10	small ↗ or—1)	
Diodone	i.v. 150	↗1)	
Mersalyl	i.v. 4 mgHg	↗6)	
Chlormerodrin	i.v. 4 mgHg	↗6)	
Other mercurial diuretics	i.v. 4 mgHg	↗6)	
p-Chloromercuribenzoate	i.v. 3 mgHg	—6)	
Chlorothiazide	i.v. 25	↗↘1) ↗2)	In 1) Initially increased FE, followed by a decrease probably not explained by dehydration
Pyrazinoic acid	p.o. 50	↘9)	
	i.v. 25	↘2)	Inhibition localized in proximal
	i.v. 50	↘9)	11)
Nicotinic acid	p.o. 25	↘9)	
PAH	i.v. < 40	—9)	
	i.v. 150	↘9)	
Dinitrophenol	i.v. 10	↘9)	
β-Hydroxybutyric acid	i.v. 100–200	↘9)	
	i.v. 1 + 0.03/min	↘2)	
Lactate	i.v. 5–20/min	↘2) 9)	

↗ Increase. ↘ Decrease. —No change.

1) FANELLI et al. (1970c); 2) SKEITH and HEALEY (1968); 3) FANELLI and WEINER (1975); 4) BLANCHARD et al. (1972); 5) MAY and WEINER (1971); 6) FANELLI et al. (1973b); 7) LEMIEUX et al. (1973a); 8) LEMIEUX et al. (1973b); 9) FANELLI et al. (1970c); 10) ROCH-RAMEL and WEINER (1973); 11) ROCH-RAMEL and WEINER (1975).

increased urinary urate excretion by increasing the metabolic production of urate and its plasma concentration (SIMKIN, 1972b).

As shown in Table 9, all mercurial diuretics were uricosuric in Cebus monkeys, while the nondiuretic and antinatriuretic compound p-chloromercuribenzoate had no effect. The mercurial diuretics, however, were less effective as uricosuric agents than in the chimpanzee. This difference cannot be explained by differences in the urinary pH (FANELLI et al., 1973b).

III. Apes

Only the chimpanzee has been studied and, for obvious reasons, only clearance-type studies have been done. Like man, chimpanzees have no uricase activity (FANELLI et al., 1970a, 1971a) and essentially excrete only uric acid as a purine metabolite. They have high urate blood levels $(2-5 \text{ mg-}\% = 110-300 \mu M)$. FE_{urate} averages 10% (FANELLI et al., 1971a); this indicates a net tubular reabsorption.

The fact that small doses of pyrazinoic acid depress FE_{urate} (FANELLI et al., 1971a; FANELLI and WEINER, 1973, 1974) demonstrates that net reabsorption represents the sum of a very large reabsorptive and of a fairly large secretory transport. In contrast, large doses of pyrazinoic acid were uricosuric (FANELLI and WEINER, 1973). Pyrazinoic acid in the chimpanzee had a "paradoxical effect" similar to that of salicylate in man (YÜ and GUTMAN, 1959); though the difference in doses inducing an uricosuric or an antiuricosuric effect was much larger for pyrazinoic acid in the chimpanzee than for salicylate in man. The presence of a secretory transtubular transport of urate in chimpanzees is also demonstrated by the observation that mercurial diuretics may transform net reabsorption into net secretion (FANELLI et al., 1973a). Changes of urine pH over a large range had no influence on FE_{urate} in the chimpanzee (FANELLI et al., 1977a).

Data on the effects of drugs and metabolites on the urinary urate excretion in the chimpanzee are summarized in Table 10. Chimpanzees are generally more sensitive to uricosuric agents than man (FANELLI and WEINER, 1975). Data on the influence of the drugs on the renal excretion of PAH in the chimpanzee have also been included. The comparison shows that the transport systems for urate and for PAH in the chimpanzee are probably separate (FANELLI and WEINER, 1973; WEINER and FANELLI, 1974, 1975).

Infusions of glucose at a high rate $(500 \text{ mg/kg} + 50 \text{ mg/kg} \cdot \text{min})$ in the chimpanzee considerably increased FE_{urate}, although mannitol infused at a comparable rate had a much lesser effect (FANELLI et al., 1971a). The uricosuric effect of glucose appeared to be intraluminal since phloridzin also proved to be uricosuric (FANELLI et al., 1971a).

IV. Conclusion

Nonhuman primates are of interest for studies on uricosuric and antiuricosuric drugs, which in Cebus monkeys are generally less potent, and in chimpanzees more potent (and more effective) than in man. Most new-world monkeys and apes mainly reabsorb urate. Neither secretory nor reabsorptive transport mechanisms for urate are identical with transport mechanisms for PAH.

K. Isolated Data on Other Species of Mammals

The urinary excretion of urate has been studied in a few goats and calves after urate loading (MUDGE et al., 1973); net secretion has been shown to occur in these species. In stop-flow experiments in the goat (MUDGE, quoted by FANELLI, 1976), net secretion

Table 10. Effects of drugs and metabolites on renal urate excretion in chimpanzees

Drug	Dose mg/kg	FE_{urate}	FE_{PAH} Low P_{PAH}	High P_{PAH}
Carinamide	p.o. 50	↗2)		
Probenecid	i.v. 25	↗1) 2)	—1)	↘2)
	p.o. 1–50	↗2)	—2)	
Salicylate	Low doses	—2)		
	i.v. 40	↗2)	—2)	
Sulfinpyrazone	p.o. 5–10	↗2)	↗2) Small	
	i.v. 14	↗2) Large	↘2)	
Zoxazolamine	p.o. 5–10	↗2) Abolishes net reabsorption	—2)	
Halofenate	i.v. 1–5	↗5)	—5)	
Diodone	i.v. 150	↗2)	—2)	
ᵃ Pyrazinoic acid	p.o. 15–20	↘1) 5)	↗1) 5)	
	i.v. 20	↘1)	Small	
PAH	i.v. 180	↗2) 6)		
Phloridzin	i.v. 100	↗1)	↘1) Small	
Glucose	i.v. 500	↗1)		
Mersalyl	i.v. 1.5 mgHg/kg	↗3) To net secretion	—3)	↘4)
Mercaptomerin or metalluride or mercumatilin or chlormerodrin	i.v. 2 mgHg/kg	↗3)	—3)	↘3)
Indanylacetic acid (MK 196)	p.o. 0.06–10	↗6) 7)		
	i.v. 1	↗6) 8)	—8)	
Furosemide	p.o. 1–5	↘6) 7)		
	i.v. 1	↘6)		
Etacrynic acid	i.v. 1	ᵇ ↗↘6)		
Chlorothiazide	i.v. 10	↗2)	—2)	
	p.o. 10	—2)		
Hydrochlorothiazide	i.v. 1	↘2)		
	p.o. 5	↘7)		

↗ Increase. ↘ Decrease. — No change.

ᵃ At high concentration in plasma ($P_{PZA} = 700\,\mu g/ml$) PZA induces uricosuria, see Table 8.

ᵇ Transient uricosuria for 15 min, followed by uric acid retention.

1) FANELLI et al. (1971a); 2) FANELLI et al. (1971b); 3) FANELLI et al. (1973a); 4) FANELLI et al. (1972b); 5) FANELLI et al. (1972a); 6) FANELLI et al. (1977a); 7) CRAGOE et al. (1975); 8) FANELLI et al. (1977b).

was observed to occur in the proximal tubules and to be inhibited by probenecid. In the cat, net proximal reabsorption and net overall reabsorption were observed in stop-flow experiments. Probenecid did not exert any clear-cut effect on urate excretion in this species (see FANELLI, 1976). Data on spontaneous urate excretion in a number of otherwise not investigated mammalian species have been published by HUNTER and GIVENS (1914a, 1914b). Badgers *(Taxidia taxus)* excreted ~4.5 mmol allantoin and 89 μmol urate/day, the urate representing 2% of the total purine metabolite excretion. The corresponding figures for the coyote *(Canis latrans)* were 2.6 mmol allantoin and 125 μmol urate, the latter representing 5% of total purine excretion. Two raccoons *(Procyon lotor)* excreted 1.4 mmol allantoin and 89 μmol urate, i.e., 6% of total purine metabolites as urate. In the opossum *(Didelphys virginiana)*, urate excretion (179 μmol/day) accounted for 22% of total purine metabolites, the excretion of allantoin being rather small (630 μmol/day).

L. Conclusions

Uric acid which is nearly 98% ionized at the pH of blood, is generally not bound to any notable extent to plasma proteins at the body temperature of mammals. A higher fraction of protein binding found in vitro at much lower temperatures has been proposed to be a protective mechanism against precipitation in blood vessels or tissues of the extremities, which tend to have a lower-than-average mean body temperature (GREGER et al., 1976).

In all mammalian species investigated (with the possible exception of pigs), urate is both reabsorbed from and secreted into tubular fluid. The quantitatively major transport in both directions occurs in the convoluted and, to a certain extent, also in the straight portion of the proximal tubules. Distal convoluted tubules appear to be generally impermeable to urate, although reabsorption of minor significance may occur from collecting ducts. There is no evidence that the tubular transport of urate differs between superficial and juxtamedullary nephrons, though this possibility cannot be excluded.

In proximal convoluted tubules, reabsorption and secretion of urate occur at the same sites. Observations made in urate-loaded rats suggest that secretion may dominate over reabsorption in the first parts of the proximal convoluted tubules but not in the lower parts.

With respect to the straight portion of the proximal tubule, net secretion occurs at this site in the rabbit and in the dalmatian coach hound. In these species, the possible occurrence of reabsorption from the pars recta has not been investigated. It is thus unknown whether net secretion is the result of secretion dominating over reabsorption, or of the absence of a reabsorptive mechanism. On the other hand in rats there is some reabsorption from "Henle's loops," possibly from the straight portion of the proximal tubules. Again, there are no data suggesting that secretion could occur in the straight portion of this species. Transtubular movements of urate in the pars recta could thus be unidirectional, the direction differing in different species.

In proximal convoluted tubules, net reabsorption or net secretion of urate represents the sum of reabsorptive and secretory movements, which appear to take place simultaneously. Reversal of the direction of net movement by pharmacologic inhibitors of urate transport argues against the other possible interpretation, i.e., that there might be a single transport mechanism across tubular walls, the direction of which changes under the influence of intrarenal or extrarenal control mechanisms. Hence, changes seen to occur in the direction of flow of urate across the walls of proximal convoluted tubules must be interpreted as being due to either enhancement or depression of transport in either the secretory or the reabsorptive direction. While reversal induced by pharmacologic agents may be assumed a priori to be due to inhibition of one of the two fluxes rather than to enhancement, the interpretation of changes brought about by physiologic metabolites are more ambiguous.

The fact that in several mammalian species increases of the plasma-urate concentration favor the proximal secretory over the reabsorptive process cannot be due to a depression of reabsorption resulting from a less favorable electrochemical gradient for reabsorptive transport. They require the assumption that there is actually a secretory mechanism, which is either enhanced at or becomes operational only at higher than normal levels of P_{urate}.

A tendency to decreased reabsorption or increased secretion through tubular walls with increasing plasma levels, and conversely, to increased reabsorption and decreased secretion at low plasma levels suggests that P_{urate} is controlled to some extent in most mammalian species. Nothing is known about the control mechanisms, which could be renal or extrarenal. Known hormonal systems do not appear to play any role in the regulation of urate transport. In view of the fact that urate is a metabolite apparently meant to be excreted, and that there is no evidence for a metabolic reutilization of urate, the possible purposes of a control mechanism maintaining constant P_{urate} levels are unclear.

It is also obscure why the phylogenetic selection should have entailed the survival of mammalian species in which urate is transported in both directions at the same sites of proximal tubules, presumably often at the expense of energy.

Proximal tubular walls appear to be able to transport urate both in the reabsorptive and in the secretory direction against electrochemical gradients. This statement does not mean that transport consistently occurs against an electrochemical gradient; active transport in one direction may very often be accompanied by opposing transport in the direction of an electrochemical gradient. Uphill transport of urates could, of course, represent "countertransports" of facilitated diffusion systems. There is, however, no evidence that this explanation applies to the transport of uric acid, and such an explanation would presumably require identification of a substance countertransported against urate.

Most of the secretory transtubular transport of urate does not appear to be mediated by the nonspecific organic anion secretory system since it is not, or at best only weakly, inhibited by PAH. It is conceivable, however, and some evidence argues in favor of this assumption, that part of the secretory transport of urates occurs through this nonspecific system, particularly at high plasma levels.

Nothing is known about the sites and the mechanisms of urate transport in both directions within tubular cells. Pumping mechanisms for the secretory transport may be assumed to be located at the contraluminal surface of tubular cells in those species in which slices actively concentrate urate, since slices may be assumed to present to the medium more contraluminal than luminal cell surfaces. Secretory transport has, however, been demonstrated to occur in species in which slices do not concentrate urate or, under conditions in which an uptake of urate into renal tissue in vivo from the peritubular side cannot be demonstrated. Since the urate concentration in tubular cells has not been investigated to any extent, the possibility cannot be ruled out that the pumping mechanisms for secretory transport may be situated at the luminal border of tubular cells. As to the reabsorptive transport, pumping mechanisms could be situated at either the luminal or the contraluminal surface. Though it is too early in the development of our knowledge of transtubular transport of urate to develop valid models, the data available suggest that such models could consist of pumping mechanisms for transport in both directions at the luminal surface of cells and a pumping mechanism, possibly only secretory, at the contraluminal surface, as well as a carrier that could be the same for transport in both directions.

References

Abramson, R. G., Levitt, M. F.: Micropuncture study of uric acid transport in rat kidney. Amer. J. Physiol. **228**, 1597—1605 (1975)

Abramson, R. G., Levitt, M. F.: Use of pyrazinamide to assess renal uric acid transport in the rat: a micropuncture study. Amer. J. Physiol. **230**, 1276—1283 (1976)

Abramson, R. G., Levitt, M. F., Maesaka, J. K., Katz, J. H.: A simple radioisotopic technique for the study of urate transport in the rat kidney. J. appl. Physiol. **36**, 500—505 (1974)

Afzelius, B. A.: The occurence and structure of microbodies: a comparative study. J. Cell Biol. **26**, 835—843 (1965)

Alexander, J. A., Wheeler, G. P., Hill, D. D., Morris, H. P.: Effects of 4-hydroxypyrazolo(3,4-d) pyrimidine upon the catabolism of purines by various tissues of the rat and upon the rate of growth of Morris 5123-C hepatoma. Biochem. Pharmacol. **15**, 881—889 (1966)

Alvsaker, J. O.: Uric acid in human plasma. III. Investigations on the interaction between the urate ion and human albumin. Scand. J. clin. Lab. Invest. **17**, 467—475 (1965)

Andreini, P. H., Decker, R. H., Tauxe, W. N., Ward, L. E.: Increased uricolysis in liver homogenates from Dalmatian as compared to non-Dalmatian dogs: further evidence supporting a cellular transport defect in the Dalmatian. Arthr. and Rheum. **9**, Abstr., 845 (1966)

Appleman, R. M., Hallenbeck, G. A., Shorter, R. G.: Effect of reciprocal allogeneic renal transplantation between Dalmatian and non-Dalmatian dogs on urinary excretion of uric acid. Proc. Soc. exp. Biol. (N. Y.) **121**, 1094—1097 (1966)

Bass, A. D., Tepperman, J., Richert, D. A., Westerfeld, W. W.: Excretion of uric acid and allantoin by rats depleted of liver xanthine oxidase. Proc. Soc. exp. Biol. (N. Y.) **73**, 687—689 (1950)

Beechwood, E. C., Berndt, W. O., Mudge, G. H.: Stopflow analysis of tubular transport of uric acid in rabbits. Amer. J. Physiol. **207**, 1265—1272 (1964)

Benedict, S. R.: Uric acid in its relations to metabolism. Harvey Lect. **11**, 346—365 (1915—16)

Berger, L., Yü, T. F.: Urinary excretion of uric acid after instantaneous intra-renal-arterial injection in mongrel and Dalmatian dogs. Mt Sinai J. Med. N. Y. **37**, 351—358 (1970)

Berger, L., Yü, T. F., Atsmon, A., Kupfer, S., Gutman, A. B.: Effect of reducing renal arterial blood pressure by balloon catheter on urate excretion in the dog. Proc. Soc. exp. Biol. (N. Y.) **115**, 58—61 (1964)

Berliner, R. W., Hilton, J. G., Yü, T. F., Kennedy, T. J.: The renal mechanisms for urate excretion in man. J. clin. Invest. **29**, 396—401 (1950)

Berndt, W. O.: The efflux of urate from rabbit renal cortex slices. J. Pharmacol. exp. Ther. **150**, 414—419 (1965)

Berndt, W. O., Beechwood, E. C.: Influence of inorganic electrolytes and ouabain on uric acid transport. Amer. J. Physiol. **208**, 642—648 (1965)

Bernheim, F., Bernheim, M. L. C.: The purine metabolism of rat liver and kidney slices in vitro. Arch. Biochem. **12**, 249—255 (1947)

Beyer, K. H.: Factors basic to the development of useful inhibitors of renal transport mechanisms. Arch. int. Pharmacodyn. **98**, 97—115 (1954)

Beyer, K. H., Russo, H. F., Tillson, E. K., Miller, A. K., Verwey, W. F., Gass, S. R.: "Benemid", p-(di-n-propylsulfamyl)-benzoic acid: its renal affinity and its elimination. Amer. J. Physiol. **166**, 625—640 (1951)

Blanchard, K. C., Maroske, D., May, D. G., Weiner, I. M.: Uricosuric potency of 2-substitued analogs of probenecid. J. Pharmacol. exp. Ther. **180**, 397—410 (1972)

Bloch, P. L., Lata, G. F.: Fluorescence assay for picomole quantities of uric acid: a new enzyme-coupled approach. Analyt. Biochem. **38**, 1—19 (1970)

Bluestone,R., Waisman,J., Klinenberg,J.R.: Chronic experimental hyperuricemic nephropathy: biochemical and morphologic characterization. Lab. Invest. **33**, 273—279 (1975)

Boda,D., Háry,J., Szinay,Gy.: Acute renal failure induced by urate infusion in the rabbit. Acta med. Acad. Sci. hung. **23**, 69—80 (1966)

Boda,D., Penzes,P., Gecse,A., Streitman,K., Zsilinszky,E., Karady,I.: Uric acid nephropathy in shocked rats after blocking of uricase activity with triazine compounds. Can. J. Physiol. Pharmacol. **51**, 496—498 (1973)

Bollman,J.L., Mann,F.C.: Studies on the physiology of the liver. XXV. Allantoin and uric acid following total removal of the liver. Amer. J. Physiol. **104**, 242—246 (1933)

Boudry,J.F.: Mécanismes de l'excrétion d'acide urique chez le rat. Pflügers Arch. **328**, 265—278 (1971a)

Boudry,J.F.: Effet d'inhibiteurs des transports transtubulaires sur l'excrétion rénale d'acide urique chez le rat. Pflügers Arch. **328**, 279—291 (1971b)

Bowman,W.: On the structure and use of the Malpighian bodies of the kidney with observations on the circulation through that gland. Phil. Trans. roy. Soc. Lond. [Biol. Sci.] **132**, 57—80 (1842)

Braun,W.: Über die Wirkung der Harnsäure auf die Phenolrotakkumulation in Schnitten von Vogel- und Säugernieren. Arch. int. Pharmacodyn. **133**, 365—377 (1961)

Burg,M.B.: Perfusion of isolated renal tubules. Yale J. Biol. Med. **45**, 321—326 (1972)

Burg,M.B., Orloff,J.: Oxygen consumption and active transport in separated renal tubules. Amer. J. Physiol. **203**, 327—330 (1962)

Byers,S.O., Friedman,M.: Rate of entrance of urate and allantoin into the cerebrospinal fluid of the Dalmatian and non-Dalmatian dog. Amer. J. Physiol. **157**, 394—400 (1949)

Byers,S.O., Friedman,M., Garfield,M.M.: The blood uric acid and allantoin of the rat after nephrectomy and hepatectomy. Amer. J. Physiol. **150**, 677—681 (1947)

Cannon,P.J., Symchych,P.S., Demartini,F.E.: The distribution of urate in human and primate kidney. Proc. Soc. exp. Biol. (N.Y.) **129**, 278—284 (1968)

Cho,K.C., Cafruny,E.J.: Renal tubular reabsorption of *p*-aminohippuric acid (PAH) in the dog. J. Pharmacol. exp. Ther. **173**, 1—12 (1970)

Chonko,A.M., Dellasega,M., Varney,D.: Mechanism of uric acid secretion by proximal straight tubules of rabbit nephron. Kidney int. **6**, Abstr., 580 (1976)

Chonko,A.M., Lowe,C.M., Grantham,J.J.: Uric acid secretion in isolated perfused rabbit kidney tubules: comparison of proximal convoluted, proximal straight and cortical collecting segments. Clin. Res. **23**, Abstr., 538A (1975)

Christen,P., Peacock,W.C., Christen,A.E., Wacker,W.E.C.: Urate oxidase in primate phylogenesis. Europ. J. Biochem. **12**, 3—5 (1970a)

Christen,P., Peacock,W.C., Christen,A.E., Wacker,W.E.C.: Urate oxidase in primates. Folia primatol. (Basel) **13**, 35—39 (1970b)

Conger,J.D., Falk,S.A., Guggenheim,S.J., Burke,T.J.: A micropuncture study of the early phase of acute urate nephropathy. J. clin. Invest. **58**, 681—689 (1976)

Cook,M.A., Adkinson,J.T., Lassiter,W.E., Gottschalk,C.W.: Uric acid excretion by the rat kidney. Amer. J. Physiol. **229**, 586—591 (1975)

Cowsert,M.K., Carrier,O., Crowell,J.W.: The effect of hemorrhagic shock on blood uric acid level. Can. J. Physiol. Pharmacol. **44**, 861—864 (1966)

Cragoe,E.J., Schultz,E.M., Schneeberg,J.D., Stokker,G.E., Woltersdorf,O.W.,Jr., Fanelli,G.M.,Jr., Watson,L.S.: (1-oxo-2-substituted-5-indanyloxy) acetic acids, a new class of potent renal agents possessing both uricosuric and saluretic activity. A reexamination of the role of sulfhydryl binding in the mode of action of acylphenoxyacetic acid saluretics. J. med. Chem. **18**, 225—228 (1975)

Cross,R.J., Taggart,V.: Renal tubular transport: accumulation of *p*-aminohippurate by rabbit kidney slices. Amer. J. Physiol. **161**, 181—190 (1950)

Cushny,A.R.: The Secretion of the Urine. London: Longmans Green & Co. 1917

Davis,B.B., Field,J.B., Rodnan,G.P., Kedes,L.H.: Localization and pyrazinamide inhibition of distal transtubular movement of uric acid-2-C^{14} with a modified stop-flow technique. J. clin. Invest. **44**, 716—721 (1965)

Deetjen,P., Silbernagl,S.: Some new developments in continuous microperfusion technique. Yale J. Biol. Med. **45**, 301—306 (1972)

Despopoulos, A.: Renal excretory transport of organic acids: inhibition by oxypurines. Amer. J. Physiol. **197**, 1107—1110 (1959)

Duncan, H., Wakim, K. G., Ward, L. E.: The effects of intravenous administration of uric acid on its concentration in plasma and urine of Dalmatian and non-Dalmatian dogs. J. Lab. clin. Med. **58**, 876—883 (1961)

Ebstein, W., Nicolaier, A.: Über die Ausscheidung der Harnsäure durch die Nieren. Arch. path. Anat. Physiol. klin. Med. **143**, 337—368 (1896)

Eckert, A.: Experimentelle Untersuchungen über geformte Harnsäureausscheidung in den Nieren. Arch. exp. Path. Pharmakol. **72**, 244—297 (1913)

Elion, G. B., Yü, T. F., Gutman, A. B., Hitchings, G. H.: Renal clearance of oxipurinol, the chief metabolite of allopurinol. Amer. J. Med. **45**, 69—77 (1968)

Epstein, F. H., Pigeon, G.: Experimental urate nephropathy: studies of the distribution of urate in renal tissue. Nephron **1**, 144—157 (1964)

Fanelli, G. M., Jr.: Drugs affecting renal handling of uric acid. In: Martinez-Maldonado, M. (Ed.): Methods in Pharmacology. Vol. IV A: Renal Pharmacology, pp. 269—292. New York-London: Plenum Press 1976

Fanelli, G. M., Jr., Beyer, K. H., Jr.: Uric acid in nonhuman primates with special reference to its renal transport. Ann. Rev. Pharmacol. **14**, 355—364 (1974)

Fanelli, G. M., Bohn, D. L., Russo, H. F.: Renal clearance of uric acid in nonhuman primates. Comp. Biochem. Physiol. **33**, 459—464 (1970a)

Fanelli, G. M., Bohn, D., Stafford, S.: Functional characteristics of renal urate transport in the Cebus monkey. Amer. J. Physiol. **218**, 627—636 (1970b)

Fanelli, G. M., Jr., Bohn, D. L., Reilly, S. S.: Renal effects of uricosuric agents in the Cebus monkey. J. Pharmacol. exp. Ther. **175**, 259—266 (1970c)

Fanelli, G. M., Jr., Bohn, D. L., Reilly, S. S.: Renal urate transport in the chimpanzee. Amer. J. Physiol. **220**, 613—620 (1971a)

Fanelli, G. M., Jr., Bohn, D. L., Reilly, S. S.: Renal effects of uricosuric agents in the chimpanzee. J. Pharmacol. exp. Ther. **177**, 591—599 (1971b)

Fanelli, G. M., Jr., Bohn, D. L., Baer, J. E., Reilly, S. S.: Renal excretion and uricosuric properties of halofenate, a hypolipidemic-uricosuric agent, in the chimpanzee. J. Pharmacol. exp. Ther. **180**, 377—396 (1972a)

Fanelli, G. M., Jr., Bohn, D. L., Reilly, S. S.: Effects of mercurial diuretics on the renal tubular transport of p-aminohippurate and diodrast in the chimpanzee. J. Pharmacol. exp. Ther. **180**, 759—766 (1972b)

Fanelli, G. M., Jr., Bohn, D. L., Reilly, S. S., Weiner, I. M.: Effects of mercurial diuretics on renal transport of urate in the chimpanzee. Amer. J. Physiol. **224**, 985—992 (1973a)

Fanelli, G. M., Jr., Bohn, D. L., Reilly, S. S.: Effects of mercurial diuretics on renal transport of urate and p-aminohippurate in the Cebus monkey. Amer. J. Physiol. **224**, 993—996 (1973b)

Fanelli, G. M., Jr., Bohn, D. L., Scriabine, A., Beyer, K. H., Jr.: Saluretic and uricosuric effects of (6,7-dichloro-2-methyl-1-oxo-2-phenyl-5-indanyloxy) acetic acid (MK-196) in the chimpanzee. J. Pharmacol. exp. Ther. **200**, 402—412 (1977a)

Fanelli, G. M., Jr., Bohn, D. L., Zacchei, A. G.: Renal excretion of a saluretic-uricosuric agent (MK-196) and interaction with a urate-retaining drug, pyrazinoate, in the chimpanzee. J. Pharmacol. exp. Ther. **200**, 413—419 (1977b)

Fanelli, G. M., Jr., Weiner, I. M.: Pyrazinoate excretion in the chimpanzee: relation to urate disposition and the actions of uricosuric drugs. J. clin. Invest. **52**, 1946—1957 (1973)

Fanelli, G. M., Weiner, I. M.: Bidirectional renal urate transport in the chimpanzee. In: Edwards, K. D. G. (Ed.): Drugs and the Kidney. Prog. Biochem. Pharmacol., Vol. IX, pp. 163—173. Basel: Karger 1974

Fanelli, G. M., Jr., Weiner, I. M.: Species variations among primates in responses to drugs which alter the renal excretion of uric acid. J. Pharmacol. exp. Ther. **193**, 363—375 (1975)

Florkin, M., Duchateau, G.: Les formes du système enzymatique de l'uricolyse et l'évolution du catabolisme purique chez les animaux. Arch. int. Physiol. **53**, 267—307 (1943)

Folin, O., Berglund, H., Derich, C.: The uric acid problem: an experimental study on animals and man, including gouty subjects. J. biol. Chem. **60**, 361—471 (1924)

Folin, O., Denis, W.: A new (colorimetric) method for the determination of uric acid in blood. J. biol. Chem. **13**, 469—475 (1912)

Forster, R.P.: Renal transport mechanisms. Fed. Proc. **26**, 1008—1019 (1967)

Foulkes, E.C.: Peritubular transport of urate in rat kidneys. Pflügers Arch. **360**, 1—6 (1975)

Fridovich, I.: The competitive inhibition of uricase by oxonate and by related derivatives of s-triazines. J. biol. Chem. **240**, 2491—2494 (1965)

Friedman, M.: The effect of glycine on the production and excretion of uric acid. J. clin. Invest. **26**, 815—819 (1947)

Friedman, M.: Observations concerning the effects of (1) sodium salicylate and (2) sodium salicylate and glycine upon the production and excretion of uric acid and allantoin in the rat. Amer. J. Physiol. **152**, 302—308 (1948)

Friedman, M., Byers, S.O.: Observations concerning the causes of the excess excretion of uric acid in the Dalmatian dog. J. biol. Chem. **175**, 727—735 (1948a)

Friedman, M., Byers, S.O.: Effect of sodium salicylate upon the uric acid clearance of the Dalmatian dog. Amer. J. Physiol. **154**, 161—169 (1948b)

Friedman, M., Byers, S.O.: Distribution of uric acid in rat tissues and its production in tissue homogenates. Amer. J. Physiol. **172**, 29—32 (1953)

Garrod, A.B.: The Nature and Treatment of Gout and Rheumatic Gout. London: Walton and Maberly 1859

Grabfield, G.P., Swanson, D.: The uricosuric effects of certain polyhydric alcohols and saccharides. J. Pharmacol. exp. Ther. **74**, 106—113 (1942)

Graham, R.C., Karnovsky, M.J.: The histochemical demonstration of uricase activity. J. Histochem. Cytochem. **13**, 448—453 (1965)

Greger, R.: Purine excretion by the rat kidney. In: Silbernagl, S., Lang, F., Greger, R. (Eds.): Amino Acid Transport and Uric Acid Transport. Symposium Innsbruck, June 1975, pp. 192—201. Stuttgart: G. Thieme 1976

Greger, R., Lang, F., Deetjen, P.: Handling of uric acid by the rat kidney. I. Microanalysis of uric acid in proximal tubular fluid. Pflügers Arch. **324**, 279—287 (1971)

Greger, R., Lang, F., Deetjen, P.: Urate handling by the rat kidney. IV. Reabsorption in the loops of Henle. Pflügers Arch. **352**, 115—120 (1974a)

Greger, R., Lang, F., Deetjen, P.: Renal excretion of purine metabolites, urate and allantoin, by the mammalian kidney. In: Thurau, K. (Ed.): Kidney and Urinary Tract Physiology, 2, (International Review of Physiology; Vol. XI) pp. 257—281. Baltimore: University Park Press 1976

Greger, R., Lang, F., Puls, F., Deetjen, P.: Urate interaction with plasma proteins and erythrocytes: possible mechanism for urate reabsorption in kidney medulla. Pflügers Arch. **352**, 121—133 (1974b)

Gremels, H., Bodo, R.: The excretion of uric acid by the kidney. Proc. roy. Soc. Lond. (Biol.) **100**B, 336—359 (1926)

Gutman, A.B., Yü, T.F.: Renal mechanisms for regulation of uric acid excretion, with special reference to normal and gouty man. Semin. Arthr. and Rheum. **2**, 1—46 (1972)

Harvey, A.M., Christensen, H.N.: Uric acid transport system: apparent absence in erythrocytes of the Dalmatian coach hound. Science **145**, 826—827 (1964)

Hashimoto, S.: A new spectrophotometric assay method of xanthine oxidase in crude tissue homogenate. Analyt. Biochem. **62**, 426—435 (1974)

Heidenhain, R., Neisser, A.: Versuche über den Vorgang der Harnabsonderung. Pflügers Arch. **9**, 1—27 (1874)

Hewitt, W.R., Clark, R.L., Hook, J.B.: Investigations on metabolic modulation of p-amino-hippurate accumulation by rabbit renal cortical slices. J. Pharmacol. exp. Ther. **199**, 498—509 (1976)

Hughes, T.R., Klotz, I.M.: Analysis of metal-protein complexes. Methods Biochem. Anal. **3**, 265—299 (1956)

Hunter, A., Givens, M.H.: Studies in the comparative biochemistry of purine metabolism. II. The excretion of purine catabolites in the urine of ungulates. J. biol. Chem. **18**, 403—416 (1914a)

Hunter, A., Givens, M.H., Guion, C.M.: Studies in the biochemistry of purine metabolism. I. The excretion of purine catabolites in the urine of marsupials, rodents and carnivora. J. biol. Chem. **18**, 387—401 (1914b)

Imbs,J.L., Parrenin, A., Spach,M.O., Schwartz,J., Batzenschlager,A.: Effets du clopamide et du furosémide sur l'urée et la créatinine sanguines du rat insuffisant rénal. Thérapie **30**, 125—135 (1975)

Iwata,H., Yamamoto,I., Gohda,E., Morita,K., Nakamura,M., Sumi,K.: Potent competitive uricase inhibitors-2,8-diazahypoxanthine and related compounds. Biochem. Pharmacol. **22**, 2237—2245 (1973)

Johnson,D.R., Foulkes,E.C.: Localization of urate and phosphate reabsorption in the mongrel dog kidney. Proc. Soc. exp. Biol. (N.Y.) **143**, 1180—1182 (1973)

Johnson,W.J., Stavric,B., Chartrand,A.: Uricase inhibition in the rat by *s*-triazines: an animal model for hyperuricemia and hyperuricosuria. Proc. Soc. exp. Biol. (N.Y.) **131**, 8—12 (1969)

Jones,C.E., Crowell,J.W., Smith,E.E.: Significance of increased blood uric acid following extensive hemorrhage. Amer. J. Physiol. **214**, 1374—1377 (1968)

Jones,V.D., Despopoulos,A.: Is uric acid transported by the hippurate transport system? Pflügers Arch. **349**, 183—190 (1974)

Keilin,J.: The biological significance of uric acid and guanine excretion. Biol. Rev. **34**, 265—296 (1958)

Kessler,R.H., Hierholzer,K., Gurd,R.S.: Localization of urate transport in the nephron of mongrel and Dalmatian dog kidney. Amer. J. Physiol. **197**, 601—603 (1959)

Kippen,I., Klinenberg,J.R.: Characteristics of uric acid uptake by separated renal cortical tubules of the rabbit. J. clin. Chem. clin. Biochem. **14**, Abstr., 300—301 (1976a)

Kippen,I., Klinenberg,J.R.: Effect of drugs in uric acid uptake by separated renal cortical tubules of the rabbit. J. clin. Chem. clin. Biochem. **14**, Abstr., 301 (1976b)

Klemperer,F.W., Trimble,H.C., Hastings,A.B.: The uricase of dogs, including the Dalmatian. J. biol. Chem. **125**, 445—449 (1938)

Knapowski,J., Adam,W., Arasimowicz,C., Weiss,K.: Intestinal excretion of uric acid in dogs. Acta med. pol. **4**, 201—207 (1963)

Kramp,R.A., Lassiter,W.E., Gottschalk,C.W.: Urate-2-^{14}C transport in the rat nephron. J. clin. Invest. **50**, 35—48 (1971)

Kramp,R.A., Lenoir,R.: Distal permeability to urate and effects of benzofuran derivatives in the rat kidney. Amer. J. Physiol. **228**, 875—883 (1975a)

Kramp,R.A., Lenoir,R.H.: Characteristics of urate influx in the rat nephron. Amer. J. Physiol. **229**, 1654—1661 (1975b)

Kuster,G., Shorter,R.G., Dawson,B., Hallenbeck,G.A.: Effect of allogeneic hepatic transplantation between Dalmatian and mongrel dogs on urinary excretion of uric acid. Surg. Forum **18**, 360—362 (1967)

Kuster,G., Shorter,R.G., Dawson,B., Hallenbeck,G.A.: Uric acid metabolism in Dalmatians and other dogs: role of the liver. Arch. intern. Med. **129**, 492—496 (1972)

Lang,F.: Parameters and mechanisms of urate transport in the rat kidney. In: Silbernagl,S., Lang,F., Greger,R. (Eds.): Amino Acid Transport and Uric Acid Transport. Symposium Innsbruck, June 1975, pp. 217—227. Stuttgart: Thieme 1976

Lang,F., Greger,R., Deetjen,P.: Handling of uric acid by the rat kidney. II. Microperfusion studies on bidirectional transport of uric acid in the proximal tubule. Pflügers Arch. **335**, 257—265 (1972)

Lang,F., Greger,R., Deetjen,P.: Handling of uric acid by the rat kidney. III. Microperfusion studies on steady state concentration of uric acid in the proximal tubule. Consideration of free flow conditions. Pflügers Arch. **338**, 295—302 (1973)

Lang,F., Greger,R., Deetjen,P.: In vivo studies on uricase activity in the rat. Pflügers Arch. **351**, 323—330 (1974)

Lassiter,W.E.: Kidney. Ann. Rev. Physiol. **37**, 371—393 (1975)

Lathem,W., Davis,B.B., Rodnan,G.P.: Renal tubular secretion of uric acid in the mongrel dog. Amer. J. Physiol. **199**, 9—12 (1960)

Lauterburg,B., Sautter,V., Herz,R., Colombo,J.P., Roch-Ramel,F., Bircher,J.: The defect of uric acid metabolism in Eck-fistula rats. J. Lab. clin. Med. **90**, 92—100 (1977)

Lemieux,G., Gougoux,A., Vinay,P., Michaud,G.: Uricosuric effect of benziodarone in man and laboratory animals: a comparative study. Amer. J. Physiol. **224**, 1431—1439 (1973a)

Lemieux,G., Kiss,A., Gougoux,A., Vinay,P.: Tienilic acid (ticrynafen): a new diuretic with uricosuric properties in man and dog. J. clin. Chem. clin. Biochem. **14**, Abstr., 306 (1976)

Lemieux,G., Plante,G.E.: The effect of starvation in the normal dog including the Dalmatian coach hound. Metabolism **17**, 620—˙630 (1968)

Lemieux,G., Vinay,P., Gougoux,A., Michaud,G.: Nature of the uricosuric action of benziodarone. Amer. J. Physiol. **224**, 1440—1449 (1973b)

Logan,D.C., Wilson,D.E., Flowers,C.M., Sparks,P.J., Tyler,F.H.: Uric acid catabolism in the woolly monky. Metabolism **25**, 517—522 (1976)

Lucas-Heron,B., Fontenaille,C.: Uric acid transport characteristics in human red blood cells. J. clin. Chem. clin. Biochem. **14**, Abstr., 307 (1976)

Ludwig,C.: Nieren und Harnbereitung. In: Wagner,R. (Ed.): Handwörterbuch der Physiologie, Vol. II, pp. 628—640. Braunschweig: F. Vieweg 1844

Maroske,D., Weiner,I.M.: The renal handling of zoxazolamine (Flexin). J. Pharmacol. exp. Ther. **159**, 409—415 (1968)

Martin,G.J.: The effect of various agents on the excretion of uric acid and allantoin. Exp. Med. Surg. **6**, 24—27 (1948)

Martinez-Maldonado,M., Stavroulaki-Tsapara,A., Tsaparas,N., Suki,W.N., Eknoyan,G.: Renal effects of lithium administration in rats: alterations in water and electrolyte metabolism and the response to vasopressin and cyclic-adenosine monophosphate during prolonged administration. J. Lab. clin. Med. **86**, 445—461 (1975)

Marzani,P.C.: Iperuricemia sperimentale. Ricerche sul coniglio (allantoina e acido urico). Arch. Sci. med. (Torino) **116**, 169—180 (1964a)

Marzani,P.C.: Ulteriori ricerche sull'iperuricemia sperimentale nel coniglio. Arch. Sci. med. (Torino) **116**, 215—225 (1964b)

May,D.G., Weiner,I.M.: The renal mechanisms for the excretion of m-hydroxybenzoic acid in Cebus monkeys: relationship to urate transport. J. Pharmacol. exp. Ther. **176**, 407—417 (1971)

McKenzie,R., Knight,T., Weinman,E.J.: The effects of indanyloxyacetic acid (MK 196) on electrolyte excretion in the rat kidney. Proc. Soc. exp. Biol. (N.Y.) **153**, 202—204 (1976)

McMaster,P.D., Drury,D.R.: The production of partial liver insufficiency in rabbits. J. exp. Med. **49**, 745—758 (1929)

Miller,G.E., Danzig,L.S., Talbott,J.H.: Urinary excretion of uric acid in the Dalmatian and non-Dalmatian dog following administration of diodrast, sodium salicylate and a mercurial diuretic. Amer. J. Physiol. **164**, 155—158 (1951)

Minkowski,O.: Untersuchungen zur Physiologie und Pathologie der Harnsäure bei Säugethieren. Arch. exp. Path. Pharmakol. **41**, 375—420 (1898)

Møller,J.V.: The effects of D- and L-lactate and osmotic diuretics on uric acid clearance in the rabbit. Acta physiol. scand. **54**, 30—36 (1962)

Møller,J.V.: The tubular site of urate transport in the rabbit kidney, and the effect of probenecid on urate secretion. Acta pharmacol. toxicol. (Kbh.) **23**, 329—336 (1965a)

Møller,J.V.: Tubular site of urate secretion in the rabbit. Nature (Lond.) **208**, 492—493 (1965b)

Møller,J.V.: The excretion of urate at various plasma concentration and during osmotic diuresis in the rabbit. Acta physiol. scand. **66**, 419—426 (1966a)

Møller,J.V.: Clearance experiments on the effect of probenecid on urate excretion in the rabbit. Acta pharmacol. toxicol. (Kbh.) **23**, 321—328 (1966b)

Møller,J.V.: The renal accumulation of urate and p-aminohippurate in the rabbit. J. Physiol. (Lond.) **192**, 519—527 (1967a)

Møller,J.V.: The relation between secretion of urate and p-aminohippurate in the rabbit kidney. J. Physiol. (Lond.) **192**, 505—517 (1967b)

Møller,J.V., Sheikh,M.I.: A review on the renal excretion of urate in the rabbit. In: Silbernagl,S., Lang,F., Greger,R. (Eds.): Amino Acid Transport and Uric Acid Transport. Symposium Innsbruck, June 1975, pp. 163—168. Stuttgart: Thieme 1976

Morgan,E.J.: The distribution of xanthine oxidase I. Biochem. J. **20**, 1282—1291 (1926)

Mudge,G.H., McLary,B., Berndt,W.O.: Renal transport of uric acid in the guinea pig. Amer. J. Physiol. **214**, 875—879 (1968a)

Mudge,G.H., Cucchi,J., Platts,M., O'Connell,J.M.B., Berndt,W.O.: Renal excretion of uric acid in the dog. Amer. J. Physiol. **215**, 404—410 (1968b)

Mudge,G.H., Berndt,W.O., Valtin,H.: Tubular transport of urea, glucose, phosphate, uric acid, sulfate, and thiosulfate. In: Orloff,J., Berliner,R.W. (Eds.): Handbook of Physiology. Sect. 8: Renal Physiology, pp. 587—652. Washington: American Physiological Society 1973

Musil, J., Sandow, J.: The effect of ethynylestradiol and estrogen on renal excretion of uric acid. In: Silbernagl, S., Lang, F., Greger, R. (Eds.): Amino Acid Transport and Uric Acid Transport. Symposium Innsbruck, June 1975, pp. 227—236. Stuttgart: Thieme 1976

Mwasi, L. M., Waisman, J., Bluestone, R., Klinenberg, J. R.: A brief note on the ultrastructure of renal glomeruli in acutely hyperuricemic rats. Invest. Urol. **13**, 321—324 (1976)

Nakajima, Y., Bourne, G. H.: Histochemical studies on urate oxidase in several mammals with special reference to uricolytic ability of primates. Histochemie **22**, 20—24 (1970)

Nolan, R. P., Foulkes, E. C.: Studies on renal urate secretion in the dog. J. Pharmacol. exp. Ther. **179**, 429—437 (1971)

Noll, R. M., Duggan, D. E.: Purine catabolism in subhuman primates; experimental uricogenesis and xanthine oxidase inhibition. Pharmacologist **13**, Abstr. 095, 208 (1971)

O'Connell, J. M. B., Romeo, J. A., Mudge, G. H.: Renal tubular secretion of creatinine in the dog. Amer. J. Physiol. **203**, 985—990 (1962)

Oelert, H., Baumann, K., Gekle, D.: Permeabilitätsmessungen einiger schwacher organischer Säuren aus dem distalen Konvolut der Rattenniere. Pflügers Arch. **307**, 178—189 (1969)

Overgaard-Hansen, K., Lassen, U. V.: Active transport of uric acid through the human erythrocyte membrane. Nature (Lond.) **184**, 553—554 (1959)

Plante, G. E., Lemieux, G.: L'excrétion rénale de l'acide urique. Union méd. Can. **97**, 1629—1635 (1968)

Platts, M. M., Mudge, G. H.: Accumulation of uric acid by slices of kidney cortex. Amer. J. Physiol. **200**, 387—392 (1961)

Poulsen, H.: Inhibition of uric acid excretion in rabbits given probenecid or salicylic acid. Acta pharmacol. toxicol. (Kbh.) **11**, 277—286 (1955)

Poulsen, H., Praetorius, E.: Tubular excretion of uric acid in rabbits. Acta pharmacol. toxicol. (Kbh.) **10**, 371—378 (1954)

Quebbemann, A. J., Cumming, J. D., Shideman, J. R., Toledo-Pereyra, L.: Synthesis of uric acid in isolated normothermic perfused mongrel and Dalmatian dog kidneys. Amer. J. Physiol. **228**, 959—963 (1975)

Reem, G. H., Vanamee, P.: Effect of sodium lactate on urate clearance in the Dalmatian and in the mongrel. Amer. J. Physiol. **207**, 113—117 (1964)

Richert, D. A., Westerfeld, W. W.: Xanthine oxidases in different species. Proc. Soc. exp. Biol. (N. Y.) **76**, 252—254 (1951)

Roch-Ramel, F., Boudry, J. F.: Tubular fate of 2-C^{14} urate: microperfusion experiments. Fed. Proc. **30**, Abstr. 819, 338 (1971)

Roch-Ramel, F., Diezi, J., Chométy, F., Michoud, P., Peters, G.: Disposal of large urea overloads by the rat kidney: a micropuncture study. Amer. J. Physiol. **218**, 1524—1532 (1970)

Roch-Ramel, F., Diezi-Chométy, F., de Rougemont, D., Tellier, M., Widmer, J., Peters, G.: Renal excretion of uric acid in the rat: a micropuncture and microperfusion study. Amer. J. Physiol. **230**, 768—776 (1976a)

Roch-Ramel, F., de Rougemont, D., Peters, G., Weiner, I. M.: Micropuncture study of urate excretion by the kidney of the rat, the Cebus monkey and the rabbit. In: Silbernagl, S., Lang, F., Greger, R. (Eds.): Amino Acid Transport and Uric Acid Transport. Symposium Innsbruck, June 1975, pp. 188—192. Stuttgart: Thieme 1976b

Roch-Ramel, F., Weiner, I. M.: Excretion of urate by the kidneys of Cebus monkeys: a micropuncture study. Amer. J. Physiol. **224**, 1369—1374 (1973)

Roch-Ramel, F., Weiner, I. M.: Inhibition of urate excretion by pyrazinoate: a micropuncture study. Amer. J. Physiol. **229**, 1604—1608 (1975)

Roch-Ramel, F., Wong, N. L. M., Dirks, J. H.: Renal excretion of urate in mongrel and Dalmatian dogs: a micropuncture study. Amer. J. Physiol. **231**, 326—331 (1976c)

De Rougemont, D., Henchoz, M., Roch-Ramel, F.: Renal urate excretion at various plasma concentrations in the rat: a free-flow micropuncture study. Amer. J. Physiol. **231**, 387—392 (1976)

Schaffer, N. K., Dill, L. V., Stander, H. J.: The effect of renin on the uric acid metabolism of the pregnant and non-pregnant Dalmatian dog. Endocrinology **29**, 243—249 (1941)

Schultz, A.: Experimentelle Studien zur Harnsäureausscheidung. Verh. dtsch. path. Ges. **26**, 174—180 (1931)

Sheikh, M. I., Møller, J. V.: Binding of urate to proteins of human and rabbit plasma. Biochim. biophys. Acta (Amst.) **158**, 456—458 (1968)

Sheikh,M.I., Møller,J.V.: The mechanism of urate transport in rabbit kidney tubules in vitro. Pflügers Arch. **325**, 235—246 (1971)

Silverman,M., Aganon,M.A., Chinard,F.P.: D-glucose interactions with renal tubule cell surfaces. Amer. J. Physiol. **218**, 735—742 (1970)

Simeone,F.A., Abraham,J., Hopkins,R.W., Damewood,C.A.: Levels of allantoin and uric acid in dogs subjected to hemorrhagic shock. J. surg. Res. **19**, 373—380 (1975)

Simkin,P.A.: Uric acid metabolism in Cebus monkeys. Amer. J. Physiol. **221**, 1105—1109 (1971)

Simkin,P.A.: Uric acid binding to serum proteins: differences among species. Proc. Soc. exp. Biol. (N.Y.) **139**, 604—606 (1972a)

Simkin,P.A.: Hexose infusions in Cebus monkeys: effects on uric acid metabolism. Metabolism **21**, 1029—1036 (1972b)

Simmonds,H.A., Hatfield,P.J., Cameron,J.S., Cadenhead,A.: Uric acid excretion by the pig kidney. Amer. J. Physiol. **230**, 1654—1661 (1976)

Skeith,M.D., Healey,L.A.: Urate clearance in Cebus monkeys. Amer. J. Physiol. **214**, 582—584 (1968)

Sonnenberg,H., Oelert,H., Baumann,K.: Proximal tubular reabsorption of some organic acids in the rat kidney in vivo. Pflügers Arch. **286**, 171—180 (1965)

Stavric,B., Johnson,W.J., Grice,H.C.: Uric acid nephropathy: an experimental model. Proc. Soc. exp. Biol. (N.Y.) **130**, 512—516 (1969)

Stavric,B., Nera,E.A., Johnson,W.J., Salem,F.A.: Uric acid kidney stones induced in rats by oxonic acid, a uricase inhibitor. Invest. Urol. **11**, 3—8 (1973)

Stavric,B., Johnson,W.J., Clayman,S., Gadd,R.E.A., Chartrand,A.: Effect of fructose administration on serum urate levels in the uricase inhibited rat. Experientia (Basel) **32**, 373—374 (1976)

Steele,T.H., Underwood,J.L.: Renal urate transport during variations in urate synthesis in the rat. Pflügers Arch. **367**, 183—188 (1976)

Steele,T.H., Underwood,J.L., Dudgeon,K.L.: Urate excretion and urine flow in a lithium-induced diabetes insipidus rat model. Pflügers Arch. **346**, 205—213 (1974)

Straus,W.: Concentration of acid phosphatase, ribonuclease, desoxyribonuclease, β-glucuronidase, and cathepsin in "droplets" isolated from the kidney cells of normal rats. J. biophys. biochem. Cytol. **2**, 513—521 (1956)

Swanson,R.E., Hakim,A.A.: Stop-flow analysis of creatinine excretion in the dog. Amer. J. Physiol. **203**, 980—984 (1962)

Taggart,J.V., Silverman,M., Trayner,E.M.: Influence of renal electrolyte composition on the tubular excretion of p-aminohippurate. Amer. J. Physiol. **173**, 345—350 (1953)

Thoenes,W., Langer,K.H.: Relationship between cell structures of renal tubules and transport mechanisms. In: Thurau,K., Jahrmärker,H. (Eds.): Renal Transport and Diuretics, pp. 37—65. Berlin-Heidelberg-New York: Springer 1969

Thuillier,G., Laforest,J., Cariou,B., Bessin,P., Bonnet,J., Thuillier,J.: Dérivés hétérocycliques d'acides phénoxyacétiques, synthèse et étude préliminaire de leurs activités diurétique et uricosurique. Europ. J. med. Chem., Chim. Ther. **9**, 625—633 (1974)

Tisher,C.C., Finkel,R.M., Rosen,S., Kendig,E.M.: Renal microbodies in the Rhesus monkey. Lab. Invest. **19**, 1—6 (1968)

Tompkins,R.B., Andreini,P.H., McCall,J.T., Ward,L.E.: Comparison of serum urate clearance by Dalmatian dog, a non-Dalmatian and a Dalmatian with a transplanted non-Dalmatian liver. Arthr. and Rheum. **10**, Abstr., 318 (1967)

Toribara,T.Y., Terepka,A.R., Dewey,P.A.: The ultrafiltrable calcium of human serum. I. Ultrafiltration methods and normal values. J. clin. Invest. **36**, 738—748 (1957)

Torretti,J., Weiner,I.M.: The renal excretion of drugs. In: Martinez-Maldonado,M. (Ed.): Methods in Pharmacology. Vol. IVA: Renal Pharmacology, pp. 357—379. New York-London: Plenum Press 1976

Truszkowski,R., Goldmanówna,C.: Uricase and its action. VI. Distribution in various animals. Biochem. J. **27**, 612—614 (1933)

Tune,B.M., Burg,M.B., Patlak,C.S.: Characteristics of p-aminohippurate transport in proximal renal tubules. Amer. J. Physiol. **217**, 1057—1063 (1969)

Ungar, H.: Transformation of the hepatic vasculature of rats following protracted experimental poisoning with carbon tetrachloride. Its possible relation to the formation of urate calculi in the urinary tract. Amer. J. Pathol. **27**, 871—883 (1951)

Waisman, J., Bluestone, R., Klinenberg, J. R.: A preliminary report of nephropathy in hyperuricemic rats. Lab. Invest. **30**, 716—722 (1974)

Weiner, I. M., Fanelli, G. M., Jr.: Bidirectional transport: urate and other organic anions. In: Wesson, L. G., Fanelli, G. M. (Eds.): Recent Advances in Renal Physiology and Pharmacology, pp. 53—68. Lancaster: Medical and Technical Publ. Co. 1974

Weiner, I. M., Fanelli, G. M., Jr.: Renal urate excretion in animal models. Nephron **14**, 33—47 (1975)

Weiner, I. M., Tinker, J. P.: Pharmacology of pyrazinamide: metabolic and renal function studies related to the mechanism of drug-induced urate retention. J. Pharmacol. exp. Ther. **180**, 411—434 (1972)

Weinman, E. J., Eknoyan, G., Suki, W. N.: The influence of the extracellular fluid volume on the tubular reabsorption of uric acid. J. clin. Invest. **55**, 283—291 (1975)

Weinman, E. J., Steplock, D., Suki, W. N., Eknoyan, G.: Urate reabsorption in proximal convoluted tubule of the rat kidney. Amer. J. Physiol. **231**, 509—515 (1976a)

Weinman, E. J., Knight, T. F., McKenzie, R., Eknoyan, G.: Dissociation of urate from sodium transport in the rat proximal tubule. Kidney int. **10**, 295—300 (1976b)

Wells, H. G.: The purine metabolism of the Dalmatian coach hound. J. biol. Chem. **35**, 221—225 (1918)

Wesson, L. G.: Physiology of the Human Kidney. Chap. 9: Aromatic acids, pp. 165—205. New York-London: Grune & Stratton 1969

Wolfson, W. Q., Cohn, C., Shore, C.: The renal mechanism for urate excretion in the Dalmatian coach-hound. J. exp. Med. **92**, 121—128 (1950)

Yü, T. F., Gutman, A. B.: Quantitative analysis of uric acid in blood and urine. Methods and interpretation. Bull. rheum. Dis. **7**, Suppl., 17—20 (1957)

Yü, T. F., Gutman, A. B.: Study of the paradoxical effects of salicylate in low, intermediate and high dosage on the renal mechanisms for excretion of urate in man. J. clin. Invest. **38**, 1298—1315 (1959)

Yü, T. F., Berger, L., Kupfer, S., Gutman, A. B.: Tubular secretion of urate in the dog. Amer. J. Physiol. **199**, 1199—1204 (1960)

Yü, T. F., Berger, L., Gutman, A. B.: Suppression of tubular secretion of urate by pyrazinamide in the dog. Proc. Soc. exp. Biol. (N.Y.) **107**, 905—908 (1961)

Yü, T. F., Gutman, A. B., Berger, L., Kaung, C.: Low uricase activity in the Dalmatian dog simulated in mongrels given oxonic acid. Amer. J. Physiol. **220**, 973—979 (1971)

Zins, G. R., Weiner, I. M.: Bidirectional urate transport limited to the proximal tubule in dogs. Amer. J. Physiol. **215**, 411—422 (1968)

Urate Excretion in Man, Normal and Gouty

T. H. STEELE

A. Introduction

Because of its existence in man as a sparingly soluble end-product of purine metabolism, the elimination of uric acid from the body has assumed special significance in human physiology and medicine (SORENSEN and LEVINSON, 1975). Urate excretion is normally partitioned between the kidney and intestine. The ratio of renal-to-extrarenal urate elimination is approximately 2:1 in normal persons stabilized on a low dietary purine intake, under steady-state conditions, when uric acid turnover reflects the rate of de novo purine biosynthesis (SORENSEN, 1960; SORENSEN, 1965). Under conditions of normal dietary purine intake, however, exogenous purine is also metabolized to uric acid (ZÖLLNER, 1973). The extent to which such exogenous purine may alter the ratio of renal-to-intestinal urate elimination has not been characterized in detail. However, based on studies in hypouricemic patients with Wilson's disease who manifested defective renal urate reabsorption, the available evidence suggests that intestinal uric acid elimination may fall to very low values in hypouricemic states, with the kidney concomitantly excreting a much greater fraction of the urate turnover (SORENSEN and KAPPAS, 1966). This situation can reverse following successful treatment of the renal lesions of Wilson's disease with penicillamine. Conversely, intestinal elimination assumes a greater role in uric acid elimination in patients with advanced chronic renal insufficiency, in whom the urinary urate excretion may be greatly depressed (SORENSEN and LEVINSON, 1975). These considerations suggest that the amount of intestinal uric acid elimination is an important factor in determining the amount of urate that must be excreted in the urine in order to avoid hyperuricemia. Extrarenal urate elimination is discussed in detail in another chapter of this volume.

In this chapter, an attempt will first be made to somewhat sequentially discuss the development of our present concepts of renal urate handling in humans. Following that, several factors that have been proposed as important in the regulation of urate excretion will be considered individually. Finally, information gained from the study of normals will be related to current concepts of renal urate excretion in gouty patients.

B. Development of Concepts of Renal Urate Handling

Early observations indicated that the urinary urate in normal man was considerably less than the amount expected in the urine if its glomerular filtration were complete and no tubular transport occurred (BERGLUND and FRISK, 1935). The relationship between the glomerular filtration of urate and its apparent reabsorption was examined in detail by BERLINER et al. (1950). Taking urate reabsorption as the difference between the filtered load and urinary excretion, they utilized lithium urate infusions to increase the amount of filtered urate. Their results indicated that net urate reabsorption initially increased with the plasma urate and filtered load but subsequently plateaued by the time the plasma urate had attained a value of approximately 15 mg/dl. Using the most economical explanation of the data, BERLINER et al. (1950) suggested that urate underwent glomerular filtration and partial reabsorption by the tubules of the human kidney. That reabsorption attained an apparent maximum value could be explained on the basis of saturability of the reabsorptive transport system at greatly elevated intratubular urate concentrations.

Although filtration and carrier-mediated reabsorption could satisfactorily explain the early data, a concept of bidirectional renal transport of urate subsequently evolved, largely through the pioneering work of the late Alexander Gutman and his associates, in a series of experiments designed to further elucidate the pathogenesis of gout (GUTMAN and YÜ, 1957). Along with clearance studies in which they were able to demonstrate net tubular secretion of urate in the dog (YÜ et al., 1960), GUTMAN et al. (1959) also demonstrated net tubular secretion of urate in man. This, however, could only be achieved under highly contrived experimental conditions, requiring the use of individuals with modest renal insufficiency, as well as the employment of urate infusions, osmotic diuretics and sulfinpyrazone, the latter being an agent that probably blocks the tubular reabsorption of urate rather selectively at the dose used. Under those conditions, urate excretion rates of approximately 20% greater than the concomitant filtered urate loads could be elicited, thereby demonstrating the existence of tubular secretion of urate.

PRAETORIUS and KIRK (1950) published data describing a hypouricemic patient whose urinary excretion of endogenous urate greatly exceeded the filtered load. In that patient, a reabsorptive defect in urate transport apparently had unmasked tubular secretion. Other patients with similar reabsorptive defects and demonstrable net secretion have been described (KHACHADURIAN and ARSLANIAN, 1973; SIMKIN et al., 1973), further strengthening the concept of bidirectional urate transport. In the patient described by SIMKIN et al. (1973), urate excretion was approximately 40% greater than the filtered load.

Following their demonstration of tubular secretion of urate in man, and using analogies to lower animals, GUTMAN and YÜ (1961) enunciated their "three-component hypothesis" describing bidirectional tubular transport as an integral feature of renal urate handling in man. According to that hypothesis, urate is initially freely filtered at the glomerulus and subsequently undergoes both reabsorption and secretion within the renal tubule. They did not speculate regarding the sequence of urate secretory and reabsorptive sites within nephrons (GUTMAN and YÜ, 1957; GUTMAN, 1964). However, many investigators originally felt that extensive reabsorption of filtered urate was the initial intratubular event, and that this was followed by the tubular secretion of urate. Such a schema encompassed the data available at the time most economically (STEELE and RIESELBACH, 1967a; GUTMAN et al., 1969).

The relative importance of tubular secretion of urate in maintaining uric acid excretion in man was surmised largely from the results of experiments employing pharmacologic inhibitors of urate secretion. In particular, pyrazinamide (PZA) was

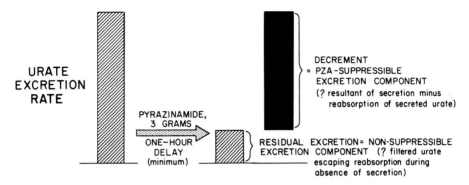

Fig. 1. Schema of a "pyrazinamide suppression test." After control measurements of the urinary urate excretion, pyrazinamide (PZA) is administered as a single 3-g dose. Following a delay of at least 1 h, specimens for subsequent clearance periods are obtained. The specimens obtained when the urinary urate is at a minimum constitute the maximum (antisecretory) action following PZA. Under those conditions, the residual urate excretion (i.e., nonsuppressible urate excretion) may reflect the amount of filtered urate escaping reabsorption. Similarly, the PZA-suppressible component of the urinary urate is the difference between control urate excretion and the residual (nonsuppressible) excretion. This PZA-suppressible component of the urinary urate appears to be a resultant of the amount of urate secretion minus the reabsorption of secreted urate. Format adapted from that of STEELE and RIESELBACH (1967a)

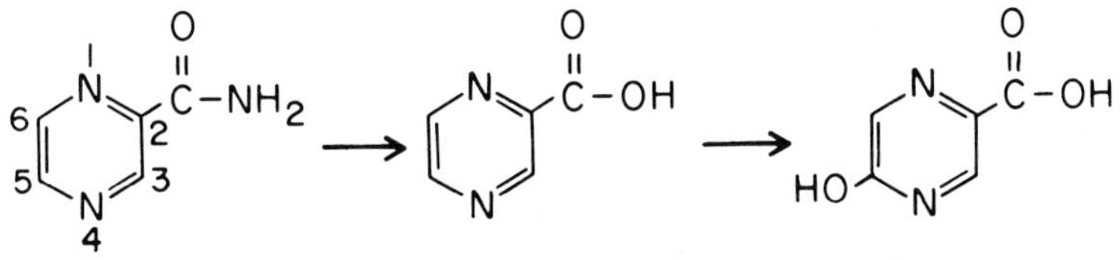

Fig. 2. Metabolism of pyrazinamide *(left)* to pyrazinoic acid (center), the renally active metabolite. Pyrazinoate appears to inhibit the tubular secretion of urate rather selectively at low plasma concentrations but inhibits urate reabsorption at high plasma concentrations in the dog (WEINER and TINKER, 1972) and chimpanzee (FANELLI and WEINER, 1973). Pyrazinoate then is hydroxylated to 5-hydroxypyrazinoic acid *(right)* through a xanthine oxidase-mediated pathway (WEINER and TINKER, 1972). 5-hydroxypyrazinoate appears to be the chief metabolite of pyrazinoate and probably is biologically inactive

used extensively as an agent, which resulted in the selective inhibition of urate secretion (YÜ et al., 1957a, 1961). This agent subsequently was used in a so-called "PZA suppression test," diagrammed in Figure 1. Recent work in several species has indicated that PZA is metabolized to pyrazinoic acid (PZO), as shown in Figure 2, and that low plasma concentrations of PZO appear to rather selectively inhibit the tubular secretion of urate; PZO also inhibits urate reabsorption at high plasma concentrations (WEINER and TINKER, 1972; FANELLI and WEINER, 1973). Because the administration of 3 g PZA to normal man always resulted in a striking decrease in urate excretion—often by more than 80%—it seemed that the plasma PZO concentrations generated following oral PZA probably remain sufficiently low to inhibit urate secretion selectively (STEELE and RIESELBACH, 1967a; GUTMAN et al., 1969).

Recent data in seven normal persons have confirmed this, in that the administration of PZA at a dosage of 3 g resulted in plasma PZO levels ranging from 12 to 18 µg/ml (PRASAD et al., 1977), values which (at least in the chimpanzee) appear to inhibit urate secretion selectively (FANELLI and WEINER, 1973). The decrease in urate excretion following PZA, as well as after low doses of salicylates (YÜ and GUTMAN, 1959) and a number of other pharmacologic agents known to be excreted via renal organic anion transport systems, together with the observation that PZO elicits an abrupt and substantial decrease in urate excretion during exogenously induced hyperuricemia (YÜ et al., 1962), suggested that tubular secretion of urate is necessary in order to maintain urate excretion at levels sufficient to prevent urate retention and, ultimately, hyperuricemia. Indeed, the chronic use of PZA in the treatment of tuberculosis has frequently produced hyperuricemia and occasionally articular gout (CULLEN et al., 1957; SHAPIRO and HYDE, 1957).

Although the importance of tubular secretion of urate seems established, a quantitative assessment of the magnitude of urate secretion has remained elusive. Unless secretory transport of urate is saturated at low plasma urate concentrations, it seems likely that urate secretion is probably a function both of plasma urate concentration and the postglomerular renal plasma flow—perhaps the superficial renal cortical component of the latter. Although precession studies have provided direct evidence for the existence of urate secretion in man (PODEVIN et al., 1968a, b), the precession technique does not well lend itself to quantification. At present, the magnitude of urate secretion cannot be measured in normal man by any available means (STEELE, 1973; STEELE, 1975a, b). The evidence for this and its ramifications will be discussed subsequently. However, the earlier concept that the tubular secretion of urate is vital in maintaining an adequate rate of urinary uric acid excretion remains valid.

C. Factors Thought to Affect Urate Excretion in Normal Man

I. Sequence of Renal Reabsorptive and Secretory Transport Sites

Data from extensive studies in the chimpanzee, a species devoid of uricase activity and whose renal urate transport resembles man's in many respects, have indicated that the intrarenal reabsorptive and secretory transport fluxes for urate are far greater than the values suggested by the decrement in urate excretion produced by PZA or PZO administration (FANELLI et al., 1971; FANELLI et al., 1973). The most compelling evidence for the partial reabsorption of secreted urate was gathered from studies in the chimpanzee using mersalyl. Administration of this mercurial diuretic to the chimpanzee elicited urate excretion rates far in excess of the filtered load (FANELLI et al., 1973). Specifically, although the urate clearance normally approximates 10% of the glomerular filtration rate (GFR) in the chimpanzee, mersalyl increased the urate clearance to values almost twice the GFR in some experiments. Two important conclusions could be formulated from these observations. Firstly, the magnitude of tubular secretion of urate in the chimpanzee is far greater than the normal rate of uric acid excretion. Secondly, the amount of urate reabsorbed by the kidneys in the chimpanzee greatly exceeds the amount of urate filtered by the glomeruli. Thus, some of the urate which is secreted in that species must subsequently be reabsorbed. Attempts to duplicate the experiments with mersalyl in man, however, met with failure (FANELLI and HITZENBERGER, 1974), probably reflecting a diminished sensitivity of man to uricosuric agents in comparison to the chimpanzee (FANELLI and WEINER, 1975).

In man, there is also evidence that a portion of the secreted urate is reabsorbed, but unfortunately the data are less direct. This evidence derives from experiments using PZA (Fig. 1) or low doses of salicylates to block the tubular secretion of urate and then noting the response to uricosuric agents. Specifically, the uricosuric response to probenecid is diminished significantly or completely eliminated by PZA (STEELE and BONER, 1973) or low-dose salicylates (DIAMOND and PAOLINO, 1973). Similar observations had also been made in the chimpanzee previously (FANELLI et al., 1971). PZA also diminishes the acute uricosuric response to chlorothiazide i.v. (STEELE and BONER, 1973). Similar observations have been made using benziodarone (LEMIEUX et al., 1973). If all urate reabsorption occurred prior to secretion, and if all secreted urate escaped into the urine, one would expect that the inhibition of tubular secretion of urate after PZA or salicylate administration would leave the uricosuric responses to pharmacologic agents intact. Specifically, the increment in urate excretion produced by a given uricosuric agent should not be diminished by the prior inhibition of urate secretion unless a portion of the secreted urate is reabsorbed. The fact that increments in urate excretion produced by probenecid and chlorothiazide were reduced by prior treatment with PZA or salicylate suggested that a portion of the secreted urate is reabsorbed.

The experiments cited above required the administration of two pharmacologic agents that affect urate transport. Several types of drug interactions could occur that might invalidate the concept that the attenuation of uricosuric responses by pharmacologic secretory inhibition provides evidence for the reabsorption of secreted urate. Firstly, the uricosuric agent itself might inhibit the tubular secretion of urate. This may occur with probenecid (SIMKIN et al., 1973), although such an inhibitory effect has not been clearly demonstrated in normal man (MUDGE et al., 1973; YÜ and GUTMAN, 1955). A second type of interaction at a pharmacologic level could result if the uricosuric agent blocked the tubular secretion of PZO. That this may occur has been demonstrated in studies using the new uricosuric natriuretic agent ticrynafen, or tienilic acid (REESE and STEELE, 1976). PZA pretreatment diminished the uricosuric response to ticrynafen by about 30% (PRASAD et al., 1977). After ticrynafen, the plasma PZO concentration increased and the PZO clearance diminished, suggesting that ticrynafen had inhibited the tubular secretion of PZO. However, urinary PZO concentrations and excretion rates remained constant, suggesting that diminished urinary PZO could not explain the residual uricosuric response to ticrynafen after PZA (Fig. 3). A third type of pharmacologic interaction could exist if PZO inhibited the renal secretion of the uricosuric agent. Because probenecid and many other uricosuric agents are strongly protein-bound, they must undergo tubular secretion in order to gain access to luminal transport sites, where they can inhibit urate reabsorption (WEINER et al., 1960; WEINER, 1967). In the case of ticrynafen (tienilic acid) or i.v. chlorothiazide, PZA pretreatment did not diminish the natriuretic action of the diuretics, thereby indirectly suggesting that ticrynafen or chlorothiazide secretion was not impaired by PZA or PZO (PRASAD et al., 1977; STEELE and BONER, 1973). Finally, recent results of MEISEL and DIAMOND (1977) indicated that PZA administration does not affect probenecid excretion, thereby suggesting that PZA or PZO

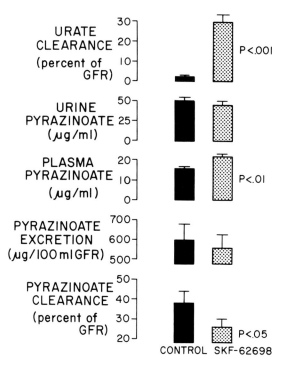

Fig. 3. Urate excretion after ticrynafen or tienilic acid (SKF-62698) in pyrazinamide-pretreated persons. Note that the urate clearance increased significantly but that urine pyrazinoate (the active metabolite of pyrazinamide) remained unchanged. The plasma pyrazinoate increased and pyrazinoate excretion remained unchanged. Thus, ticrynafen (SKF-62698) appeared to decrease the clearance of pyrazinoate. It had no discernible effect upon pyrazinamide. Data are from PRASAD et al. (1977)

does not inhibit probenecid secretion sufficiently to affect the amount available at intraluminal sites where urate reabsorption takes place (WEINER et al., 1960).

A type of experiment that did not employ two pharmacologic agents involved the use of 3% sodium chloride infusion to elicit a uricosuric response (MANUEL and STEELE, 1974). In normal persons manifesting a uricosuric response to 3% NaCl, pretreatment with PZA significantly diminished the NaCl-induced increment in urate excretion. Those experiments precluded any type of pharmacologic interaction and further strengthened the argument that a portion of the secreted urate in man is reabsorbed before it gains access to the urine. This concept is illustrated diagrammatically in Figure 4.

Other indirect evidence favoring the existence of significant reabsorption of secreted urate in normal man involves studies employing PZA administration in hypouricemic persons with renal "urate wastage" (i.e., elevated urate-to-GFR clearance ratios). These have included patients with Wilson's disease (WILSON et al., 1973), Hodgkin's disease (BENNET et al., 1972), and sickle cell anemia (DIAMOND et al., 1975). In all these instances, PZA administration decreased urate excretion to extremely low levels, and the decrement in urate excretion produced after PZA was

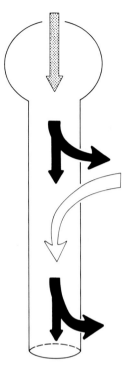

Fig. 4. Schematic representation of urate transport within human nephrons. Following filtration at the glomerulus (top), a portion of the filtered urate is reabsorbed. The remainder traverses the nephron, joined by an additional amount contributed by tubular secretion *(unshaded arrow)*. Finally, a portion of the intraluminal urate is again reabsorbed prior to its gaining access to the urine. Note that both presecretory and postsecretory reabsorption of urate occur according to this model (see text). Although evidence exists for each reabsorptive modality as well as for urate secretion, the relative magnitudes of each are not presently known. For example, the amount of filtered urate remaining unreabsorbed prior to secretion cannot be determined by available techniques. Adapted from STEELE, 1973

greater than that which would be expected in normals. Although this could be interpreted as suggesting increased tubular secretion of urate in these patients, an alternative explanation is that they may have manifested defective reabsorption of secreted urate. The latter explanation is in accord with multiple deficiencies of renal tubule function found in some of these individuals.

II. Plasma Urate and GFR

Experiments employing urate infusions have indicated that both the clearance and excretion of urate increase rapidly as the plasma urate concentration is elevated (YÜ et al., 1962; BERLINER et al., 1950; LATHEM and RODNAN, 1962). Other studies employing either short- or long-term loading with urate precursors in order to enhance urate synthesis have also demonstrated that urate excretion increases with the plasma urate (NUGENT and TYLER, 1959; NUGENT et al., 1964; STEELE and

RIESELBACH, 1967a; GUTMAN et al., 1969). Conversely, allopurinol has been employed to decrease the rate of urate synthesis. In doing so, it depressed the urate clearance and excretion together with the plasma urate (STEELE and RIESELBACH, 1967a; GUTMAN et al., 1969). On the other hand, the data indicate that at normal endogenous urate levels plasma urate concentrations in normals do not correlate significantly with urate excretion (STEELE and RIESELBACH, 1967a; GUTMAN et al., 1969). In view of the changes accompanying urate infusion, RNA or allopurinol noted above, this observation seems surprising. Perhaps, over the relatively narrow range of normal endogenous plasma urate concentrations, the failure of plasma urate to correlate with urate excretion may reflect variations in renal function among individuals.

The plasma urate concentration directly affects the amount of urate filtered by renal glomeruli. However, there is little evidence to suggest that the amount of filtered urate per se affects the urinary uric acid excretion in any significant or predictable manner. Studies by JENKINS and RIESELBACH (1974) have suggested that the capacity for the reabsorption of filtered urate by the human kidney is extremely great. They administered PZA concomitantly with RNA to normal individuals. Although th plasma urate increased to more than twice the normal values after several days, the urinary uric acid excretion did not change significantly. In fact, at any plasma urate concentration or filtered urate load that can be attained physiologically, the capacity for reabsorption of filtered urate may remain nearly complete. Studies in dogs, employing experimentally compromised renal blood flow, have also suggested that urate excretion does not decrease in proportion to the GFR (BERGER et al., 1964). On the other hand, the postglomerular renal blood flow and delivery of urate to tubule secretory sites could affect the magnitude of urate secretion. Indeed, the available evidence suggests that changes in the renal plasma flow influence urate excretion more importantly than do minor alterations in GFR.

III. Urate Binding by Plasma Proteins

The subject of urate binding by plasma proteins has remained controversial for many years (YÜ and GUTMAN, 1953; CAMPION et al., 1975). The significance of any putative urate binding could be several-fold. Firstly, bound urate might be unavailable for glomerular filtration. However, evidence that the filtered urate is not an important determinant of urate excretion has been summarized in the previous section. Secondly, the extent of the inhibition of urate binding or *displacement* of urate from plasma proteins by certain pharmacologic agents has been a good indicator or predictor of the potential efficacy of these compounds as uricosuric agents (BLUESTONE et al., 1969; BLUESTONE et al., 1970; WHITEHOUSE et al., 1971; SCHLOSSTEIN et al., 1973). Indeed, one report indicated that such displacement might enhance urate removal during hemodialysis (POSTLETHWAITE et al., 1974). Interactions between urate and albumin or alpha-globulins have been postulated to be of importance in the pathogenesis of gout (ALVSAKER, 1965; ALVSACKER and SEEGMILLER, 1972). Finally, tightly bound urate might be unavailable for renal tubular secretion.

Much evidence for urate binding has come from equilibrium dialysis experiments conducted at 4° C (KLINENBERG and KIPPEN, 1970). Using that methodology, plasma is dialyzed against a bath containing a high concentration of urate. After prolonged dialysis, the binding of urate to plasma proteins is computed from the urate concentration difference between that in the dialysis bag and the bath outside. In equilibrium dialysis apparatus (KLINENBERG and KIPPEN, 1970) or conventional ultrafiltration systems (SHEIKH and MØLLER, 1968), urate binding to plasma or serum proteins declines as the temperature is increased. In fact, in the hands of several investigators, urate binding to serum proteins has been negligible at physiologic temperatures using either type of apparatus or continuous ultrafiltration techniques (KOVARSKY et al., 1976).

Studies of FARRELL et al. (1971a) indicated that the use of lithium urate, when added to plasma, artifactually increases apparent binding of urate. In addition, in other extensive studies by FARRELL et al. (1971b, 1976) and FARRELL (1974) using an elaborate ultrafiltration system, only negligible binding of urate to plasma proteins could be demonstrated under physiologic conditions of temperature and medium composition.

In contrast, CAMPION et al. (1973) reported that solutions of urate and defatted human serum albumin stabilized with phosphate buffer showed substantial binding of urate to albumin at 37° C. Those studies were performed in an ultrafiltration cell that included a magnetic stirrer on the high-pressure side of a synthetic polymer membrane (CAMPION and OLSEN, 1974). The results indicated that considerably more than 10% of the urate in solution could bind to albumin at physiologic temperatures. However, the binding energy of urate to albumin was weak. Subsequent studies using a similar apparatus demonstrated binding of urate to protein in plasma samples (CAMPION et al., 1975), displacement of urate from binding sites by uricosuric drugs (WHITEHOUSE et al., 1973; CAMPION et al., 1974), and diminished binding in renal insufficiency (RESS et al., 1975). Thus, studies on urate binding have yielded markedly different results, depending on the techniques employed.

We have reinvestigated the problem of urate ultrafilterability, using an apparatus similar to that employed by CAMPION et al. (1973), in which a magnetic stirrer continually mixes the protein-containing solution (STEELE, 1976). Plasma or serum samples were gassed with 5% carbon dioxide for pH adjustment. Ultrafiltration was then accomplished through Amicon PM-10 membranes (Amicon Corp., Hartwell, MA, USA) by applying 5% carbon dioxide to the ultrafiltration cell. Equivalent results were obtained using serum or heparinized plasma at ultrafiltration pressures ranging from 100 to 1000 torr. Neither the ultrafiltration cells nor the magnetic stirring bars bound measurable amounts of urate. Increasing the ultrafiltration temperature from 24° C to 37° C increased ultrafilterable urate from 78% to 87% in eight specimens ($p < 0.001$).

Using plasma from normal volunteers, paired simultaneous studies were done in stirred and unstirred ultrafiltration cells under identical ultrafiltration pressures. In almost all instances, the apparent ultrafilterability of plasma urate was substantially greater in the unstirred filtration cells than in their paired stirred cells (STEELE, 1976). Only about 20% of the original plasma sample was filtered, corresponding to the filtration fraction of the normal human kidney. In cells without rotating magnetic stirrers, the concentration of urate in ultrafiltrate averaged 92% of the total plasma urate concentrations at 25° C in 15 specimens. When ultrafiltration of the same samples was accomplished in stirred cells, the ultrafiltrate urate concentrations averaged 74% of the total plasma concentrations. This difference in ultrafilterability was manifest in most samples and was highly significant on paired testing ($p < 0.001$).

Because the buildup of a protein layer on the retentate side of the membrane in unstirred cells might have affected binding, other experiments were done using sodium urate in solutions containing defatted human serum albumin (STROMBERG and STEELE, unpublished observations). The albumin concentration was varied systematically 2–10 g/dl. Urate binding to albumin was very modest (less than 10%) under these conditions. Surprisingly, the modest degree of urate binding varied *inversely* with the albumin concentration ($r = -0.86$, $p < 0.001$). In 17 other studies, ultrafilterable urate was measured on plasma specimens before and after extensive ultrafiltration. Initially, with the plasma albumin averaging 5 g/dl ultrafilterable urate averaged 80% of the total urate concentrations when stirred (unstirred values averaged 85%; $p < 0.02$). After extensive sample ultrafiltration, plasma albumin averaged 10 g/dl; at that time, the concentration of urate in the ultrafiltrates had increased to 88% of the total plasma urate, a highly significant increase ($p < 0.001$). In other studies, urate ultrafilterability was not found to be pH-dependent. Furthermore, ultrafiltration at the isoelectric pH of albumin did not alter the disparity in urate filterability between stirred and unstirred samples.

These results indicate that the matter of urate ultrafilterability is complex and point out the hazards encountered in using measurements of urate binding in vitro as estimates of the amount of urate prohibited in vivo from traversing the walls of glomerular capillaries. Conceivably, the results can be explained using a model of ultrafiltration similar to that proposed by TEREPKA et al. (1970). Although urate concentrations in glomerular ultrafiltrate cannot be measured in man, ROCH-RAMEL et al. (1976) have published data from the Munich-Wistar rat indicating that the concentration of urate in filtrate from surface glomeruli in that species is essentially equal to that in plasma.

IV. Extracellular Fluid Volume and the Renal Circulation

Urate excretion increases during rapid expansion of the extracellular fluid volume by hypertonic sodium chloride infusion (CANNON et al., 1970; MANUEL and STEELE, 1974; DIAMOND and MEISEL, 1975). Much of the increment in urate excretion produced by hypertonic sodium chloride infusion can be suppressed by pretreatment with PZA (MANUEL and STEELE, 1974). That the uricosuric response to sodium chloride occurs within the PZA-suppressible component of the urinary urate suggests that volume expansion results in the diminished reabsorption of secreted urate. In addition, because sodium chloride infusion still elicits some uricosuric response in PZA-treated subjects (STEELE, 1969), volume expansion probably also inhibits the reabsorption of *filtered* urate (although not necessarily at a different site within the nephron). This interpretation depends upon the degree of completeness and specificity with which PZO at low concentrations blocks the tubular secretion of urate. Irrespectively, urate reabsorption is diminished following vigorous expansion of the extracellular fluid volume, as is true for many other solutes.

Conversely, extracellular volume *depletion* with i.v. furosemide or ethacrynic acid rapidly results in a diminished urate excretion and clearance (STEELE and OPPENHEIMER, 1969), as illustrated in Figure 5. In subjects pretreated with PZA, rapid extracellular volume depletion with i.v. ethacrynic acid also results in diminished urate excretion and clearance (STEELE, 1969). Thus, volume depletion may enhance the

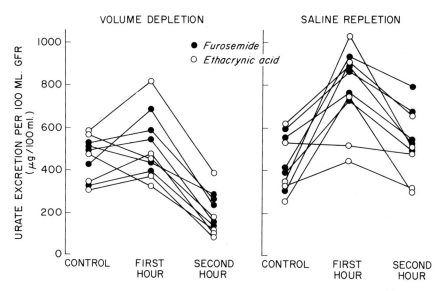

Fig. 5. The action of furosemide *(solid circles)* or ethacrynic acid *(open circles)* injection upon urate excretion. Each normal person received 50 mg ethacrynic acid or 40 mg furosemide as a single i.v. dose. In most cases, both caused an immediate uricosuric response. In those receiving continuous replacement of salt and water losses with i.v. saline, *(right)* no net change in urate excretion ultimately occurred. In contrast, the lack of salt and water replacement *(left)* uniformly decreased urate excretion within 2 h. These findings suggest that diuretic-induced urate retention results from salt depletion occurring as a result of the diuretic action. Data are those of Steele and Oppenheimer (1969)

fractional reabsorption of filtered urate. However, the major portion of the decrement in urate excretion produced by "loop-active" diuretic agents resides within the PZA-suppressible component of urate excretion. This is compatible with the interpretation that diuretic administration could inhibit urate secretion or, alternatively, could result in the enhanced reabsorption of secreted urate. Pharmacologically inhibited secretion of urate by ethacrynic acid or furosemide seems unlikely, however, because the replacement of urinary salt and water losses by i.v. saline after the administration of these diuretics prevents any decrease in urate excretion or clearance (Steele and Oppenheimer, 1969). Similar observations have been made in man during chronic studies by Suki et al. (1967) and Hull et al. (1967), using a thiazide diuretic. In their studies, diuretic administration was accompanied by a decrease in the urate clearance and an increase in the plasma urate as the subjects lost weight. When urinary electrolyte losses were replaced, however, the urate clearance remained unchanged. In summary, these and other acute and chronic observations suggest that extracellular volume contraction following diuretic administration is responsible for urate retention (Steele, 1977).

The means by which extracellular volume expansion and contraction affect renal urate transport is not understood. Indeed, urate excretion is often not rigidly correlated with sodium excretion. For example, the infusion of isotonic sodium chloride in normal persons may result in the increased excretion of sodium as well as several

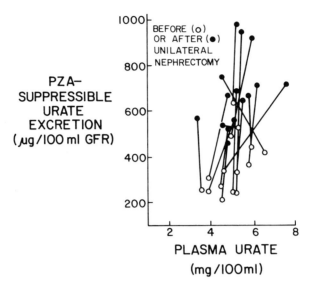

Fig. 6. PZA-suppressible urate excretion in patients before and after unilateral nephrectomy for transplant donation purposes. A brisk increase in PZA-suppressible urate excretion occurred, rapidly following contralateral nephrectomy, before compensatory renal hypertrophy occurred. Similar changes in total urate excretion following nephrectomy occurred. Note that for very little change in the plasma urate concentration PZA-suppressible urate excretion almost doubled. These data suggest that hemodynamic influences are important in the regulation of either urate secretion or postsecretory reabsorption. Data are from SHELP and RIESELBACH (1968)

other solutes but with no significant change in urate excretion (STEELE, 1974). A likely possibility is that volume expansion and contraction could affect the renal circulation and indirectly influence urate transport. Speculatively, altered renal blood flow or a redistribution of renal blood flow might affect urate secretion by changing the amount delivered to tubule secretory sites.

Diazoxide, a nondiuretic thiazide derivative is used for its antihypertensive effect and regularly promotes sodium and urate retention in clinical settings. However, when given at a very low dosage by JOHNSON (1971), diazoxide did not affect the arterial pressure and produced no changes in GFR or renal plasma flow. Yet, there was a decrease in sodium excretion, and this was accompanied by a diminished urate excretion. That the enhanced sodium reabsorption did not result from a direct stimulatory pharmacologic effect of diazoxide upon ion transport is suggested from other observations by FINE and WEBER (1975), indicating that the intrarenal infusion of diazoxide produces a natriuresis rather than sodium retention in the rat. Thus, the sodium retention accompanying low-dose diazoxide in man probably resulted from changes in intrarenal hemodynamics, possibly occurring secondary to systemic vasodilatation, and might account for the changes in urate excretion.

Conversely, renal hyperemia might result in an increased urate clearance, possibly secondary to the delivery of more urate to tubule secretory sites. Under those circumstances, one would expect an increase in the PZA-suppressible component of the urinary urate. In fact, the latter was observed in hyperuricosuric patients with 'sickle-cell disease who also manifested an increase in effective renal plasma flow (DIAMOND et al., 1975). Additionally, the extremely brisk increase in urate excretion per nephron following contralateral nephrectomy bears no relationship to kidney size and could be mediated through intrarenal circulatory adjustments. Studies of SHELP and RIESELBACH (1968) indicated that the uricosuric response to removal of the contralateral kidney occurs almost exclusively as a result of an increase in the PZA-suppressible urate excretion (Fig.6). Nevertheless, the mechanisms through which changes in the renal circulation and extracellular volume affect urate transport remain poorly characterized.

V. Urine Flow

BRØCHNER-MORTENSON (1937) originally demonstrated a flow-dependent increase in urate excretion at very low rates of urine flow, but not after flow exceeded 2 ml/min. Thus, in normal man, a transition from hydropenia to water diuresis is accompanied by a significant increase in both urate excretion and clearance. More recently, DIAMOND et al. (1972) have suggested that urate excretion may be flow-related over a wide range of urine flow rates. In their studies, hydropenic subjects were hydrated to various degrees and the urate clearance then measured. The results indicated that urate elimination increased progressively, even after urine flow exceeded 5 ml/min.

Since changes in urine flow relate per se primarily to differences in water reabsorption by collecting tubules and ducts, the degree of change in solute excretion related purely to flow is determined by the degree of passive back-diffusion of the solute in terminal nephron segments (WALSER, 1966). Experiments by OELERT et al. (1969) originally suggested that the distal nephron of the rat is relatively impermeable to urate, and other studies employing animals with lithium-induced diabetes insipidus provided no evidence for flow-dependence of urate excretion in the rat (STEELE et al., 1974). Indeed, vasopressin facilitates the movement of urate across anuran membranes (LEVINE et al., 1976), and recent clearance studies by MEISEL and DIAMOND (1976) have demonstrated that vasopressin administration in man produces a slight decrease in urate excretion.

Because the studies of DIAMOND et al. (1972) had involved different degrees of hydration of subjects from an initially hydropenic state, the observed changes in urate excretion with flow could have represented urate transport alterations reflecting the correction of overnight extracellular volume depletion. In order to examine this question further, ENGLE and STEELE (1976) conducted studies in normal volunteers, sufficiently hydrated to produce a urine flow averaging 14 ml/min. Following the establishment of control conditions during water diuresis, a single injection of only 4 or 8 milliunits of vasopressin was administered. Urine flow declined to 8.6 ml/min and then returned toward control values. Very slight changes in urate excretion and clearance occurred in parallel with the changes in flow. Those data suggest that urine flow per se is not an important determinant of urate excretion in man, tending to confirm the work in the rat of OELERT et al. (1969). Instead, changes in the extracellular volume probably constitute a far more important influence. For example, a decrease in urine flow and urate excretion may both occur as a consequence of extracellular fluid volume contraction.

VI. Urine pH

The degree of pH-dependence for the excretion of a weak acid depends upon greater permeability and hence greater back-diffusion of its lesser charged (usually nonionized) moiety. Somewhat analogous to flow-dependence, however, pH-dependence of solute excretion can occur only to the extent that tubule epithelium is permeable to the substance. Because the first ionization constant of uric acid is approximately 5.5 in urine, pH-dependence of urate excretion could occur if tubule epithelium were significantly more permeable to uric acid than to monovalent urate. As indicated above, however, studies on the effect of flow on urate excretion have suggested that the permeability of terminal nephron segments to both uric acid and urate is relatively limited.

Consistent with the above, the available data suggest that the influence of urine pH upon urate excretion is exceedingly modest. Early studies by GUTMAN et al. (1956) indicated that alkalinization of the urine did not increase total uric acid excretion appreciably, and a recent reexamination of the problem has confirmed these results (STEELE et al., 1975). Although the urate clearance does increase very modestly during urinary alkalinization, the change in urate excretion is quantitatively insignificant. This is in accord with the observation that the uricosuric response to acetazolamide, a diuretic which produces a bicarbonate-rich alkaline urine, is exceedingly modest (AYVAZIAN and AYVAZIAN, 1961; STEELE et al., 1975).

VII. Angiotensin and Other Vasoactive Substances

Although FERRIS and GORDEN (1968) demonstrated that the infusion of angiotensin II at pressor dosages results in a rapid decrease in the excretion and clearance of urate, any physiologic role of the renin-angiotensin system in the maintenance of urate homeostasis is still far from certain. For example, in untreated hypertensives, there is apparently no correlation between the plasma urate concentration and renin activity (BRUNNER et al., 1972). On the other hand, a direct relationship of these two parameters apparently develops following treatment of the hypertension with diuretics (AMES, 1974). Perhaps it is not surprising, however, that diuretic-induced volume contraction could simultaneously activate the renin-angiotensin system and induce renal urate retention.

Another item of at least associative interest is the characterization of Bartter's syndrome as a hyperuricemic disorder (MODLINGER et al., 1973; MEYER et al., 1975). This normotensive hyper-reninemic condition can be treated successfully with pharmacologic inhibitors of prostaglandin synthetase (VERBERCKMOES et al., 1976; GILL et al., 1976; FICHMAN et al., 1976). It is not yet reported if indomethacin-induced normalization of plasma renin in this syndrome is associated with amelioration of hyperuricemia. The data in Bartter's Syndrome are of interest, however, in that they raise the possibility that the renin-angiotensin system and renal prostaglandin synthesis may play a significant role in the renal regulation of urate homeostasis.

VIII. Relation of Urate Transport to Other Organic Compounds

Certain endogenously produced weak acids, such as lactate (YÜ et al., 1957b), beta-hydroxybutyrate, and acetoacetate (GOLDFINGER et al., 1965), acutely decrease the excretion and clearance of urate, probably by inhibiting urate secretion. In fact, lactate has been implicated by SCHIRMEISTER et al. (1969) in the pathogenesis of furosemide-induced hyperuricemia. Presently, it is unclear whether or not these substances compete with urate for tubular secretion. Their antiuricosuric actions may be sufficient to result in hyperuricemia in certain disease states, as will be discussed in another chapter. However, the degree to which lactate, beta-hydroxy-butyrate, and acetoacetate may modulate urate excretion in health is unknown at present, even though the latter substances probably cause urate retention during brief fasting (FOX et al., 1976). Conversely, uricosuric substances have been isolated from the serum of patients with renal insufficiency by BOUMENDIL-PODEVIN et al. (1975). Two of these substances are indoxyl sulfate and hippurate.

Many pharmacologic agents compete with urate both for tubular secretion and reabsorption (GUTMAN, 1966; STEELE and RIESELBACH, 1976). Such agents include salicylate (YÜ and GUTMAN, 1959), sulfinpyrazone (YÜ et al., 1963), and a host of other agents. They often exert so-called "paradoxical" actions upon urate transport. At low plasma concentrations, they predominantly inhibit the tubular secretion of urate, whereas at higher plasma levels they inhibit both urate secretion and reabsorption. Based upon studies using isolated tubules from snake (DANTZLER, 1973) and rabbit (CHONKO et al., 1976) kidneys, it seems likely that competition for tubular secretion must occur at a binding site located at the contraluminal cell surface. In contrast, because of extensive protein binding and a consequent lack of filterability, many uricosuric agents can gain access to tubule fluid only through tubular secretion (WEINER, 1967). Once in tubule fluid, it is likely that they may inhibit urate reabsorption by binding at luminal transport carrier sites, as suggested by extensive studies with probenecid (WEINER et al., 1960).

In several nonhuman species, substituted hippurates such as para-amminohip-purate (PAH) appear to compete with urate for tubule transport sites. In the chimpanzee (FANELLI et al., 1971) and man (BONER and STEELE, 1973), however, there is evidence that the secretion of PAH and of uric acid may involve separate transport systems. The relationship between substrate specificities of these putatively different transport systems is complex; different types of interactions may occur, depending on the species.

IX. Possibility of Intrarenal Urate Synthesis

Limited data have indicated that the human kidney contains the enzymes necessary for the synthesis of uric acid, at least from nucleotide degradation (WATTS et al., 1965). If quantitatively significant intrarenal urate synthesis occurred, then considerations of urate transport would become exceedingly complex, because renally derived urate might simulate either secretion or reabsorption, depending upon its exit from the luminal or contraluminal side of the tubule cell. Definite intrarenal urate synthesis appears to occur in the chicken (QUEBBEMANN, 1973; ZMUDA and QUEBBE-MANN, 1975) and has also been reported in the isolated perfused dog kidney (QUEB-BEMANN et al., 1975). In the latter, however, the quantitative contribution of intrarenal synthesis to the total urinary urate content is difficult to ascertain. In addition, urate synthesis has been reported in isolated perfused rat kidney preparations (QUEBBEMANN, 1973; COULSON, 1976), although experience in our laboratory with

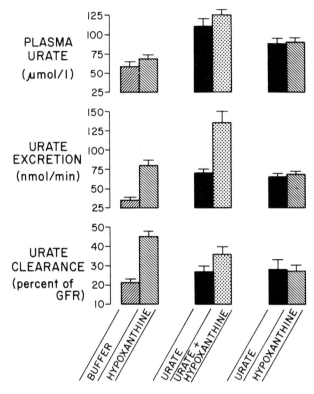

Fig. 7. Urate excretion during hypoxanthine infusion in the rat. Systemic hypoxanthine infusion increased the plasma urate and the excretion and clearance of urate *(left)*. Urate infusion throughout, combined with hypoxanthine, had the same effect *(center)*. However, when the hypoxanthine was *preceded* by urate infusion in order to maintain a constant plasma urate *(right)*, hypoxanthine had no effect on urate elimination. Data are means and S.E.M., taken from STEELE and UNDERWOOD (1977)

such a preparation has as yet failed to demonstrate chemically measurable urate senthesis in preparations perfused with nucleotide-free solutions and possessing optimal GFR and sodium reabsorption (UNDERWOOD and STEELE, unpublished observations). Also, pharmacologic data in the chimpanzee (WEINER and FANELLI, 1975) and intact rat (STEELE and UNDERWOOD, 1977) have failed to provide evidence for significant intrarenal urate synthesis (Figs. 7 and 8). Based upon the divergent findings in these studies with animal kidneys, the possibility and significance of intrarenal urate synthesis in man is entirely questionable at present.

If intrarenal urate synthesis occurred, however, the results could have broad significance. For example, the addition of cyclic nucleotides in large amounts to the perfusate utilized in an isolated rat kidney preparation results in the conversion of a large portion of the nucleotide to uric acid, most of which is released into the renal venous effluent (COULSON, 1976). If a portion of renally synthesized cAMP were converted to uric acid, this would provide a link between the action of many hormones and uric acid metabolism. It might, for example, explain the hyperuricemia

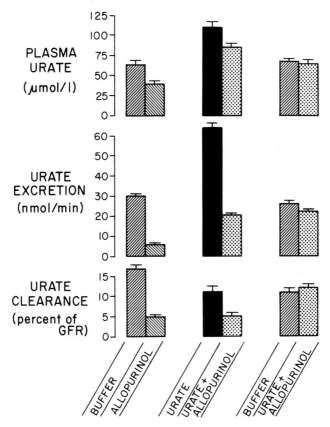

Fig. 8. Urate excretion during allopurinol infusion in the rat. Allopurinol, administered systemically, decreased the plasma urate, and the excretion and clearance of urate *(left)*. Urate infusion throughout, combined with allopurinol, had the same effect *(center)*. However, when a decrease in plasma urate was prevented by infusing urate with the allopurinol *(right)*, there was no change in urate elimination. Data from this and the preceding figure suggest that decreasing urate synthesis (with allopurinol) or increasing it (with hypoxanthine) has no measurable effect on urate excretion. The implication is that intrarenally synthesized urate has little effect on renal urate elimination in the rat under normal circumstances. Data are from STEELE and UNDERWOOD (1977)

sometimes associated with hyperparathyroidism (AURBACH et al., 1973). In clearance studies, parathyroid hormone injection failed to elicit a uniform uricosuric response but did result in large increases in urate excretion in several subjects (SHELP et al., 1969). At our present state of knowledge, however, any physiologic relationship between cAMP metabolism and uric acid excretion is speculative.

X. Red Cell Uptake and Renomedullary Accumulation

GREGER et al. (1974) have recently reported significant transport of urate into rat and human red blood cells, which is accelerated when the suspending medium is acid and reverses at alkaline pH. They hypothesized that accelerated urate uptake by red cells in an environment with lowered pH may play an important role in facilitating urate reabsorption within the renal medulla of the rat, presumably by the loop of Henle (GREGER et al., 1974). In man, however, "loop-active" diuretic agents that eliminate renomedullary hypertonicity and urinary concentrating ability do not exhibit substantial or protracted uricosuric actions (STEELE and OPPENHEIMER 1969). LANG et al. (1975) have reported that the red cell uptake of urate is diminished in gouty patients. Although red cell urate transport has been known for many years (LASSEN, 1961), it has not been studied extensively in health or disease. Therefore, it is presently difficult to evaluate the significance of red cell urate transport as it might relate to renal urate reabsorption or to urate homeostasis in general.

Postmortem studies have indicated that urate is sequestered within the human renal medulla (CANNON et al., 1968). Since evaluated medullary urate concentrations were present after death, it is likely that it had precipitated, probably as monosodium urate. A tendency toward monosodium urate precipitation in the hyperosmotic renal medulla can be explained on the basis of a diminished solubility of urate in the presence of increased medullary concentrations of the sodium ion (WILCOX et al., 1972). Thus, the ion activity product of monosodium urate could exceed its solubility or formation product in that region (KLINENBERG et al., 1973). As already indicated, it is not clear whether medullary urate sequestration affects urate reabsorption appreciably. However, it does seem likely that intramedullary monosodium urate precipitation could constitute an early step in the pathogenesis of urate-induced abnormalities of renal function (VERGER et al., 1967; ÖSTBERG, 1968).

D. Urate Excretion in Gout

I. Classification of Gout

The role of the kidney in the pathogenesis of gout has been a subject of considerable controversy for many years. Many observers since the time of GARROD (1850) have commented upon an apparent sluggishness of urate excretion in the gouty, as compared to normals. However, in many gouty patients with a normal GFR, the urinary urate excretion lies within the normal range (GUTMAN, 1973). On the other hand, because of concomitant hyperuricemia, it might seem more appropriate if the kidneys were to excrete *supranormal* amounts of urate until the plasma urate concentration decreased to normal.

NUGENT and TYLER (1959) produced hyperuricemia in normals by oral loading with urate and purine precursors. In their results, exogenously hyperuricemic normals had greater absolute urate excretion rates and fractional urate clearances than did a group of gouty patients at similar degrees of hyperuricemia. Because those studies could have been criticized on the basis of the short duration of hyperuricemia, NUGENT et al. (1964) subsequently performed other studies in which prolonged yeast RNA loading was used. Again, the results indicated that urate excretion and fractional clearance values tended to be greater in normals than in gouty patients at similar plasma urate values. LATHEM and RODNAN (1962) employed lithium urate infusions to study urate excretion at a variety of plasma urate concentrations and filtered urate loads. In their studies, conducted over a wide range of plasma and filtered urate values, the fractional urate clearances were substantially less in gouty

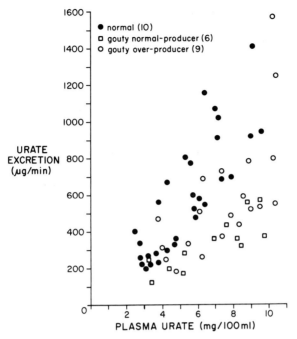

Fig. 9. Urate excretion, plotted as a function of plasma urate concentration in normal persons *(solid circles)*, gouty normal-producers of uric acid *(squares)*, and gouty over-producers of uric acid *(open circles)*. Each normal was studied at his own endogenous plasma urate concentration, following a decrease in plasma urate with allopurinol and after an increase in plasma urate secondary to RNA ingestion. The gouty patients were studied both at their normal (hyperuricemic) plasma urate concentrations and after allopurinol administration in order to normalize these values. Note that at any plasma urate level urate excretion was especially sluggish in some gouty normal-producers. Data from the normals taken from STEELE and RIESELBACH (1967a). Data from the gouty patients taken from RIESELBACH et al. (1970)

patients than in normals. As a group, all these studies suggested that an increase in the excretion and clearance of urate is the appropriate renal response to hyperuricemia in normal persons, and that this response is blunted in some gouty individuals.

Using the results from uric acid pool and turnover studies, SEEGMILLER et al. (1962) pioneered in the development of a physiologic classification of gout. Those investigators were able to classify gouty patients in three groups—those with normal urate production, moderate urate overproduction, and excessive urate overproduction. In five gouty patients who had normal urate production values, there was a diminished fractional urate clearance. On the other hand, the patients with excessive overproduction exhibited mixed renal responses, in that fractional urate clearance values ranging from normal to subnormal were encountered. However, differences in plasma urate concentrations between different groups of patients made interpretation of the data difficult.

Using the approach of SEEGMILLER and associates, RIESELBACH et al. (1970) classified a group of gouty patients with normal GFR values as "normal-producers" or "over-producers" of uric acid. Each patient was studied at his own endogenously

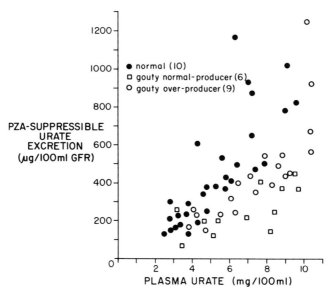

Fig. 10. The pyrazinamide-suppressible component of urate excretion, plotted as a function of the plasma urate concentration, in the same persons as in the previous figure. Note that there is very little change in the relationships between the three groups. Although there was a tendency for diminished PZA-suppressible urate excretion to occur in the gouty normal-producers, broad overlap occurred. The PZA-suppressible component of urate excretion is an index of the amount of secreted urate minus its postsecretory reabsorption. This parameter probably is the most sensitive one reflecting the role of the kidney in the pathogenesis of gout. Data of STEELE and RIESELBACH (1967a) and RIESELBACH et al. (1970)

elevated plasma urate concentration, as well as while normouricemic following allo-purinol administration (Fig. 9). The results were compared with values obtained in a group of normal persons, each of whom had been studied at three plasma urate concentrations, using allopurinol or RNA loading to produce diminished or increased plasma urate values, respectively (STEELE and RIESELBACH, 1967a). Regression analyses of urate excretion per unit GFR, the PZA-suppressible component of urate excretion, or fractional urate clearance as functions of the plasma urate indicated that these parameters describing urate elimination were significantly greater in gouty over-producers than in normal-producers of uric acid. Although there was a considerable degree of overlap of values in normal and gouty persons, the PZA-suppressible component of urate excretion during hyperuricemia was significantly diminished in the normal-producer gouty group (Fig. 10). These results indicated that differences in urate elimination between gouty over-producers and normal-producers of uric acid resided within the PZA-suppressible component of the urinary urate, suggesting that either urate secretion itself could have been impaired or that the reabsorption of secreted urate could have been accelerated. The results also suggested that renal urate handling in most of the over-producers studied was normal (Fig. 11). Parenthetically, a defect in the tubular secretion of urate appears to be responsible for urate retention in a strain of gouty chickens (AUSTIC and COLE, 1972; AUSTIC and COLE, 1976; ZMUDA and QUEBBEMANN, 1975).

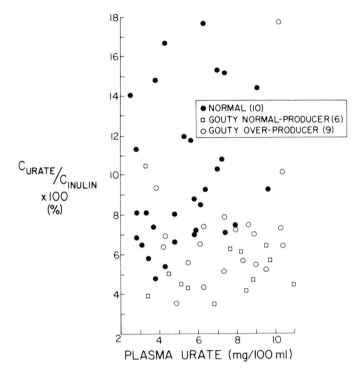

Fig. 11. Fractional urate clearance (C_{urate}/C_{inulin}) as a function of the plasma urate in the same persons as Figures 9 and 10. Note that similar relationships exist but are somewhat exaggerated with the use of the clearance parameter. Sources same as Figures 9 and 10

GUTMAN et al. (1969) also studied urate transport in gouty patents using PZA and compared the results with values in normals—but did not group their patients according to urate production. Although a general correlation between urate clearance or excretion and the plasma urate seems evident on visual inspection of their data, the correlation between these two parameters was lost when data points having plasma urate concentrations greater than 9 mg/dl were omitted from calculation. GUTMAN et al. (1969) concluded that no abnormality of urate transport could be documented in their gouty patients, although some of the urate clearance values encountered were very low. One explanation for the discrepancy is that their population may have been a heterogeneous one with respect to endogenous urate production and renal urate handling.

II. Chronic Renal Disease with Gout

In most nongouty patients with chronic renal insufficiency, urate excretion per unit GFR tends to increase progressively with advancing severity of disease (BRØCHNER-MORTENSEN, 1938; STEELE and RIESELBACH, 1967b). This increase in urate excretion per nephron results from increases in both the PZA-suppressible and nonsuppressi-

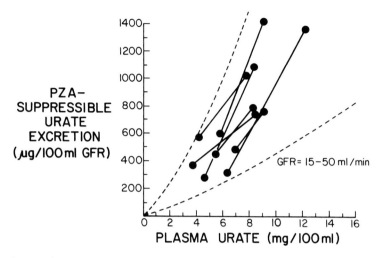

Fig. 12. The pyrazinamide-suppressible component of urate excretion, plotted as a function of the plasma urate concentration, in gouty patients with renal insufficiency. The data are those of RIESELBACH et al. (1967). All the gouty patients had normal urate turnover (production) rates. Each patient was studied at his own endogenous plasma urate level and following allopurinol administration, in order to decrease the plasma urate. The dotted lines outline the 95% tolerance limits of PZA-suppressible urate excretion in normal persons (STEELE and RIESELBACH, 1967a). In these gouty patients with GFR values between 15 and 50 ml/min, PZA-suppressible urate excretion always lay within normal limits. These data suggest that hyperuricemia and gout in many patients with chronic renal insufficiency may occur primarily as a result of a diminished nephron population and not secondary to a maladaptation of nephron function

ble components of the urinary urate in moderate renal insufficiency. In far-advanced disease, the PZA-suppressible component of the urinary urate usually declines, and the nonsuppressible component increases (STEELE and RIESELBACH, 1967b). These observations are compatible with the hypothesis that in far-advanced disease, tubular secretion of urate per nephron fails and the fraction of filtered urate reabsorbed also declines. However, in patients with lead nephropathy (EMMERSON et al., 1971) and in certain other individuals with far-advanced chronic renal disease (DANOVITCH, 1972; DANOVITCH et al., 1972), the PZA-suppressible component of the urinary urate excretion per nephron can increase to supranormal values. Abnormalities of urate transport in various disease states will be considered in greater detail in a separate chapter of this volume.

In seven patients with gout who also suffered moderate chronic insufficiency, RIESELBACH et al. (1967) found that urate production was normal. Both the total urate excretion per unit GFR and the PZA-suppressible component were normal or increased (Fig. 12). Furthermore, the regression values for PZA-suppressible urate excretion per unit GFR, as a function of plasma urate, were significantly greater in this group than in the normal-producer gouty patients without renal insufficiency. These results, taken together, indicate that urate excretion per nephron can proceed at a rate commensurate with the plasma urate value (i.e., similar to exogenously hyperuricemic normals) in many gouty individuals with renal insufficiency. Presumably, hyperuricemia and gout occur in patients with a greatly diminished GFR primarily because of the greatly diminished number of functioning nephrons, in most instances.

On the other hand, the role of hyperuricemia or hyperuricosuria (per nephron) in initiating and exacerbating progressive chronic renal disease currently is controversial (SEEGMILLER and FRAZIER, 1966; EMMERSON and ROW, 1975). Indeed, urate deposits have been described within the kidneys of nongouty patients succumbing to chronic renal insufficiency (VERGER et al., 1967; ÖSTBERG, 1968). In contrast, evidence already discussed suggests that renal involvement in gout worsens extremely slowly compared to most other nephropathies (BERGER and YÜ, 1975).

E. Conclusion

In man, renal urate transport processes are complex and still remain poorly understood. However, the available evidence indicates that bidirectional tubule transport processes for urate are greater in magnitude than conventional clearance computations would suggest, and that the urinary urate is the resultant of opposing reabsorptive and secretory transport movements. Substantial pharmacologic evidence, albeit indirect, suggests that urate secretion is normally vital for the maintenance of a normal rate of urate excretion and for avoiding hyperuricemia.

Numerous factors affect renal urate transport. These include changes in the extracellular fluid or plasma volume and resultant changes in the renal circulation, as well as numerous endogenous substances and exogenous pharmacologic agents. Many drugs affecting urate transport appear primarily to inhibit urate secretion at a low dosage but inhibit both reabsorption and secretion at a higher dosage—probably because of the necessity for their transport into the renal tubule lumen before they can bind to reabsorptive transport sites. In the transition from hydropenia to a water diuresis, an increase in urate excretion accompanies the increase in urine flow; urate excretion, however, does not increase substantially with further increases in flow. Likewise, urate excretion is largely independent of the urine pH. Finally, the effects of urate uptake by red blood cells and of a putative component of intrarenal urate synthesis upon renal urate transport in man are entirely speculative at present.

In persons with hyperuricemia and gout, renal urate transport may appear normal. This has been the case in most patients with endogenous urate overproduction thus far studied. In gouty persons with normal urate turnover rates, however, urate excretion often seems inappropriately sluggish for the elevated plasma urate concentrations. Although available evidence suggests that this may be due to a defect in urate secretion, the data can be explained equally well by an accelerated rate of reabsorption of secreted urate. Finally, in many gouty patients with moderate renal insufficiency, the rate of urate elimination per nephron appears normal or supranormal. In these patients, hyperuricemia probably occurs as the result of a diminished number of functioning nephrons.

Acknowledgments. The ultrafiltration experiments were done by Barbara A. Stromberg, supported in part by a grant from The Kroc Foundation.

References

Alvsaker, J. O.: Uric acid in human plasma. III. Investigations on the interaction between the urate ion and human albumin. Scand. J. clin. Lab. Invest. **17**, 467—475 (1965)

Alvsaker, J. O., Seegmiller, J. E.: Plasma concentrations of the urate-binding alpha-1-2-globulin in patients with different types of primary gout as compared to control subjects. Europ. J. clin. Invest. **2**, 66—71 (1972)

Ames, R. P.: Relation of serum uric acid to plasma renin activity and the response of primary hypertension to treatment. Amer. Soc. Nephrol. Abstr. **7**, 2 (1974)

Aurbach, G. D., Mallette, L. E., Patten, B. M., Heath, D. A., Dappman, J. L., Bilezikian, J. P.: Hyperparathyroidism: recent studies. Ann. intern. Med. **79**, 566—575 (1973)

Austic, R. E., Cole, R. K.: Impaired renal clearance of uric acid in chickens having hyperuricemia and articular gout. Amer. J. Physiol. **223**, 525—530 (1972)

Austic, R. E., Cole, R. K.: Hereditary variation in uric acid transport by anion kidney slices. Amer. J. Physiol. **231**, 1147—1151 (1976)

Ayvazian, J. H., Ayvazian, L. F.: A study of the hyperuricemia induced by hydrochlorothiazide and acetazolamide separately and in combination. J. clin. Invest. **40**, 1961—1966 (1961)

Bennet, J. S., Bond, J., Singer, I., Gottlieb, A.: Hypouricemia in Hodgkin's disease. Ann. intern. Med. **76**, 751—756 (1972)

Berger, L., Yü, T.-F.: Renal function in gout. IV. An analysis of 524 gouty subjects including long-term follow-up studies. Amer. J. Med. **59**, 605—613 (1975)

Berger, L., Yü, T.-F., Kupfer, S., Gutman, A. B.: Effect of reducing renal arterial blood pressure by balloon catheter on urate excretion in the dog. Proc. Soc. exp. Biol. (N.Y.) **115**, 58—61 (1964)

Berglund, H., Frisk, A. R.: Uric acid elimination in man. Acta med. scand. **86**, 128—135 (1935)

Berliner, R. W., Hilton, J. G., Yü, T.-F., Kennedy, Jr., T. J.: The renal mechanism for urate excretion in man. J. clin. Invest. **29**, 396—401 (1950)

Bluestone, R., Kippen, I., Klinenberg, J. R.: Effect of drugs on urate binding to plasma proteins. Brit. med. J. **4**, 590—593 (1969)

Bluestone, R., Kippen, I., Klinenberg, J. R., Whitehouse, M. W.: Effect of some uricosuric and anti-inflammatory drugs on the binding of uric acid to human serum albumin in vitro. J. Lab. clin. Med. **76**, 85—91 (1970)

Boner, G., Steele, T. H.: Relationship of urate and PAH secretion in man. Amer. J. Physiol. **225**, 100—104 (1973)

Boumendil-Podevin, E. F., Podevin, R. A., Richet, G.: Uricosuric agents in uremic sera. Identification of indoxyl sulfate and hippuric acid. J. clin. Invest. **55**, 1142—1152 (1975)

Brøchner-Mortensen, K.: Uric acid in blood and urine. Acta med. scand. [Suppl.] **84**, 1—269 (1937)

Brøchner-Mortensen, K.: Uric acid in blood and urine in Brights' disease. Acta med. scand. **96**, 438—461 (1938)

Brunner, H. R., Laragh, J. H., Baer, L., Newton, M. A., Goodwin, F. T., Krakoff, L. R., Bard, R. H., Buhler, F. R.: Essential hypertension: Renin and aldosterone, heart attack and stroke. New Engl. J. Med. **286**, 441—449 (1972)

Campion, D. S., Bluestone, R., Klinenberg, J. R.: Uric acid: characterization of its interaction with human serum albumin. J. clin. Invest. **52**, 2383—2387 (1973)

Campion, D. S., Bluestone, R., Klinenberg, J. R.: Displacement by uricosuric agents of sodium urate bound to human serum albumin. Biochem. Pharmacol. **23**, 1653—1657 (1974)

Campion, D. S., Olsen, R.: Measurement of drug displacement by continuous ultrafiltration. J. Pharm. Sci. **63**, 249—252 (1974)

Campion, D. S., Olsen, R., Bluestone, R., Klinenberg, J. R.: Binding of urate by serum proteins. Arthr. and Rheum. **18**, (Suppl.) 747—749 (1975)

Cannon, P. J., Svahn, D. S., Martini, F. E., de: The influence of hypertonic saline infusion upon the fractional reabsorption of urate and other ions in normal and hypertensive man. Circulation **41**, 97—108 (1970)

Cannon, P. J., Symchych, P. S., Martini, F. E., de: The distribution of urate in human and primate kidney. Proc. Soc. exp. Biol. (N.Y.) **129**, 278—280 (1968)

Chonko, A. M., Dellasega, M., Varney, D., Grantham, J. J.: Mechanism of uric acid secretion by proximal straight tubules of the rabbit nephron. Clin. Res. **24**, 553 A (1976)

Coulson, R.: Metabolism and excretion of exogenous adenosine 3′:5′-monophosphate and guanosine 3′:5′-monophosphate. Studies in the isolated perfused rat kidney and in the intact rat. J. biol. Chem. **251**, 4958—4967 (1976)

Cullen, J. H., Levine, M., Fiore, J. M.: Studies of hyperuricemia produced by pyrazinamide. Amer. J. Med. **23**, 587—595 (1957)

Danovitch, G. M.: Uric acid transport in renal failure. A review. Nephron **9**, 291—299 (1972)

Danovitch, G. M., Weinberger, J., Berlyne, G. M.: Uric acid in advanced renal failure. Clin. Sci. **43**, 331—341 (1972)

Dantzler, W. H.: Characteristics of urate transport by isolated perfused snake proximal renal tubules. Amer. J. Physiol. **224**, 445—453 (1973)

Diamond, H. S., Lazarus, R., Kaplan, D., Halberstam, D.: Effect of urine flow rate on uric acid excretion in man. Arthr. and Rheum. **15**, 338—346 (1972)

Diamond, H., Meisel, A.: Influence of volume expansion, serum sodium, and fractional excretion of sodium on urate excretion. Pflügers Arch. **356**, 47—57 (1975)

Diamond, H. S., Meisel, A., Sharon, E., Holden, D., Cacatian, A.: Hyperuricosuria and increased tubular secretion of urate in sickle cell anemia. Amer. J. Med. **59**, 796—802 (1975)

Diamond, H. S., Paolino, J. S.: Evidence for a post-secretory reabsorptive site for uric acid in man. J. clin. Invest. **52**, 1491—1499 (1973)

Emmerson, B. T., Mirosch, W., Douglas, J. B.: The relative contributions of tubular reabsorption and secretion to urate excretion in lead nephropathy. Aust. N.Z. J. Med. **4**, 353—362 (1971)

Emmerson, B. T., Row, P. G.: An evaluation of the pathogenesis of the gouty kidney. Kidney Int. **8**, 65—71 (1975)

Engle, J. E., Steele, T. H.: Variation of urate excretion with urine flow in normal man. Nephron **16**, 50—56 (1976)

Fanelli, Jr., G. M., Hitzenberger, G.: Uricosuric activity of intravenous mersalyl in man. Medikon Int. **30**, 2—4 (1974)

Fanelli, Jr., G. M., Weiner, I. M.: Species variations among primates in responses to drugs which alter the renal excretion of uric acid. J. Pharm. exp. Ther. **193**, 363—375 (1975)

Fanelli, Jr., G. M., Weiner, I. M.: Pyrazinoate excretion in the chimpanzee. Relation to urate disposition and the actions of uricosuric drugs. J. clin. Invest. **52**, 1946—1957 (1973)

Fanelli, Jr., G. M., Bohn, D., Reilly, S. S.: Renal urate transport in the chimpanzee. Amer. J. Physiol. **220**, 613—620 (1971)

Fanelli, Jr., G. M., Bohn, D. L., Reilly, S. S., Weiner, I. M.: Effects of mercurial diuretics on renal transport of urate in the chimpanzee. Amer. J. Physiol. **224**, 985—992 (1973)

Farrell, P. C.: Protein binding of urate ions in vitro and in vivo. In: Edwards, K. D. G. (Ed.): Drugs and the Kidney. Progr. Biochem. Pharmacology, Vol. 9, pp. 153—162. Basel: Karger 1974

Farrell, P. C., Popovich, R. P., Babb, A. L.: Binding levels of urate ions in human serum albumin and plasma. Biochim. biophys. Acta (Amst.) **243**, 49—52 (1971 a)

Farrell, P. C., Popovich, R. P., Babb, A. L.: In vitro dynamic dialysis technique to determine solute-protein binding interactions. J. Pharmac. Sci. **60**, 1471—1475 (1971 b)

Farrell, P. C., Ward, R. A., Hone, P. W., Mahoney, J. F., Stewart, J. H.: Urate ion binding levels in normal and uremic plasma. In: Silbernagl, S., Lang, F., Greger, R. (Eds.): Amino Acid Transport and Uric Acid Transport, pp. 146—152. Stuttgart: Georg Thieme 1976

Ferris, T. F., Gorden, P.: Effect of angiotensin and norepinephrine upon urate clearance in man. Amer. J. Med. **44**, 359—365 (1968)

Fine, L. G., Weber, H.: Effect of diazoxide on renal handling of sodium in the rat. Clin. Sci. molec. Med. **49**, 277—282 (1975)

Fichman, M. P., Telfer, N., Zia, P., Speckart, P., Golub, M., Rude, R.: Role of prostaglandins in the pathogenesis of Bartter's Syndrome. Amer. J. Med. **60**, 785—797 (1976)

Fox, I. H., Halperin, M. L., Goldstein, M. B., Marliss, E. B.: Renal excretion of uric acid during prolonged fasting. Metabolism **25**, 551—559 (1976)

Garrod, A. B.: Observations on certain pathological conditions of the blood and urine in gout, rheumatism and Bright's disease. Trans. Med. Chir. Soc. Edinburgh **31**, 83—97 (1848)

Gill,Jr.,J.R., Frolich,J.C., Bowden,R.E., Taylor,A.A., Keiser,H.R., Seyberth,H.W., Oates,J.A., Bartter,F.C.: Bartter's Syndrome: A disorder characterized by high urinary prostaglandins and a dependence of hyperreninemia on prostaglandin synthesis. Amer. J. Med. **61**, 43—51 (1976)

Goldfinger,S., Klinenberg,J.R., Seegmiller,J.E.: Renal retention of uric acid induced by infusion of beta-hydroxybutyrate and acetoacetate. New Engl. J. Med. **272**, 351—353 (1965)

Greger,R., Lang,F., Puls,F., Deetjen,P.: Urate interaction with plasma proteins and erythrocytes. Possible mechanism for urate reabsorption in kidney medulla. Pflügers Arch. **352**, 121—133 (1974)

Gutman,A.B.: Significance of the renal clearance of uric acid in normal and gouty man. Amer. J. Med. **37**, 833—838 (1964)

Gutman,A.B.: Uricosuric drugs with special reference to probenecid and sulfinpyrazone. Advanc. Pharmacol. Chemother. **4**, 91—142 (1966)

Gutman,A.B.: The past four decades of progress in the knowledge of gout, with an assessment of the present status. Arthr. and Rheum. **16**, 431—445 (1973)

Gutman,A.B., Yü,T.-F.: Renal function in gout. With a commentary on the renal regulation of urate excretion, and the role of the kidney in the pathogenesis of gout. Amer. J. Med. **23**, 600—622 (1957)

Gutman,A.B., Yü,T.-F.: A three-component system for regulation of renal excretion of uric acid in man. Trans. Ass. Amer. Phycns **74**, 353—365 (1961)

Gutman,A.B., Yü,T.-F., Berger,L.: Tubular secretion of urate in man. J. clin. Invest. **38**, 1778—1781 (1959)

Gutman,A.B., Yü,T.-F., Berger,L.: Renal function in gout. III. Estimation of tubular secretion and reabsorption of uric acid by use of pyrazinamide (pyrazinoic acid). Amer. J. Med. **47**, 575—592 (1969)

Gutman,A.B., Yü,T.-F., Sirota,J.H.: Contrasting effects of bicarbonate and Diamox, with equivalent alkalinization of the urine on salicylate uricosuria in man. (Abstract). Fed. Proc. **15**, 85 (1956)

Hull,A.R., Suki,W.N., Rector,F.C., Seldin,D.W.: Mechanism of diuretic-induced hyperuricemia. Amer. Soc. Nephrol. Abstr. **1**, 31 (1967)

Jenkins,P., Rieselbach,R.E.: Unique characteristics of the mechanism for reabsorption of filtered versus secreted urate. J. clin. Invest. **53**, 36a (Abstract) (1974)

Johnson,B.F.: Diazoxide and renal function in man. Clin. Pharmacol. Ther. **12**, 815—824 (1971)

Khachadurian,M.D., Arslanian,M.J.: Hypouricemia due to renal uricosuria. Ann. intern. Med. **78**, 547—550 (1973)

Klinenberg,J.R., Bluestone,R., Schlosstein,L., Waisman,J., Whitehouse,M.W.: Urate deposition disease—how is it regulated and how can it be modified. Ann. intern. Med. **78**, 99—111 (1973)

Klinenberg,J.R., Gonick,H.C., Dornfeld,L.: Renal function abnormalities in patients with asymptomatic hyperuricemia. Arthr. and Rheum. **18** (Suppl.), 725—730 (1975b)

Klinenberg,J.R., Kippen,I.: The binding of urate to plasma proteins determined by means of equilibrium dialysis. J. Lab. clin. Med. **75**, 503—510 (1970)

Klinenberg,J.R., Kippen,I., Bluestone,R.: Hyperuricemic nephropathy: Pathologic features and factors influencing urate deposition. Nephron **14**, 88—98 (1975a)

Kovarsky,J., Holmes,E.W., Kelley,W.N.: Absence of significant urate binding to human serum proteins. Clin. Res. **24**, 331A (1976)

Lang,F., Greger,R., Silbernagel,H., Günther,R., Deetjen,P.: Aufnahme von 2-Cl4 Harnsäure in die Erythrocyten von Patienten mit Hyperurikämie und Gicht. Klin. Wschr. **53**, 261—264 (1975)

Lassen,U.V.: Kinetics of uric acid transport in human erythrocytes. Biochim. biophys. Acta (Amst.) **53**, 557—569 (1961)

Lathem,W., Rodnan,G.P.: Impairment of uric acid excretion in gout. J. clin. Invest. **41**, 1955—1963 (1962)

Lemieux,G., Vinay,P., Gougoux,A.: Nature of the uricosuric action of benziodarone. Amer. J. Physiol. **224**, 1440—1449 (1973)

Levine, S. D., Franki, N., Einhorn, R., Hays, R. M.: Vasopressin-stimulated movement of drugs and uric acid across the anuran urinary bladder. Kidney Int. **9**, 30—35 (1976)

Manuel, M. A., Steele, T. H.: Changes in renal urate handling after prolonged thiazide treatment. Amer. J. Med. **57**, 741—746 (1974 a)

Manuel, M. A., Steele, T. H.: Pyrazinamide suppression of the uricosuric response to sodium chloride infusion. J. Lab. clin. Med. **83**, 417—427 (1974 b)

Mayne, J. G.: Pathological study of the renal lesions found in 27 patients with gout. Ann. Rheum. Dis. **15**, 61—62 (1956)

Meisel, A., Diamond, H.: Effect of vasopression on uric acid excretion: Evidence for distal nephron reabsorption of urate in man. Clin. Sci. molec. Med. **51**, 33—40 (1976)

Meisel, A. D., Diamond, H. S.: Inhibition of probenecid uricosuria by pyrazinamide and para-aminohippurate. Amer. J. Physiol. **32**; F222—F226 (1977)

Meyer, W. J., III., Gill, Jr., J. R., Bartter, F. C.: Gout as a complication of Bartter's Syndrome. Ann. intern. Med. **83**, 56—59 (1975)

Modlinger, R. S., Nicolis, G. L., Krakoff, L. R., Gabrilove, J. L.: Some observations on the pathogenesis of Bartter's Syndrome. New Engl. J. Med. **289**, 1022—1024 (1973)

Mudge, G. O., Berndt, W. O., Valtin, H.: Tubular transport of urea, glucose, phosphate, uric acid, sulfate and thiosulfate. In: Orloff, J., Berliner, B. W. (Eds.): Handbook of Physiology, Vol. 8, pp. 587—652. Renal Physiology. Washington: Am. Physiol. Soc. 1973

Nugent, C. A., MacDiarmid, W. D., Tyler, F. H.: Renal excretion of urate in patients with gout. Arch. intern. Med. **113**, 115—121 (1964)

Nugent, C. A., Tyler, F. H.: The renal excretion of uric acid in patients with gout and in non-gouty subjects. J. clin. Invest. **38**, 1890—1898 (1959)

Oelert, H., Baumann, K., Gekle, D.: Permeabilitätsmessungen einiger schwacher organischer Säuren aus dem distalen Konvolut der Rattenniere. Pflügers Arch. **307**, 178—189 (1969)

Östberg, Y.: Renal urate deposits in chronic renal insufficiency. Acta med. scand. **183**, 197—201 (1968)

Podevin, R., Ardaillou, R., Paillard, F., Fontanelle, J., Richet, G.: Etude chez l'homme de la cinétique d'apparition dans l'urine de l'acide urique-2-¹⁴C. Nephron **5**, 134—140 (1968 a)

Podevin, R., Paillard, F., Hornych, A., Ardaillou, R., Fontanelle, J., Richet, G.: Cinétique d'apparition dans l'urine de l'acide para-aminohippurique (P.A.H.) et de l'acide urique-2-¹⁴C chez l'homme. Rev. franc. Etud. clin. Biol. **13**, 513—522 (1968 b)

Postlethwaite, A. E., Gutman, R. A., Kelley, W. N.: Salicylate mediated increase in uric acid removal during hemodialysis: evidence for urate binding to protein in vivo. Metabolism **23**, 771—777 (1974)

Praetorius, E., Kirk, J. E.: Hypouricemia: with evidence for tubular elimination of uric acid. J. Lab. clin. Med. **35**, 856—868 (1950)

Prasad, D. R., Weiner, I. M., Steele, T. H.: Diuretic-induced uricosuria: Interaction with pyrazinoate transport in man. J. Pharm. exp. Ther. **200**, 58—64 (1977)

Quebbemann, A. J.: Renal synthesis of uric acid. Amer. J. Physiol. **224**, 1398—1402 (1973)

Quebbemann, A. J., Cumming, J. D., Shideman, J. R., Toledo-Pereyra, L.: Synthesis of uric acid in isolated normothermic perfused mongrel and Dalmation dog kidneys. Amer. J. Physiol. **228**, 959—963 (1975)

Reese, Jr., O. G., Steele, T. H.: Renal transport of urate during diuretic-induced hypouricemia. Amer. J. Med. **60**, 973—979 (1976)

Ress, R. M., Campion, D. S., Bluestone, R., Llach, F., Olsen, R. W., Klinenberg, J. R.: Binding of urate to plasma proteins in normal subjects and patients with renal insufficiency. Clin. Res. **23**, 122 A (1975)

Rieselbach, R. E., Sorensen, L. B., Shelp, W. D., Steele, T. H.: Tubular secretion of urate per unit GFR in gout. J. clin. Invest. **47**, 1108 (1967)

Rieselbach, R. E., Sorensen, L. B., Shelp, W. D., Steele, T. H.: Diminished renal urate secretion per nephron as a basis for primary gout. Ann. intern. Med. **73**, 359—366 (1970)

Rieselbach, R. E., Steele, T. H.: Influence of the kidney upon urate homeostasis in health and disease. Amer. J. Med. **56**, 665—675 (1974)

Rieselbach, R. E., Steele, T. H.: Intrinsic renal disease leading to abnormal renal urate excretion. Nephron **14**, 81—87 (1975)

Roch-Ramel, F., Diezi-Chomety, F., Rougemont, D., de, Tellier, M., Widmer, J., Peters, G.: Renal excretion of uric acid in the rat: a micropuncture and microperfusion study. Amer. J. Physiol. **230**, 768—776 (1976)

Schirmeister, J., Man, N. K., Hallauer, W.: Study on renal and extrarenal factors involved in the hyperuricemia induced by furosemide. In: Peters, G., Roch-Ramel, F. (Eds.): Progr. Nephrol, pp. 59—63. Berlin-Heidelberg-New York: Springer 1969

Schlosstein, L. H., Kippen, I., Whitehouse, M. W., Bluestone, R., Paulus, H. E., Klinenberg, J. R.: Studies with some novel uricosuric agents and their metabolites: correlation between clinical activity and drug-induced displacement of urate from its albumin-binding sites. J. Lab. clin. Med. **82**, 412—418 (1973)

Seegmiller, J. E., Frazier, P. D.: Biochemical considerations of the renal damage of gout. Ann. Rheum. Dis. **25**, 668—672 (1966)

Seegmiller, J. E., Grayzel, A. I., Howell, R. R., Plato, C.: The renal excretion of uric acid in gout. J. clin. Invest. **41**, 1094—1098 (1962)

Shapiro, M., Hyde, L.: Hyperuricemia due to pyrazinamide. Amer. J. Med. **23**, 596—599 (1957)

Sheikh, M. I., Møller, J. V.: Binding of urate to proteins of human and rabbit plasma. Biochim. biophys. Acta (Amst.) **158**, 456—458 (1968)

Shelp, W. D., Rieselbach, R. E.: Increased bidirectional urate transport per nephron following unilateral nephrectomy. Amer. Soc. Nephrol. Abstr. **2**, 24 (1968)

Shelp, W. D., Steele, T. H., Rieselbach, R. E.: Comparison of urinary phosphate, urate and magnesium excretion following parathyroid hormone administration to normal man. Metabolism **18**, 63—70 (1969)

Simkin, P. A., Skeith, M. D., Healey, L. A.: Suppression of uric acid secretion in a patient with renal hypouricemia. Israel J. med. Sci. **9**, 1113 (1973)

Sorensen, L. B.: The elimination of uric acid in man studied by means of C^{14}-labelled uric acid. Uricolysis. Scand. J. clin. Lab. Invest. **12** (Suppl. 54), 1—214 (1960)

Sorensen, L. B.: Role of the intestinal tract in the elimination of uric acid. Proc. Conf. Gout and Purine Metabolism. New York: Grune and Stratton 1965

Sorensen, L. B., Kappas, A.: The effects of penicillamine therapy on uric acid metabolism in Wilson's disease. Trans. Ass. Amer. Phycns **39**, 157—162 (1966)

Sorensen, L. B., Levinson, D. J.: Origin and extrarenal elimination of uric acid in man. Nephron **14**, 7—20 (1975)

Steele, T. H.: Evidence for altered renal urate reabsorption during changes in volume of the extracellular fluid. J. Lab. clin. Med. **74**, 288—299 (1969)

Steele, T. H.: Urate secretion in man—the pyrazinamide suppression test. Ann. intern. Med. **79**, 734—737 (1973)

Steele, T. H.: Studies on urate handling in man utilizing pyrazinamide. In: Wesson, L. G., Fanelli, G. M., Jr. (Eds.): Recent Advances in Renal Physiology and Pharmacology, pp. 361—373. Baltimore: University Park Press 1974

Steele, T. H.: Renal excretion of uric acid. Arthr. and Rheum. **18** (Suppl.), 793—804 (1975a)

Steele, T. H.: Notes on the use of pyrazinamide. Arthr. and Rheum. **18** (Suppl.), 817—821 (1975b)

Steele, T. H.: Pyrazinamide suppressibility of urate excretion in health and disease: relationship to urate filtration. In: Silbernagl, S., Lang, F., Greger, R. (Eds.): Amino Acid Transport and Uric Acid Transport, pp. 248—253. Stuttgart: Georg Thieme 1976

Steele, T. H.: Diuretic-induced hyperuricemia. In: Kelley, W. N. (Ed.): Clinics in Rheumatic Disease. London: Saunders **3**, 37—50 (1977)

Steele, T. H., Boner, G.: Origins of the uricosuric response. J. clin. Invest. **52**, 1368—1375 (1973)

Steele, T. H., Manuel, M. A., Boner, G.: Diuretics, urate excretion, and sodium reabsorption: effect of acetazolamide and urinary alkalinization. Nephron **14**, 48—61 (1975)

Steele, T. H., Oppenheimer, S.: Factors affecting urate excretion following diuretic administration in man. Amer. J. Med. **47**, 564—574 (1969)

Steele, T. H., Rieselbach, R. E.: The renal mechanism for urate homeostasis in normal man. Amer. J. Med. **43**, 868—875 (1967a)

Steele, T. H., Rieselbach, R. E.: The contribution of residual nephrons within the chronically diseased kidney to urate homeostasis in man. Amer. J. Med. **43**, 876—886 (1967b)

Steele, T. H., Rieselbach, R. E.: Renal urate excretion in normal man. Nephron **14**, 21—32 (1975)

Steele, T. H., Rieselbach, R. E.: Renal handling of urate and other organic anions. In: Brenner, B. M., Rector, F. C., Jr. (Eds.): The Kidney, Vol. I, Chap. 12, pp. 442—476. Philadelphia: B. Saunders Co. 1976

Steele, T. H., Underwood, J. L.: Renal urate transport during variations in urate synthesis in the rat. Pflügers Arch. **367**, 183—188 (1976)

Steele, T. H., Underwood, J. L., Dudgeon, K. L.: Urate excretion and urine flow in a lithium-induced diabetes insipidus rat model. Pflügers Arch. **346**, 205—213 (1974)

Suki, W. N., Hull, A. R., Rector, F. C., Seldin, D. W.: Mechanism of the effect of thiazide diuretics on calcium and uric acid. J. clin. Invest. **46**, 1121 (1967)

Talbott, J. H., Terplan, K. L.: The kidney in gout. Medicine **39**, 405—462 (1960)

Terepka, A. R., Chen, Jr., P. S., Toribara, T. Y.: Ultrafiltration: a conceptual model and a study of sodium, potassium, chloride, and water distribution in normal human sera. Physiol. Chem. Physics **2**, 59—78 (1970)

Verberckmoes, R., Damme, B., Van, Clement, J., Amery, A., Michielsen, P.: Bartter's syndrome with hyperplasia of renomedullary cells: successful treatment with indomethacin. Kidney Int. **9**, 302—307 (1976)

Verger, D., Leroux-Robert, C., Ganter, P., Richet, G.: Les toph'us goutteux de la médullaire rénale des urémiques chroniques. Nephron **4**, 356—370 (1967)

Walser, M.: Mathematical aspects of renal function. The dependence of solute reabsorption on water reabsorption and the mechanism of osmotic natriuresis. J. theor. Biol. **10**, 307—326 (1966)

Watts, R. W. E., Watts, J. E. M., Seegmiller, J. E.: Xanthine oxidase activity in human tissues and its inhibition by allopurinol (4-hydroxy-pyrazolo[3,4-d]pyrimidine). J. Lab. clin. Med. **66**, 688—697 (1965)

Weiner, I. M.: Mechanisms of drug absorption and excretion. The renal excretion of drugs and related compounds. Ann. Rev. Pharmacol. **7**, 39—56 (1967)

Weiner, I. M., Fanelli, Jr., G. M.: Renal urate excretion in animal models. Nephron **14**, 33—47 (1975)

Weiner, I. M., Tinker, J. P.: Pharmacology of pyrazinamide: metabolic and renal function studies related to the mechanism of drug-induced urate retention. J. Pharmacol. exp. Ther. **180**, 411—434 (1972)

Weiner, I. M., Washington, J. A., II., Mudge, G. H.: On the mechanism of action of probenecid on renal tubular secretion. Johns Hopkins med. J. **106**, 333—346 (1960)

Whitehouse, M. W., Kippen, I., Klinenberg, J. R.: Biochemical properties of anti-inflammatory drugs. XII. Inhibition of urate binding to human albumin by salicylate and phenylbutazone analogues and some novel anti-inflammatory drugs. Biochem. Pharmacol. **20**, 3309—3320 (1971)

Whitehouse, M. W., Kippen, I., Klinenberg, J. R., Schlosstein, L., Campion, D. S., Bluestone, R.: Increasing excretion of urate with displacing agents in man. Ann. N. Y. Acad. Sci. **226**, 309—318 (1973)

Wilcox, W. R., Khalaf, A., Weinberger, A., Kippen, I., Klinenberg, J. R.: Solubility of uric acid and monosodium urate. Med. Biol. Engl. **10**, 522—531 (1972)

Wilson, D. M., Goldstein, N. P.: Renal urate excretion in patients with Wilson's disease. Kidney Int. **4**, 331—336 (1973)

Yü, T.-F., Berger, L., Kupfer, S., Gutman, A. B.: Tubular secretion of urate in the dog. Amer. J. Physiol. **199**, 1199—1204 (1960)

Yü, T.-F., Berger, L., Gutman, A. B.: Suppression of tubular secretion of urate by pyrazinamide in the dog. Proc. Soc. exp. Biol. (N.Y.) **107**, 905—908 (1961)

Yü, T.-F., Berger, L., Gutman, A. B.: Renal function in gout. II. Effect of uric acid loading on renal excretion of uric acid. Amer. J. Med. **33**, 829—844 (1962)

Yü, T.-F., Berger, L., Stone, D. J., Wolf, J., Gutman, A. B.: Effect of pyrazinamide and pyrazinoic acid on urate clearance and other discrete renal functions. Proc. Soc. exp. Biol. (N.Y.) **96**, 264—267 (1957a)

Yü, T.-F., Dayton, P. G., Gutman, A. B.: Mutual suppression of the uricosuric effects of sulfinpyrazone and salicylate: a study in interactions between drugs. J. clin. Invest. **42**, 1330—1339 (1963)

Yü,T.-F., Gutman,A.B.: Ultrafilterability of plasma urate in man. Proc. Soc. exp. Biol. (N.Y.) **84**, 21—24 (1953)

Yü,T.-F., Gutman,A.B.: Paradoxical retention of uric acid by uricosuric agents in low dosage. Proc. Soc. exp. Biol. (N.Y.) **90**, 542—547 (1955)

Yü,T.-F., Gutman,A.B.: A study of the paradoxical effects of salicylate in low, intermediate and high dosage on the renal mechanism for excretion of urate in man. J. clin. Invest. **38**, 1298—1315 (1959)

Yü,T.-F., Sirota,J.H., Berger,L., Halpern,M., Gutman,A.B.: Effect of sodium lactate infusion on urate clearance in man. Proc. Soc. exp. Biol. (N.Y.) **96**, 809—813 (1957b)

Zmuda,M.J., Quebbemann,A.J.: Localization of renal tubular uric acid transport defect in gouty chickens. Amer. J. Physiol. **229**, 820—825 (1975)

Zöllner,N.: Influence of various purines on uric acid metabolism. Nutr. Diet. **19**, 34—43 (1973)

CHAPTER 11

Abnormal Urate Excretion Associated with Renal and Systemic Disorders, Drugs, and Toxins

B. T. EMMERSON

A. Introduction

Abnormalities of renal excretion of urate may result in either hyperuricemia or hypouricemia, or an increase or reduction in the elimination of uric acid by the renal tract. These four abnormalities may also be found in various combinations, the most common being hyperuricemia and reduced renal excretion of urate. However, abnormalities of plasma urate may occur without apparent abnormality of renal excretion, and abnormalities of excretion may be present with normal serum urate concentrations.

Ultimately, there are four principal factors that affect the amount of uric acid which is eliminated from the body by the kidney, viz: 1. dietary consumption of purines; 2. endogenous urate production; 3. extrarenal urate disposition; and 4. renal excretory mechanisms.

Uric acid appearing in the urine is a flexible parameter subject to many influences. Urate entering the kidney is subject to filtration, reabsorption, and secretion before it appears in the urine, and each of these processes is subject to separate controls and separate disturbances. Thus, the renal factors determining the ultimate concentration of urate in the urine are many and varied.

A reduction in renal blood flow causes a reduction in renal urate excretion. Such a reduction is also associated with a reduction in glomerular filtration rate, and, as the fall in urate excretion is roughly proportional to the degree of reduction in the glomerular filtration rate (BERGER et al., 1964), this may be the more important parameter. Because of the obvious difficulties, there has been very little study of the effect on urate excretion of redistribution of blood flow to different parts of the kidney. However, it has been established that the redistribution of renal blood flow to the inner cortical nephrons following administration of a renal vasodilator results in an alteration in sodium excretion that leads to a natriuresis (STEIN et al., 1971), and it is thought that the reduction in urate clearance by angiotensin and norepinephrine (FERRIS and GORDEN, 1968) may be due to the associated decrease in effective renal blood flow.

A reduction in the glomerular filtration rate GFR will also lead to a reduction in the renal excretion of urate. Such reductions may be due to renal disease (as will be discussed) or may be physiologic, related to the considerable fluctuations in GFR that occur from day to day over any 24-h period (DAVIES and SHOCK, 1950).

Renal excretion of urate also changes with variations in the urine flow rate. It has long been appreciated that the urate clearance falls when the urine flow rate is less than 1 ml/min (BRØCHNER-MORTENSEN, 1937) but is not greatly increased with moderate increases above this value. There is, however, considerable variation between individuals in the response of their urate clearance to a diuresis. While the augmentation of the urate clearance with a diuresis is almost always less than the augmentation of the urea clearance, there is usually a moderate increase in the urate clearance associated with an increase in urine flow rate (DIAMOND et al., 1972; EMMERSON et al., 1976b). Part of this effect may be due to redistribution of renal blood flow, resulting in an increase in medullary perfusion. Reduction in urine flow rate following the administration of vasopressin was found to cause a significant reduction in urate excretion; excretion also correlated with flow rate, and the effect could be distinguished from that of plasma volume expansion (MEISEL and DIAMOND, 1976). These findings are of particular significance in those who habitually pass relatively small volumes of urine, a not inconsiderable group in warm climates.

A variety of experiments both in man and animals (SUKI et al., 1967; STEELE, 1969; WEINMAN et al., 1975) have suggested that urate transport in the proximal tubule tends to parallel that of sodium. Thus, in states of plasma volume contraction, where proximal tubular reabsorption of sodium is considerable, there is a tendency toward elevation of the plasma urate concentration with reduction in renal excretion of urate. In states of plasma volume expansion, such as occur in saline loading and salt administration, there is reduced reabsorption of urate in the proximal tubule, with an increased renal elimination (CANNON et al., 1970). The effect does not appear to be a specific one and applies to many other components of the glomerular filtrate, such as phosphate (SUKI et al., 1969). Thus, the state of contraction and expansion of the plasma volume exerts an important influence on the ultimate excretion of uric acid in the urine.

B. Renal Response to Increased Urate Production

I. Over-Excretion with Over-Production of Urate

Urate excretion by the kidney normally increases when there is an increase in the urate load or an increase in the serum urate concentration. This was confirmed by the increase in tubular secretion of urate with an increase in the serum urate concentration (STEELE and RIESELBACH, 1967). Thus, a high urinary uric acid is an early manifestation of urate over-production, such as may occur in myeloproliferative disorders, lymphomas, chronic hemolysis (DIAMOND et al., 1975), or active psoriasis. It is a regular association of enzyme mutations leading to over-production of urate (such as HGPRT deficiency or mutations of PRPP synthetase).

Over-excretion of urate could be indicated by an increase in the urate clearance beyond the normal range. However, over-excretion due to over-production is most easily demonstrated by an increase in the 24-h renal excretion of urate on a purine free diet (SEEGMILLER et al., 1961). Thus, a mean 24-h urinary urate excretion exceeding 600 mg/24 h (3.6 mmol/24 h) is indicative of underlying over-production of urate. In the early stages of urate over-production and while renal excretion of urate can increase sufficiently to cope with the increased delivery of uric acid to the kidney, the serum urate may remain within the normal range. However, if renal disease develops due to uric acid nephropathy (as discussed subsequently) or to other causes, the capacity of the kidney to excrete urate will decline, resulting in an increase in the serum urate concentration. Such a sequence has been deduced from studies of congenital over-producers with HGPRT deficiency (EMMERSON et al., 1976a).

II. Over-Excretion of Uric Acid Due to Dietary Variables, Especially Purine Consumption

Dietary purines are degraded to uric acid and result in an increased renal elimination of uric acid. Hence, in attempting to assess the balance between urate production and excretion by measuring the 24-h renal excretion of urate, a patient must be on a purine-free diet for a sufficient period to eliminate the effects of dietary purines. This is between 3 and 5 days. Dietary purine consumption varies enormously and may contribute a surprisingly large amount to urate excretion. On average, elimination of purines from the diet will lead to a fall in the serum urate concentration of 1 mg/100 ml (0.06 mmol/liter). Dietary components can also modify the extent of purine synthesis, and an increase in the dietary intake of purine-free protein can effect an increase in the urinary excretion of urate (BOWERING et al., 1970). Perhaps this is a reflection of the increased urate excretion observed with glycine feeding (FRIEDMAN, 1947; YÜ et al., 1970).

The most common cause of hyperuricosuria in patients with renal calculi is the ingestion of an unusually high proportion of their calories as purine-containing foods (the "purine gluttons" of COE and KAVALACH, 1974), and this hyperuricosuria can be reduced by substituting foods of relatively low purine content. In this group of hyperuricosuric patients with renal calculi, these workers also found two other abnormalities, viz: 1) Up to 30% had evidence of overproduction of urate on a purine-free diet and 2) most tended to have a high urate clearance, i.e., they over-excreted urate at lower serum urate levels than normal subjects. The authors regarded this latter finding as a distinctive disturbance, although they were uncertain as to whether it was a primary phenomenon or the result of tubular adaptation to chronic purine loading.

III. Over-Production with Under-Excretion of Urate

A combination such as this can lead to extreme disorders of urate homeostasis. It is commonly seen clinically when any of the conditions listed as causing urate under-excretion are associated with an increase in urate production. Such a combination is regularly seen together in patients with Type I glycogen storage disease (glucose-6-phosphatase deficiency), a condition in which hyperuricemia is associated with elevated serum concentrations of lactate, triglycerides, and free fatty acids.

C. Renal Causes of Abnormal Urate Metabolism

I. Abnormal Renal Excretion of Urate not Associated with Chronic Disease

1. Genetic Tubular Dysfunction

a) Urate-Losing Disorders

In 1950, PRAETORIUS and KIRK reported a patient whose urate clearance exceeded the glomerular filtration rate (GFR). There was no evidence of other renal dysfunction, and they concluded that this patient demonstrated not only a defect in reabsorption of urate but clear evidence for tubular secretion of urate as well. The case was looked upon as a curiosity and a second case was not reported until 1973 (SIMKIN et al., 1974). This patient demonstrated a urate clearance which varied between 1.2 and 2.3 times the GFR. The absence of a response to uricosuric drugs led these authors to conclude that at least their patient lacked a normal capacity for urate reabsorption. An additional patient whose urate clearance was 48% higher than the creatinine clearance has also been reported (KHACHADURIAN and ARSLANI-AN, 1973). None of these patients showed evidence of phosphaturia, glycosuria, or amino aciduria, and all had very low serum urate concentration.

Other patients with less severe hypouricemia have been reported in whom the ratio of urate clearance to GFR was less than 1, being between 0.4 and 0.7 instead of the normal 0.1 (GREENE et al., 1972; SPERLING et al., 1974; AKAOKA et al., 1975). Some other family members were similarly affected and in two families, there was associated hypercalciuria.

b) Urate-Retaining Disorders

Hyperuricemia and gout due to an isolated renal tubular lesion, resulting in reduced renal excretion of urate, is a well-established entity (RIESELBACH et al., 1970). This will be considered in more detail during the consideration of gout of renal origin. It is a functional rather than a structural problem and is often inherited.

2. Reversible Tubular Dysfunction

a) Metabolites

The renal excretion of urate is influenced in a reversible fashion by the presence of a wide variety of metabolites, drugs, and toxins. The renal handling of urate is subject to modification by normal metabolites in all persons at some time or other. Some of these metabolites, such as lactate and ketone bodies, are readily identified and of major importance, but other as yet undefined metabolites may also play a role. The importance of the pattern of organic acid excretion on urate excretion has yet to be defined (KRAMER et al., 1972), and there is also evidence that branched-chain keto-acids reduce urate excretion (SHULMAN et al., 1970).

As far back as 1923, GIBSON and DOISY showed that the ingestion of sodium lactate by normal human subjects resulted in a marked decrease in the renal excretion of uric acid, associated with a slight elevation of the plasma urate concentration. This dramatic decline in urate clearance was later confirmed by YÜ et al. (1957), who also showed that lactate administration could neutralize drug-induced uricosuria. No other natural metabolite was known to act as intensively to reduce the renal excretion of urate, and lactate is probably still the most important metabolite to do so (BURCH and KURKE, 1968). Its importance will be emphasized on many occasions when considering systemic disorders associated with abnormal renal excretion of urate. A consideration of all the factors which may lead to an elevation of the plasma lactate concentration would be a major separate consideration, but in general these are due either to relative oxygen lack in tissues from any cause or to a wide variety of other factors, one of which may be drug therapy (COHEN and WOODS, 1976). Although the lactate concentration is usually measured in a sample from a peripheral vein, it is usually assumed that it is the concentration of lactate in renal arterial blood that is the factor which may modify the renal excretion of urate.

It has been known since early this century that fasting or starvation leads to hyperuricemia, which is due to renal under-excretion of urate. This was accompanied by ketonuria and a fall in the plasma bicarbonate concentration. The return to food, either carbohydrate or protein, was associated with a remission of the ketonuria, some correction of the acidosis, and a return of the serum urate towards normal levels. As the ketosis associated with a high-fat diet also promoted hyperuricemia, and the administration of sodium bicarbonate did not prevent the development of urate retention, ketone bodies were incriminated in this renal retention of urate. SCOTT et al. (1964) induced ketosis without acidosis by infusing sodium beta-hydroxybutyrate, and this was associated with a clear reduction in the renal excretion of urate, thereby establishing a direct effect of beta-hydroxybutyrate upon renal excretion of urate. This was confirmed by infusions of various ketone bodies (GOLDFINGER et al., 1965). Severe hyperuricemia, often with gouty arthritis, has been observed in patients undergoing prolonged starvation as treatment for severe obesity, but this hyperuricemia can be reversed or prevented by feeding relatively small amounts of calories (DRENICK et al., 1964). There is also some suggestion of an increase in uric acid production as well as decreased renal excretion of urate during total caloric deprivation (PABLICO et al., 1965).

FOX et al. (1976) confirmed the initial urate retention during prolonged fasting but noted that it tended to subside considerably with sustained ketonemia. They suggested a biphasic renal urate response to ketones, such as is seen with some drugs. Thus, lactate and β-hydroxybutyrate remain the most common and important metabolites to have a significant effect upon renal handling of urate.

The effect of two other metabolites, angiotensin and norepinephrine, upon the urate clearance has also been studied in man (FERRIS and GORDEN, 1968). Both result in a marked reduction in urate clearance that is not mediated by lactate or ketoacids. Their effect appears to be more related to an associated reduction in renal blood flow than to any associated fall in glomerular filtration rate (GFR). Of the two, angiotensin appears to be more potent.

Whereas acute and prolonged exercise results in increases in the serum urate due to a fall in the urate clearance to values as low as 20–30% of the pre-exercise values (NICHOLS et al., 1951), physical training tends to lower the serum urate concentration (BOSCO et al., 1970). The rise with acute exercise appears due in part to a reduction in the renal blood flow and in part to a more sustained elevation of the serum lactate concentration (NICHOLS et al., 1951). The tendency to a lower serum urate with prolonged exercise training has been attributed to the effect of an increasing plasma volume and an increasing renal excretion of urate (BOSCO et al., 1970). The reduced tendency to elevation of the plasma lactate and ketone-body concentrations with exercise in athletes in comparison with nonathletes may also be an important contributory factor (JOHNSON et al., 1969). The complexity of the multitude of factors affecting urate metabolism during physical training (e.g., muscle injury contributing to urate over-production, oliguria, impairment of GFR, and alteration in extracellular volume) are illustrated in a study of exercise in hot climates (KNOCHEL et al., 1974).

b) Drugs

Alterations to the renal excretion of urate are caused by a wide variety of drugs, all of which produce their effects by modification of the processes of reabsorption and secretion of urate by the renal tubules. Many drugs have a biphasic action so that at a particular blood concentration, their net effect may be quite the reverse of that seen at a different concentration. This can best be illustrated by aspirin which is uricosuric in high dosage but tends to retain urate in low dosage (YÜ and GUTMAN, 1959). In low dosage, urate-retaining effects predominate, and these must be due either to a reduction in the secretion of urate or an increase in reabsorption of urate. In high dosage, on the other hand, to this low dosage effect must be added an increase in renal elimination of urate due either to reduction in urate reabsorption or an increase in active tubular secretion. The variety of drugs which can alter urate handling by the kidneys will be considered subsequently (Section C).

c) Toxins

As much reabsorption of filtered urate occurs in the proximal renal tubule, it might be expected that lesions in this region, such as the Fanconi syndrome, might result in uricosuria and hypouricemia. Recent studies have confirmed this, along with glyco-suria, generalized aminoaciduria, phosphaturia, and vitamin D-resistant rickets (LEE et al., 1972). Although there are many etiologies for the Fanconi syndrome, the general pattern as far as urate excretion is concerned appears to be that of an increase in the fractional excretion of urate. However, even in the Fanconi syndrome sometimes seen in the acute nephropathy due to heavy metals, there are very few reports of an associated increase in renal excretion of urate. One such report in a patient with acute cadmium nephropathy (EMMERSON, 1967) was associated with hypouricemia and uricosuria, although the phosphate clearance in this case was reduced rather than increased. When the Fanconi syndrome is associated with renal failure, it is more difficult to demonstrate an effect on renal handling of urate because of the generalized tendency in this situation to an increased fractional excretion of a large number of different solutes. Little is published concerning the effect of an acute lead nephropathy on urate excretion, although personal experience suggests a reduction in urate clearance with hyperuricemia in such cases rather than the pattern of hypouricemia, which might have been expected.

On the other hand, hypouricemia is a very common feature of Wilson's disease (hepatolenticular degeneration) (BISHOP et al., 1954; WILSON and GOLDSTEIN, 1973), in which the renal lesion is attributed to the deposition of copper. The increase in renal excretion of urate and the increased clearance of urate in this condition is reversed when the excessive deposition of copper is corrected. Thus, there is good evidence that the Fanconi syndrome related to the deposition of copper within the kidney is associated with excessive renal excretion of urate.

II. Abnormal Renal Excretion of Urate Associated with Chronic Renal Disease

As the kidney is the major route of elimination of urate, it would be expected that renal dysfunction would have some consequential effect upon urate metabolism.

However, as primary disorders of urate metabolism are also known to have second-ary effects upon the kidney (see chapter by TALBOTT in this volume), it is essential for studies of the effect of renal disease upon urate metabolism to differentiate patients with both hyperuricemia and renal disease into two groups, viz: 1) those in whom the hyperuricemia or gout is the primary condition and the renal disease a secondary development, and 2) those in whom the renal disease is primary.

Acceptance into the second group would require evidence that the renal disease was present before the development of gout, as well as precise definition of the nature of the renal disease.

Whereas, in former times primary gout used to be a severe and progressive disease often complicated by renal insufficiency, the common clinical picture seen today presents gout more as an inconvenience and is complicated by renal insuffi-ciency in only a minority of cases. At the same time as this change in the clinical pattern of gout was occurring, primary renal disease was coming to be diagnosed clinically at an early rather than a late stage, and patients with chronic renal disease were living in reasonable health for periods of many years. Simultaneously, the mean serum urate concentration in healthy subjects in developed countries was tending to become higher. Thus, prolonged hyperuricemia secondary to intrinsic renal disease, sometimes complicated by gouty arthritis, is now seen frequently, although the precise frequency of development of gout will depend in part upon how intensively it is sought. Thus, the first consideration in this problem should concern the effect of primary renal disease upon the serum and urine urate concentrations.

Even in health, the urate clearance tends to parallel the creatinine clearance (RAMSAY et al., 1975). With the development of chronic renal disease, there is an initial rise in the plasma urate as part of the general nitrogen retention (CAMERON, 1973), and hyperuricemia is often seen early in chronic renal insufficiency (EMMER-SON, 1965). In such patients, a positive correlation between the serum urate and the serum creatinine concentrations has been shown (GRESHAM et al., 1971). However, although many patients with early chronic renal disease demonstrate hyperuricemia, other nonrenal factors that would independently promote hyperuricemia are also often found to coexist, so that it is often difficult to determine the precise contribu-tion that the renal disease is making to the hyperuricemia. MCPHAUL (1968) studied renal handling of urate in three groups, 1. normal subjects, 2. patients with renal disease but with a normal glomerular filtration rate, and 3. patients with renal dis-ease in whom the glomerular filtration rate was reduced. He showed that the devel-opment of kidney disease led to a rise in the serum urate concentration and that there was further rise as the glomerular filtration rate fell. In the presence of renal disease at a time when the glomerular filtration rate was normal, the urate clearance was reduced, and there was a further reduction with fall in the filtration rate. When the urate clearance was related to the inulin clearance, the urate/inulin clearance ratio initially fell with the development of renal disease (in the absence of impaired glomerular filtration rate) but subsequently increased significantly as functioning nephrons were lost. Thus, although hyperuricemia was observed early in the course of chronic renal disease, compensatory tubular function tends to minimize its rate of increase as renal disease progresses. With progressive renal disease, the rise in the serum urate concentration is always proportionately less than the rise in the blood urea or serum creatinine concentrations. Although the miscible pools increase in renal insufficiency, the relative increase in the urate pool is very much less than that of other retained nitrogenous substances (RICHET, 1968; CLARKSON, 1966).

Studies of renal excretion of urate with progressive renal insufficiency have uniformly shown that with a reduction in the glomerular filtration rate, there is a progressive increase in urate excretion per nephron (SARRE and MERTZ, 1965; STEELE and RIESELBACH, 1967). This was particularly striking when the inulin clearance had fallen to less than 15 ml/min, at which level the ratio of UV urate: GFR had increased five times, whereas the plasma urate concentrations had less than doubled. This was attributed to an increased fractional excretion of filtered urate by the tubules. Similar results were obtained by DANOVITCH et al. (1972) in the presence of advanced renal failure. Likewise, studies of renal function in transplant donors undergoing nephrectomy demonstrated that urate homeostasis could usually be maintained by a proportional increase in urate excretion per nephron (SHELP and RIESELBACH, 1968) and such an adaptation would act to minimize the elevation of the serum urate concentration with destruction of nephrons by persistent disease.

However, the fact that an increase in urate excretion per nephron is occurring should not cause one to overlook the fact that there is a reduction in the absolute excretion of uric acid in the urine per 24 h (EMMERSON and Row, 1975). Similar information can be deduced from the data of STEELE and RIESELBACH (1967), where a significant regression of the urinary excretion of urate on the inulin clearance may be demonstrated. Their data shows that at an inulin clearance of 100 ml/min, urinary excretion of urate amounts to about 600 µg/min, whereas it falls to about 300 µg/min at an inulin clearance of 10 ml/min. There is relatively little information concerning the effect of renal failure on nonrenal aspects of urate kinetics, although it is thought that there is a proportionate increase in urate excretion by extrarenal (chiefly alimentary) routes, and it is possible that urate production might be decreased (CLARKSON, 1966). In practice, most patients with stable chronic renal insufficiency are found to have serum urate concentrations which rarely exceed 0.6 mmol/liter (10 mg/100 ml), unless there is evidence of additional complicating factors promoting hyperuricemia, such as an acute deterioration of renal function, plasma volume contraction, severe hypertension, diuretic therapy, or a high-purine diet.

The study of the changes in urate metabolism due to renal failure has been further complicated by the demonstration of microtophi in the renal medulla in a few patients dying with chronic uremia (VERGER et al., 1967; OSTBERG, 1968). Even though they have been reported so infrequently, their very existence causes concern that the hyperuricemia secondary to renal disease may lead to urate crystal deposition within the renal medulla with the formation of microtophi and a secondary aggravation of the renal disease. The potential importance of such a process is emphasized by the knowledge that a urate gradient exists between the renal cortex and the medulla, and that this gradient increases during antidiuresis, and the extent of the accumulation of urate in the medulla is in some way related to the serum urate concentration (EPSTEIN and PIGEON, 1964; CANNON et al., 1968). These considerations have led many physicians to consider that drug treatment of the hyperuricemia of chronic renal failure is justified. However, such a philosophy has not received support from those therapeutic trials that have been undertaken to date. An extensive study from Israel of hyperuricemic patients with mild-to-moderate degrees of renal insufficiency showed that prolonged therapy with allopurinol did not have any effect upon the rate of deterioration of renal function (ROSENFELD, 1974). However, the hyperuricemia in the group studied was not severe. Further support for the lack of nephrotoxicity from hyperuricemia in many patients has been presented by BERGER and YÜ (1975), whose detailed studies over a 12-year period did not demonstrate any deterioration of renal function in gouty patients with plasma urate concentrations persistently between 8 and 10 mg/100 ml (0.48–0.60 mmol/liter). It appears, therefore, that sustained concentrations of urate in serum of up to 10 mg/100 ml (0.6 mmol/liter) are not necessarily damaging to renal function. The risk of microtophus formation in the renal medulla is more likely to be determined predominantly by local factors, and the serum urate concentration is only one of many influences. It would seem that the prevention of medullary hypertonicity is probably one of the most important measures to prevent the formation of medullary microtophi, and such therapy is basic to the good management of most patients with chronic renal disease.

Several specific varieties of renal disease have been identified that appear to be associated with disproportionate hyperuricemia and an increased incidence of gout. The first of these is chronic lead nephropathy. This condition was originally documented in Queensland, Australia, following an extensive epidemic of lead poisoning in childhood that was followed some 10–30 years later by renal failure, from which patients died with granular-contracted kidneys. Half of the persons so affected developed gouty arthritis (EMMERSON, 1963). At all levels of renal function studied, the mean serum urate concentration in patients with chronic lead nephropathy was significantly higher than that for patients whose renal disease was not produced by lead. This disproportionate hyperuricemia was attributable to lower urate clearances in relation to corresponding creatinine clearances (EMMERSON, 1965). A similar finding of a high incidence of gout with disproportionate hyperuricemia and renal disease has also been reported from the southern states of the USA in subjects who have chronically ingested illicitly distilled "moonshine" contaminated with lead (MORGAN et al., 1966). Detailed studies of urate kinetics in such subjects, who showed signs of persisting lead intoxication, demonstrated renal under-excretion of urate as the cause of their hyperuricemia. Impaired renal function was identified as the cause of the hyperuricemia and gout in these subjects (BALL and SORENSEN, 1969). Similarly, patients with chronic industrial lead intoxication in Paris showed a selective impairment of urate excretion by the kidney, with a high incidence of gouty arthritis (RICHET et al., 1964). Thus, in chronic lead nephropathy of various origins, we have one particular variety of chronic renal disease in which a specific impairment of urate excretion has been demonstrated.

In studying 17 cases in which gout appeared during the course of, and therefore presumably secondary to, chronic renal failure, RICHET et al. (1965) found three cases of renal amyloidosis. They regarded the gout as being premature in its appearance and noted that it occurred in the absence of hypertension. NEWCOMBE (1973) found gout in over one-third of patients with polycystic disease of the kidney, an association which had been reported by MARTINEZ-MALDONADO in 1974 from Puerto Rico. This latter study, however, was confined to one family, whereas the study of NEWCOMBE (1973) included 11 families. Reports from GULATI et al. (1974) claim disproportionate hyperuricemia due to reduced urate clearance in patients with bilateral hydronephrosis. This suggested the possibility that disproportionate hyperuricemia

might be a function of those types of renal disease in which there was disproportionate damage to the renal tubules, such as occurs in polycystic disease of the kidney,
and that such a distal nephron type of renal disease tends to be associated with less
severe proteinuria, a sodium-losing tendency and less-severe hypertension. It is
therefore interesting to find a report of gout in 21% of patients with analgesic
nephropathy (NANRA, 1976). However, much further study will be needed to establish whether disproportionate hyperuricemia is a common feature of all renal disease, which predominantly affects the distal nephron.

It seems that gouty arthritis may well be a complication of much primary renal
disease when hyperuricemia is unusually severe or prolonged (SARRE and MERTZ,
1965). Personal experience suggests that this may be not unfrequent. The difficulty in
determining its true incidence lies in documenting the role and contribution of many
of the environmental factors that promote hyperuricemia. It is also difficult to define
when a serum urate concentration is elevated disproportionately to the renal disease.
Some progress has been made, however, and a table has been prepared which gives
the theoretical upper limit of average serum urate concentrations for hypertensive
patients according to sex, the plasma urea concentration, and whether or not the
patient is receiving a thiazide diuretic (BULPITT, 1975).

D. Drugs Affecting Urate Excretion

A wide variety of therapeutic agents can alter renal handling of urate, resulting either
in uricosuria and lowered serum urate or a reduced renal excretion of urate and
hyperuricemia. The main factor that determines the ultimate amount of urate in the
urine is the balance between tubular reabsorption and tubular secretion of urate.
Precise sites in the nephron, where these functions occur in man, have not been
localized, and, although much reabsorption of urate occurs in the proximal tubule,
evidence obtained from the effects of different drugs, both singly and in combination,
upon the renal handling of urate suggests that urate reabsorption may also occur
distal to the main site of tubular secretion of urate. This review will therefore consider predominantly the over-all effect of drugs upon renal excretion of urate with
less emphasis upon the intrarenal mechanisms mediating the net effect. Thus, an
increase in the urinary excretion of urate can either be due to a dominant inhibition
of reabsorption or a stimulation of secretion, whereas a reduction in renal excretion
of urate can be attributed to impairment of urate secretion or to an increase in
tubular reabsorption of urate or both.

I. Drugs that have a Biphasic Action on Renal Excretion of Urate

Just as urate transport in the renal tubule is bidirectional, the effects of many drugs
on urate transport are biphasic, i.e., the net effect upon the renal excretion of urate is
different at high concentrations of the drug from that which applies at low concentrations. Although this review will emphasize the biphasic action of some drugs,
there is a strong body of opinion that believes all drugs that affect urate excretion
would have a biphasic action if it were possible to study the action at appropriate
drug concentrations.

1. Uricosuric Drugs

In 1955, YÜ and GUTMAN demonstrated that salicylate, phenylbutazone, and probenecid, all of which in high drug concentrations increased the urate clearance, could be shown to depress the urate clearance at low drug concentrations. They noted that all of these drugs produced an initial fall in the urate clearance with a later rise. They interpreted this paradoxical effect as indicating a change in the tubular transport mechanism. They postulated two more-or-less distinct systems of tubular transport: 1. one responsible for tubular reabsorption of urate, thought normally to have a considerably greater capacity and which was suppressed only by a high concentration of the drug, and 2. another concerned with tubular secretion of urate, normally having a limited capacity that could be inhibited by low as well as by high concentrations of a drug.

2. Aspirin

In 1959, these same workers studied further the paradoxical effect of various salicylate dosages on renal excretion of urate. They confirmed that daily doses of aspirin of between 1 and 2 g/24 h produced a reduction in urinary urate excretion, whereas doses between 3 and 5 g/day produced a significant increase in urate excretion. Dissociation of the plasma and urinary salicylate concentrations by altering the pH of the urine showed that the determining factor was the concentration of free salicylate in the tubular urine. Thus, alkalinization of the urine promoted the renal excretion of free salicylate and resulted in a considerable increase in urate excretion. They interpreted these results as showing that low concentrations of free salicylates in the tubular urine depressed tubular secretion and that intermediate concentrations depressed both tubular secretion and reabsorption to result in no net change, whereas high concentrations of free salicylate in tubular fluid suppressed both reabsorption and secretion, the net effect being a considerable uricosuria.

3. Diuretics

The early studies of oral diuretics also showed a biphasic effect upon urate excretion. Intravenous administration of chlorothiazide produced a significant increase in the urate clearance (HEINEMANN et al., 1959; DUARTE and BLAND, 1965), whereas the usual doses given orally resulted in reduced urate excretion. Moreover, the effect of oral thiazide diuretics on the serum urate is dose-related, so that large doses tend to retain more urate than do lower doses (BENGTSSON et al., 1975). Several mechanisms have been invoked to explain the urate retention following oral thiazide diuretics. Firstly, plasma volume contraction due to the diuresis promoted increased urate reabsorption from the renal tubule. To some extent, the administration of additional salt can correct the resultant hyperuricemia (SUKI et al., 1967). Secondly, altered renal blood flow due to the plasma volume contraction, with a reduction in filtration rate, has been implicated (STEELE and OPPENHEIMER, 1969). The possibility of angiotensin release was also invoked. A third possible factor would be a specific effect upon the urate transport mechanisms in the kidney. The above studies imply that correction of plasma volume contraction and any impairment of glomerular filtration rate would restore the serum urate to normal. However, the observation of uricosuria following the i.v. administration of thiazide diuretics in high dosage suggests the possibility of a specific effect of the drugs, which promote urate retention when given in low doses, on urate transport mechanisms. The recent development of diuretics that are also uricosuric in low dosage indicates that it is possible for the uricosuric action of a drug to override the urate-retaining action due to the associated diuretic effect upon plasma volume or glomerular filtration rate (REESE and STEELE, 1976; EMMERSON et al., 1976c; LEMIEUX et al., 1976).

Ethacrynic acid has also been shown to have a biphasic effect upon urate excretion, an initial transient increase in urate excretion at the time of maximum diuresis, followed by a decrease in both renal clearance and renal excretion of urate persisting for several hours. A consideration of urate excretion in relation to osmolar clearance suggests that this drug has a specific effect upon urate transport (BOURKE et al., 1966). Acetazolamide also tends to induce hyperuricemia (AYVAZIAN and AYVAZIAN, 1961), although its action too can be biphasic (STEELE et al., 1975).

4. Pyrazinamide

When used as an antibiotic in patients with tuberculosis, this drug has long been known to be associated with the development of hyperuricemia (YÜ et al., 1957; CULLEN et al., 1957; SCHNEEWEISS and POOLE, 1960). The marked reduction in urate excretion was originally attributed to the specific effect of inhibition of tubular secretion of urate. Hence, the response to this drug was used in an attempt to quantitate secreted urate and separate it from urinary urate that had not been reabsorbed (STEELE and RIESELBACH, 1967). A reevaluation of the specificity of its effect on secretion of urate alone has led to a reduced confidence in such an interpretation (HOLMES et al., 1972). It has been suggested that the pyrazinamide suppression test may considerably underestimate the magnitude of the various urate transport processes within the kidney (STEELE, 1973). Further studies have demonstrated that the effect of pyrazinamide, while predominantly an inhibition of urate secretion at usual dose levels, may result in uricosuria when considerably higher drug concentrations are reached (WEINER and TINKER, 1972). Thus, under appropriate circumstances it has been demonstrated once again that a drug that may have predominantly a single effect at usual concentrations may have an opposite net effect at a different concentration.

II. Drugs that Increase Renal Excretion of Urate

Therapeutic use is made of this effect when the uricosuric group of drugs is used for the treatment of hyperuricemia and gout (KIPPEN et al., 1974). The two most commonly used are probenecid and sulphinpyrazone, although zoxazolamine, benziodarone, and benzbromarone are potent uricosurics used in some countries. Many drugs used primarily for other purposes also have a uricosuric action, some of which have already been discussed. High doses of aspirin (greater than 5 g/day), especially if the urine is alkalinized with an equal amount of sodium bicarbonate, or high-dosage phenylbutazone also promotes renal excretion of urate (see Table 1). Two drugs that also reduce plasma lipids, namely chlorphenoxyisobutyric acid and halofenate, promote renal excretion of urate (TREVAKS and LOVELL, 1965; ARONOW et al., 1973;

Table 1. Drugs that increase renal excretion of urate

(1)	Uricosuric drugs	
	Probenecid	SIROTA et al. (1952)
		BISHOP and PFAFF (1955)
	Sulphinpyrazone	BURNS et al. (1957)
	Zoxazolamine	BURNS et al. (1958)
	Benziodarone	LEMIEUX et al. (1973)
	Benzbromarone	SORENSEN and LEVINSON (1976)
(2)	Aspirin in high dosage	YÜ and GUTMAN (1955)
(3)	Phenylbutazone in high	YÜ et al. (1953)
	dosage	WYNGAARDEN (1955)
(4)	Chlorphenoxyisobutyric acid	TREVAKS and LOVELL (1965)
(5)	Halofenate	RAVENSCROFT et al. (1973)
		ARONOW et al. (1973)
		DUJOVNE et al. (1976)
(6)	Diodrast	BONSNES et al. (1944)
(7)	Radiocontrast media	POSTLETHWAITE and KELLEY (1971)
	sodium diatrizoate	
	iopanoic acid	
	calcium ipodate	
	meglumine iodipamide	
(8)	Orotic acid	FALLON et al. (1961)
		KELLEY et al. (1970)
(9)	Ascorbic acid	STEIN et al. (1976)
(10)	Adrenal steroids	INGBAR et al. (1951)
(11)	Anticholinergic agents	POSTLETHWAITE et al. (1974)
	Glycopyrrolate	RAMSDELL et al. (1974)
	Tridihexethyl chloride	
(12)	Anticoagulants	SOUGIN-MIBASHAN and HORWITZ (1955)
	Ethyl biscoumacetate	THOMPSON et al. (1959)
	Dicoumarol	
	Phenindione	
(13)	Glyceryl guaiacolate	RAMSDELL et al. (1974)
(14)	Phlorhidzin	SKEITH et al. (1970)
(15)	Osmotic diuretics, mannitol	SKEITH et al. (1967)
(16)	Acetoheximide	YÜ et al. (1968)
(17)	6-Azauridine	FALLON et al. (1961)
	Diflumidone	SCHLOSSTEIN et al. (1973)
	Sulfaethylthiadiazole	
(18)	Glycine	YÜ et al. (1970)

RAVENSCROFT et al., 1973; DUJOVNE et al., 1976). Also, radiographic contrast media, both the original iodopyracet (BONSNES et al., 1944) and several of the newer radiocontrast agents, will promote uricosuria for the duration of their excretion by the kidney (POSTLETHWAITE and KELLEY, 1971). The increased excretion of urate induced by adrenal steroids was detected soon after their discovery (INGBAR et al., 1951). Similarly, high doses of ascorbic acid, sometimes taken for upper respiratory infections, induce a significant increase in urate excretion (STEIN et al., 1976). Orotic acid, particularly after i.v. administration, is significantly uricosuric, although it has the additional effect of depleting 5-phosphoribosyl pyrophosphate (PRPP) in man (FALLON et al., 1961; KELLEY et al., 1970). A variety of other agents, such as oral antico-

Table 2. Drugs that reduce renal excretion of urate

Pyrazinamide, pyrazinoic acid	YÜ et al. (1957)
	CULLEN et al. (1957)
Uricosuric agents in low dosage	YÜ and GUTMAN (1955)
Aspirin in low dosage	YÜ and GUTMAN (1959)
Thiazide diuretics—orally	MANUEL and STEELE (1974)
Ethambutol	POSTLETHWAITE and KELLEY (1972)
Nicotinic acid	GAUT et al. (1971)
	GERSHON and FOX (1974)

agulants (SOUGIN-MIBASHAN and HORWITZ, 1955; THOMPSON et al., 1959), anticholinergic agents (POSTLETHWAITE et al., 1974), the antidiabetic agent acetohexamide (YÜ et al., 1968), and osmotic diuretics (SKEITH et al., 1967), also promote renal excretion of urate (Table 1).

III. Drugs that Reduce the Renal Excretion of Urate

As mentioned in the consideration of drugs with a biphasic action, oral diuretics are the most common therapeutic agents to illustrate the net effect of lowering the urinary excretion of urate (Table 2). Low-dosage aspirin (less than 2 g/24 h) will have a similar effect, and the dominant effect of pyrazinamide in most therapeutic doses is to reduce the renal excretion of urate, resulting in hyperuricemia. The antituberculous agent ethambutol causes hyperuricemia by reducing the fractional excretion of urate (POSTLETHWAITE and KELLEY, 1972). A comparison of the effects on ethambutol-induced urate retention of a variety of agents that can modify renal excretion of urate suggested that the action of ethambutol was a distinctive one, different from that of diuretics, lactate, pyrazinamide, or low-dosage aspirin. Nicotinic acid in doses of 1.5 g three times daily also reduces renal excretion of urate and may cause hyperuricemia (GAUT et al., 1971). More precise study of its effect was undertaken by GERSHON and FOX (1974), who demonstrated a considerable decrease in the fractional clearance of urate and its ability to inhibit the uricosuria induced by sulphinpyrazone. They also demonstrated an 80% reduction in the PRPP concentration of erythrocytes. Thus, numerically fewer drugs act by reducing the renal excretion of urate, but several of these are used so extensively that renal retention of urate due to drugs has become a significant therapeutic problem.

IV. Drugs that Alter Urate Excretion by Altering Urate Production

1. Drugs that Increase Urate Production

Many cytotoxic drugs causing cellular damage in patients with leukaemia, lymphoma, or polycythemia vera result in an increase in urate production due to nucleoprotein degradation. The body's response to such a urate load has already been considered, together with the potential risk of a uric acid nephropathy. However, some 2-substituted thiadiazoles in man, particularly 2-ethylamino-1,3,4-thiadiazole, have the unique property of causing an increase in uric acid production that is not related to tissue destruction. Drugs in this group have been shown to increase de novo purine synthesis, an effect that is blocked by the administration of nicotinamide. The mechanism whereby these drugs increase urate production (which is then likely to result in an increase in renal excretion of urate) has not been elucidated (KRAKOFF and BALIS, 1959).

2. Drugs that Reduce Purine Production

Part of the effect of allopurinol, which is considered in detail by Dr. Elion in Chapter 21 is due to inhibition of overall purine synthesis. In addition, the drug azathioprine, which is largely metabolized to 6-mercapto-purine, also inhibits purine synthesis, an effect that is dependent on the presence of HGPRT enzyme activity (SORENSEN and BENKE, 1967).

E. Systemic Conditions Leading to Abnormal Urate Metabolism

I. Hypertension

Hyperuricemia is a frequent finding in patients with hypertension. Its incidence in untreated hypertensive patients has been reported to vary between 20 and 32% (DOLLERY et al., 1960; KINSEY, 1963; BRECKENRIDGE, 1966; GARRICK et al., 1972). This hyperuricemia increases in patients receiving hypotensive agents, and the incidence of hyperuricemia increases to about 60% (GARRICK et al., 1972). While thiazide diuretics are the most common agents causing this increase in serum urate concentration, other hypotensive agents also contribute significantly. The incidence and severity of the hyperuricemia does not appear to increase in proportion to the blood pressure until malignant levels are reached, although GARRICK et al. (1972) found a correlation between the serum urate concentration and the diastolic blood pressure.

Interpretation of these findings is further complicated by the difficulty of determining the coexistence of renal disease, particularly minor degrees of renal disease. However, when renal disease, as evidenced by an increase in the serum creatinine or serum urea concentration, is present there is good evidence that a further increase in the serum urate concentration occurs (SIMON et al., 1969; GARRICK et al., 1972; BULPITT et al., 1975). GARRICK et al. (1972) for instance, found that the mean serum urate concentration was at least 1 mg/100 ml higher in their patients with renal hypertension than in those with nonrenal hypertension. Theoretical upper limits of average serum urate concentrations in hypertensive patients that make allowance for sex, plasma urea concentration, and whether or not a thiazide diuretic is being administered, have been prepared (BULPITT, 1975). This should permit the determination of whether or not a given level of serum urate in a hypertensive patient is excessive. This author found that the administration of long-term diuretic therapy increased the serum urate by an average of 0.04 mmol/liter (approximately 0.7 mg/100 ml). Despite the reported high incidence of hyperuricemia in hypertensive patients, actual gouty arthritis appeared to be a problem in less than 10% (GARRICK et al., 1972). In some of these, the gout was thought to be the primary condition and hypertension a secondary development.

The studies of BRECKENRIDGE (1966) in patients with hypertension demonstrated reduced renal tubular excretion of urate, leading to a lowered urate clearance; subsequent studies have confirmed the renal basis for this hyperuricemia. Limited studies of urate production have shown this to be normal (BRECKENRIDGE, 1966). Comparative studies of urate clearance in the two kidneys of patients with hypertension due to renal artery stenosis have shown that urate excretion per unit of GFR is reduced on the side of the stenosis (SIMON et al., 1969). This defective excretion reverted to normal following surgical correction of the renal artery stenosis. The precise mechanism causing this has not been fully elucidated, although the effect of local accumulation of lactate (? due to local renal ischemia) or the effect of angiotensin have been invoked. It must be remembered that the blood pressure in the kidney affected by the renal artery stenosis may not be elevated, whereas the systemic hypertension will be affecting the kidney with the normal vasculature. Hence, factors other than the hypertension itself must be involved in this reduction in urate excretion by the ischemic kidney. The answer may lie in the response of the kidney to a reduction in renal blood flow. The studies of BULLPITT (1975) suggested that the mechanism for increasing the serum urate was the same as that which caused an increase in the plasma urea concentration, and he suggested that this may be related to a reduction in renal blood flow. Such a mechanism would explain the situation in renal artery stenosis as well as the rise in serum urate that occurs with the use of some drugs that induce a fall in blood pressure chiefly in the upright posture, such as pempidine, mecamylamine (DOLLERY et al., 1960), und guanethidine (BULLPITT, 1974). This seems to be the most likely explanation, although the precise role of metabolites in contributing to hyperuricemia in hypertension has not been fully elucidated.

II. Obesity

One of the strongest associations of the serum urate concentration is with the various parameters of body size, of which body weight is the simplest. In the Tecumseh Health Survey, the incidence of hyperuricemia in groups steadily increased as relative weight increased (MYERS et al., 1968). Classically, patients with gout have been depicted as obese, and surveys of patients with primary gout have shown that about half of them average between 15% and 20% above the desirable weight for height (GRAHAME and SCOTT, 1970; EMMERSON and KNOWLES, 1971). Recently, it has been suggested that subjects with gout place an unusually high value on the flavor of food and that most find eating and drinking to be one of the great pleasures of life (KAHN, 1976). In this study, a group of gouty subjects and a control group of comparable weight were asked whether they liked sauces and spices and were given a choice of four answers—no, yes, very much, and extremely much. A significantly greater number of gouty patients indicated either great or enormous pleasure in these flavors, and the author postulated that gouty subjects were uncommonly sensitive to the stimuli of taste and smell.

Many population surveys have demonstrated a positive correlation between serum urate and body weight (HOLLISTER et al., 1967), and this has been confirmed in a variety of Caucasian groups (ACHESON and FLOREY, 1969; KATZ et al., 1973; TRAN et al., 1973; GRIEBSCH and ZOLLNER, 1973). Similar findings have also been made in several Polynesian groups, many of whom have a tendency to both hyperuricemia and obesity (EVANS et al., 1968). Another aspect concerning the relation between serum urate and body size has been the defining of the normal range of urate production in relation to body surface area (RIESELBACH et al., 1970). Such a relationship implies a dependency of one upon the other and that urate production would be greater in subjects with a greater surface area. In studying the etiology of hyperuricemia among patients in a general hospital, either obesity or degenerative vascular disease was present in over half of those studied (VAN PEENEN, 1971).

It has been more difficult to determine the mechanism whereby body size affects the serum urate concentration. Weight loss by dieting led to a mean decrease of 0.8 mg/100 ml in the serum urate concentration in 12 of 15 obese subjects who lost between 4 and 22 kg (NICHOLLS and SCOTT, 1972). These authors were unable to demonstrate any increase in the urate clearance to account for this fall in serum urate concentration. Elucidation of mechanisms in this area is complex because of the simultaneous operation of several dependent factors that cannot be controlled or modified independently. Nonetheless, urate metabolism has been documented in one subject both during obesity and subsequently after weight loss (EMMERSON, 1973). In this study, a weight loss of 18 kg was associated with a significant fall in the serum urate concentration but no change in the mean 24-h urinary excretion of urate. However, there was a significant increase in the renal clearance of urate without any significant change in the renal clearance of creatinine. In addition, the miscible urate

Table 3. Studies of urate metabolism in a gouty subject on two occasions, while obese and after weight reduction

	First study	Second study	Significance of difference
Weight (kg)	99	81	
Surface area (m^2)	2.12	1.94	
Blood pressure (mm Hg)	170/110	140/80	
Serum urate (mg/100 ml)	7.0±0.2	5.3±0.3	$p < .001$[a]
Urine urate (mg/24 h)	494±46	487±46	N.S.[a]
Renal clearance urate (ml/min)	5.3±0.5	8.0±0.9	$p < .01$[a]
Renal clearance creatinine (ml/min)	141±13	132±10	N.S.[a]
Miscible urate pool (mg)	2050	1419	$p < .001$[b]
(95% range)	(1956–2148)	(1304–1545)	
Urate turnover (pools/24 h)	0.43	0.49	$p < .001$[b]
Urate production (mg/24 h)	885	696	
I.V. urate excreted 7 days (%)	51.7	72.3	
$\dfrac{\text{24-h urinary urate excretion}}{\text{24-h urate production}}$ (%)	55.8	70.0	
Extrarenal disposal (mg/24 h)	391	209	
^{14}C-glycine incorporation into urinary urate 7 days (% dose)	0.29	0.25	
^{14}C-glycine incorporation into produced urate 7 days (% dose)	0.56	0.34	

[a] Student's 't' test.
[b] Statistical comparison of the intercepts and slopes of the regression lines of ^{15}N-urate enrichment on time for the two studies.
This table reproduced with permission from the Aust. N.Z.J. Med. 3, 411 (1973).

pool fell significantly, and there was a fall in urate production from 885 mg/24 h to just under 700 mg/24 h. The apparent fall in urate production was confirmed by a reduced incorporation of glycine into urate. Thus, the improvement in urate metabolism in this patient (see Table 3) could be attributed to two changes: 1. a rise in the urate clearance without change in glomerular filtration rate; the remission of his hypertension with his weight reduction could have contributed to this; 2. a reduction in the amount of urate produced.

This study demonstrates the complexity of elucidating the many factors that determine the etiology of the hyperuricemia. It reflects some of the difficulties in determining the precise etiology of the hyperuricemia found in many systemic disorders.

III. Regular Alcohol Consumption

Gout has been traditionally associated with the regular consumption of a variety of alcoholic beverages. Although the validity of this association has been questioned, the higher prevalence of gout among regular drinkers has been confirmed in many recent studies (SAKER et al., 1967; PELL and D'ALONZO, 1968). GIBSON and GRAHAM (1974) found that 42% of their gouty subjects in England were excessive drinkers of alcohol and this would also be the experience of many other gout clinics.

Ethanol is oxidized by alcohol dehydrogenase to acetaldehyde, which is continuously and irreversibly removed by an aldehyde dehydrogenase (LIEBER, 1976). During this oxidation, there is a considerable increase in the concentration of NADH at the expense of NAD, resulting in an increase in the NADH:NAD ratio; in turn, this disturbs the balance between the redox pairs, lactate:pyruvate and β-hydroxybutyrate and acetoacetate, leading to a shift in the equilibrium towards lactate and β-hydroxybutyrate. Thus, alcohol consumption readily leads to the increased formation of metabolites known to impair the renal excretion of urate. Apart from this potential increase in hepatic formation of lactate, there is also evidence of decreased lactate disposal following ethanol consumption, with significant inhibition of lactate incorporation into glucose (KREISBERG et al., 1971). It can also induce hyperlipemia and hypoglycemia (GEBBIE and PRIOR, 1967).

The effect of acute alcoholic intoxication upon uric acid metabolism has been studied by LIEBER et al. (1962). These authors demonstrated hyperuricemia in half of a group of patients intoxicated with ethanol, with significant falls in serum urate concentration in all subjects during recovery from intoxication. This hyperuricemia was associated with a decrease of renal excretion of urate and of the urate clearance, without change in the creatinine clearance, changes resembling those produced by lactate. Subsequently, the administration of sufficient amounts of ethanol to produce serum levels exceeding 200 mg/100 ml was shown to result in steady rises in the serum lactate and urate concentrations and a steady fall in the uric acid to creatinine clearance ratio. Thus, there is good evidence in acute alcoholic intoxication that hyperuricemia is due to renal under-excretion of urate.

Smaller doses of alcohol (up to 100 g) taken over a longer period may produce only minor changes in the serum urate concentration (MACLACHLAN and RODNAN, 1967). Larger amounts of alcohol than this were needed to raise blood lactate concentrations, with consequent changes in serum and urine urate. However, these authors found that even small amounts of alcohol (less than 100 g) taken during a brief period of fasting had much greater effects than those produced by alcohol alone or by fasting alone, and small amounts of alcohol during fasting were accompanied by increases in both serum lactate and the β-hydroxybutyrate concentrations.

Thus, many factors contribute to the tendency to hyperuricemia and gout in regular drinkers of alcohol:

1. Purine content. Few alcoholic beverages contain significant amounts of purines, but beer does contain sufficient to add to the dietary purine load. Its contribution to hyperuricemia will be magnified if the beer consumption is considerable or if the renal ability to eliminate urate is reduced.

2. Obesity. This has already been considered, but obesity is also a common association of regular alcohol consumption and may also be an important contributory factor to the persistent hyperuricemia.

3. Intermittent episodes of hyperlactatemia. Although the serum lactate concentration is very variable, and dietary factors may also be involved (MACLACHLAN and RODNAN, 1967), intermittent elevation of the serum lactate concentration in regular drinkers may contribute to the hyperuricemia. In addition, the hepatic uptake of circulating lactate is reduced during the metabolism of ethanol by the liver, so that reduced use of lactate may compound the effect of increased production (KREISBERG et al., 1971).

4. Alcoholic hyperlipemia. Ethanol has been directly implicated in the production of hyperlipemia (JONES et al., 1963; SCHAPIRO et al., 1965; OSTRANDER et al., 1974), and hyperuricemia is a regular feature of this condition (LOSOWSKY et al., 1963; GEBBIE and PRIOR, 1967). GINSBERG et al. (1974) found that this response to alcohol is much greater in persons with preexisting hypertriglyceridemia; it has been suggested that alcohol induces the hepatic secretion of lipoprotein (CHAIT et al., 1972) particularly, in predisposed individuals having a relatively poor ability to clear triglycerides from plasma.

5. Alcoholic hypoglycemia. This occurs chiefly when hepatic gluconeogenesis is impaired in malnourished persons with depleted glycogen stores and presumably induces hyperuricemia by the associated ketonemia.

6. Fat-dependent ketogenic effect. Significant ketonemia and ketonuria have been observed in alcoholics, being most easily induced by alcohol in subjects taking a diet containing moderate amounts of fat (LEFEVRE et al., 1970). The effect is not an immediate one, however, and results from changes in intermediate metabolism characterized by an increased production of ketone bodies from fatty acids. This in turn may be related to glycogen depletion and depression of citric acid cycle activity induced by the alcohol (LEFEVRE et al., 1970).

7. Poor nutritional status, leading to starvation and ketosis.

8. Muscular hyperactivity such as may occur during delirium tremens and some of the alcohol withdrawal seizures (NEWCOMBE, 1972).

9. The possibility of chronic plasma volume contraction due to the diuretic effect of alcohol (inhibition of ADH secretion) has been suggested and may well contribute (NEWCOMBE, 1972).

Thus, there are many factors in the alcoholic acting together to promote hyperuricemia. In almost all of these situations, the dominant mechanism appears to be by reduction in renal excretion of urate.

IV. Hyperlipidemia

When the importance of abnormalities of lipid metabolism came to be recognized, initial reports in subjects with gout suggested the frequent finding of elevated levels of serum cholesterol (HARRIS-JONES, 1957). Subsequently, more extensive studies did not confirm this, and, conversely, the serum urate was shown generally to be normal in familial hypercholesterolemia (JENSEN et al., 1966). However, increasing numbers of studies suggested a strong association between hypertriglyceridemia and gout (FELDMAN and WALLACE, 1964). BENEDEK (1967) noted this association in gouty subjects together with obesity but found that the urate and triglycerides varied independently of each other. BARLOW (1968) found a variety of hyperlipidemias in 77% of his patients with primary gout, although only 15% had evidence of occlusive vascular disease. He found no one type of hyperlipidemia to predominate. Many other studies, however, have confirmed the high incidence of Type IV hyperlipopro-teinemia in gout, although many of the studies also showed that the mean weight in the gouty group was higher than in the control group (KUNTZ et al., 1969; CAMUS et al., 1969; RONDIER et al., 1970; BLUESTONE et al., 1971; DARLINGTON and SCOTT, 1972; MIELANTS et al., 1973). Thus, the persistent unanswered question is the mecha-nism of the association between the hyperuricemia and hypertriglyceridemia in gouty patients. Hyperuricemia was noted in 40% of patients with either type IV or type V hyperlipoproteinemia (FREDRICKSON and LEVY, 1972), usually in the absence of gout, so that the problem has wider implications. EMMERSON and KNOWLES (1971), in comparing groups of patients with primary and secondary gout, found that al-though obesity and greater alcohol consumption were more marked in the primary gout group; the presence of these factors in the individual patients did not correlate well with the presence of hypertriglyceridemia. Even when due allowance was made for their weight and alcohol intake, greater hypertriglyceridemia was found in the gouty subjects. MERTZ et al. (1972) also confirmed that the hyperlipoproteinemia in gouty patients did not necessarily depend upon nutrition, alcohol consumption, or glucose intolerance. On the other hand, GIBSON and GRAHAME (1974) have inter-preted their data as suggesting that the hypertriglyceridemia may be attributed to the coincident obesity and alcohol consumption. However, WIEDEMANN et al. (1972) studied lipid metabolism, glucose tolerance, and insulin responsiveness in gouty subjects, and weight and age matched groups without gout. They found type IV hyperlipoproteinemia in six out of 14 gouty subjects and one out of 14 control subjects and significantly greater insulin secretion after oral glucose toler-ance in the hypertriglyceridemic gouty patients. They concluded that a direct rela-tionship between gout and type IV hyperlipoproteinemia existed independent of obesity and carbohydrate intolerance.

Type IV hyperlipoproteinemia in patients with gout probably has protean caus-es, just as it does in nongouty subjects (SCHONFELD and KUDZMA, 1973). In some gouty subjects, therefore, obesity, carbohydrate or fat induction, hyperinulinism (OLEFSKY et al., 1974), or renal insufficiency (LOSOWSKY and KENWARD, 1968) can be involved, whereas in others, none of these factors can be detected and no specific abnormality can be determined. In some cases, the lipid abnormality may be the primary disorder, and the patient may be seen because the associated hyperuricemia, presenting as gouty arthritis, induces symptoms first. Such a case (AMIDI, 1972) would be regarded as primary gout unless the familial hyperlipoproteinemia was recognized. Presumably, the most likely cause of the moderate degrees of hypertriglyceridemia, such as are seen in gout, is an increase in the hepatic secretion of triglycerides (KAYE and GALTON, 1975). In a situation such as this, with such a wide diversity of causes for the hypertriglyceridemia, there has been no definitive study done to determine the relative roles of urate over-production and/or renal under-excretion in the genesis of the hyperuricemia of this condition. However, there has been no increased association with hyperlipidemia seen in over-producers of urate. It is perhaps notable that abnormalities of both mechanisms operate in patients with the severe hypertriglyceridemia of type I glycogen storage disease (glucose-6-phosphatase deficiency).

V. Degenerative Vascular Disease

Hyperuricemia is commonly seen in patients with vascular disease and has been recorded as a risk factor in coronary heart disease. It has been difficult to assess the mechanism of this association. Age and sex may contribute to such hyperuricemia as may hypertension, obesity, and hypertriglyceridemia (MYERS et al., 1968; BLACKET et al., 1973). In a group of patients with peripheral vascular disease, adjustment of urate and lipid values for the effect of age and obesity left no residual evidence of association (BALLANTYNE et al., 1976). In addition, in a group of over 2000 men with a previous myocardial infarction, an association was shown between serum urate and other recognized risk factors for cardiovascular disease. However, when allowance was made for the effect of the administration of diuretic drugs, the serum urate had no value with regard to prediction of mortality (Coronary Drug Project Research Group). Gouty arthritis tended to occur in persons with serum urate concentrations greater than 9 mg/100 ml (0.54 mmol/liter). It seems, therefore, that until more information is obtained the hyperuricemia associated with vascular disease can best be attributed to the influence of one or more of the following conditions, viz: obesity, hypertension, diuretic therapy, or hypertriglyceridemia.

VI. Acute Myocardial Infarction

Hyperuricemia has long been recognized after myocardial infarction (GERTLER et al., 1951), but the mechanism has only recently been studied. Definition of urate metabolism shortly after myocardial infarction showed an expansion of the urate pool but also an increased rate of urate turnover (DOSMAN et al., 1975). There was no elevation of the serum lactate concentration and, although the creatinine clearance exceeded 80 ml/min, the authors could not assess the effects of the abnormal circulatory hemodynamics after infarction. A more recent assessment has suggested that in individual patients the rise in the plasma urate correlated well with rises in the plasma urea and plasma creatinine concentrations, and that there were associated reductions in the creatinine clearance. This suggests that diminished renal perfusion and reduced renal excretion of urate are important in the development of hyperuricemia after myocardial infarction.

VII. Diabetes

About 1% of patients with diabetes suffer from gout (WHITEHOUSE and CLEARY, 1966). Of patients with both gout and diabetes mellitus, about 80% do not require insulin and the great majority of these are obese. In addition, many are hyperlipidemic and some are hypertensive. It is, therefore, difficult to separate the role of the diabetes from the role of these other factors that may influence the serum urate concentration independently. In addition, whenever ketoacidosis occurs, there will be an increased tendency to hyperuricemia due to reduced renal excretion of urate (PADOVA and BENDERSKY, 1962). The incidence of diabetes in groups of gouty subjects, on the other hand, depends largely upon the criteria used for diagnosing diabetes in asymptomatic individuals, criteria which can be controversial in obesity, already a common finding in subjects with gout (DENIS and LAUNAY, 1969).

It has long been known that hyperglycemia is associated with an increase in the renal clearance of urate (BONSNES and DANA, 1946), the resulting increment in urate clearance being much greater than the associated increase in the urea or the creatinine clearance. No abnormality of the handling of urate has been demonstrated in mild diabetes (PADOVA et al., 1964), although increased urate clearances were observed when blood sugars reached levels which would result in glycosuria. There have been several studies of glucose tolerance and plasma insulin responses in groups of patients with gout. Some investigators have concluded that obesity and hyperlipidemia can account for most of the metabolic defects resulting in hyperuricemia in diabetes (BOYLE et al., 1969), whereas others have interpreted their data as indicating that additional factors over and above obesity and hyperlipidemia are responsible for the altered urate excretion (DIAMOND et al., 1974). Thus, two factors may affect urate excretion in diabetes in opposite directions: 1. reduced renal excretion of urate as a result of altered metabolic processes, obesity, hyperlipidemia, and ketosis; and 2. increased renal excretion of urate associated with hyperglycemia and glycosuria (SKEITH et al., 1967). It is, therefore, not surprising that no uniform pattern of change in urate excretion is seen in diabetics.

VIII. Myxedema

Hyperuricemia in myxedema has been attributed to reduced renal excretion of urate (LEEPER et al., 1960). Replacement therapy sufficient to return the basal metabolic rate to normal caused an increase in the renal excretion of urate and a fall in the serum urate concentration. The mean change in serum urate with replacement therapy was 2 mg/100 ml. The precise renal mechanism causing this under-excretion of urate was not elucidated, although the authors noted moderate increases in blood urea nitrogen in the myxedematous patients, which were corrected when euthyroidism was achieved. Thus, the hyperuricemia may be part of a generalized impairment of renal excretory function rather than a specific one relating only to urate.

IX. Parathyroid Disease

Hyperuricemia, apparently of renal origin, has been frequently reported in hyperparathyroidism (MINTZ et al., 1961; SCOTT et al., 1964; JACKSON and HARRIS, 1965). No effect of parathyroid extract has been demonstrated on urate clearance (SHELP et al., 1969), and the mechanism for the association of hyperuricemia with hyperparathyroidism has not been unequivocally demonstrated. Most of the patients studied have had some associated impairment of renal excretory function with elevation of the blood urea concentration. In view of the frequency of renal damage in hyperparathyroidism (sometimes showing as nephrocalcinosis), it is not surprising that few remissions of the hyperuricemia following parathyroidectomy have been documented. Thus, although further studies may demonstrate other mechanisms, the present evidence attributes the hyperuricemia of hyperparathyroidism to the associated renal disease. In some cases of hyperparathyroidism, the synovial fluid has contained both urate and calcium pyrophosphate crystals (JACKSON and HARRIS, 1965), so that the association of an acute arthritis with hyperparathyroidism does not necessarily establish the diagnosis as one of gout.

A case has also been recorded of hyperparathyroidism associated with hypouricemia due to a markedly increased urate clearance (48.9 ml/min/1.73 m^2) (GIBSON et al., 1976). The authors were unable to adduce any evidence of an etiologic relationship between the increased urate clearance and the hyperparathyroidism, and it is possible that the hypouricemia was due to an isolated renal tubular defect unrelated to the hyperparathyroidism.

Hyperuricemia has also been reported in patients with hypoparathyroidism (DUBIN et al., 1956), apparently due to a reduction in the urate clearance. Changes in serum urate parallelled changes in serum phosphate, and these authors postulated a common tubular excretory mechanism for both urate and phosphate. Further support for this postulate has not been found subsequently.

X. Glycogen Storage Disease

An almost invariable ultimate development in glycogen storage disease type I (glucose-6-phosphatase deficiency) is hyperuricemia and gout. Other associated features include increased concentrations of both lactate and ketones in blood, as well as an increase in a number of lipid components, particularly the free fatty acids and triglycerides (HOWELL et al., 1962). This regular association with an elevated serum lactate concentration caused the hyperuricemia to be attributed entirely to this associated feature, which was confirmed by the demonstration of reduced renal clearances of urate (FINE et al., 1966). However, when urate kinetics were studied in detail by measurement of the urate pool and turnover rate, evidence of increased de novo purine biosynthesis was also found (ALEPA et al., 1967; JAKOVCIC and SORENSEN, 1967; KELLEY et al., 1968). Thus, the hyperuricemia in this condition appears to be due to a combination both of reduced renal excretion of urate and of increased urate production. The cause of the increased purine biosynthesis has been attributed to an increased production of phosphoribosyl pyrophosphate (PRPP) due to increased diversion of glucose-6-phosphate through the pentose-phosphate pathway (HOWELL et al., 1962; ALEPA et al., 1967). The associated hyperlipidemia may be related to the finding of an increased capacity for de novo synthesis of fatty acids from citrate in the liver of patients with glucose-6-phosphatase deficiency (HÜLSMANN et al., 1970). Studies of urate production in heterozygotes for glucose-6-phosphatase deficiency who showed levels of enzyme activity in their platelets intermediate between normal and affected individuals have been shown to be normal (STORMONT et al., 1976).

Special interest, therefore, has been shown in the report of a mild variety of glycogen storage disease due to a mutation of glucose-6-phosphatase, resulting in only a partial deficiency of enzyme activity in the liver (STAMM and WEBB, 1975). In this case, the manifestations of the glycogen storage disease were mild and unrecognized, and the presenting symptom was of attacks of gout that had been recurring since age 14 and which developed into gout nephropathy by the age of 40. Apart from the gout, the patient's only symptoms were of malaise and fatigue. Estimation of enzyme activity in the liver demonstrated a reduction of glucose-6-phosphatase activity to approximately half normal levels. Thus, in this condition the gout and its complications may be the dominant overt sign of the enzyme deficiency.

XI. Fructose Administration

The rapid i.v. administration of fructose results in a rise in both the serum urate and the urinary urate concentrations (PERHEENTUPA and RAIVIO, 1967). The most likely cause of this is an increase in urate production that has been attributed to the rapid dephosphorylation of adenine nucleotides resulting from the rapid phosphorylation of the administered fructose. Dephosphorylation of these nucleotides, particularly in the liver, causes an increase in production of purine bases, many of which are degraded to uric acid (MAENPAA et al., 1968; WOODS et al., 1970). The amount of urate produced following such parenteral administration of fructose in man depends upon the rate of administration of the fructose (HEUCKENKAMP and ZOLLNER, 1971; SAHEBJAMI and SCALETTAR, 1971), and any rises which occur in the serum or urine urate concentrations depend upon the renal response to this urate load.

From the time of the first report, it was recognized that the parenteral administration of fructose was also associated with a rapid rise in the serum lactate concentration (PERHEENTUPA and RAIVIO, 1967). This has been attributed to a block in the gluconeogenetic pathway due to inhibition of glucose phosphate isomerase by fructose-1-phosphate, which ultimately promotes generation of lactate. The parenteral administration of fructose to man is also associated with a decrease in the erythrocyte concentration of both phosphoribosylpyrophosphate (PRPP) and ribose-5-phosphate (FOX and KELLEY, 1972). Although depletion of tissue nucleotide phosphates has been observed in animal studies, no decrease in erythrocyte ATP concentration was observed. Thus, the i.v. administration of fructose to man is potentially hazardous with its resulting increase in the formation of both lactate and urate and its depletion of high energy phosphate compounds. Caution has been recommended before using large amounts of i.v. fructose in conditions that could be associated with lactic acidosis, such as hepatic disease, anoxic states, and diabetic ketoacidosis (WOODS and ALBERTI, 1972). An increase in the serum ammonia has also been reported (BRODAN et al., 1975).

The effect on urate production of a diet containing a large amount of fructose (approximately 250 g/day) has also been studied and compared with urate metabolism in the same individual on an isocaloric diet containing comparable amounts of glucose (EMMERSON, 1974). The high-fructose diet induced increases in both the serum and urine urate and also an increase in the daily production of urate. This diet was also associated with increases in the incorporation of glycine into urate, indicating greater de novo purine biosynthesis during the fructose administration. The pool and turnover of urate have also been studied in subjects who were given a single rapid infusion of between 125 and 200g fructose over 3h during day 1 of study. In each case, the urate pool increased as did the daily production and renal excretion of urate and the incorporation of labeled glycine into urinary uric acid (RAIVIO et al., 1975). In both of these studies of urate kinetics in man, it has not been possible to determine whether the increase in glycine incorporation into urate, usually taken as a reflection of de novo purine synthesis, is secondary to reduced re-utilization of purine bases, or whether it is a primary phenomenon due to altered activity of the pentose phosphate pathway resulting in a primary stimulation of purine biosynthesis.

XII. Toxemia of Pregnancy

During normal pregnancy, both the urate and inulin clearances are consistently elevated to up to 1.5 times the postpartum values. This results in the serum urate being lower than normal during pregnancy, with a slight rise towards more normal values at the puerperium (SEMPLE et al., 1974). Hyperuricemia has thus been reported to be a useful indicator of the development of toxemia of pregnancy. However, one difficulty in studying urate excretion in this condition is that of precise diagnosis of toxemia. Using both clinical and renal biopsy criteria, POLLAK and NETTLES (1960) established a higher incidence of hyperuricemia in patients with preeclampsia and eclampsia than is found in either a normal pregnancy or during pregnancy in a patient with hypertensive vascular disease. They also showed a correlation between the severity of the hyperuricemia and the grade of the histologic lesion in the glomerulus. Although hyperuricemia may be seen in most patients with eclampsia, it is a less uniform feature in patients with preeclampsia (CONNON and WADSWORTH, 1968). Raised plasma prolactin levels have been found in preeclamptic toxemia, the elevation being most significant in women with rising plasma urate concentrations (REDMAN et al., 1975).

Urate production has been shown to be normal in this condition (SEITCHIK et al., 1958), and the hyperuricemia is due to reduced renal excretion of urate. This reduction in urate excretion is disproportionate to the impairment of glomerular filtration rate, and additional tubular factors are thought to be responsible (CHESLEY and WILLIAMS, 1945). Many possible causes have been implicated in this reduced renal excretion of urate. Although an increased plasma lactate concentration was originally implicated, recent studies (FADEL et al., 1976) have shown no tendency to an increased plasma lactate concentration in this condition so that this simple explanation has had to be discarded. Some authors have suggested that there is an increased local release of angiotensin, possibly related to a heightened activity of the renin system (GORDON et al., 1973; HODARI et al., 1967), while other investigators have suggested the possibility of an increased local action by norepinephrine due to reduction in monoamine oxidase production by an ischemic placenta (DEMARIA and SEE, 1966; SANDLER and BALDOCK, 1963). Other possible contributory factors are the associated use of diuretics and contraction of the plasma volume. Thus, again one of the difficulties of determining the mechanism of hyperuricemia in a condition is complicated by our lack of complete understanding of the underlying condition itself.

The children of mothers with toxemia of pregnancy also tend to be hyperuricemic. The severity of the hyperuricemia gives some indication of the fetal prognosis, and fetal perinatal mortality was shown to increase greatly with maternal hyperuricemia, possibly a reflection of early preeclampsia (MONKUS et al., 1970; REDMAN et al., 1976). On the other hand, REDMAN et al. (1976) found that maternal hypertension without hyperuricemia did not adversely affect fetal prognosis. When it is related to pregnancy toxemia, the hyperuricemia in both mother and child usually remits within several days of parturition (MONKUS et al., 1970; SCHAFFER et al., 1943), and it is wise to allow at least 3 days for it to subside before assuming any continuing disorder of urate metabolism.

XIII. Liver Disease

As the liver is the major site of de novo purine synthesis in the body (LAJTHA and VANE, 1958), it is functionally important in purine metabolism. Rarely, however, does liver dysfunction become severe enough to affect urate production. Many patients with gout demonstrate liver disease or abnormal tests of liver function. In some cases this has been attributed to a fatty liver (KLEIN, 1971; MERTZ, 1972). In others, the liver disease has been attributed to alcohol consumption (GRAHAME et al., 1968).

Hypouricemia was a common finding during impaired hepatic function, and the recovery from jaundice has been shown to be associated with an increase (about 1.2 mg/100 ml) in the serum urate concentration and a reduction (about 3 ml/min) in the urate clearance (SCHLOSSTEIN et al., 1974). Similarly, in cirrhosis, the mean serum urate was reduced and was associated with an increase in the urate clearance/creatinine clearance ratio (MICHELIS et al., 1974). In addition, these authors found a significant inverse correlation between the serum bilirubin levels and the serum urate concentrations. We have noted excessive uricosuria in some patients with liver disease, with the urinary urate concentration exceeding the urinary concentration of creatinine. This appeared to be associated with the syndrome of inappropriate antidiuretic hormone secretion, which has been documented as causing elevation of the urate clearance (DORHOUT-MEES et al., 1971).

Remission of gout and hyperuricemia has been reported following a portacaval shunt in a patient with alcoholic cirrhosis (LEFKOVITS et al., 1968), but as there were associated changes in alcohol consumption, diet, and fluid intake, it is not possible to assess the role of the portacaval shunt in the improvement of this patient.

XIV. Sarcoidosis and Chronic Beryllium Disease

Hyperuricemia has been described in up to 50% of patients with sarcoidosis (ZIMMER and DEMIS, 1966), but the mechanism of its association has not been established.

Hyperuricemia has also been noted in about 40% of patients with chronic beryllium poisoning, a condition that closely resembles sarcoidosis in some of its clinical manifestations (KELLEY et al., 1969). Attempts have also been made to define the mechanism of this association (KELLEY et al., 1969). In a group of 15 patients with the disease, four or five hyperuricemic patients showed evidence of pulmonary alveolar-capillary block, an incidence much higher than that in the normouricemic patients.

Although the results did not reach significance, the trend of the results suggested that the serum lactate concentrations were higher, and the urate clearance in relation to the creatinine clearance was lower in the hyperuricemic group. There was no clear evidence of specific renal tubular dysfunction. Thus, although the evidence is not conclusive, current concepts suggest that hyperuricemia in berylliosis results from reduced renal excretion of urate due to low-grade chronic lactic acidosis resulting from tissue anoxia due to the associated lung disease.

XV. Respiratory Acidosis

Urate metabolism was studied in patients with respiratory acidosis (ISOMAKI and KREUS, 1968). These authors found that the severe hyperuricemia returned to normal after correction of the carbon dioxide retention, and this was associated with an increase in renal excretion of urate. It was not possible to determine the relative contribution of lactic acid and other organic acids in producing this renal excretion of urate, but both are probably increased in these patients. As already mentioned, lactic acidosis is a common feature of most conditions associated with tissue anoxia, particularly diseases of the heart or the lungs (FULOP et al., 1973). Extreme obesity may also contribute to such anoxia by permitting intermittent obstruction of the upper airway during sleep, thereby aggravating chronic respiratory failure (HENSLEY and READ, 1976).

XVI. Psoriasis

The etiology of the hyperuricemia found in between 30 and 40% of patients with psoriasis (ZIMMER and DEMIS, 1966) was studied by EISEN and SEEGMILLER (1961). In five patients with active psoriasis, they showed a pattern of urate over-production which accounted for the hyperuricemia and the high levels of urinary urate excretion. In one patient, the over-incorporation of labeled glycine into urate returned to normal when his psoriasis remitted. They concluded that the abnormality was related to the active psoriatic process, the implication being that it was due to the accelerated cellular turnover in the skin in active psoriasis.

XVII. Infectious Mononucleosis

Hyperuricemia is a regular feature of chronic myeloproliferative disorders or the massive degradation of nuclear material, so that a similar situation might be expected in patients with infectious mononucleosis. This has in fact been demonstrated (COWDREY, 1966), with the hyperuricemia tending to parallel the period of maximal abnormal lymphocytosis. Excessive renal excretion of urate, which might be expected to accompany this over-production, has not been sought.

XVIII. Estrogen Therapy

All studies have confirmed that the serum urate concentration is higher in postpubertal males than in postpubertal females. The administration of estrogens to males produces a fall in the plasma urate concentration and a significant rise in the ratio of the urate clearance to the creatinine clearance (NICHOLLS et al., 1973). It seems likely that estrogen production at puberty is responsible for the lower serum urate concentration in the female during the years of fertility, and that the rise in the female at the menopause is due to reduced estrogen production. The site of action of the estrogen appears to be the kidney.

XIX. Down's Syndrome

Among the various metabolic abnormalities noted in patients with Down's syndrome has been the consistent finding of a significant hyperuricemia when compared with well-matched controls. This difference has persisted, even when allowance has been made for weight and sex and environmental variables (KAUFMAN, 1967). Associated with this hyperuricemia has been slight, but significant increases in the serum concentrations of xanthine and hypoxanthine (APPLETON et al., 1969) and also of urea and creatinine (COBURN et al., 1967). Studies of urate kinetics in patients with Down's syndrome demonstrated no increase in urate production (COBURN et al., 1968). The results have rather indicated that the hyperuricemia is renal in origin, with the renal clearances of urate, creatinine, and urea being significantly lower (COBURN et al., 1967). These workers emphasized the importance of the reduction in the endogenous creatinine clearance and postulated that normal urate excretion is maintained in these subjects by a compensatory hyperuricemia.

XX. Hodgkin's Disease and Other Malignancies

Patients with neoplastic disease frequently show hyperuricemia, which is usually attributed to the excessive degradation of nucleoproteins. However, hypouricemia due to excessive renal loss of urate has been reported in some patients with lung carcinoma (WEINSTEIN et al., 1965) and also in patients with Hodgkin's disease (BENNETT et al., 1972). In the cases with bronchogenic carcinoma, increased renal clearance of urate was associated with a generalized renal aminoaciduria, suggestive of a proximal tubular lesion. In one case, the urate clearance was 84 ml/min, and the ratio of the urate to inulin clearance was 0.59. In these cases, no unequivocal etiologic relationship was demonstrated between the uricosuria and the carcinoma. Rather more extensive data are available concerning Hodgkin's disease, however, where therapy leading to a remission of the Hodgkin's disease caused a subsidence of the uricosuria and the hypouricemia. When a relapse of the Hodgkin's disease occurred, there was recurrence of the hypouricemia. The mechanism whereby Hodgkin's disease leads to excessive renal loss of urate in the absence of significant other abnormality of renal tubular function has not been elucidated. BENNETT et al. (1972) postulated the existence of a product of tumor metabolism that promoted renal tubular excretion of uric acid.

References

Acheson, R. M., Florey, C. V.: Body weight, AB0 blood-groups, and altitude of domicile as determinants of serum-uric-acid in military recruits in four countries. Lancet **1969** II, 391—394

Akaoka, I., Nishizawa, T., Yano, E., Takeuchi, A., Nishida, Y.: Familial hypouricaemia due to renal tubular defect of urate transport. Ann. clin. Res. **7**, 318—324 (1975)

Alepa, F. P., Howell, R. R., Klinenberg, J. R., Seegmiller, J. E.: Relationships between glycogen storage disease and tophaceous gout. Amer. J. Med. **42**, 58—66 (1967)

Amidi, M.: Type IV hyperlipoproteinaemia in a consanguineous family. Circulation **45**, 988—990 (1972)

Appleton, M. D., Haab, W., Burti, U., Orsulak, P. J.: Plasma urate levels in mongolism. Amer. J. ment. Defic. **74**, 196—199 (1969)

Aronow, W. S., Vangrow, J. S., Nelson, W. H., Pagano, J., Papageorge's, N. P., Khursheed, M., Harding, P. R., Khemka, M.: Halofenate: an effective hypolipemia- and hypouricemia-inducing drug. Curr. ther. Res. **15**, 902—906 (1973)

Ayvazian, J. H., Ayvazian, L. F.: A study of the hyperuricaemia induced by hydrochlorothiazide and acetazolamide separately and in combination. J. clin. Invest. **40**, 1961—1966 (1961)

Ball, G. V., Sorensen, L. B.: Pathogenesis of hyperuricemia in saturnine gout. New Engl. J. Med. **280**, 1199—1202 (1969)

Ballantyne, D., Strevens, E. A., Lawrie, T. D. V.: Relationship of plasma uric acid to plasma lipids and lipoproteins in subjects with peripheral vascular disease. Clin. chim. Acta **70**, 323—328 (1976)

Barlow, K. A.: Hyperlipidemia in primary gout. Metabolism **17**, 289—299 (1968)

Benedek, T. G.: Correlations of serum uric acid and lipid concentrations in normal, gouty and atherosclerotic men. Ann. intern. Med. **66**, 851—861 (1967)

Bengtsson, C., Johnsson, G., Sannerstedt, R., Werkö, L.: Effect of different doses of chlorthalidone on blood pressure, serum potassium and serum urate. Brit. med. J. **1975** I, 197—199

Bennett, J. S., Bond, J., Singer, I., Gottlieb, A. J.: Hypouricemia in Hodgkin's disease. Ann. intern. Med. **76**, 751—756 (1972)

Berger, L., Yü, T. F.: Renal function in gout. IV. An analysis of 524 gouty subjects including long term follow-up studies. Amer. J. Med. **59**, 605—613 (1975)

Berger, L., Yü, T. F., Atsmon, A., Kupper, S., Gutman, A. B.: Effect of reducing renal arterial blood pressure by balloon catheter on urate excretion in the dog. Proc. Soc. exp. Biol. (N.Y.) **115**, 58—61 (1964)

Bishop, C., Pfaff, W.: Immediate uricosuric effect of probenecid in normal humans. Proc. Soc. exp. Biol. (N.Y.) **87**, 346—348 (1955)

Bishop, C., Zimdahl, W. T., Talbott, J. H.: Uric acid in two patients with Wilson's disease (hepatolenticular degeneration). Proc. Soc. exp. Biol. (N.Y.) **86**, 440 (1954)

Blacket, R. B., Leelarthaepin, B., Palmer, A. J., Woodhill, J. M.: Coronary heart disease in young men: a study of 70 patients with a critical review of etiological factors. Aust. N.Z. J. Med. **3**, 39—62 (1973)

Bluestone, R., Lewis, B., Mervart, I.: Hyperlipoproteinaemia in gout. Ann. rheum. Dis. **30**, 134—137 (1971)

Bonsnes, R. W., Dana, E. S.: On the increased uric acid clearance following the intravenous infusion of hypertonic glucose solutions. J. clin. Invest. **25**, 386—388 (1946)

Bonsnes, R. W., Dill, L. V., Dana, E. S.: The effect of Diodrast on the normal uric acid clearance. J. clin. Invest. **23**, 776 (1944)

Bosco, J. S., Greenleaf, J. E., Kaye, R. L., Averkin, E. G.: Reduction of serum uric acid in young men during physical training. Amer. J. Cardiol. **25**, 46—52 (1970)

Bourke, E., Ledingham, J. G. G., Stokes, G. S.: Effects of intravenous ethacrynic acid on the renal handling of citrate and urate in man. Clin. Sci. **31**, 231—246 (1966)

Bowering, J., Calloway, D. H., Margen, S., Kaufmann, N. A.: Dietary protein level and uric acid metabolism in normal man. J. Nutr. **100**, 249—261 (1970)

Boyle, J. A., McKiddie, M., Buchanan, K. D., Jasani, M. K., Gray, H. W., Jackson, I. M. D., Buchanan, W. W.: Diabetes mellitus and gout. Blood sugar and plasma insulin responses to oral glucose in normal weight, overweight and gouty patients. Ann. rheum. Dis. **28** (Suppl. 1), 374—378 (1969)

Breckenridge, A.: Hypertension and hyperuricaemia. Lancet **1966 I**, 15—18

Brøchner-Mortensen, K.: Uric acid in blood and urine. Acta med. scand. [Suppl. 1] 84 (1937)

Brodan, V., Brodanov, A., Kuhn, E., Filip, J., Pechar, J.: Ammonia and uric acid formation after rapid intravenous fructose administration to healthy subjects and patients with compensated cirrhosis of the liver. Nutr. Metab. **19**, 233—241 (1975)

Bulpitt, C. J.: Blood urea changes in hypertensive patients according to therapy given, blood pressure control, and serum potassium levels. Brit. Heart J. **36**, 383—386 (1974)

Bulpitt, C. J.: Serum uric acid in hypertensive patients. Br. Heart J. **37**, 1210—1215 (1975)

Burch, R. E., Kurke, N.: The effect of lactate infusion on serum uric acid. Proc. Soc. exp. Biol. (N.Y.) **127**, 17—20 (1968)

Burns, J. J., Yü, T. F., Berger, L., Gutman, A. B.: Zoxazolamine-physiological disposition and uricosuric properties. Amer. J. Med. **25**, 401—408 (1958)

Burns, J. J., Yü, T. F., Ritterband, A., Perel, J. M., Gutman, A. B., Brodie, B. B.: A potent new uricosuric agent, the sulfoxide metabolite of the phenylbutazone analogue, G 25671. J. Pharmacol. exp. Ther. **119**, 418—426 (1957)

Cameron, J. S.: Uric acid and the kidney. Proc. roy. Soc. Med. **66**, 900—902 (1973)

Camus, J. P., Ghata, J., Guillien, P.: Etude de quelques fractions lipidiques du plasma dans la goutte. J. méd. liban. **3**, 261—269 (1969)

Cannon, P. J., Symchych, P. S., Martini, F. E., de: The distribution of urate in human and primate kidney. Proc. Soc. exp. Biol. (N.Y.) **129**, 278—284 (1968)

Cannon, P. J., Svahn, D. S., Martini, F. E., de: The influence of hypertonic saline infusions upon the fractional reabsorption of urate and other ions in normal and hypertensive man. Circulation **41**, 97—108 (1970)

Chait, A., Mancini, M., February, A. W., Lewis, B.: Clinical and metabolic study of alcoholic hyperlipidaemia. Lancet **1972 II**, 62—64

Chesley, L. C., Williams, L. O.: Renal glomerular and tubular function in relation to hyperuricemia of pre-eclampsia and eclampsia. Amer. J. Obstet. Gynecol. **50**, 367—375 (1945)

Clarkson, B. A.: Uric acid related to uraemic symptoms. Proceedings of the European Dialysis and Transplant Association, pp. 3—7. Amsterdam: Excerpta Medica 1966

Coburn, S. P., Seidenberg, M., Mertz, E. T.: Clearance of uric acid, urea and creatinine in Down's syndrome. J. appl. Physiol. **24**, 579—580 (1967)

Coburn, S. P., Sirlin, E. M., Mertz, E. T.: Metabolism of N^{15} labelled uric acid in Down's syndrome. Metabolism **17**, 560—562 (1968)

Coe, F. L., Kavalach, A. G.: Hypercalciuria and hyperuricosuria in patients with calcium nephrolithiasis. New Engl. J. Med. **291**, 1344—1350 (1974)

Cohen, R. D., Woods, H. F.: Clinical and biochemical aspects of lactic acidosis. Oxford-London: Blackwell 1976

Connon, A. F., Wadsworth, R. J.: An evaluation of serum uric acid estimations in toxemia of pregnancy. Aust. N.Z. J. Obstet. Gynaec. **8**, 197—201 (1968)

Coronary Drug Project Research Group: Serum uric acid: Its association with other risk factors and with mortality in coronary heart disease. J. chron. Dis. **29**, 557—569 (1976)

Cowdrey, S. C.: Hyperuricemia in infectious mononucleosis. J. Amer. med. Ass. **196**, 319—321 (1966)

Cullen, J. H., Levine, M., Fiore, J. M.: Studies of hyperuricaemia produced by pyrazinamide. Amer. J. Med. **32**, 587—596 (1957)

Danovitch, G. M., Weinberger, J., Berlyne, G. M.: Uric acid in advanced renal failure. Clin. Sci. **43**, 331—341 (1972)

Darlington, L. G., Scott, J. T.: Plasma levels in gout. Ann. rheum. Dis. **31**, 487—489 (1972)

Davies, D. F., Shock, N. W.: The variability of measurement of inulin and diodrast tests of kidney function. J. clin. Invest. **29**, 491—495 (1950)

Denis, G., Launay, M. P.: Carbohydrate intolerance in gout. Metabolism **18**, 770—775 (1969)

Diamond, H. S., Carter, A. C., Feldman, E. B.: Abnormal regulation of carbohydrate metabolism in primary gout. Ann. rheum. Dis. **33**, 554—562 (1974)

Diamond, H. S., Lazarus, R., Kaplan, D., Halberstam, D.: Effect of urine flow rate on uric acid excretion in man. Arthr. and Rheum. **15**, 338—346 (1972)

Diamond, H. S., Meisel, A., Sharon, E., Holden, D., Cacatian, A.: Hyperuricosuria and increased tubular secretion of urate in sickle cell anemia. Amer. J. Med. **59**, 796—802 (1975)

Dollery, C. T., Duncan, H., Schumer, B.: Hyperuricaemia related to treatment of hypertension. Brit. med. J. **1960 II**, 832—835

Dorhout Mees, E. J., Assendelft, P. B., Niewenhus, M. G.: Elevation of uric acid clearance caused by inappropriate antidiuretic hormone secretion. Acta. med. scand. **189**, 69—72 (1971)

Dosman, J. A., Crawhall, J. C., Klassen, G. A.: Uric acid kinetic studies in the immediate post-myocardial infarction period. Metabolism **24**, 473—480 (1975)

Drenick, E. J., Swendseid, M. E., Blahd, W. H., Tuttle, S. G.: Prolonged starvation as a treatment for severe obesity. J. Amer. med. Ass. **187**, 100—105 (1964)

Duarte, C. G., Bland, J. H.: Calcium, phosphorus and uric acid clearances after intravenous administration of chlorothiazide. Metabolism **14**, 211—219 (1965)

Dubin, A., Kushner, D. S., Bronsky, D., Pascale, L. R.: Hyperuricemia in hypoparathyroidism. Metabolism **5**, 703—709 (1956)

Dujovne, C. A., Azarnoff, D. L., Huffman, D. H., Pentiklainen, P., Hurwitz, A., Shoeman, D. W.: One-year trials with halofenate, clofibrate and placebo. Clin. Pharmacol. Ther. **19**, 352—359 (1976)

Eisen, A. Z., Seegmiller, J. E.: Uric acid metabolism in psoriasis. J. clin. Invest. **40**, 1486—1494 (1961)

Emmerson, B. T.: Chronic lead nephropathy: the diagnostic use of calcium EDTA and the association with gout. Aust. Ann. Med. **12**, 310—324 (1963)

Emmerson, B. T.: The renal excretion of urate in chronic lead nephropathy. Aust. Ann. Med. **14**, 295—303 (1965)

Emmerson, B. T.: Metals and the kidney. In: Black, D. A. K. (Ed.): Renal Disease, 2nd Ed., p. 575. Oxford: Blackwell 1967

Emmerson, B. T.: Alteration of urate metabolism by weight reduction. Aust. N.Z. J. Med. **3**, 410—412 (1973)

Emmerson, B. T.: Effect of oral fructose on urate production. Ann. rheum. Dis. **33**, 276—280 (1974)

Emmerson, B. T., Gordon, R. B., Johnson, L. A.: Urate kinetics in hypoxanthineguanine phosphoribosyltransferase deficiency: their significance for the understanding of gout. Quart. J. Med. **45**, 49—61 (1976a)

Emmerson, B. T., Knowles, B. R.: Triglyceride concentrations in primary gout and gout of chronic lead nephropathy. Metabolism **20**, 721—729 (1971)

Emmerson, B. T., Ravenscroft, P. J., Williams, G.: The effect of urine flow rate on urate clearance. Z. klin. Chem. Biochem. **14**, 285—286 (1976b)

Emmerson, B. T., Row, P. G.: An evaluation of the pathogenesis of the gouty kidney. Kidney Int. **8**, 65—71 (1975)

Emmerson, B. T., Thompson, L., Mitchell, K.: Dose response relationship of a uricosuric diuretic. J. clin. Chem. Biochem. **14**, 286 (1976c)

Epstein, F. H., Pigeon, G.: Experimental urate nephropathy: studies of the distribution of urate in renal tissue. Nephron **1**, 144—157 (1964)

Evans, J. G., Prior, I. A. M., Harvey, H. P. B.: Relation of serum uric acid to body bulk, haemoglobin, and alcohol intake in two South Pacific Polynesian populations. Ann. rheum. Dis. **27**, 319—325 (1968)

Fadel, H. E., Northrop, G., Misenhimer, H. R.: Hyperuricemia in pre-eclampsia. A reappraisal. Amer. J. Obstet. Gynec. **125**, 640—647 (1976)

Fallon, H. J., Frei, E. M., III., Block, J., Seegmiller, J. E.: The uricosuria and orotic aciduria induced by 6-Azauridine. J. clin. Invest. **40**, 1906—1914 (1961)

Feldman, E. B., Wallace, S. L.: Hypertriglyceridaemia in gout. Circulation **29**, 508—513 (1964)

Ferris, T. F., Gorden, P.: Effect of angiotensin and norepinephrine upon urate clearance in man. Amer. J. Med. **44**, 359—365 (1968)

Fine, R. N., Strauss, J., Donnell, G. N.: Hyperuricemia in glycogen-storage disease type I. Amer. J. Dis. Child. **112**, 572—576 (1966)

Fox, I. H., Halperin, M. L., Goldstein, M. B., Marliss, E. B.: Renal excretion of uric acid during prolonged fasting. Metabolism **25**, 551—559 (1976)

Fox, I. H., Kelley, W. N.: Studies on the mechanism of fructose-induced hyperuricemia in man. Metabolism **21**, 713—721 (1972)

Fredrickson, D. S., Levy, R. I.: Familial hyperlipoproteinaemia. In: Stanbury, J. B., Wyngaarden, J. B., Fredrickson, D. S. (Eds.): The Metabolic Basis of Inherited Disease, 3rd Ed., pp. 545—614. New York: McGraw Hill 1972

Friedman, M.: The effect of glycine on the production and excretion of uric acid. J. clin. Invest. **26**, 815—819 (1947)

Fulop, M., Horowitz, M., Jaffe, A. A.: Lactic acidosis in pulmonary edema due to left ventricular failure. Ann. intern. Med. **79**, 180—186 (1973)

Garrick, R., Bauer, G. E., Ewan, C. E., Neale, F. C.: Serum uric acid in normal and hypertensive Australian subjects. Aust. N.Z. J. Med. **2**, 351—356 (1972)

Gaut, Z. N., Pocelinko, R., Solomon, H. M., Thomas, G. B.: Oral glucose tolerance, plasma insulin, and uric acid excretion in man during chronic administration of nicotinic acid. Metabolism **20**, 1031—1035 (1971)

Gebbie, T., Prior, I. A. M.: Alcoholic hyperlipaemia. Med. J. Aust. **2**, 769—772 (1967)

Gershon, S. L., Fox, I. H.: Pharmacologic effects of nicotinic acid on human purine metabolism. J. Lab. clin. Med. **84**, 179—186 (1974)

Gertler, M. M., Garn, S. M., Levine, S. A.: Serum uric acid in relation to age and physique in health and in coronary heart disease. Ann. intern. Med. **34**, 1421—1431 (1951)

Gibson, H. V., Doisy, E. A.: A note on the effect of some organic acids upon the uric acid excretion of man. J. biol. Chem. **55**, 605 (1923)

Gibson, T., Grahame, R.: Gout and hyperlipidaemia. Ann. rheum. Dis. **33**, 298—303 (1974)

Gibson, T., Sims, H. P., Jimenez, S. A.: Hypouricaemia and increased renal urate clearance associated with hyperparathyroidism. Ann. rheum. Dis. **35**, 372—376 (1976)

Ginsberg, H., Olefsky, J., Farquhar, J. W., Reaven, G. M.: Moderate ethanol ingestion and plasma triglyceride levels. A study in normal and hypertriglyceridemic persons. Ann. intern. Med. **80**, 143—149 (1974)

Goldfinger, S., Klinenberg, J. R., Seegmiller, J. E.: Renal retention of uric acid induced by infusions of β-hydroxy-butyrate and acetoacetate. New Engl. J. Med. **272**, 351—355 (1965)

Gordon, R. D., Symonds, E. M., Wilmshurst, E. G., Pawsey, C. G. K.: Plasma renin activity, plasma angiotensin and plasma and urinary electrolytes in normal and toxemic pregnancy, including a prospective study. Clin. Sci. molec. Med. **45**, 115—127 (1973)

Grahame, R., Scott, J. T.: Clinical survey of 354 patients with gout. Ann. rheum. Dis. **29**, 461—468 (1970)

Greene, M. L., Marcus, R., Aurbach, G. D., Kazam, E. S., Seegmiller, J. E.: Hypouricemia due to isolated renal tubular defect. Amer. J. Med. **53**, 361—367 (1972)

Gresham, G. E., Keller, M. D.: Hyperuricaemia and chronic renal disease. J. Chron. Dis. **23**, 755—762 (1971)

Griebsch, A., Zollner, N.: Normalwerte der Plasmaharnsäure in Süddeutschland. Z. Klin. Chem. Biochem. **11**, 346—356 (1973)

Gulati, O. P.: Cited in Editorial: Renal Disease and Urate Excretion. J. Ass. Phycns India **22**, 349—351 (1974)

Harris-Jones, J. N.: Hyperuricaemia and essential hypercholesterolaemia. Lancet **1957 I**, 857

Heinemann, H. O., Martini, F. E., de, Laragh, J. H.: The effect of chlorothiazide on renal excretion of electrolytes and free water. Amer. J. Med. **26**, 853—861 (1959)

Hensley, M. J., Read, D. J. C.: Intermittent obstruction of the upper airway during sleep causing profound hypoxaemia. Aust. N.Z. J. Med. **6**, 481—486 (1976)

Heuckenkamp, P.-U., Zollner, N.: Fructose-induced hyperuricaemia. Lancet **1971 I**, 808—809

Hodari, A. A., Smery, R., Bumpus, F. M.: A renin-like substance in the human placenta. Obstet. Gynec. **29**, 313—317 (1967)

Hollister, L. E., Overall, J. E., Snow, H. L.: Relationship of obesity to serum triglyceride, cholesterol and uric acid and to plasma glucose levels. Amer. J. clin. Nutr. **20**, 777—782 (1967)

Holmes, E. W., Kelley, W. N., Wyngaarden, J. B.: The kidney and uric acid excretion in man. Kidney Int. **2**, 115—118 (1972)

Howell, R. R., Ashton, D. M., Wyngaarden, J. B.: Glucose-6-phosphatase deficiency glycogen storage disease. Studies on the interrelationships of carbohydrate, lipid and purine abnormalities. Pediatrics **29**, 553—565 (1962)

Hülsmann, W. C., Eijkenboom, W. H. M., Koster, J. F., Fernandes, J.: Glucose-6-phosphatase deficiency and hyperlipidaemia. Clin. chim. Acta **30**, 775—778 (1970)

Ingbar,S.H., Kass,E.H., Burnett,C.N., Relman,A.S., Burrows,B.A., Sesson,J.H.: Effects of ACTH and cortisone on renal tubular transport of uric acid, phosphorus and electrolytes in patients with normal renal and adrenal function. J. Lab. clin. Med. **38**, 533—541 (1951)

Isomaki,H., Kreus,K.-E.: Serum and urinary uric acid in respiratory acidosis. Acta med. scand. **184**, 293—296 (1968)

Jackson,W.P.U., Harris,F.: Gout with hyperparathyroidism: Report of case with examination of synovial fluid. Brit. med. J. **1965 II**, 211

Jakovcic,S., Sorensen,L.B.: Studies of uric acid metabolism in glycogen storage disease associated with gouty arthritis. Arthr. and Rheum. **10**, 129—134 (1967)

Jensen,J., Blankenhorn,D.H., Kornerup,V.: Blood-uric-acid levels in familial hypercholesterolaemia. Lancet **1966 I**, 298—300

Johnson,R.H., Walton,J.L., Krebs,H.A., Williamson,D.H.: Metabolic fuels during and after severe exercise in athletes and non-athletes. Lancet **1969 I**, 452—455

Jones,D.P., Losowsky,M.S., Davidson,C.S., Lieber,C.S.: Effects of ethanol on plasma lipids in man. J. Lab. clin. Med. **62**, 675—682 (1963)

Kahn,M.F.: Goutte, obésité et plaisirs de la table. (Comparison entre 40 goutteux et 40 témoins). Nouv. Presse méd. **5**, 1897—1898 (1976)

Katz,J.L., Weiner,H., Gutman,A., Yü,T.-F.: Hyperuricemia, gout, and the executive suite. J. Amer. med. Ass. **224**, 1251—1257 (1973)

Kaufman,J.M.: Hyperuricemia in mongolism. New Engl. J. Med. **276**, 953—956 (1967)

Kaye,J.P., Galton,D.J.: Triglyceride production rates in patients with type IV hypertriglyceridaemia. Lancet **1975 I**, 1005—1007

Kelley,W.N., Goldfinger,S.E., Hardy,H.L.: Hyperuricemia in chronic beryllium disease. Ann. intern. Med. **70**, 977—983 (1969)

Kelley,W.N., Greene,M.L., Fox,I.H., Rosenbloom,R.M., Levy,R.I., Seegmiller,J.E.: Effects of orotic acid on purine and lipoprotein metabolism in man. Metabolism **19**, 1025—1053 (1970)

Kelley,W.N., Rosenbloom,F.M., Seegmiller,J.E.: The effects of azathioprine (Imuran) on purine synthesis in clinical disorders of purine metabolism. J. clin. Invest. **46**, 1518—1529 (1967)

Kelley,W.N., Rosenbloom,F.M., Seegmiller,J.E., Howell,R.R.: Excessive production of uric acid in type I glycogen storage disease. J. Pediat. **72**, 488—496 (1968)

Khachadurian,A.K., Arslanian,M.J.: Hypouricemia due to renal uricosuria. Ann. intern. Med. **78**, 547—550 (1973)

Kinsey,D.: Gout and hyperuricaemia in hypertensive patients 15–25 years following lumbodorsal sympathectomy. Arthr. and Rheum. **6**, 778—779 (1963)

Kippen,J., Whitehouse,M.W., Klinenberg,J.R.: Pharmacology of uricosuric drugs. Ann. rheum. Dis. **33**, 391—396 (1974)

Klein,W.W.: Leberfunktion bei Gicht und asymptomatischer Hyperurikämie. Z. Rheumaforsch. **30**, 230—235 (1971).

Knochel,J.P., Dotin,L.N., Hamburger,R.J.: Heat stress, exercise and muscle injury: Effects on urate metabolism and renal function. Ann. intern. Med. **81**, 321—328 (1974)

Krakoff,I.H., Balis,M.E.: Studies on the uricogenic effect of 2-substituted thiadiazoles in man. J. clin. Invest. **38**, 907—915 (1959)

Kramer,H.J., Lu,E., Gonick,H.E.: Organic acid excretion patterns in gout. Ann. rheum. Dis. **31**, 137—144 (1972)

Kreisberg,R.A., Owen,W.C., Siegal,A.M.: Ethanol-induced hyperlactic-acidemia: Inhibition of lactate utilization. J. clin. Invest. **50**, 166—185 (1971)

Kuntz,D., Roques,C., Paolaggi,F., Ryckewaert,A.: Étude comparative de la triglycéridémie, de la lipidémie, de la glycémie et de l'index pondéral chez les hyperuricémiques et les normo-uricémiques. Path. et Biol. (Paris) **17**, 399—403 (1969)

Lajtha,L.G., Vane,J.R.: Dependence of bone marrow cells on the liver for purine supply. Nature (Lond.) **182**, 191—192 (1958)

Lee,D.B., Drinkard,J.P., Rosen,V.J., Gonick,H.C.: The adult Fanconi syndrome. Observations on etiology, morphology, renal function and mineral metabolism in three patients. Medicine (Baltimore) **51**, 107—138 (1972)

Leeper,R.D., Benua,R.S., Brener,J.L., Rawson,R.W.: Hyperuricemia in myxedema. J. clin. Endocr. **20**, 1457—1466 (1960)

Lefèvre,A., Adler,H., Lieber,C.S.: Effect of ethanol on ketone metabolism. J. clin. Invest. **49**, 1775—1782 (1970)

Lefkovits,A.M., Herman,J.T., Irving,C.C.: Cessation of gout following portacaval shunt. J. Amer. med. Ass. **205**, 213—214 (1968)

Lemieux,G., Kiss,A., Gougoux,A., Vinay,P.: Tienilic acid (Ticrynafen): a new diuretic with uricosuric properties in man and dog. J. clin. Chem. Biochem. **14**, 306 (1976)

Lemieux,G., Vinay,P., Gougoux,A., Michaud,G.: Nature of the uricosuric action of benziodarone. Amer. J. Physiol. **224**, 1440—1449 (1973)

Lieber,C.S.: The metabolism of alcohol. Sci. Amer. **234**, 25—33 (1976)

Lieber,C.S., Jones,D.P., Losowsky,M.S., Davidson,C.S.: Interrelation of uric acid and ethanol metabolism in man. J. clin. Invest. **41**, 1863—1870 (1962)

Losowsky,M.S., Jones,D.P., Davidson,C.S., Lieber,C.S.: Studies of alcoholic hyperlipemia and its mechanism. Amer. J. Med. **35**, 794—803 (1963)

Losowsky,M.S., Kenward,D.H.: Lipid metabolism in acute and chronic renal failure. J. Lab. clin. Med. **71**, 736—743 (1968)

MacLachlan,M.J., Rodnan,G.P.: Effects of food, fast, and alcohol on serum uric acid and acute attacks of gout. Amer. J. Med. **42**, 38—57 (1967)

McPhaul,J.J.: Hyperuricaemia and urate excretion in chronic renal disease. Metabolism **17**, 430—438 (1968)

Maenpaa,P.H., Raivio,K.O., Kekomaki,M.P.: Liver adenine nucleotides: Fructose-induced depletion and its effect on protein synthesis. Science **161**, 1253—1254 (1968)

Manuel,M.A., Steele,T.H.: Changes in renal urate handling after prolonged thiazide treatment. Amer. J. Med. **57**, 741—746 (1974)

Maria,F.J., de, See,H.Y.C.: Role of the placenta in pre-eclampsia. Amer. J. Obstet. Gynec. **94**, 471—476 (1966)

Martinez-Maldonado,M.: Polycystic kidney disease and hyperuricemia. Ann. intern. Med. **80**, 116 (1974)

Meisel,A., Diamond,H.: Effect of vasopressin on uric acid excretion: evidence for distal nephron reabsorption of urate in man. Clin. Sci. molec. Med. **51**, 33—40 (1976)

Mertz,D.P.: Gicht, Diabetes Mellitus und Fettleber. Münch. med. Wschr. **5**, 180—185 (1972)

Mertz,D.P., Schwoerer,P., Babucke,G.: On the classification of hyperlipoproteinaemia in primary gout. Dtsch. med. Wschr. **15**, 600—604 (1972)

Michelis,M.F., Warms,P.C., Fusco,R.P., Davis,B.B.: Hypouricemia and hyperuricosuria in Laennec cirrhosis. Arch. intern. Med. **134**, 681—683 (1974)

Mielants,H., Veys,E.M., Weerat,A., de: Gout and its relation to lipid metabolism. I. Serum uric acid, lipid and lipoprotein levels in gout. II. Correlation between uric acid, lipid, and lipoprotein levels in gout. Ann. rheum. Dis. **32**, 501—509 (1973)

Mintz,D.H., Canary,J.J., Carreon,G., Kyle,L.H.: Hyperuricemia in hyperparathyroidism. New Engl. J. Med. **265**, 112—115 (1961)

Monkus,E., Nyhan,W.L., Fogel,B.J., Yankow,S.: Concentrations of uric acid in the serum of neonatal infants and their mothers. Amer. J. Obstet. Gynec. **108**, 91—97 (1970)

Morgan,J.M., Hartley,M.W., Miller,R.E.: Nephropathy in chronic lead poisoning. Arch. intern. Med. **118**, 17—29 (1966)

Myers,A.R., Epstein,F.H., Dodge,H.J., Mikkelsen,W.M.: The relationship of serum uric acid to risk factors in coronary heart disease. Amer. J. Med. **45**, 520—528 (1968)

Nanra,R.S.: Personal communication (1976)

Newcombe,D.S.: Ethanol metabolism and uric acid. Metabolism **21**, 1193—1203 (1972)

Newcombe,D.S.: Gouty arthritis and polycystic kidney disease. Ann. intern. Med. **79**, 605—606 (1973)

Nicholls,A., Scott,J.T.: Effect of weight loss on plasma and urinary levels of uric acid. Lancet **1972 II**, 1223—1224

Nicholls,A., Snaith,M.L., Scott,J.T.: Effect of oestrogen therapy on plasma and urinary levels of uric acid. Brit. med. J. **1973 I**, 449—451

Nichols,J., Miller,A.T., Hiatt,E.P.: Influence of muscular exercise on uric acid excretion in men. J. appl. Physiol. **3**, 501—507 (1951)

Olefsky,J.M., Farquhar,J.W., Reaven,G.M.: Reappraisal of the role of insulin in hypertriglyceridemia. Amer. J. Med. **57**, 551—560 (1974)

Ostberg, Y.: Renal urate deposits in chronic renal insufficiency. Acta med. scand. **183**, 197—201 (1968)

Ostrander, L. D., Lamphiear, D. E., Block, W. D., Johnson, B. C., Ravenscroft, C., Epstein, F. H.: Relationship of serum lipid concentrations to alcohol consumption. Arch. intern. Med. **134**, 451—456 (1974)

Pablico, R. C., Canfield, C. J., Barry, K. G.: The effects of acute total caloric starvation on uric acid metabolism in obese human subjects. Clin. Res. **13**, 45 (1965)

Padova, J., Bendersky, G.: Hyperuricemia in diabetic ketoacidosis. New Engl. J. Med. **267**, 530—534 (1962)

Padova, J., Patchefsky, A., Onesti, G., Faludi, G., Bendersky, G.: The effect of glucose loads on renal uric acid excretion in diabetic patients. Metabolism **13**, 507—512 (1964)

Peenen, H. J., Van: The causes of nonazotemic hyperuricemia. Amer. J. clin. Pathol. **55**, 698—700 (1971)

Pell, S., D'Alonzo, C. A.: The prevalence of chronic disease among problem drinkers. Arch. environ. Hlth. **16**, 679—684 (1968)

Perheentupa, J., Raivio, K.: Fructose-induced hyperuricaemia. Lancet **1967 II**, 528—531

Pollak, V. E., Nettles, J. B.: The kidney in toxemia of pregnancy. A clinical and pathological study based on renal biopsies. Medicine (Baltimore) **39**, 469—526 (1960)

Postlethwaite, A. E., Kelley, W. N.: Uricosuric effect of radio contrast agents. A study in man of four commonly used preparations. Ann. intern. Med. **74**, 845—852 (1971)

Postlethwaite, A. E., Kelley, W. N.: Studies on the mechanism of ethambutol-induced hyperuricemia. Arthr. and Rheum. **15**, 403—409 (1972)

Postlethwaite, A. E., Ramsdell, M., Kelley, W. N.: Uricosuric effect of an anticholinergic agent in hyperuricemic subjects. Arch. intern. Med. **134**, 270—275 (1974)

Praetorius, E., Kirk, J. E.: Hypouricaemia: with evidence for tubular elimination of uric acid. J. Lab. clin. Med. **35**, 865—868 (1950)

Raivio, K. O., Becker, M. A., Meyer, L. J., Greene, M. L., Nuki, G., Seegmiller, J. E.: Stimulation of human purine synthesis de novo by fructose infusion. Metabolism **24**, 861—869 (1975)

Ramsay, L., Levine, D., Shelton, J., Branch, R., Auty, R.: Alkalosis and urate clearance. Ann. intern. Med. **83**, 903—904 (1975)

Ramsdell, C. M., Postlethwaite, A. E., Kelley, W. N.: Uricosuric effect of glyceryl guaiacolate. J. Rheumatol. **1**, 114—116 (1974)

Ravenscroft, P. J., Sands, J. M., Emmerson, B. T.: Studies of the uricosuric action of the hypolipidemic drug halofenate. Clin. Pharmacol. Ther. **14**, 547—551 (1973)

Redman, C. W., Beilin, L. J., Bonnar, J., Wilkinson, R. H.: Plasma-urate measurements in predicting fetal death in hypertensive pregnancy. Lancet **1974 I**, 1370—1373

Redman, C. W., Bonnar, J., Beilin, L. J., McNeilly, A. S.: Prolactin in hypertensive pregnancy. Brit. med. J. **1976 I**, 304—306

Reese, O. G., Steele, T. H.: Renal transport of urate during diuretic-induced hypouricemia. Amer. J. Med. **60**, 973—978 (1976)

Richet, G.: Some aspects of uric acid metabolism in chronic renal failure. In: Berlyne, G. M. (Ed.): Nutrition in Renal Disease. Edinburgh: Livingstone 1968

Richet, G., Albahary, C., Ardaillou, R., Sultan, C., Morel-Maroger, A.: Le rien du saturnisme chronique. Rev. franc. Étud. clin. biol. **9**, 188—196 (1964)

Richet, G., Mignon, F., Ardaillou, R.: Goutte secondaire des néphropathies chroniques. Presse méd. **73**, 633—638 (1965)

Rieselbach, R. E., Sorensen, L. B., Shelp, W. D., Steele, T. H.: Diminished renal urate secretion per nephron as a basis for primary gout. Ann. intern. Med. **73**, 359—366 (1970)

Rondier, J., Truffert, J., Go, A., le, Brouilhet, H., Saporta, L., Gennes, J. L., de, Delbarre, F.: Goutte et hyperlipidémies (étude portant sur 50 goutteux et sur 50 sujets non gouttes). Rev. europ. Étud. clin. biol. **15**, 959—968 (1970)

Rosenfeld, J. B.: Effect on long term allopurinol administration on serial GFR in normotensive and hypertensive hyperuricaemic subjects. In: Sperling, O., De Vries, A., Wyngaarden, J. B. (Eds.): Purine Metabolism in Man. Advances in Experimental Medicine and Biology, Vol. XLI B, pp. 581—596. New York: Plenum 1974

Sahebjami, H., Scalettar, R.: Effects of fructose infusion on lactate and uric acid metabolism. Lancet **1971 I**, 366—369

Saker, B. M., Tofler, O. B., Burvill, M. J., Reilly, K. A.: Alcohol consumption and gout. Med. J. Aust. **1**, 1213 (1967)

Sandler, M., Baldock, E.: In vivo monamine oxidase activity in toxaemia of pregnancy. J. Obstet. Gynaec. **70**, 279—283 (1963)

Sarre, H., Mertz, D. P.: Sekundäre Gicht bei Niereninsuffizienz. Klin. Wschr. **43**, 1134—1140 (1965)

Schaffer, N. K., Dill, L. V., Cadden, J. F.: Uric acid clearance in normal pregnancy and pre-eclampsia. J. clin. Invest. **22**, 201—206 (1943)

Schapiro, R. H., Scheig, R. L., Drummey, G. D., Mendelson, J. H., Isselbacher, K. J.: Effect of prolonged ethanol ingestion on the transport and metabolism of lipids in man. New Engl. J. Med. **272**, 610—615 (1965)

Schlosstein, L., Kippen, I., Bluestone, R., Whitehouse, M. W., Klinenberg, J. R.: Association between hypouricemia and jaundice. Ann. rheum. Dis. **33**, 308—312 (1974)

Schlosstein, L. H., Kippen, I., Whitehouse, M. W., Bluestone, R., Paulus, H. E., Klinenberg, J. R.: Studies with some novel uricosuric agents and their metabolites: correlation between clinical activity and drug-induced displacement of urate from its albumin-binding sites. J. Lab. clin. Med. **82**, 412—418 (1973)

Schneeweiss, J., Poole, G. W.: Hyperuricaemia due to pyrazinamide. Brit. med. J. **1960 II**, 830—832

Schonfeld, G., Kudzma, D. J.: Type IV hyperlipoproteinemia: a critical appraisal. Arch. Intern. Med. **132**, 55—62 (1973)

Scott, J. T., McCallum, F. M., Holloway, V. P.: Starvatin, ketosis and uric acid excretion. Clin. Sci. **27**, 209—221 (1964)

Scott, J. T., Dixon, A. St. J., Bywaters, E. G. L.: Association of hyperuricaemia and gout with hyperparathyroidism. Brit. med. J. **1964 I**, 1070—1073

Seegmiller, J. E., Grayzel, A. I., Laster, L., Liddle, L.: Uric acid production in gout. J. clin. Invest. **40**, 1304—1314 (1961)

Seitchik, J., Szutka, A., Alper, C.: Further studies on the metabolism of N^{15}-labelled uric acid in normal and toxemic pregnant women. Amer. J. Obstet. Gynec. **76**, 1151—1155 (1958)

Semple, P. F., Carswell, W., Boyle, J. A.: Serial studies of the renal clearance of urate and inulin during pregnancy and after the puerperium in normal women. Clin. Sci. molec. Med. **47**, 559—565 (1974)

Shelp, W. P., Rieselbach, R. E.: Increased bidirectional urate transport per nephron following unilateral nephrectomy. Amer. Soc. Nephrol. Abst. 24 (1968)

Shelp, W. D., Steele, T. H., Rieselbach, R. E.: Comparison of urinary phosphate, urate and magnesium excretion following parathyroid hormone administration to normal man. Metabolism **18**, 63—70 (1969)

Shulman, J. D., Lustberg, T. J., Seegmiller, J. E.: Hyperuricemia in branched chain ketoaciduria (maple syrup urine disease). Arthr. and Rheum. **13**, 347 a (1970)

Simkin, P. A., Skeith, M. D., Healy, L. A.: Suppression of uric acid secretion in a patient with renal hypouricaemia. Advanc. exp. med. Biol. [B] **41**, 723—728 (1974)

Simon, N. M., Smucker, J. E., O'Connor, V. J., Greco, F., del: Differential uric acid excretion in essential and renal hypertension. Circulation **39**, 121—125 (1969)

Sirota, J. H., Yü, T.-F., Gutman, A. B.: Effect of benemid (p-[di-n-propyl-sulfamyl]benzoic acid) on urate clearance and other discrete renal functions in gouty subjects. J. clin. Invest. **31**, 692—701 (1952)

Skeith, M. D., Healey, L. A., Cutler, R. E.: Urate excretion during mannitol and glucose diuresis. J. Lab. clin. Med. **70**, 213—220 (1967)

Skeith, M. D., Healey, L. A., Cutler, R. E.: Effect of phloridzin on uric acid excretion in man. Amer. J. Physiol. **219**, 1080—1082 (1970)

Sorensen, L. B., Benke, P. J.: Biochemical evidence for a distinct type of primary gout. Nature (Lond.) **213**, 1122—1123 (1967)

Sorensen, L. B., Levinson, D. J.: Clinical evaluation of benzbromarone. A new uricosuric drug. Arthr. and Rheum. **19**, 183—190 (1976)

Sougin-Mibashan, R., Horwitz, M.: The uricosuric action of ethyl biscoumacetate. Lancet **1955 I**, 1191—1197

Sperling, O., Weinberger, A., Oliver, I., Liberman, U. A., Vries, A., de: Hypouricemia, hypercalciuria and decreased bone density. A new hereditary syndrome. Advanc. exp. med. Biol. **41**, 717—721 (1974)

Stamm, W. E., Webb, D. I.: Partial deficiency of hepatic glucose-6-phosphatase in an adult patient. Arch. intern. Med. **135**, 1107—1109 (1975)

Steele, T. H.: Evidence for altered renal urate reabsorption during changes in volume of the extracellular fluid. J. Lab. clin. Med. **74**, 288—299 (1969)

Steele, T. H.: Urate secretion in man: The pyrazinamide suppression test. Ann. intern. Med. **79**, 734—737 (1973)

Steele, T. H., Manuel, M. A., Boner, G.: Diuretics, urate excretion and sodium reabsorption: Effect of acetazolamide and urinary alkalinization. Nephron **14**, 49—61 (1975)

Steele, T. H., Oppenheimer, S.: Factors affecting urate excretion following diuretic administration in man. Amer. J. Med. **47**, 564—574 (1969)

Steele, T. H., Rieselbach, R. E.: The renal mechanism for urate homeostasis in normal man. Amer. J. Med. **43**, 868—875 (1967a)

Steele, T. H., Rieselbach, R. E.: The contribution of residual nephrons within the chronically diseased kidney to urate homeostasis in man. Amer. J. Med. **43**, 876—886 (1967b)

Stein, J. H., Ferris, T. F., Huprich, J. E., Smith, T. C., Osgood, R. W.: Effect of renal vasodilatation on the distribution of cortical blood flow in the kidney of the dog. J. clin. Invest. **50**, 1429—1438 (1971)

Stein, H. B., Hasan, A., Fox, I. H.: Ascorbic acid-induced uricosuria. A consequence of megavitamin therapy. Ann. intern. Med. **84**, 385—388 (1976)

Stormont, D., Davies, C., Emmerson, B. T.: Urate production in heterozygotes for glucose-6-phosphatase deficiency. Clin. chim. Acta **71**, 303—308 (1976)

Suki, W. N., Hull, A. R., Rector, F. C., Seldin, D. W.: Mechanism of the effect of thiazide diuretics on calcium and uric acid. J. clin. Invest. **46**, 1121 (1967)

Suki, W. N., Martinez-Maldonado, M., Rouse, D., Terry, A.: Effect of expansion of extracellular fluid volume on renal phosphate handling. J. clin. Invest. **48**, 1888—1894 (1969)

Thompson, G. R., Mikkelsen, W. M., Willis III, P. W.: The uricosuric effect of certain oral anticoagulant drugs. Arthr. and Rheum. **2**, 383—388 (1959)

Tran, M. H., Lellouch, J., Richard, J. L.: Fat body mass. II. Its relationships with some biological parameters, blood pressure and physical training in a population of 8660 men aged 20 to 55. Biomedicine **18**, 499—506 (1973)

Trevaks, G., Lovell, R. R. H.: Effect of atromid and its components on uric acid excretion and on gout. Ann. rheum. Dis. **24**, 572—575 (1965)

Verger, D., Leroux-Robert, C., Ganter, P., Richet, G.: Les tophus goutteux de la médullaire rénale des urémiques chroniques. Nephron **4**, 356—370 (1967)

Weiner, I. M., Tinker, J. P.: Pharmacology of pyrazinamide; metabolic and renal function studies related to the mechanism of drug-induced urate retention. J. Pharmacol. exp. Ther. **180**, 411 (1972)

Weinman, E. J., Eknoyan, G., Suki, W. N.: The influence of the extracellular fluid volume on the tubular reabsorption of uric acid. J. clin. Invest. **55**, 283—291 (1975)

Weinstein, B., Irrevere, F., Watkin, D. M.: Lung carcinoma, hypouricemia and aminoaciduria. Amer. J. Med. **39**, 520—526 (1965)

Whitehouse, F. W., Cleary, W. J.: Diabetes mellitus in patients with gout. J. Amer. med. Ass. **197**, 73—76 (1966)

Wiedemann, E., Rose, H. B., Schwartz, E.: Plasma lipoproteins, glucose tolerance and insulin response in primary gout. Amer. J. Med. **53**, 299—307 (1972)

Wiener, K.: Uraemia and hyperuricaemia in acute myocardial infarction. Clin. Chim. Acta **73**, 45—50 (1976)

Wilson, D. M., Goldstein, N. P.: Renal urate excretion in patients with Wilson's Disease. Kidney Int. **4**, 331—336 (1973)

Woods, H. F., Alberti, K. G. M. M.: Dangers of intravenous fructose. Lancet **1972 II**, 1354—1356

Woods, H. F., Eggleston, L. V., Krebs, H. A.: The cause of hepatic accumulation of fructose loading. Biochem. J. **119**, 501—510 (1970)

Wyngaarden, J. B.: The effect of phenylbutazone on uric acid metabolism in two normal subjects. J. clin. Invest. **34**, 256—262 (1955)

Yü, T. F., Berger, L., Gutman, A. B.: Hypoglycemic and uricosuric properties of acetohexamide and hydroxyhexamide. Metabolism **17**, 309—316 (1968)

Yü, T. F., Berger, L., Stone, D. J., Wolf, J., Gutman, A. B.: Effects of pyrazinamide and pyrazinoic acid on urate clearance and other discrete renal functions. Proc. Soc. exp. Biol. **96**, 264—267 (1957)

Yü, T. F., Gutman, A. B.: Paradoxical retention of uric acid by uricosuric drugs in low dosage. Proc. Soc. exp. Biol. (N.Y.) **90**, 542 (1955)

Yü, T. F., Gutman, A. B.: Study of the paradoxical effects of salicylate in low, intermediate and high dosage on the renal mechanisms for excretion of urate in man. J. clin. Invest. **38**, 1298—1315 (1959)

Yü, T. F., Kaung, C., Gutman, A. B.: Effect of glycine loading in plasma and urinary uric acid and amino acids in normal and gouty subjects. Amer. J. Med. **49**, 352—359 (1970)

Yü, T. F., Sirota, J. H., Berger, L., Halpern, M., Gutman, A. B.: Effect of sodium lactate infusion on urate clearance in man. Proc. Soc. exp. Biol. (N.Y.) **96**, 809—813 (1957)

Yü, T. F., Sirota, J. H., Gutman, A. B.: Effects of phenylbutazone on renal clearance of urate and other discrete renal functions in gouty subjects. J. clin. Invest. **32**, 1121—1132 (1953)

Zimmer, J. G., Demis, D. J.: Associations between gout, psoriasis and sarcoidosis with consideration of their pathogenic significance. Ann. intern. Med. **64**, 786—796 (1966)

CHAPTER 12

Extrarenal Disposal of Uric Acid

L. B. SORENSEN

A. Introduction

In a marvelous book entitled *Truth and Poetry Concerning Uric Acid*, Lewellys Barker, then Physician-in-Chief to the Johns Hopkins Hospital, reviewed the state of knowledge of the subject in 1905, sifting as carefully as possible what he considered the wheat from the chaff. The 17 chapters that make up the book were originally published as editorials in *The Journal of the American Medical Association*, but the large number of requests that the editorials be united led the *Journal* to issue them as a collection. "One of the subjects," Dr. Barker wrote, "in which the growth of our conceptions has been extremely slow, but about which, today, our knowledge far outruns the general professional recognition of it, is that which has to do with uric acid. We really know a great deal about its origin, the transformations which it undergoes and the way it is excreted. We are beginning to know something of its significance, though far less, it must be admitted than many people imagine."

In discussing uric acid formation within the body, Barker points out that it would be fallacious to suppose that the amount of uric acid excreted is an index to the amount formed. Two other factors must be considered: firstly, in disease there may be marked retention of uric acid and precipitation in the tissues; secondly, and more important under normal conditions, is the fact that a certain amount of uric acid is destroyed in the body after it is formed. Although his conclusions on the mode and site of cleavage of uric acid in man did not withstand the test of time, he recognized the marked variability that existed in different animals in this regard and felt compelled to reason: "There is room for much valuable work on the ferments or catalyzers which are responsible for uric acid formation and for uric acid destruction. Only a beginning has been made in this direction, but the field is so promising a one that it will be strange if a number of investigators are not soon attracted to it."

Over the next 50 years many investigators debated the question of catabolism of uric acid in man. The evidence was derived from three sources: 1) attempts at demonstrating uricase or uricolytic activity in human tissues; 2) recovery of injected uric acid; and 3) origin of allantoin found in human urine. However, it was not until 1949, when isotopically labeled uric acid first was available, that it became possible unequivocally to define the ways in which uric acid is excreted in man. The literature antedating this era has been reviewed (SORENSEN, 1960); the reader who seeks a historic perspective of the subject should consult this source. In the following, I shall first review the components of the uricolytic enzyme system and their distribution in animals and plants. I shall then discuss the fate of isotopically labeled uric acid in man, with special emphasis on that part that is not excreted by way of the kidney.

B. The Uricolytic Enzyme System

Uric acid represents the last step of purine metabolism in which the purine ring is still intact. The breakdown of this ring, uricolysis, occurs when one or more components of the uricolytic enzyme system are operative. The terms *uricolysis* and *uricolytic ferment* were assigned by SCHITTENHELM (1905) at a time when the enzymatic oxidation product of uric acid was not known. The full complement of the uricolytic enzyme system consists of the following four enzymes: uricase, allantoinase, allantoicase, and urease. FLORKIN (1949) has surveyed the distribution of the uricolytic enzymes at various levels of the phylogenetic scale. Contrary to what might be expected, the lower forms of animal life possess all the enzymes necessary for degrading purines completely, and as one ascends the evolutionary scale, the capacity for metabolizing purines becomes, in general, increasingly deficient. Crustacea and some marine invertebrates degrade uric acid via allantoin, allantoic acid, and urea to carbon dioxide and ammonia. Marine teleosts and elasmobranchs, which require relatively high plasma concentrations of urea in order to maintain themselves hypertonic to the surrounding sea water, have lost urease and eliminate a substantial proportion of their waste nitrogen as urea. Another group of marine teleosts, lacking allantoicase, excretes large quantities of allantoic acid. In almost all ureotelic mammals purine metabolism terminates with allantoin. The only exception is man and certain monkeys and apes, who lack uricase and in whom uric acid becomes the main end product of purine metabolism. Thus, it can be seen that the evolution of purine metabolism has been attained through a process of simplification by successive loss of urease, allantoicase, allantoinase, and uricase.

It has been generally accepted that man and the anthropoid apes (fam. Pongidae) are the only mammals devoid of uricase. At least one species of the New World monkeys has been found to lack uricase activity in liver tissue (LOGAN et al., 1976). The effect of fasting on uric acid concentration in serum in this species, Humboldt's woolly monkey, was similar to the hyperuricemia observed in man, suggesting that factors affecting uric acid metabolism in man may also be expected to affect that of these New World primates. Old World monkeys were found to have low serum urate levels and to possess a highly unstable form of liver uricase, perhaps reflecting a partial degeneration of this enzyme in primate phylogenesis.

It has long been known that the Dalmatian Coach Hound excretes uric acid in large quantities, although the liver is rich in uricase. In contrast to other mammals, the Dalmatian Hound has defective tubular reabsorption of uric acid in the kidney in addition to a limited access of urate to hepatic uricase. As a consequence, a substantial amount of uric acid is excreted before it is converted to allantoin. (See GUTMAN and YÜ, 1972, for a review of the literature.)

Uric acid is the end product not only purine metabolism, but also of protein metabolism in uricotelic animals such as birds, reptiles and terrestrial insects. In terms of adaptation to the environment, there are obvious advantages for one animal in the phylogenetic scale to eliminate its excess nitrogen chiefly as uric acid (uricotelism) and for another, chiefly as urea (ureotelism). During embryonic development of the uricotelic bird and reptile in a closed environment, the cleidoic egg, there is a limited quantity of water which the embryo cannot afford to expend in the production or urine. Uric acid formed from purines and amino acids is excreted by the embryo through the kidney in a dilute solution, the water of which is then almost completely reabsorbed in the cloaca leaving the uric acid as a solid mass to be retained in the allantois. Birds and reptiles have preserved this uricotelic mechanism throughout their lives and it is generally assumed that uricolysis does not occur in uricotelic animals. In conformity with that view are the findings that uric acid made up of 93% of total excreted nitrogen in two species of lizards (KHALIL, 1951).

Data on the distribution of the uricolytic enzymes in plants are available, particularly in the French literature (BRUNEL-CAPELLE, 1950). Certain plants contain high concentrations of allantoin and allantoic acid, which have been postulated to function as the nitrogen reservoir of plants and to play a central role in protein synthesis.

Microbiologists have been engaged in innumerable studies on purine metabolism of yeasts and bacteria. Various routes of uric acid degradation by bacteria are known, but except for *Veillonella alcalescens* (WHITELEY and DOUGLAS, 1951), *Clostridium cylindrosporum*, and *Clostridium acidiurici* (BARKER, 1956), all pathways involve allantoin, allantoate, ureidoglycolate, glyoxylate, and urea as intermediates. The enzymes involved and the optical isomers of the various intermediates are different, however, in the various bacteria studied (BONGAERTS and VOGELS, 1976). The complete catabolic pathway of uric acid in bacteria is depicted in Figure 1.

Aerobacter aerogenes, which occurs in the upper part of the jejunum in man and which contains uricase, allantoinase, and urease, can decompose uric acid oxidatively. It has been generally accepted that *Escherichia* species cannot utilize uric acid as a primary source of nitrogen. BARE et al. (1966) confirmed that *Escherichia* species obtained from the intestinal contents of a variety of animals and man were unable to use uric acid as the sole source of nitrogen, but uricolysis was observed in all isolates when grown in a medium containing an additional nitrogen source. The demonstration of uricolysis by *Escherichia* in the presence of additional nitrogenous material suggests that these bacteria may also partake in the breakdown of uric acid in the animal intestinal tract.

Until recently, only one pathway had been known for degradation of allantoate by bacteria. In the reaction catalyzed by the enzyme allantoicase (allantoate amidinohydrolase), 2 mol urea and 1 mol glyoxylate are formed from 1 mol allantoate. VOGELS (1966) reported the existence of another enzyme allantoate amidohydrolase in several bacteria, e.g., *Streptococcus allanticus*, *E. coli*, and *Proteus rettgeri*. Under anaerobic conditions these organisms can grow in media containing allantoin as the sole source of carbon, nitrogen, and energy. Allantoin is converted to allantoate, which in turn yields 2 mol ammonia, 1 mol carbon dioxide, and 1 mol ureidoglycolate. The latter compound is converted into glyoxylate and urea by ureidoglycolase. The production of ammonia was not due to a combined action of allantoicase and urease, since ammonia is also formed by extracts of strains that do not contain urease. The degradation of uric acid was studied in several Bacillus strains that grow well on urate but which are unable to use adenine, guanine, hypoxanthine, or xanthine (BONGAERTS and VOGELS, 1976). The metabolic pathway for urate to glyoxylate involved uricase, allantoinase, allantoate amidohydrolase, ureidoglycolase, and in some strains urease.

Clostridium acidiurici and *C. cylindrosporum* can use uric acid under anaerobic conditions (BARKER, 1956). Even though ammonia and carbon dioxide are also end

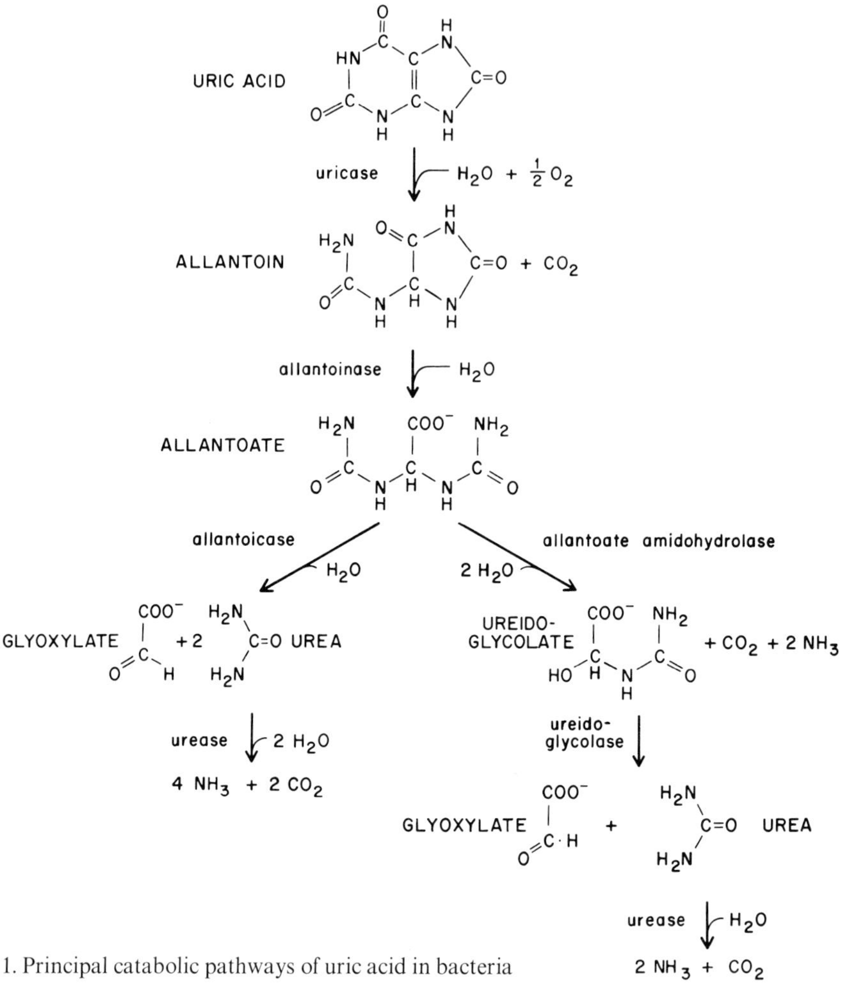

Fig. 1. Principal catabolic pathways of uric acid in bacteria

products in the anaerobic breakdown of uric acid, allantoin is not an intermediary product in the anaerobic process and cannot be used by Clostridium species.

Two other enzyme systems are capable of oxidizing uric acid in vitro at a physiologic pH, i.e., cytochrome-cytochrome oxidase (GRIFFITHS, 1952) and peroxidase (CANELLAKIS et al., 1955). The end products occurring in the cytochrome-cytochrome oxidase reaction have not been further investigated. Peroxidases are present in a variety of mammalian tissues, e.g., liver, adrenal medulla, erythrocytes, and leukocytes. Myeloperoxidase, originally called verdoperoxidase, accounts for 1% of the dry weight of human leukocytes. It is present in white blood cells of the myeloid series and has been crystallized from chloroma tumors (SCHULTZ, 1958). A large number of compounds can be produced in the peroxidase mediated destruction of uric acid, dependent on the conditions of incubation. Formation of allantoin, urea, carbon dioxide, carbamyldiurea, cyanuric acid, parabanic acid, oxaluric acid, oxonic acid, and alloxanic acid has been reported by CANELLAKIS et al. (1955). The peroxida-tive destruction of uric acid catalyzed by methemoglobin and other heme proteins in vitro has been demonstrated by HOWELL and WYNGAARDEN (1960). Incubation of uric acid, leukocyte suspension, and H_2O_2 in an acid medium resulted in formation of alloxan in quantities corresponding to 5–20% of the uric acid present (SOBERON and COHEN, 1963). It was implied that under certain conditions in vivo conversion of uric acid to alloxan might occur and, thus, could explain the lesion of the β-cells of the islands of Langerhans produced as a result of the i.p. injection of uric acid in glutathione depleted rabbits (GRIFFITHS, 1948).

The absence of uricase from human tissues predisposes man to the development of hyperuricemia, and the clinical manifestations that may arise as a consequence thereof. A number of attempts have been made to use uricase as a possible therapeu-tic agent for chronic gout with renal insufficiency and acute hyperuricemia in malig-nant blood dyscrasias (cf. Part C, 3). The model systems that have been explored include the direct injection of the enzyme (LONDON and HUDSON, 1957; KISSEL et al., 1968; BROGARD et al., 1972), uricase immobilized on glass beads within an extracor-poreal shunt (VENTER et al., 1975), and preparation of uricase-loaded human erythro-cytes (IHLER et al., 1975). The transient hypouricemic effect of treatment with uricase has been shown to be due to a stoichiometric conversion of uric acid to allantoin. Although the conversion of uric acid to the more soluble, nontoxic allantoin is theoretically desirable and elegant, repeated injections of uricase have been asso-ciated with antibody formation and resulting gradual weakening of the uricolytic activity (BROGARD et al., 1973). The question of immunogenicity of encapsulated and immobilized uricase preparations has not been finally resolved.

C. Recovery of Injected Isotopic Uric Acid

I. Recovery of Isotopic Uric Acid in Urine

The first use of isotopically labeled uric acid to determine uric acid production in man was made by BENEDICT et al. (1949). In this and subsequent studies of the miscible pool of uric acid and its daily turnover, there has been a consistent discrep-ancy between the amount of uric acid calculated to be produced per day and the amount of uric acid actually found in the urine (BUZARD et al., 1952; WYNGAARDEN and STETTEN, 1953; SORENSEN, 1959; SEEGMILLER et al., 1961; SCOTT et al., 1969; KELLEY et al., 1969). Furthermore, intravenously injected uric acid is incompletely recovered as uric acid in the urine. There is a remarkable agreement between the fraction of injected isotopic uric acid that can be recovered in the urine and the percentage that urinary uric acid constitute of the calculated turnover. Nine non-gouty subjects without overt renal disease excreted an average of 67.8% of injected ^{14}C-uric acid in the urine (SORENSEN, 1976). The deficit in excretion may be taken to represent loss of uric acid from the body by extrarenal pathways. The only situation in which this relationship is not valid is in the patient with severe tophaceous gout. In such a patient the possibility exists that isotopically labeled urate of the miscible pool exchanges with unlabeled urate of the solid phase, resulting in a falsely high dilution rate of isotope in solution. From the isotope dilution curve for such a patient it could be calculated that 800 mg of uric acid in the miscible pool exchanges each day with uric acid in a tophaceous compartment 300 times the size of the soluble pool (SORENSEN 1962). In normal subjects the daily turnover of uric acid is of the order of 600 mg; we may infer, therefore, that approximately 200 mg uric acid is normally excreted each day by extrarenal pathways.

The majority of patients with primary gout produce uric acid in normal amounts and have diminished renal urate excretion as a basis for their hyperuricemia. As a group, these patients excrete a smaller fraction of injected ^{14}C-urate in the urine than do normal subjects (RIESELBACH et al., 1970). Patients with partial or complete deficiency of hypoxanthine-guanine phosphoribosyl transferase deficiency, who have grossly exaggerated production, have no impairment in intrinsic renal handling of urate (KELLEY et al., 1969).

Patients with impaired renal tubular reabsorption of urate, either due to isolated defects in urate reabsorption or in association with the Fanconi syndrome or Wilson's disease, have abnormally high clearance of uric acid, and in such patients intravenously injected ^{14}C-uric acid can be almost quantitatively recovered in the urine (SORENSEN and KAPPAS, 1966).

In chronic renal disease, the extrarenal excretion of uric acid assumes a greater role and eventually becomes the major route of elimination of urate. We have studied uric acid metabolism in 15 patients with primary renal disease, all but one of whom had gouty arthritis. Glomerular filtration rate ranged between 3 cc/min and 66 cc/min (average 30 cc/min). The mean daily turnover was 592 mg/day, of which 209 mg were excreted in the urine. The cumulative recovery of intravenously injected ^{14}C-uric acid from the urine averaged 32%. Clearly, when renal function is compromised, there is a compensatory increase in extrarenal elimination of uric acid.

II. Recovery of Isotopic Uric Acid in Degradation Products

After i.v. administration of uric acid-^{15}N, BENEDICT et al. (1949) found small, but significant concentrations of ^{15}N in urea and ammonia in several urines collected at random. This finding certainly suggested that a portion of uric acid had been degraded to smaller fragments. However, the minute concentration of isotope in these products precluded a precise evaluation of the extent of this conversion of uric acid. The problem was reinvestigated by WYNGAARDEN and STETTEN (1953), who administered 1000 mg uric acid-1,3-^{15}N intravenously in the hope of obtaining high isotope concentration in degradation products. They found 76% of the injected uric acid excreted unchanged in the urine, 17% degraded to urea, and 1% to ammonia. Three months later, after pretreatment with phthalylsulphathiazole for the purpose of obtaining intestinal bacteriostasis, the experiment was repeated. No significant changes in the analytical results were obtained. This was taken to mean that uricolysis does take place in man, but that the intestinal flora was unlikely to play an essential role in the breakdown of uric acid. BUZARD et al. (1954) examined the extent to which uric acid is converted to allantoin in man. Upon i.v. administration of uric acid-^{15}N to one normal and to one gouty subject, they were unable to demonstrate any incorporation of ^{15}N into allantoin isolated from the urine. On the basis of these results, they concluded that uricolysis does not take place in man. POLLYCOVE et al. (1957) used uric acid-^{14}C to determine the total amount of uric acid in the body, the daily turnover as well as the quantity of uric acid that was degraded to carbon dioxide in two normal subjects and four patients with gout or polycythemia. In two normal subjects, 10% and 16% of the uric acid was broken down to carbon dioxide. In the patients with hyperuricemia, still more uric acid was degraded to carbon dioxide.

Although the composite impression one gains from reading these earlier reports clearly pointed to degradation of uric acid, there was sufficient uncertainty in regard to the mode and site of this breakdown to warrant reinvestigation of the problem. To this end we studied uric acid degradation in six subjects (SORENSEN, 1960). Following i.v. injection of uric acid-2-^{14}C, a portion of the isotopic label could be recovered in urinary allantoin, allantoic acid, and urea as well as in carbon dioxide of expired air. In two normal subjects, 2.1 and 3.9% of the injected uric acid-^{14}C was recovered in urinary allantoin after days 5 and 2, respectively, while two gouty patients excreted 4.7 and 0.4% of the isotope in allantoin after days 5 and 2, respectively. Thus, at least part of the urinary allantoin arises from uricolysis. Another part may well originate from preformed allantoin ingested with the diet. It is possible to approximate the amount of urinary allantoin that arises from breakdown of uric acid. Knowing the total amount of ^{14}C in urinary allantoin and the isotope concentration in urinary uric acid, one could calculate that on the average 24 mg allantoin arose from uric acid each day. Incorporation of ^{14}C into allantoic acid was demonstrated in the urine from two of four subjects, indicating that allantoic acid is an intermediary product in the breakdown of uric acid. Allantoic acid is inconsistently found in the urine, undoubtedly due to its tendency to degrade spontaneously into glyoxylic acid and urea, especially at a pH lower than 7. Significant concentrations of ^{14}C were found in urea in all five subjects in whom this conversion was looked for. The cumulative recovery of ^{14}C in urea ranged from 1.6 to 2.5% of the injected isotope. ^{14}C was constantly found in expired air. Two normal persons excreted 4% and 11% of the injected ^{14}C through the lungs in 1 and 4 days, respectively, while 7% of the dose was recovered from a gouty subject over a period of 48 h. A greater amount of ^{14}C was recovered in carbon dioxide than in any other degradation product, indicating that CO_2 and ammonia are the principal uricolytic products in man. By the action of uricase, allantoinase, allantoicase, and urease, part of the uric acid is degraded to the simplest end products, carbon dioxide and ammonia.

Moreover, significant quantities of uric acid-2-^{14}C injected intravenously were recovered in feces. One normal subject excreted 7.1% of the administered dose over the next 5 days, and a patient with gout excreted 3.8% in 4 days. This was a clear indication that uric acid had entered the gastrointestinal tract, and the question which needed to be answered next was: In which form does ^{14}C appear in feces? By the enzymatic spectrophotometric method uric acid could not be demonstrated at all in two patients, while in a third case only 1.5 mg uric acid was present in 23 g dry feces. By relating total ^{14}C recovered to the quantity of uric acid excreted in feces, it became obvious that almost all of the ^{14}C in feces had to be present in compounds other than uric acid. Actually, 3–4% of feces-^{14}C was found in bicarbonate, but much more had been assimilated by bacteria for their own metabolism. To analyze this process, supernates of fecal homogenates containing intestinal bacteria in suspension were assayed for ^{14}C before and after passage through a Seitz filter. The finding that 83–91% of the radioactivity was retained by the filter proved that most of the ^{14}C in feces had been used by bacteria.

Since patients with chronic renal disease excrete a much smaller fraction of injected ^{14}C-uric acid in the urine than do normal subjects, it was of interest to study the extent of uricolysis in three patients with nephropathy (SORENSEN, 1965). The amount of ^{14}C recovered in degradation products was 1.45, 2.06, and 3.24 times greater than that recovered in urinary uric acid. As in normal man, carbon dioxide and ammonia are the principal uricolytic products. One of the patients excreted more than 60% of intravenously administered uric acid-2-^{14}C in carbon dioxide of expired air.

D. Site of Uricolysis

The appearance of significant radioactivity in feces following i.v. injection of ^{14}C-uric acid and the observation that ingested uric acid is extensively broken down pointed to the gastrointestinal tract as a likely site of uricolysis in man. GEREN et al. (1950) found that a mere 9% of orally administered ^{15}N-uric acid was absorbed and excreted unchanged in the urine, whereas 47% of the ^{15}N appeared in urinary urea in 3 days. With ^{14}C-uric acid, we recovered a similar fraction, 11.1%, of ingested uric acid unchanged in the urine and found the following distribution of ^{14}C in degradation products: 0.4% in allantoin, 2.4% in urea, 55% in carbon dioxide of expired air and 16.3% in feces. The total recovery of ^{14}C was 86% of the dose over a period of 6 days. No radioactivity was present in expired air during the first 2 h following ingestion of uric acid; at this time the activity rose sharply, until a peak was reached at 8 h. Almost all of the ^{14}CO$_2$ formed was recovered in the first 20 h. Only traces of uric acid could be demonstrated in feces, viz., two stools with a dry weight of 28.6 and 11.1 g contained only 1.3 and 1.8 mg of uric acid, respectively (SORENSEN, 1960).

The ultimate proof of the role of the intestinal flora in man was obtained by determining the extent of breakdown of intravenously injected ^{14}C-uric acid before and during a high degree of intestinal bacteriostasis. Since it had been previously shown that the breakdown of uric acid remained unaltered during administration of phthalylsulfathiazole (WYNGAARDEN and STETTEN, 1953), it was felt that this drug was ineffective in rendering the gut bacteriostatic, and that a more effective bacteriostasis might be obtained by addition of streptomycin and neomycin. Under these experimental conditions, there was a significant decrease in uricolytic activity. Whereas 22.5% of injected uric acid-2-^{14}C was found in various degradation products during the first 5 days of the control study, this fraction fell to 3% over the same period of time during intestinal bacteriostasis. Moreover, whereas uric acid could not be found in feces in the control study, it was readily demonstrable in the drug study. A total of 930 mg uric acid was excreted over a 5-day period during intestinal bacteriostasis. This was equivalent to 26.6% of the calculated turnover. Over the same period, 30.1% of the injected ^{14}C had been recovered in the feces, indicating that essentially all of the fecal ^{14}C was still incorporated in uric acid.

The excretion of uric acid in feces during intestinal bacteriostasis shows that uric acid is not reabsorbed appreciably by the bowel, even when it is prevented from being degraded.

These studies clearly established the gastrointestinal tract as the principal site of uricolysis in man. The possibility remained, however, that trivial amounts of uric acid might be destroyed in human tissues by enzymes, e.g., peroxidase and cytochrome-cytochrome oxidase, referred to earlier in this review. Such a breakdown had been reported to occur in whole blood as well as in plasma incubated with red or white blood cells (BIEN and ZUCKER, 1955). The average decrease in uric acid concentration measured by a colorimetric method was 34% after incubation for 24 h at 37° C. Gouty patients demonstrated a lower rate of uricolysis than did normals, which led the authors to speculate that hyperuricemia in gout might be due in part to diminution in the rate of uricolysis. The capacity to destroy uric acid was attributed to the presence of peroxidase and cytochrome-cytochrome oxidase in blood cells. The finding that plasma incubated with peroxidase showed little if any disappearance of uric acid after 6 h but almost complete breakdown of urate after 20 h suggests that bacterial contamination could have been responsible for this degradation.

A different matter is the uricolysis that occurs when microcrystalline sodium urate-6-^{14}C is incubated with human leukocytes (HOWELL and SEEGMILLER, 1962). The crystals in these preparations were of similar size to those observed in synovial fluid in acute gouty arthritis and which are readily phagocytable by leukocytes. With microcrystalline preparations the uricolytic activity in leukocyte suspensions was equivalent to degradation of 0.25 μg urate/h/10^6 leukocytes. The rate of breakdown of uric acid in solution by leukocytes was 45% compared to that of microcrystalline suspensions, and uricolysis by intact erythrocytes was negligible.

In our own studies of uricolytic activity in human tissues, whole blood and homogenates of liver, kidney, pancreas, and spleen were incubated with uric acid-6-^{14}C in modified Warburg flasks equipped with a center well containing potassium hydroxide. The presence of uricolytic activity would be evidenced by formation of radioactive carbon dioxide. The amount of $^{14}CO_2$ liberated was negligible in all cases. The average value indicated a degradation of 0.2–0.3% of the incubated uric acid, but a similar degradation occurred when homogenate was replaced by Krebs-Ringer solution. No quantitative differences in rate of degradation were obtained for the various tissues. In general, the breakdown was slightly higher when the reaction was carried out at pH 9.3 than at pH 7.3. These results led us to conclude that uric acid is not enzymatically degraded in human tissues.

Although human leukocytes and other tissues contain the necessary enzymatic equipment for degrading uric acid, one would be on tenuous grounds to extrapolate the minute uricolysis observed in in vitro studies to the situation in vio; for example, if the ability of leukocytes to degrade uric acid in solution observed by HOWELL and SEEGMILLER (1962) was applied to the total population of circulating leukocytes, more than 125 mg of uric acid could be degraded by white blood cells alone each day. This figure is definitely too high, considering the limited extent of uricolysis occurring during intestinal bacteriostasis. The fact that neomycin, streptomycin, and phthalylsulfathiazole altered the intestinal flora in such a way that degradation was lowered to less than 15% of the control value is in itself remarkable and suggests that the residual breakdown likewise takes place in the gut.

E. Extrarenal Excretion of Uric Acid

Earlier studies on the contents of uric acid in digestive juices and feces were hampered by the lack of specific methods for measruing uric acid. As a result, there was a general feeling that the extrarenal routes were not important in elimination of uric acid. A review of the earlier literature on this subject has been presented elsewhere (SORENSEN, 1960).

Reinvestigation of digestive juices for uric acid using enzymatic methods suggested to us that the amount of uric acid entering the alimentary tract is adequate to account for degradation of one-third of the uric acid turned over in normal subjects (SORENSEN, 1960). The average concentration of uric acid in mixed saliva was 3.1 mg-% in men and 1.9 mg-% in women. The daily excretion of uric acid in saliva was estimated to be between 30 and 50 mg. In patients with hyperuricemia, excretion in saliva constituted a larger part of the total elimination of uric acid. Gastric juice was found to contain small amounts of uric acid of some 5–10 mg/liter. The daily excretion of uric acid in saliva, gastric juice, and bile in normal man amounts to at least 100 mg. A similar amount of uric acid may be expected to be excreted in pancreatic and intestinal juices.

Very little direct information is available on the mechanism of transport of uric acid into the gut. Preliminary data on parotid gland excretion of uric acid under conditions that alter renal urate excretion are available (KATZ and SORENSEN, 1968). Parotid fluid was collected in the basal state and with stimulation by chewing gum (intermediate stimulus) or a sour candy (maximal stimulus). During the control period uric acid concentration in parotid fluid ranged from 0.2 to 3.6 times the concurrent value for plasma, depending on the rate of salivary flow. The salivary uric acid concentration varied inversely with flow rate in all subjects. Total fasting is associated with accumulation of ketone bodies, principally β-hydroxybutyric acid, which inhibit renal tubular secretion of uric acid. Seven obese subjects whose mean plasma urate had been elevated from a baseline of 4.9 mg-% to 11.5 mg-% by a period of 5–10 days of total fasting demonstrated consistently diminished parotid fluid uric acid excretion at all three flow rates compared to control studies. Similarly, the well-known paradoxical effect of low versus high doses of salicylate on renal excretion of uric acid is discernible in saliva. Thus, four out of seven men given a slow infusion of sodium salicylate had a decrease in parotid fluid urate clearance at low levels of plasma salicylate (below 10 mg-%) while all subjects had an increase in salivary urate clearance over control values when high plasma salicylate concentration was obtained. These studies suggest that the parotid gland may react similarly to the kidney to factors that inhibit and stimulate renal transport of urate. A more comprehensive study of this relationship should prove rewarding.

Although salivary uric acid may be diminished during total starvation, the overall extrarenal elimination is greatly augmented in this situation. This is evident from data on the fate of ^{14}C-uric acid injected intravenously into five obese subjects who were studied during prolonged fasting (unpublished data). Whereas the handling of uric acid was normal in the control period, a larger fraction of injected ^{14}C was recovered in expired carbon dioxide than in urinary uric acid during complete starvation, indicating that excretion into and degradation within the gut had become the principal excretory pathway of uric acid.

F. Conclusion

In this chapter I have reviewed the importance of the extrarenal excretion of uric acid. Approximately one-third of all uric acid is normally excreted into the gastrointestinal tract, but this pathway assumes major proportions in disease states associated with hyperuricemia, particularly when renal function is compromised. In the gastrointestinal tract uricolytic enzymes of the intestinal flora catalyze an extensive breakdown of uric acid with formation of carbon dioxide and ammonia as the principal degradation products. Part of the uricolytic intermediary products are absorbed and excreted in the urine or expired air. Another part is used by bacteria as sources of nitrogen and carbon.

Uricase is absent in man and enzymes, such as peroxidase and cytochrome-cytochrome oxidase, which can destroy uric acid in vitro in the presence of hydrogen peroxide, do not appear to cause appreciable breakdown of uric acid in the tissues of man.

The extrarenal excretion of uric acid is much more meaningful when we consider the inefficiency of the human kidney in elimination of uric acid. Were the kidney to excrete the entire amount of uric acid produced, plasma urate concentration would have to rise by almost 50%!

I believe I have accurately reviewed our present knowledge of the degradation of uric acid. Yet, new advances will be made and some of the ideas I have expressed will be recognized as fallacies. Again, I turn to LEWELLYS BARKER (1905): "No one who grows can escape the pain of being forced, now and then, to sacrifice clearly cherished opinions, but if truth be followed, a satisfaction is always gained superior to that which has been lost." EMERSON put it well: "*Heartily know, when half-gods go, the gods arrive.*"

References

Bare, L. N., Wiseman, R. F., Ruchman, I.: Uricolysis by *Escherichia* spp. Appl. Microbiol. **14**, 474 (1966)

Barker, H. A.: Bacterial fermentations. In: Ciba Lectures in Microbial Biochemistry, pp. 57—90. New York: John Wiley and Sons 1956

Barker, L. F.: Truth and Poetry Concerning Uric Acid. Chicago: American Medical Association Press 1905

Benedict, J. D., Forsham, P. H., Stetten, DeW. Jr.: The metabolism of uric acid in the normal and gouty human studied with the aid of isotopic uric acid. J. biol. Chem. **181**, 183—193 (1949)

Bien, E. J., Zucker, M.: Uricolysis in normal and gouty individuals. Ann. rheum. Dis. **14**, 409—411 (1955)

Bongaerts, G. P. A., Vogels, G. D.: Uric acid degradation by *Bacillus fastidiosus* strains. J. Bacteriol. **125**, 689—697 (1976)

Brogard, J. M., Coumaros, D., Franelshauser, J., Stahl, A., Stahl, J.: Enzymatic uricolysis: A study of the effect of a fungal urate-oxydase. Rev. europ. Etud. clin. biol. **17**, 840—895 (1972)

Brogard, J. M., Frankhauser, J., Stahl, A.: Application de l'uricolyse enzymatique au traitement des hypéruricémies d'origine rénale. Schweiz. med. Wschr. **103**, 404—410 (1973)

Brunel-Capelle, G.: Sur la mise en évidence de l'allantoïcase chez les êtres vivants (Végétaux). C. R. Acad Sci. **230**, 2224—2226 (1950)

Buzard, J., Bishop, C., Talbott, J. H.: Recovery in humans of intravenously injected isotopic uric acid. J. biol. Chem. **196**, 179—184 (1952)

Buzard, J., Bishop, C., Talbott, J. H.: The conversion of uric acid to allantoin in the normal and gouty human. J. biol. Chem. **211**, 559—564 (1954)

Canellakis, E. S., Tuttle, A. L., Cohen, P. P.: A comparative study of the end-products of uric acid oxidation by peroxidases. J. biol. Chem. **213**, 397—404 (1955)

Florkin, M.: Biochemical evolution. New York: Academic Press 1949

Geren,W., Bendich,A., Bodansky,O., Brown,G.B.: Fate of uric acid in man. J. biol. Chem. **183**, 21—31 (1950)

Griffiths,M.: Uric acid diabetes. J. Biol. Chem. **172**, 853—854 (1948)

Griffiths,M.: Oxidation of uric acid catalyzed by copper and the cytochrome-cytochrome oxidase system. J. biol. Chem. **197**, 399—407 (1952)

Gutman,A.B., Yü,T.-F.: Renal mechanisms for regulation of uric acid excretion, with special reference to normal and gouty man. Seminars in Arthr. and Rheum. **2**, 1—46 (1972)

Howell,R.R., Seegmiller,J.E.: Uricolysis by human leucocytes. Nature (Lond.) **196**, 382—483 (1962)

Howell,R.R., Wyngaarden,J.B.: On the mechanism of peroxidation of uric acid by hemoproteins. J. biol. Chem. **235**, 3544—3550 (1960)

Ihler,G., Lantzy,A., Purpura,J., Glew,R.H.: Enzymatic degradation of uric acid by uricase-loaded human erythrocytes. J. clin. Invest. **56**, 595—602 (1975)

Katz,F.H., Sorensen,L.B.: Parotid fluid uric acid (abstract). Clin. Res. **16**, 387 (1968)

Kelley,W.N., Greene,M.L., Rosenbloom,F.M., Henderson,J.F., Seegmiller,J.E.: Hypoxanthin-guanine phosphoribosyl-transferase deficiency in gout. Ann. intern. Med. **70**, 155—206 (1969)

Khalil,F.: Excretion in reptiles IV. Nitrogenous constituents of the excreta of lizards. J. biol. Chem. **189**, 443—445 (1951)

Kissel,P., Lamarche,M., Royer,R.: Modification of uricaemia and the excretion of uric acid nitrogen by an enzyme of fungal origin. Nature (Lond.) **217**, 72—74 (1968)

Logan,D.C., Wilson,D.E., Flowers,C.M., Sparks,P.J., Tyler,F.H.: Uric acid catabolism in the woolly monkey. Metabolism **25**, 517—522 (1976)

London,M., Hudson,P.B.: Uricolytic activity of purified uricase in two human beings. Science **125**, 937—938 (1957)

Pollycove,M., Tolbert,B.M., Lawrence,J.H., Harman,D.: Uric acid metabolism: The oxidation of uric acid in normal subjects and patients with gout, polycythemia and leukemia. Clin. Res. Proc. **5**, 38—39 (1957)

Rieselbach,R.E., Sorensen,L.B., Shelp,W.D., Steele,T.H.: Diminished renal urate secretion per nephron as a basis for primary gout. Ann. intern. Med. **73**, 359—366 (1970)

Schittenhelm,A.: Über das uricolytische Ferment. Z. physiol. Chem. **45**, 161—165 (1905)

Schultz,J.: Myeloperoxidase. Ann. N.Y. Acad. Sci. **75**, 22—30 (1958)

Scott,J.T., Holloway,V.P., Glass,H.I., Arnot,R.N.: Studies of uric acid pool size and turnover rate. Ann. rheum. Dis. **28**, 366—373 (1969)

Seegmiller,J.E., Grayzel,A.I., Laster,L., Liddle,L.: Uric acid production in gout. J. clin. Invest. **40**, 1304—1314 (1961)

Soberon,G., Cohen,P.P.: Peroxidatic formation of alloxan from uric acid by leucocytes. Arch. Biochem. Biophys. **103**, 331—337 (1963)

Sorensen,L.B.: Degradation of uric acid in man. Metabolism **8**, 687—703 (1959)

Sorensen,L.B.: The elimination of uric acid in man. Scand. J. clin. Lab. Invest. **12**, (suppl. 54) 1—214 (1960)

Sorensen,L.B.: The pathogenesis of gout. Arch. intern. Med. **109**, 379—390 (1962)

Sorensen,L.B.: Role of the intestinal tract in the elimination of uric acid. Arthr. and Rheum. **8**, 694—706 (1965)

Sorensen,L.B.: Excretion of uric acid in health and in disease. In: Zöllner,N., Gröbner,W. (Eds.): Handbuch der inneren Medizin, 5th Ed., Vol. 7, Part 3, pp. 142—163. Gicht. Berlin-Heidelberg-New York: Springer 1976

Sorensen,L.B., Kappas,A.: The effects of penicillamine therapy on uric acid metabolism in Wilson's disease. Trans. Ass. Amer. Physcns **79**, 157—164 (1966)

Venter,J.C., Venter,B.R., Dixon,J.E., Kaplan,N.O.: A possible role for glass bead immobilized enzymes as therapeutic agents (immobilized uricase as enzyme therapy for hyperuricemia). Biochem. Med. **12**, 79—91 (1975)

Vogels,G.D.: Reversible activation of allantoate amidohydrolase by acid-pretreatment and other properties of the enzyme. Biochim. biophys. Acta (Amst.) **113**, 277—291 (1966)

Whiteley,H.R., Douglas,H.C.: The fermentation of purines by *Micrococcus lactilyticus*. J. Bacteriol. **61**, 605—616 (1951)

Wyngaarden,J.B., Stetten,DeW. Jr.: Uricolysis in normal man. J. biol. Chem. **203**, 9—21 (1953)

CHAPTER 13

Initial Events in the Development of an Acute Attack of Gouty Arthritis

H. R. SCHUMACHER

A. Introduction

A precise description of the initial events of an episode of acute gouty arthritis as it spontaneously occurs is not possible, as there have been no sequential studies in humans beginning before the onset of acute inflammation. Part of the picture, however, can be constructed from experimental human and dog studies and from observations during spontaneous arthritis. Crystals of monosodium urate seem to be essential for induction of gouty joint inflammation. There are several possible ways in which they may do this.

B. How Do Crystals Appear in the Joint?

Two major theories have been proposed to explain the arrival of monosodium urate crystals in the joint fluid. Crystals might precipitate de novo in the synovial fluid or they might initially deposit in synovial membrane or cartilage much as they do in other connective tissues. Subsequent release into the joint space could be by either mechanical or metabolic changes.

I. Precipitation in Synovial Fluid

Some factors that might cause this precipitation have been suggested on the basis of in vitro studies (KIPPEN et al., 1974). Lowering of temperature; changes in sodium, calcium, and other ion concentrations; and lowering of albumin or glycosaminoglycan levels can decrease urate solubility. Lowering of pH has been said to enhance urate nucleation in vitro.

SIMKIN (1973) performed subcutaneous injections of urate solutions at the same concentration as plasma. He showed that this was followed by a transient increased concentration of urate in the subcutaneous fluid, because the water was absorbed out of the subcutaneous space before the urate. He suggested that minor trauma might produce a similar phenomenon in the joint that would favor crystal precipitation, He did not do similar injections into joints.

We have seen a subcutaneous tophus develop at the site of a very recent burn, showing that at least this type of tissue injury can favor local crystal deposition (SCHUMACHER, 1977a).

II. Deposition in Synovial Membrane

It seems more likely that initial crystal deposition takes place in the subcutaneous or connective tissue. Monosodium urate crystal containing tophi have occasionally

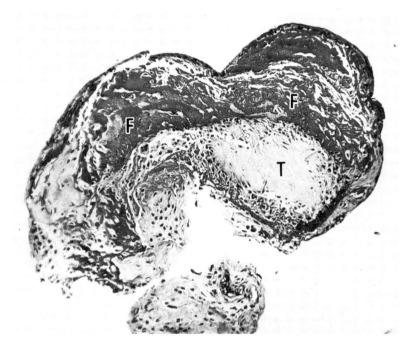

Fig. 1. Synovial tophus (*T*) surrounded by a capsule containing few histiocytes from a patient with acute gouty arthritis. In addition to the superficial tophus, the villus above the tophus is filled with fibrin (*F*), suggesting the possible explanation that crystals had been released from the deposit to initiate the attack and were now being sealed off. 90 ×. H&E

been identified in the synovial membrane at the time of initial attacks of gouty arthritis (Agudelo and Schumacher, 1973) (Fig. 1). Arthroscopists have noted synovial tophi in patients said never to have had acute gouty arthritis, but no fully documented descriptions of these patients have appeared. It is of course difficult to exclude a previous subclinical attack with subsequent sequestration of crystals in the synovium. Most experimental studies involving intra-articular injection of crystals have been done in dogs, where uricase presumably prevents any such deposits from occuring in synovium, even if they might do so in man.

If analogy with chondrocalcinosis and "pseudogout" can be used to help, it is clear that deposits in cartilage of calcium pyrophosphate crystals detectable by X-ray regularly antedate any clinically evident joint inflammation. Such deposits begin in the mid-zone of articular cartilage or meniscus and seem most unlikely to have arisen by phagocytosis from the joint fluid.

The constituents of the matrix surrounding a synovial tophus should offer some clues as to any local factors involved in the mechanisms of formation; unfortunately, they are only weak clues thus far. Immunoglobulins are concentrated at tophi more intensely than in the adjacent synovium (Hasselbacher and Schumacher, 1976). Whether these plasma constituents are an early or secondary factor is not known. Muscopolysaccharides also appear to be concentrated at tophi (Sokoloff, 1957). Since tophi occur predominantly in connective tissues that are rich in mucopolysaccharides, it is intriguing to speculate, as have KATZ and LIGOT (1972) and KIPPEN et al. (1974), that altered mucopolysaccharide matrix might favor crystal deposition. Unfortunately, there is as yet no analysis of tophus mucopolysaccharides to substantiate this. Acid phosphatase, a lysosomal enzyme that might be a factor in altering connective tissue components, has been identified in synovial tophi (SCHUMACHER, 1977a).

Many of the factors shown to alter urate solubility in vitro might also be factors in precipitation in connective tissue sites. The occurence of acute gout when plasma urate is suddenly lowered with allopurinol or uricosuric therapy might be explained by resorption or urate from a synovial tophus, leading to tophus weakening and crystal release. Attacks induced while plasma urate is low would seem difficult to explain upon new crystal deposition in joint fluid.

C. How Do Urate Crystals Induce Inflammation in the Joint?

I. Why Do Crystals not Always Seem to Produce Inflammation?

Crystals of monosodium urate in gout as well as calcium pyrophosphate crystals in "pseudogout" can often be identified in joint fluid in the interim between episodes of arthritis as well as in joints that have never been involved with known joint inflammation. Even massive numbers of crystals can be seen without any inflammatory cell reaction. No single factor seems to explain all these effusions lacking cellular exudation despite the presence of crystals. Possible factors include generation of naturally occuring antiinflammatory substances, changes in crystal coating by proteins or other materials, crystal size, rapidity of appearance or numbers of crystals, pH changes, and probably other factors.

Naturally occuring antiinflammatory substances have been described in a variety of joint diseases (CAPSTICK et al., 1975), although the authors did not specifically mention gouty arthritis. Such factors included globulins that stabilize lysosomal membranes and antiproteases. If such materials were especially profuse and/or effective, they might influence the ability of crystals to be phlogistic.

Monosodium urate crystals in tophi and in synovial fluid appear to be coated with protein (HASSELBACHER and SCHUMACHER, 1976). Some protein coatings, such as IgG, may enhance crystal phagocytosis and thus increase inflammation. These ongoing studies by KOZIN and McCARTY (1976) suggest that adsorbed albumin, lysozyme, IgA, and IgM inhibit phagocytosis of crystals by neutrophils and, thus, might prevent the phlogistic response to crystals. Unfortunately, sequential studies of the proteins associated with crystals during and after acute gouty arthritis have not yet been possible. Proteins associated with cell and phagosomal membranes may also be important in how crystals react with phagocytic cells. Proteoglycans and other materials associated with crystals in joint effusions have received little study but may also influence crystal properties and behavior (BRANDT, 1974).

Crystal size clearly influences phagocytosis, in that cells cannot ingest huge crystals. Even within the size range of crystals that can be phagocytized there appears to be greater phagocytosis with smaller crystals (SCHUMACHER et al., 1975). Very limited studies, however, suggest that, despite avid phagocytosis, monosodium urate crystals averaging only 2 µ in length may produce less cell necrosis than larger crystals. Mechanical effects of the larger crystal in the phagolysosome may account for some of the different effects of crystals of different sizes (WEISSMAN, 1971). The sizes of crystals at onset and during resolution of attacks have not been estimated. Crystals seen in tophi do tend to be longer than those seen in most effusions. If long crystals are released from tophi into joints to initiate attacks of synovitis, these may well become smaller after partial digestion in synovial fluid leucocytes by myeloperoxidase (HOWELL and SEEGMILLER, 1962).

Amounts of urates injected into joints influence the inflammation induced in dog knees. Very small numbers of crystals induce less inflammation. Rate of appearance of crystals has not been studied, but rate as well as dose may well influence the manner in which crystals are handled, including how they are coated with protein. Some unexplained variation in response of dogs to crystal injection has been seen (SEEGMILLER et al., 1962; SCHUMACHER et al., 1974).

During acute gouty arthritis, pH in the synovial fluid does fall slightly, presumably at least in part due to lactic acid production at the site of inflammation (SEEGMILLER et al., 1962). The precise effect of this on cells and crystals in vivo is not known. WILCOX et al. (1972) show some increased solubility of monosodium urate, with lowering of pH that might decrease crystal size and, thus, help slow the attack.

Among many other factors that must eventually be considered, one can mention the levels of soluble urate in synovial fluid. A very recent report, using a liposome in vitro system with silica crystals, suggests that urate in solution enhances membrane permeability by reversing the protective effect of albumin; other proteins were not studied (DiSABATINO et al., 1977). Interestingly, there appears to be very little inflammation around tophi in synovial tissue (SCHUMACHER, 1975). Whether this is due to some of the factors noted above, the relative avascularity around the crystals or other factors is not known.

II. How Can Crystals Induce Inflammation After Arrival in the Joint Fluid?

I. Intra-Articular Injection of Urates

We (SCHUMACHER et al., 1974) have examined the sequence of changes detectable after intra-articular injection of synthetic urate crystals into dog knees. The first changes seen were at 20–30 min, when vasodilation and margination of neutrophils was noted in synovial vessels, and there was mild synovial edema and prominent cytoplasmic processes on the synovial lining cells. Some neutrophils in vascular lumens were degranulating (SCHUMACHER and AGUDELO, 1972). Crystals could be identified in vacuoles of intact synovial lining cells and in large mononuclear cells in the synovial fluid after 30 min (Fig. 2A). Not until 60 min did PHELPS (1970) detect chemotactic activity in synovial fluid. At 45–60 min, intra-articular pressure elevations were noted. At 75–90 min, the synovial fluid leukocyte count began to rise, and fullblown synovitis evolved with phagocytosis of crystals by synovial fluid polymorphonuclear neutrophils. These observations still leave the initial biochemical facts unclear. Are some chemotactic and vasoactive materials generated by the mononuclear cells that phagocytize the crystals or by the intraluminal cells that degranulate without any direct contact with crystals (Fig. 2B)? Certainly further studies of possi-

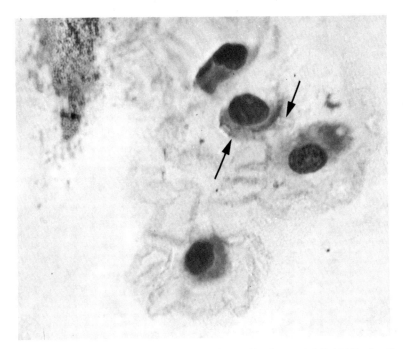

Fig. 2 A. Urate crystals *(arrows)* in large mononuclear cells of synovial fluid 30 min after injection into a dog knee joint. Wright's stain. 720 ×

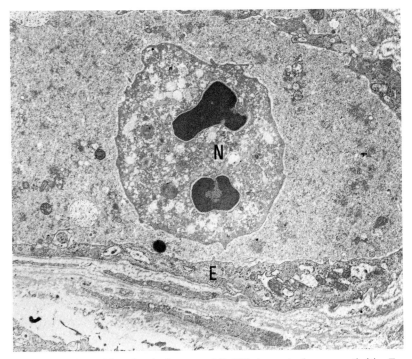

Fig. 2 B. Degranulation of intraluminal neutrophil *(N)* in acute human arthritis. E-vascular endothelium. Electron micrograph. 6000 ×

ble sources of small amounts of chemotactic materials are needed. It was of interest that animals previously injected with urate crystals had a more marked inflammatory response to subsequent injections. The time sequence was not studied in animals with repeated injections. Depletion of circulating neutrophils by vinblastine supressed but did not in all cases abolish intra-articular pressure rise after intra-articular urate injection (PHELPS and McCARTY, 1966). Neutrophils are prominent in synovial fluid and membrane in most acute gouty arthritis (AGUDELO and SCHUMACHER, 1973) (Fig. 3), but the possibility that some gouty arthritis can occur with virtual absence of synovial fluid leukocytes has also been suggested by ORTEL and NEWCOMBE (1974). In their patient with renal failure and an acute colchicine responsive effusion containing only rare leukocytes, a few strongly negatively birefringent needle-shaped crystals were seen. However, since their patient had renal failure, it must be considered possible that the crystals seen were not urates by rather other crystals, such as hydroxyapatite. Apatite is occasionally birefringent and can be seen in renal failure patients with joint effusions (SCHUMACHER, 1977a; DIEPPE et al., 1976).

2. In Vitro Studies of Crystal-Cell Interaction

Monosodium urate crystals are almost invariably seen within synovial fluid leukocytes during acute gouty arthritis. Many crystal-containing cells appear necrotic (Fig. 4).

Electron microscopic studies of urate crystal interaction with neutrophils in vitro has shown rapid crystal phagocytosis, with subsequent degranulation, phagolysosome membrane lysis, and cell necrosis of 33% of cells after 2 h (SCHUMACHER and PHELPS, 1971). That the mechanism of this neutrophil necrosis involves membranolysis is supported by the studies of WEISSMAN (1971) and of WALLINGFORD and McCARTY (1971), who showed that urate crystals can lyse erythrocyte membranes. As noted above, proteins and other materials coating the crystals and cell membranes almost certainly influence crystal effects in vivo. Certain immunoglobulins, such as IgG, may favor crystal phagocytosis but protect against membranolysis. Since urate crystals do not seem to lyse leukocytes from contact with their external cell membrane; it has been proposed (McCARTY, 1973; SCHUMACHER, 1974) that lysosomal enzymes emptied into phagosomes might need to digest off a protein or other coating before the crystals can lyse the phagosomal membrane. Routine election microscopic studies have not easily documented changes in protein coating, since lysosomal material on the crystal surface cannot be distinguished from immunoglobulins on standard transmission electron micrographs (Fig. 5). Hydrogen bonding of urates to phagosomal membranes has been proposed as the mechanism of membranolysis (WALLINGFORD and McCARTY, 1971). In addition to cell death with lactate dehydrogenase release, there is release of lysosomal enzymes after crystal phagocytosis. Thus, both cytoplasmic and lysosomal materials may contribute to the inflammatory joint-space reaction.

3. Immunologic Contributions

Some evidence suggests immunologic alterations in gouty arthritis, but none of these have been systematically studied in vivo for possible contributions to the initial

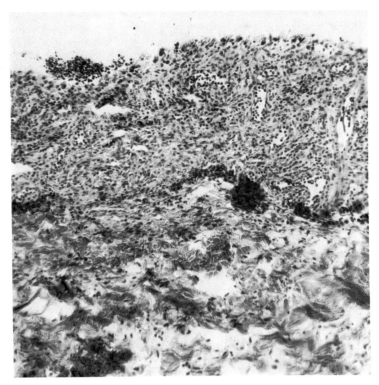

Fig. 3. Intense acute synovitis characteristic of human or experimental gouty arthritis. H&E. 90 ×

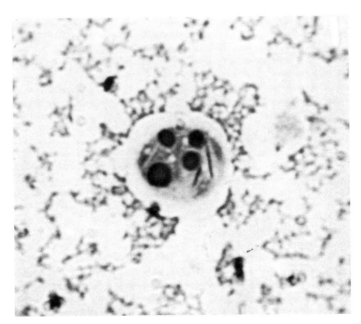

Fig. 4. Monosodium urate crystals in necrotic synovial fluid neutrophil with pyknotic nucleus. Wrights stain. 800 ×

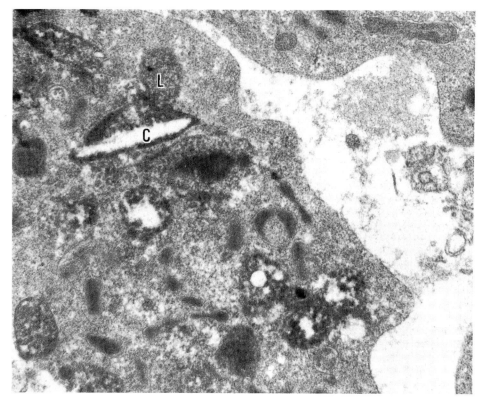

Fig. 5. Urate crystal *(C)* in phagosome surrounded by electron dense peroxidase that presumably has emptied into the vacuole from the adjacent lysosome *(L)*. Electron micrograph. 30 000 ×

events. Complement-derived chemotactic factors have been found in gouty synovial fluids (WARD and ZVAIFLER, 1971). Complement can be activated by urate crystals in vitro (NAFF and BYERS, 1973). We have noted electron dense deposits in synovial vessel walls during acute gouty arthritis (AGUDELO and SCHUMACHER, 1973). These deposits need further characterization but might conceivably include immunoglobulins and complement. Plasma cells can be seen in human gouty synovium and in dog synovial membrane after repeated intra-articular urate injections (SCHUMACHER, 1975; SCHUMACHER et al., 1974). KOZIN and MCCARTY (1976) noted rheumatoid factor in 40% of patients with chronic tophaceous gout.

D. Conclusion

Monosodium urate crystals in synovial fluid can induce the acute attack of gouty arthritis, but despite much recent research the exact sequence of events is not defined. Important factors are release into or precipitation of crystals in joint fluid; proteins, proteoglycans, and other materials associated with the crystals and cells; crystal size;

and pH and solute concentrations. Crystals are phagocytized by polymorphonuclear and mononuclear cells, and chemotactic materials are generated.

Neutrophils are lysed by a membranolytic effect of urate crystals that seems to be influenced by crystal protein coating.

References

Agudelo, C. A., Schumacher, H. R.: The synovitis of acute gouty arthritis. A light and electron microscopic study. Hum. Pathol. **2**, 265—279 (1973)

Brandt, K. D.: The effect of synovial fluid hyaluronate on the ingestion of monosodium urate crystals by leucocytes. Clin. chim. Acta **55**, 207—315 (1974)

Capstick, R. B., Lewis, D. A., Cosh, J. A.: Naturally occuring anti-inflammatory factors in the synovial fluids of patients with rheumatic disease and their possible modes of action. Ann. rheum. Dis. **24**, 213—218 (1975)

Dieppe, P. A., Crocker, P., Huskisson, E. C., Willoughby, D. A.: Apatite deposition disease. A new arthropathy. Lancet **1976 I**, 266—269

Di Sabatino, C. A., Breitenstein, M. G., Malawista, S. E.: Crystal induced membrane permeability in liposomes: Dissolved urate reverses the protective effect of albumin. (Abst.) Arthr. and Rheum. **20**, 113 (1977)

Hasselbacher, P., Schumacher, H. R.: Localization of immunoglobulin in gouty tophi by immunohistology and on the surface of monosodium urate crystals by immune agglutination. (Abst.) Arthr. and Rheum. **19**, 802 (1976)

Howell, R. R., Seegmiller, J. E.: Uricolysis by human leukocytes. Nature (Lond.) **196**, 482—483 (1962)

Katz, W., Ligot, P.: Deposition of urate crystals in gout. (Abstr.) Clin. Res. **20**, 511 (1972)

Kippen, I., Klinenberg, J. R., Weinberger, A., Wilcox, W. R.: Factors affecting urate solubility in vitro. Ann. Rheum. Dis. **33**, 313—317 (1974)

Kozin, F., McCarty, D. J.: Absorption of protein to monosodium urate (MSU) crystals: A possible mechanism of crystal-induced inflammation. (Abst.) Arthr. and Rheum. **19**, 805—806 (1976)

McCarty, D. J.: Mechanisms of crystal deposition diseases. Gout and pseudogout (Editorial). Ann. intern. Med. **78**, 767—771 (1973)

Naff, G. B., Byers, P. H.: Complement as a mediator of inflammation in acute gouty arthritis. I. Studies on the reaction between human serum complement and sodium urate crystals. J. Lab. clin. Med. **81**, 747—760 (1973)

Oertel, R. W., Newcombe, D. S.: Acute gouty arthritis and response to colchicine in the virtual absence of synovial fluid leucocytes. New Engl. J. Med. **290**, 1363—1364 (1974)

Phelps, P.: Polymorphonuclear leucocyte motility in vitro. IV. Colchicine inhibition of chemotactic activity formation after phagocytosis of urate crystals. Arthr. and Rheum. **13**, 1—9 (1970)

Phelps, P., McCarty, D. J.: Crystal induced inflammation in canine joints. II. Importance of polymorphonuclear leucocytes. J. exp. Med. **124**, 115—125 (1966)

Schumacher, H. R.: Morphologic studies of the unresolved problems in crystal-induced arthritis. Inflo. **7**, 3 (1974)

Schumacher, H. R.: Pathology of the synovial membrane in gout. Light and electron microscopic studies. Arthr. and Rheum. **18**, 771—782 (1975)

Schumacher, H. R.: Pathogenesis of crystal induced arthritis. Clin. rheum. Dis. **3**, 105—131 (1977a)

Schumacher, H. R.: Bullous tophi in gout. Ann. Rheum. Dis. **36**, 91—93 (1977b)

Schumacher, H. R., Agudelo, C. A.: Intravascular degranulation of neutrophils: An important factor in inflammation. Science **175**, 1139—1140 (1972)

Schumacher, H. R., Fishbein, P., Phelps, P., Tse, R., Krauser, R.: Comparison of sodium urate and calcium pyrophosphate crystal phagocytosis by polymorphonuclear leucocytes. Effects of crystal size and other factors. Arthr. and Rheum. **18**, 783—792 (1975)

Schumacher, H. R., Phelps, P.: Sequential changes in human polymorphonuclear leukocytes after urate crystal phagocytosis. An electron microscopic study. Arthr. and Rheum. **14**, 513—526 (1971)

Schumacher, H. R., Phelps, P., Agudelo, C. A.: Urate crystal induced inflammation in dog joints: Sequence of synovial changes. J. Rheum. **1**, 102—113 (1974)

Seegmiller, J. E., Howell, R. R., Malawista, S. E.: The inflammatory reaction to sodium urate. J. Amer. med. Ass. **180**, 469—475 (1962)

Simkin, P. A.: Local concentration of urate in the pathogenesis of gout. Lancet **1973 II**, 1295—1298

Sokoloff, L.: The pathology of gout. Metabolism **6**, 230—241 (1957)

Wallingford, W. R., McCarty, D. J.: Differential membranolytic effects of microcrystalline sodium urate and calcium pyrophosphate dihydrate. J. exp. Med. **133**, 100—112 (1971)

Ward, P. A., Zvaifler, N. J.: Complement derived chemotactic factors in inflammatory synovial fluids of humans. J. clin. Invest. **50**, 606—616 (1971)

Weissman, G.: The molecular basis of gout. Hosp. Pract. **6**, 43—52 (1971)

Wilcox, W. R., Khalaf, A., Weinberger, A., Kippen, I., Klinenberg, J. R.: Solubility of uric acid and monosodium urate. Med. Biol. Eng. **10**, 522—531 (1972)

CHAPTER 14

Role of Proteoglycans in the Development of Gouty Arthritis

W. A. KATZ

A. Introduction

Gout is defined as the deposition of urate crystals, clinically expressed by acute arthritis or tophi. It is well accepted that hyperuricemia, or at least an abnormally high total uric acid pool, is a critical precursor to the deposition phenomenon and that urate crystals, once precipitated in the joint, give rise to an intense phlogistic reaction. The mechanism of urate deposition remains enigmatic and controversial. GARROD (1876) was one of the first to recognize that gouty arthritis was caused by the precipitation of sodium urate crystals in the joints or neighboring tissues:

"Gouty inflammation is invariably attended with the deposition of urate of soda ... This fact I wish to impress forcibly upon my readers because in the constancy of such deposition lies the clue that has long been wanting; the occurrence of the deposit is at once pathognomonic and separates gout from every other disease which at first sight might appear allied to it."

Even the name gout alludes to the deposition phenomenon, being derived from the French "goutte"; in the thirteenth century it was thought that poisonous humours entered the joint drop (goutte) by drop. Furthermore, urate deposition is responsible for the pathologic changes of gout, i.e., erosive destruction of the joint. Despite its importance, the deposition phase of gout has largely been ignored and much taken for granted.

B. Historical Background

The predilection of urates to precipitate in the articular cartilages and other connective tissues has been recognized for many years. PAULUS AEGINETA (AD 625-690) recorded the following:

It is not weakness of the parts alone that occasions gouty and arthritis complaints; for then the paroxysms would be without ceasing, insomuch as the debility is always present in the weak parts ... When the disease is protracted in the joints, and humours become thick and viscid, so as to form what are called tophi or chalk-stones.

PARACELSUS (1493–1541) called attention to the association of urate and synovial fluid:

... the gluten which was called synovia by the old wound surgeons, is sticky and gelatinous like egg white. Now when the salty matter comes into contact with and mixes itself with this, it coagulates at once into a solid ... The gout of the feet, hands, and knees has its origin in this coagulation, depending on the location of the gluten from which the inflammation comes ... (RODNAN, 1965).

One of the earliest accounts of urate deposition is in CHEYNE's (1724) book entitled "An Essay of the True Nature and Due Method of Treating the Gout":

Hence we may learn the Reason why, on the first Attacks of the Gout, in otherwise healthy People, the Humours generally fall on the Joints of the Limbs: Because, in the Joints, the smallest vessels are more compressed by the larger Heads or Protuberancy of the Bones, and are thereby render'd narrower and more readily obstructed ... By the smallness of the Glands in the Joints, the natural Coldness of these Parts, their Distance from the Heart, their Compression by the larger Extremities of the Bones ... The Joints become more liable to gouty Indispositions.

Here is found probably the first allusion to avascularity as a cause of urate deposition. The avascularity theory, never proven, was taught for many years. As late as 1969, in the Fourth Edition of COPEMAN's *Textbook of the Rheumatic Diseases*, nonvascularity was given as an explanation of the apparent predilection of urates for surface types of articular cartilage. The affinity of urates for cartilage was probably first proven by Sir WILLIAM ROBERTS (1892). He noted the encrustation of tophaceous material on the cartilagenous articulating surfaces of pig tarsal bones that were incubated in a saturated solution of sodium biurate for 3 days. Sir WILLIAM proposed that the precipitation was caused by the relatively high sodium concentration in connective tissue as compared to the parenchymal organs. This theory of "common ion effect" (that a salt containing a given cation will diminish the solubility of another salt with the same cation) was later to be expounded by PETERS and VAN SLYKE (1946). Indeed, sodium chloride added to a saturated solution of sodium urate will cause the precipitation of the latter. McCARTY (1965) suggested that polymorphonuclear leukocytes, as they ingested urate crystals during the acute gouty attack, elaborated increased lactic acid, causing a fall in local pH which fostered the precipitation of more urate. He offered no explanation of how the first urate crystal precipitated from hyperuricemic body fluids. SEEGMILLER (1965) demonstrated that sodium urate crystals added to saturated solutions triggered crystallization of urates. He speculated "that the essential difference between the gouty patient and his equally hyperuricemic brother may be the chance formation of the first crystal of sodium urate." HOWELL (1965) supported this hypothesis by detecting lower pHs in the synovial fluid and tophi of patients with gout when compared to their whole blood. However, SPILBERG (1977) has disputed that such a low magnitude of hydrogen ion change could indeed precipitate urates in tissue. SIMKIN (1973, 1977) recently examined the permeability of the synovium to a number of small molecules. He noted that the mean permeability of synovium to urate was approximately 50% that of the smaller molecule of water.

When a synovial effusion resolves, water will leave the joint more rapidly than urate, causing a transient increase in the concentration of urate within the residual synovial fluid ... I believe that the more rapid diffusion of water causes the intrasynovial concentratin of urate to rise above the saturation point, leading to the nocturnal precipitation of urate crystals that in turn incites the inflammatory response that we recognize as acute podagra.

Several investigators have pointed to the serum and tissue proteins as solubilizing agents that prevent precipitation of urates from saturated body solutions. Irreversible binding of urate to serum protein could not be demonstrated by equilibrium dialysis, ultrafiltration, or electrophoresis (ADLERSBERG et al., 1942; MORRIS, 1958; YÜ and GUTTMAN, 1953). Recent studies, however, have suggested that plasma proteins may bind urate reversibly. α-globulin and β-globulin fractions markedly solubilize urate whereas albumin and γ-globulin have little such effect (KATZ and EHRLICH, 1968). In another study, three patients with chronic tophaceous gout could not bind urate normally (KLINENBERG and KIPPEN, 1970). ALVSAKER (1965) detected a diminished α_1/α_2 binder of urate in patients with gout. It is too simplistic to suggest that the loss of the ability of the protein to bind urate would result in precipitation, and this explanation would not account for the obvious fact that urates, with few exceptions, fail to deposit in the bloodstream.

C. The Deposition Phenomenon: Modern Connective Tissue Concepts

SOKOLOFF (1957), in a systematic review of the morbid anatomy of gout, reemphasized the predisposition of urate crystals to deposit in articular cartilage of gouty patients, and others have pointed to the predilection of urates for all connective tissues—cartilage, tendon sheaths, synovium, synovia, and the subcutaneous tissues of the skin. Urates rarely appear in the parenchymal organs such as brain, liver, or spleen. There are reports of tophi in the heart, but these are seen only in the connective tissue portions, i.e., the valves, conduction system, and pericardium. Any apparent infiltration of the myocardium by tophi is by secondary extension only. Uric acid, of course, deposits in the renal parenchyma, but it is primarily found in the tubules where the relatively high acidity renders the substance less soluble. Monosodium urate crystals were reported by FRAZIER and SEEGMILLER (1966) developing in the interstitial areas of the kidney. These, however, are the same tissues found by FARBER et al. (1962) to be rich in acid mucopolysaccharides (proteoglycans and glycosaminoglycans).

VON GREILING (1962) attempted to show by titration studies that chondroitin sulfate caused the conversion of monosodium urate to uric acid by serving as a cation exchanger and replacing the sodium ion. He proposed that uric acid, being less soluble, would then precipitate in polysaccharide-rich connective tissue. However, although uric acid is, indeed, less soluble in distilled water, it is actually more soluble in tissue fluids at physiologic pH. Also in contradiction to VON GREILING'S hypothesis is the fact that X-ray diffraction studies show the deposits to be composed of monosodium urate and not uric acid. Furthermore, chondroitin sulfate is not present in a form that would render it an ion exchanger, i.e., a free acid.

LAURENT (1964) demonstrated that chondroitin-4-sulfate reduced the solubility of monosodium urate when solutions of progressively higher concentrations of chondroitin sulfate were agitated with excess urate for 48 h. An inverse relationship between the dissolved urate and the polysaccharide in solution was found, i.e., the higher the chondroitin sulfate concentration, the lower the urate solubility. He attributed this phenomenon to the ability of polysaccharides to exclude part of the water from participating effectively in a solution of the urate. These conclusions were subject to question because it was more likely that the uricase action of certain bacterial contaminants, not an excluded volume effect, accounted for the changes. KATZ and SCHUBERT (1970) suggested that the excluded volume effect of protein-polysaccharides to a smaller molecule like urate would be neglible unless the urate were bound to a larger molecule.

I. Solubility of Monosodium Urate in Bovine Tissues

In order to affirm the apparent affinity of urates for connective tissue, the solubilizing effect of bovine nasal cartilage on urate was investigated.

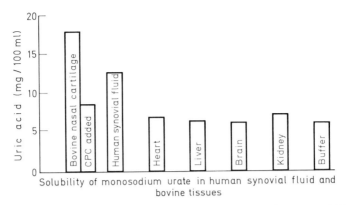

Fig. 1. Solubilizing effect of bovine tissue homogenates on monosodium urate (pH 7.4, 0.61 *M*, phosphate saline buffer). Note that solubility diminishes after addition of cetyl pyridinium chloride (CPC) to bovine nasal cartilage!

Acetone dried homogenates of bovine nasal cartilage, heart, liver, brain, and kidney were dialyzed against 0.021 *M* potassium phosphate buffer containing 0.130 *M* sodium chloride for 3 days at 4° C. The homogenates were then suspended in an aliquot of the buffer, the final pH being 7.40 ± 0.03. Monosodium urate (MSU) crystals (10 mg) were prepared (SEEGMILLER, 1962) and added to the homogenates. The resultant mixture was placed in a sealed ampul and agitated continuously for 24 h at 4° C. After the excess urate was removed by centrifugation at 3500 rpm for 15 min, the uric acid of the supernatant was determined. The supernatants were then incubated at 4° C for 16–20 h, centrifuged and analyzed again for uric acid.

The solubility of MSU in phosphate saline solution not containing homogenates was 5.7 mg/100 ml measured as uric acid. Solutions of bovine nasal cartilage contained 25.5 mg/100 ml whereas homogenates of the other organs caused minimal augmentation of urate solubility (Fig. 1). Following the incubation of a solution of urate-saturated bovine nasal cartilage with trypsin, the uric acid concentration of the supernatant after centrifugation fell to 5.7 mg/100 ml, a value identical to that of the control buffer. Trypsin, when added to solutions containing homogenates of heart, liver, brain, or kidney, did not change the uric acid concentration, nor did visible urate precipitation occur.

Bovine nasal cartilage, as a prototype of connective tissue, markedly solubilized MSU.

II. Detection of a Urate-Solubilizing Substance in Connective Tissue

The basic components of cartilage and other connective tissues are cells (fibroblasts and chondroblasts), fibers, and matrix or ground substance. Other than the organelles, the components of cells are similar to those of the ground substance in which they bathe. Fibers, notably collagen, elastin, and reticulin, are relatively insoluble. The ground substance is composed of substances similar to that found in serum as well as macromolecular proteinpolysaccharides. These polysaccharides were formerly referred to as acid mucopolysaccharides and under the new nomenclature are called glycosaminoglycans (GAG); when bound to protein they are labeled proteoglycans (PG). An ultracentrifically light fragment (PPL) was, at the time these studies were performed, the polysaccharide most easily purified and placed into solution. Proteoglycans are heavy, highly polymerized molecules which tend to interdigitate with similar molecules to form a meshlike network that is largely responsible for the viscosity and elasticity of connective tissues. These substances are readily precipitated by cetyl pyridinium chloride.

Homogenates of bovine nasal cartilage were dialyzed against running tap water or frequent washes of phosphate saline solution for 5 days in order to eliminate electrolytes, hexosamines, and other substances that could conceivably be responsible for urate solubilization. The level of polysaccharide was measured using the uronic acid method of BITTER and MUIR (1962), and urate solubility studies were performed before and after prolonged dialysis. Polysaccharides were precipitated by cetyl pyridinium chloride at the end of dialysis. Urate solubility studies were again performed.

Prolonged dialysis did not either alter the concentration of uronic acid in the bovine nasal cartilage mixture, or significantly affect urate solubility. On the other hand, precipitation of polysaccharides with cetyl pyridinium chloride completely obviated the solubilizing effect so that the final solubility level of urate was 5.6 mg/100 ml.

III. Solubility of Monosodium Urate in Polysaccharide Solutions

Proteoglycans and unbound chondroitin sulfate were studied in order to compare their solubilizing effect on urate. Excess amounts of MSU (equivalent to 2 mg/ml) were weighed into ampuls and then sterilized by dry heat at 100° C overnight in order to eliminate growth of uricase-producing bacterial organisms. Varying concentrations of proteoglycans prepared by either the ultracentrifugation method of PAL et al. (1966) or the method of SAJDERA and HASCALL (1969) were added to ampuls. Chondroitin sulfate was either prepared by the method of EINBINDER and SCHUBERT (1950) or obtained commercially (pentex Biochemical, Kankakee, Ill.). The polysaccharides were sterilized by dry heat; biochemical properties were not affected. Sterilized potassium phosphate saline buffer was added to the vessels. The specimens were agitated continuously for periods extending to 4 days. The supernatant uric acid was determined. No excessive urate crystals were identified in the supernatant by polarizing microscopy. A similar study was performed using albumin (120 mg/ml) in saline phosphate buffer and buffer alone.

Proteoglycans greatly enhanced urate solubility. At higher concentrations of proteoglycans, more urate entered the solution. At relatively lower concentrations the relationship between urate solubility and proteoglycans concentration was linear. That is, the greater the concentration of proteoglycans, the greater the urate solubility. At proteoglycan concentrations in excess of 8 mg/ml, the uric acid solubility was 16.8 mg/100 ml. Unbound chondroitin sulfate in concentrations as high as 80 mg/ml, ten times that of proteoglycans, produced only a slight augmentation of urate solubility (Fig. 2). Similar minor changes in urate solubility occurred with albumin. Proteoglycans obtained from bovine humeral articular cartilage, used in a limited number of experiments, caused solubilization of urates similar to that of

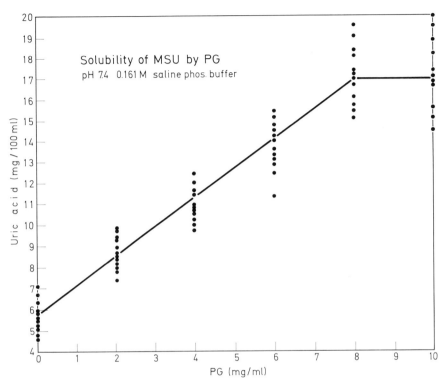

Fig. 2. Direct relationship between the concentration of proteoglycans (PG) and the degree of urate solubility in phosphate buffer solutions in vitro. (Reproduced with permission of The Journal of Clinical Investigation and the J. B. Lippincott Co.)

cartilage from bovine nasal septum. Proteoglycans, predigested with trypsin, failed to increase urate solubility. Following the addition of cetyl pyridinium chloride to saturated solutions of the proteoglycans-urate solution, urate crystallization was observed with a corresponding diminution in urate concentration after only a few minutes (KATZ and SCHUBERT, 1970).

IV. Inhibition of Urate Crystallization by Polysaccharides

Given the hypothesis that proteoglycans markedly augment urate solubility, it would follow that proteoglycans inhibit urate crystallization from supersaturated solutions. Supersaturated solutions of urate were prepared by dissolving 350 mg/100 ml(MSU) in 0.01 M potassium phosphate buffer pH 7.4 on a boiling water bath. Sodium chloride was added to give a final concentration of 0.161 M. After the solutions cooled to room temperature, varying amounts of heat-sterilized proteoglycans, chondroitin sulfate, or albumin were added. Maximum concentrations of proteoglycans, chondroitin sulfate 10 mg/ml, and albumin 100 mg/ml were used. The solutions were kept at 4° C and agitated for 1 h 4 times daily. They were then centrifuged until maximal separation of crystals took place (approximately 10 min). Although the solution containing proteoglycans remained opalescent after centrifugation, urate crystals in excess could not be identified microscopically in the supernatant. Opalescence disappeared when the solution was warmed to room temperature, despite the fact that further crystallization did not take place.

After 6 days of agitation, the solutions containing buffer alone exhibited a urate concentration of 5.7 mg/100 ml, a quantity identical to the solubility level of urate in buffer. On the other hand, proteoglycans inhibited the complete crystallization of urates, its solubility being approximately 15 mg/100 ml. Predigested proteoglycans, chondroitin sulfate, and albumin failed to significantly inhibit urate crystallization. Thus, proteoglycans inhibited the precipitation of urates from supersaturated buffer solutions.

V. Induction of Urate Crystallization from Polysaccharide Solutions Saturated with Urate

Connective tissue components seemingly prevent urate crystallization, a concept that on first inspection would be inconsistent with the observation that tophaceous deposits are the result of decreased, not increased solubility of urate. It has been noted, however, that proteoglycans are subject to enzymatic degradation. These experiments were designed to show that disruption of the proteoglycans molecule would indeed obviate the inhibition of crystallization by these polysaccharides.

Supersaturated solutions were again prepared by dissolving excessive amounts of MSU in a saline phosphate buffer. Bovine nasal cartilage proteoglycans, 10 mg/ml, were added to the cooled solutions which were in turn agitated for 6 days. The supernatants obtained by centrifugation were warmed to room temperature so that there was no opalescence. The specimen of urate solution without proteoglycans served as a control. Trypsin or hyaluronidase was added to an aliquot of each, incubated at room temperature (higher temperatures induced bacterial overgrowth) and gently stirred for 4 h. The specimens were observed closely for urate crystallization. After centrifugation, the supernatants were analyzed under a polarizing microscope for evidence of crystallization and were tested for the level of uric acid. Enzyme was not added either to a control solution of proteoglycans saturated with urate or to another of saturated urate without proteoglycans.

No visible or significant changes in uric acid content were noted in the solutions of urate without polysaccharides whether or not enzymes had been added. Visible precipitation of urate crystals from previously clear proteoglycans-urate solutions occurred within 1–2 h; this precipitation was complete in 3 h (Fig. 3). The uric acid level of the supernatant contained 5.5 mg/100 ml, the approximate value of the control specimens.

VI. Induction of Urate Crystallization from Human Synovial Fluid

Proteoglycans content and type varies from species to species. Furthermore, the previously performed experiments called for dissolving proteoglycans sometimes obtained by harsh methods and stored for considerable periods of time. The following experiments called for the use of a readily available human connective tissue already containing large amounts of proteoglycans.

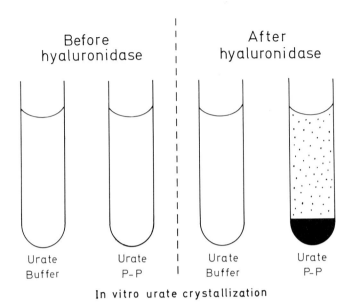

Fig. 3. Crystallization in vitro of urate crystals from supersaturated solutions of protein polysaccharide (P-P) after hyaluronidase. (Reproduced with permission of the J. B. Lippincott Co.)

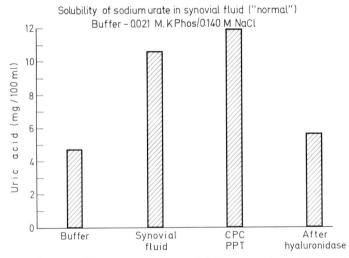

Fig. 4. Solubility of monosodium urate by synovial fluid preparations. The cetyl pyridinium chloride (CPC) precipitate represents concentrated proteoglycans

Viscous, clear osteoarthritic synovial fluid containing less than 1000 polymorphonuclear leukocytes/mm^3 was dialyzed against pH 7.4 salinephosphate buffers overnight at 4° C. Some of the fluid was subjected to ultrafiltration through millipore filters of varying porosity. This procedure yielded a protein-free fluid (synovial "water") and a markedly viscous synovial fluid concentrate. Whole synovial fluid, synovial fluid water, synovial fluid concentrate, and a control pH 7.4 salinephosphate buffer were saturated with MSU as described above. Hyaluronidase was added to each of the urate-saturated solutions which were then observed for urate crystallization and tested for urate concentration.

Urate crystallization was not observed in the specimen of synovial fluid water or saline-phosphate buffer. Visible precipitation was noted in the whole synovial fluid specimen (Fig. 4). Some crystals were noted in the concentrate but observations were not clear cut because of a sludgelike formation. Uric acid concentration in the whole synovial fluid specimen after treatment with hyaluronidase was only slightly greater than that in the saline-phosphate and serum water controls. This hyaluronidase-induced crystallization of urate may have a counterpart in clinical gout.

D. Speculations on Altered Connective Tissue Metabolism in Gout

I. Normal Connective Tissue Metabolism

Connective tissue physiology has in the past been considered an inert process, but recent studies have indicated that the metabolism is actually quite dynamic. Proteoglycans are formed, degraded, and then reformed. The glycosaminoglycans (GAG) of connective tissue ground substances are macromolecules composed of linear heteropolysaccharide chains linked to a protein core by covalent bonds. Hexosamine (glucosamine or galactosamine) alternating with another sugar (glucuronic acid, induronic or galactose) comprise the polysaccharide chains. Various combinations of hexosamines and other sugars determine whether the end product is one of the following:

hyaluronic acid	heparin
chondroitin-4-sulfate	heparatin
chondroitin-6-sulfate	keratosulfate
dermatan-4-sulfate	

Each of the glycosaminoglycans is sulfated except hyaluronic acid.

Polysaccharide synthesis proceeds through glycosal esters of nucleotides (sugar nucleotides), e.g.:

Glucose-1-phosphate + uridine triphosphate (UTP)

↓   UDPG pyrophosphorylase

Uridine diphosphoglucose (UDPG) + pyrophosphate

Several different enzymes enable the sugar nucleotides to undergo a variety of reactions, some of which involve the transfer of the sugar component to form glycosides, oligosaccharides, or polysaccharides. Certain hormones and drugs control the biosynthesis of polysaccharides. For example, corticosteroids seemingly inhibit polysaccharide formation (SCHUBERT and HAMERMAN, 1968).

Sulfate esters comprise a large portion of the polysaccharide molecule. Through a series of reactions catalyzed in part by the enzyme ATP sulfurylase, the sulfated polysaccharide is formed:

$ATP + SO_4 \Rightarrow$ adenosine 5'-phosphosulfate (APS) + pyrophosphate

$ATP + APS \Rightarrow$ 3-phosphoadenosine 5'-phosphosulfate (PAPS) + ADP.

$PAPS + ROH \rightarrow ROSO_3^- +$ 3',5'-diphosphoadenosine (where ROH is a polysaccharide, i.e., chondroitin).

Radioactive sulfate uptake studies indicate that sulfate passes rapidly into cartilage and that it is then accumulated in the chondrocytes. It is eventually slowly
released into the surrounding matrix. It is uncertain at which stage activated sulfate
is transfered into the synthesis of the sulfated polysaccharides, nor is the order
incorporation of the sugar units understood. It still is not known definitely whether
the polysaccharides are first synthesized and then attached to a growing protein
chain or whether they grow out of a protein chain. It seems that protein and polysaccharide synthesis are simultaneous.

It is thought that the proteinpolysaccharide degradation is controlled by enzymatic action in the extracellular tissue spaces. Unquestionably, proteases can disrupt
protein polysaccharide molecules. THOMAS (1956) showed that crude papain injected
into young rabbits under proper conditions produced within several hours droopy
ears which became erect again after several days. Histologic examination of the ears
showed that the polysaccharides disappeared from the cartilage and simultaneously
appeared in the blood plasma. High doses of vitamin A, causing lysosomal disruption, produced a similar effect in rabbits. Turnover of tissue proteoglycans may come
about as a result of polysaccharidases such as hyaluronidase.

Accelerated breakdown of connective tissue does indeed occur in diseases where
activated lysosomes release a number of hydrolytic enzymes (i.e., cathepsin D) (DIN-
GLE, 1965). The cell also releases nonlysosomal enzymes such as lysozyme. Abnormalities in the synthesis or degradation of glycosaminoglycans are seen in certain
heritable diseases of connective tissue (the mucopolysaccharidoses), osteoarthritis,
and rheumatoid arthritis. Accelerated connective tissue destruction is associated
with an increased plasma and urine free glycosaminoglycans (BRYANT et al., 1958).
Apparently the glycosaminoglycans molecules, smaller than proteoglycans, more
readily find their way into the bloodstream and urine.

II. Accelerated Connective Tissue Metabolism as a Cause of Urate Deposition

KATZ (1975) proposed that connective tissue turnover was related to the deposition
of urate crystals in cartilage and other connective tissues. Recognizing the constant
turnover of proteoglycans, he postulated that proteoglycans entrapped urate molecules, rendering them supersaturated in the hyperuricemic subject and thereby preventing the deposition of urates as in the in vitro studies described above. However,
as part of the normal metabolic turnover of connective tissues, lysosomal and other
enzymes released into small packets or microcosms digest the adjacent proteoglycans, so altering the complex that it can no longer solubilize; urate deposition results
just as crystallization takes place from supersaturated solutions in vitro (Fig. 5). It
was proposed that over a period of years the urate crystals coalesce to form tophi.
This scheme would account for gout being dependent upon the duration of disease
and the degree of hyperuricemia.

If, however, normal connective tissue turnover was the only factor operative in
the deposition of urates, then we would expect that all patients with hyperuricemia
would develop gout sooner or later. Yet less than 15% of patients with hyperuricemia ever develop gout in the form of either acute arthritis or tophi. This observation
led KATZ (1975) to suggest that, in patients with gout, connective tissue metabolism

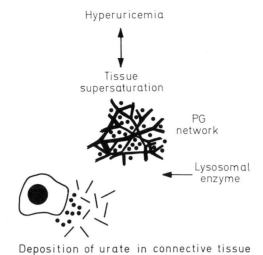

Fig. 5. Proposed mechanism of urate deposition in connective tissues of patients with gout. (Reproduced with permission of Arthritis and Rheumatism.)

was accelerated and that urate deposition was caused by the fortuitous or related assocation between elevated tissue uric acid and rapid turnover of connective tissue. He therefore studied serum glycosaminoglycans in patients with gout and compared them to patients with hyperuricemia or no abnormalities.

The glycosaminoglycans, chondroitin sulfate, have been recognized as a normal component of serum. Until recently it was thought that glycosaminoglycan was entirely free in serum. CALATRONI et al. (1969), however, have now shown that about 25% is bound to protein. The proteoglycans complex, which was successfully isolated from serum, migrated electrophoretically with the α- and β-globulins. Both these protein fractions moderately augmented urate solubility during in vitro studies (KATZ and EHRLICH, 1968). Chondroitin sulfate has been found elevated in patients with rheumatoid arthritis, cancer, and other conditions. The precise significance of proteoglycans and glycosaminoglycans in gout is unclear. In one study by SHETLAR et al. (1950), chondroitin sulfate was elevated in patients with gout. They thought this to be an acute phase reactant. ALVSAKER (1965) found that an α_1/α_2-globulin fraction was deficient in patients with gout. Preliminary studies have shown that a serum proteoglycans exhibiting the electrophoretic mobility of the α_1/α_2-globulin could indeed augment urate solubility.

That increased serum glycosaminoglycans is the reflection of increased connective tissue turnover has already been demonstrated by the famous rabbit experiments of THOMAS (1956). Capitalizing on this classic investigation, KATZ (1975) suspected that if connective tissue turnover in gout were rapid, the serum glycosaminoglycans would be increased.

Ecteola column chromatography makes it possible to measure relatively small amounts of proteoglycans or glycosaminoglycans without interference from proteins and hexoses. Total polysaccharide (i.e., glycosaminoglycans and proteoglycans) in 20 normal individuals ranging in age from 18 to 70 was 329 µg/100 ml $\pm$ 70. These

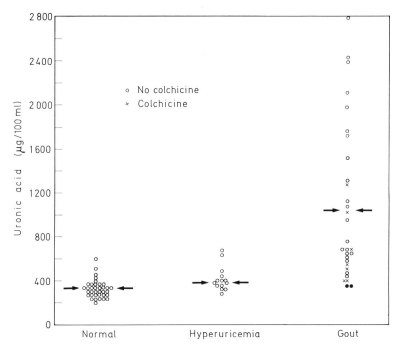

Fig. 6. Serum glycosaminoglycans (polysaccharides) in normals and patients with gout

results compared favorably with similar determinations by CALATRONI et al. (1969). Of the total polysaccharides, 30% was in the bound form. Normal serum glycosaminoglycans values are stable from one day to another. They tend to be slightly higher in men. Fifteen patients with hyperuricemia but with no clinical evidence of gout exhibited slightly elevated total polysaccharide levels—421 ± 78. Minimal elevations were detected in some patients with osteoarthritis and rheumatoid arthritis. Investigations are currently underway to determine the mechanism of hyperpolysaccharidemia.

Serum proteoglycans and glycosaminoglycans were analyzed in 30 patients with gout, the diagnosis having been established by the demonstration of urate crystals in synovial fluid, urate tophi (biopsy proven), or a classic history of podagra clearly responsive to colchicine administration. Total polysaccharide levels in 20 of the patients who were untreated at the time of initial study were elevated (Fig. 6). One patient exhibited a value in the top normal range. Values ranged from 380 to 2970 µg/100 ml while the mean was 1060 µg/100 ml (KATZ, 1975). The degree of binding to protein was significantly diminished to 14%. We interpreted this to mean that increased amounts of free glycosaminoglycans were split off from proteoglycans and found their way into the general circulation. In nine additional patients, total polysaccharide levels were within normal limits at the time of initial testing; however, all these patients had been taking varying amounts of colchicine (Fig. 6).

No positive correlation could be found between the level of serum polysaccharides and the degree of hyperuricemia. In some instances, marked hyperpolysaccharidemia was detected in patients with normal serum uric acid levels. Some authors questioned whether hyperuricemia might somehow stimulate connective tissue metabolism. Indeed, one might inquire whether the phenomena of hyperuricemia and hyperpolysaccharidemia are two fortuitous independent processes or whether they are somehow interrelated. The answers are not yet known, but the lack of correlation between accelerated connective tissue metabolism and the size of the uric acid pool would tend to refute such a hypothesis. Ingestion of allopurinol, probenecid, or sulfinpyrazone did not apparently affect serum glycosaminoglycans even though uric acid concentration was altered considerably. Anti-inflammatory drugs such as aspirin, indomethacin, or phenylbutazone did not have any effect on connective tissue metabolism.

Although some of the patients were in the midst of an acute attack when first studied, there was no evidence to indicate that hyperpolysaccharidemia was related to an acute attack. Polysaccharides have been found elevated in the serum of patients with carcinoma, arthritis, and various infections (SHETLAR et al., 1950). KERBY (1958), when evaluating a group of patients with inflammation unrelated to rheumatoid disease, noted that the level of serum polysaccharides was elevated when compared to the normal control group to an extent comparable to that found in rheumatoid arthritis. In both instances, the hyperpolysaccharidemia paralleled the increase in plasma euglobulins which has been noted in the presence of any inflammatory process, including rheumatoid arthritis. Thus, one might suspect that elevated glycosaminoglycans in gout were nothing more than a reflection of the acute attack. Yet no correlation could be detected either between the intensity of the acute attack and serum polysaccharides or between the Westergren erythrocyte sedimentation rate and serum polysaccharides. The latter remained at the same level (without treatment) even though in some cases several weeks had elapsed since the acute attack. On the other hand, many untreated patients who had not had acute attacks for several years showed marked elevations of serum glycosaminoglycans.

E. Effect of Colchicine on Connective Tissue Metabolism

At the time of initial study 20 other patients were taking colchicine in varying amounts. For the most part, these patients exhibited considerably lower serum polysaccharides than did the untreated patients. A positive correlation between the amount of colchicine taken and the depression of serum glycosaminoglycans was established. Untreated patients with elevated serum glycosaminoglycans were given colchicine in varying amounts. Colchicine caused a return of the serum glycosaminoglycans to normal levels in each of the four patients given 1.95 mg daily, whereas in 75% of those patients who took only 0.65 mg colchicine daily the serum glycosaminoglycans fell to normal levels. In one patient, 0.65 mg colchicine had no effect whatsoever on serum polysaccharides. Doubling the dose caused a rapid fall to normal levels. The phenomenon of colchicine suppression of serum glycosaminoglycans was not only doserelated but timerelated as well. Significant suppression had occurred following 1–2 weeks of colchicine administration, and all patients on larger doses were within the normal range by week 6 (Fig. 7). The serum glycosaminoglycans remained at normal levels as long as the dose of colchicine remained stable. In an additional five individuals, withdrawal of colchicine caused a reversal of previously suppressed levels to elevated values. Increased serum glycosaminoglycans

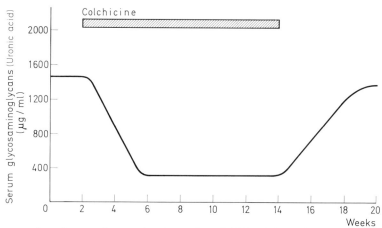

Fig. 7. Suppression of serum glycosaminoglycans by colchicine (schematic)

concentrations after withdrawal of colchicine presaged acute attacks of gout in five patients who had been entirely asymptomatic when the serum glycosaminoglycans levels were normal. The fluctuations of serum glycosaminoglycans correlating with the dose of colchicine were predictable. For example, a 69 year old black man who had had chronic tophaceous gout for more than 20 years had been well controlled on 1.3 mg colchicine daily as well as on 400 mg allopurinol daily. Over a period of 3 years the size of a tophus at the right elbow shrunk from 7 cm to 1.5 cm. Serum glycosaminoglycans were 310 µg/100 ml with no greater than 15% variation in re-peat determinations. Colchicine was completely withdrawn while the patient was maintained on allopurinol. The serum glycosaminoglycans rose to 2050 µg/100 ml and remained at this level for approximately 2 weeks. When colchicine was reini-tiated at the previous dose, the serum glycosaminoglycans levels fell to less than 300 µg/100 ml. After several weeks the colchicine was again withdrawn; the serum glycosaminoglycans rose and the patient developed an attack of acute gouty arthritis in the first metatarsal phalangeal joint. Colchicine was restarted. The attack abated, and serum glycosaminoglycans levels once again fell to normal values. Another patient, a 54 year old woman who had developed chronic tophaceous gout 4 years after a hysterectomy at age 40, continued to have multiple attacks of gout despite up to 1.3 mg colchicine daily and 100 mg allopurinol daily. The uric acid level was 11.6 mg/100 ml. Additional amounts of allopurinol or probenecid could not be toler-ated. Serum glycosaminoglycans were consistently in excess of 2000 µg/100 ml. When the dose of colchicine was adjusted to 1.95 mg daily, mild intermittent diar-rhea ensued, but the serum glycosaminoglycans levels fell to nearly normal values (452 µg/100 ml), and the patient became asymptomatic.

F. Diagnostic Value of Serum Glycosaminoglycans Determination

Gout is in most instances not difficult to diagnose by clinical means. However, some cases present problems in differentiation from other rheumatic and nonrheumatic disorders for the following reasons:

1. Gout is not always present as an acute, monoarticular inflammation of the first metatarsal phalangeal joint. The course may be subacute or protracted. Multiple joints may be involved simultaneously, and gouty arthritis may occur in joints not usually involved in this disease, e.g., the hips, sacroiliac joints, and shoulders.

2. Gout may on rare occasions be seen in an unexpected age and sex, for example, in a 32-year-old woman.

3. Rheumatoid nodules may closely resemble tophi, especially when they occur in the hand. Differentiation by clinical means is sometimes impossible.

4. Gout may coexist with other diseases which may overshadow acute urate crystal disease. Notable examples are rheumatoid arthritis, osteoarthritis, and infectious arthritis.

5. All too often, the diagnosis of gout is based on hyperuricemia; yet many patients with acute gout do not have elevated serum uric acid levels. Conversely, most patients with hyperuricemia never have gout.

6. The detection of urate crystals in synovial fluid and tophi is pathognomonic of gout, but fluid and tophaceous materials are not always obtainable because of a variety of clinical conditions which might prevail.

7. Roentgenographic changes of advanced disease are usually quite typical; however, early in the course of gout there are no radiographic features. Even the classical finding of a marginal erosion with an overhanging edge may be seen in diseases other than gout.

8. A rapid response to colchicine administered within 24 h of onset of acute arthritis is strongly suggestive but not diagnostic of gout. Other rheumatic diseases such as acute sarcoid arthropathy may also respond to colchicine.

Preliminary studies have indicated that hyperpolysaccharidemia provides an additional means of differentiating gout from those diseases that mimic it. Of course, elevated serum glycosaminoglycans, even in excess of 2000 µg/100 ml, are not diagnostic of gout but rather serve as an additional tool for establishing the diagnosis in difficult cases. While rheumatoid arthritis, osteoarthritis, and other rheumatic or nonrheumatic disorders may also produce modest elevations in serum glycosaminoglycans, only in gout, Paget's disease, and systemic lupus erythematosus have marked elevations of serum glycosaminoglycans been noted. On the other hand, with the exception of one case, all patients with gout not treated with colchicine have exhibited high serum glycosaminoglycans. In 11 patients where the diagnosis was not clearcut because of one or more of the reasons stated above, hyperpolysaccharidemia was a helpful finding in either establishing the diagnosis of gout or in heightening our clinical suspicions of gout.

Case Report:

A 49-year-old male laborer presented to the Arthritis Clinic with a 6-year history of periodic pain and swelling of the left knee. The current episode had begun gradually several days earlier. The pain was mild and not disabling. These were the characteristics of pre-existing attacks. Physical examination showed the knee to be slightly warm, slightly tender and moderately swollen. Quadriceps muscle atrophy was present and the patient walked with a barely perceptible limp. The remainder of the rheumatologic examination was within normal limits. The complete blood count was normal. The Westergren erythrocyte sedimentation rate was 28 mm/hr and the latex fixation test for rheumatoid factor was negative. Serum uric acid was 4.8 mg/100 ml (normal: less than 7.2 mg/100 ml). Synovial fluid was aspirated from the joint and initially described as moderately cloudy. The specimen was apparently lost on the way to the laboratory, so no crystal examination was performed. Because of the indolent nature of the arthritis and the normal serum uric acid, a diagnosis of gout was not seriously entertained. Serum that had remained after the uric acid determination had been routinely analyzed for serum glycosaminoglycans; a value of 2450 μg/100 ml was noted, the highest found in our laboratory at that time. The attending rheumatologist was asked to reaspirate synovial fluid at the next visit and provide an additional serum specimen. Intracellular and extracellular urate crystals were abundantly present in the synovial fluid. The serum uric acid was again well within normal limits, but the serum glycosaminoglycans were markedly elevated. The diagnosis of gout, suspected from the finding of hyperpolysaccharidemia, was confirmed by synovial fluid analysis, and appropriate treatment was instituted.

The reader is cautioned that serum glycosaminoglycans determinations are not routinely performed and that the diagnostic value of this test has yet to be borne out through the analysis of large numbers of patients.

G. Conclusion

Serum glycosaminoglycans levels were significantly elevated in patients with gout, presumably because of accelerated connective tissue metabolism. Colchicine reduced the values to the normal range, probably by interfering with connective tissue turnover mediated by lysosomal enzyme-producing cells. Further investigation using different techniques will be required to elucidate the mechanism of urate deposition. I suspect that altered connective tissue metabolism is but one phenomenon responsible for the deposition of urate crystals in man.

The connective tissue metabolism studies are of potential value in that:

1. They provide basic knowledge of the deposition phenomenon in gout.

2. They may have predictive value in determining which patients with hyperuricemia will develop gout and which will not.

3. They are likely to establish a parameter for improved prophylactic control of gout.

4. They may be of value in cases where the diagnosis of gout is not clearcut.

5. They may shed light on how gout is related to other diseases such as hypertension, diabetes mellitus, and atherosclerosis.

McCARTY (1977) ties together the existing theories of the pathogenesis of gout in the following outline:

1. Hyperuricemia—supersaturation of extracellular fluids

2. Elevated serum glycosaminoglycans levels—found only in patients with gout

3. Physical properties of uric acid solutions—low temperature, selective clearance, trauma, degenerative arthritis, and altered thermodynamic equilibrium between urate in crystals and urate in solution

4. Chemical (enzymatic) changes in articular tissue

The building blocks of the urate story have been started. The full story has yet to unfold.

References

Adlersberg,D., Grisham,E., Sobotka,H.: Uric acid partition in gout and hepatic disease. Arch. intern. Med. **70**, 101—120 (1942)

Alvsaker,J.O.: Uric Acid in human plasma IV. Investigations on the interactions between urate and the macromolecular fraction in plasma from healthy individuals and patients with diseases associated with hyperuricemia. Scand. J. clin. Lab. Invest. **18**, 227—239 (1965)

Bitter,T., Muir,H.M.: A modified uronic acid carbazole reaction. Anal. Biochem. **4**, 330—334 (1962)

Bryant,J.H., Leder,I.G., Stetten,D.: The release of chondroitin sulfate from rabbit cartilage following the intravenous injection of crude papain. Arch. Biochem. Biophys. **76**, 122—130 (1958)

Bunim,J.J., McEwen,C.: Tophus of mitral valve in gout. Arch. Path. **29**, 700—704 (1940)

Calatroni,A., Donnelly,P.V., Di Ferrante,N.: The glycosaminoglycans of human plasma. J. clin. Invest. **48**, 332—343 (1969)

Cheyne,G.: An essay of the true nature and due method of treating the gout. London: Strahan 1724

Copeman,W.S.C.: Textbook of rheumatic diseases. Edinburgh: Livingstone 1969

Dingle,J.T.: Synthesis and degradation of connective tissue in organ cultures. In: Structure and Function of Connective and Skeletal Tissue. London: Butterworths 1965

Einbinder,J., Schubert,M.: Separation of chondroitin sulfate from cartilage. J. biol. Chem. **185**, 725 (1950)

Faires,J.S., McCarty,D.J.: Acute arthritis in man and dog produced by intrasynovial injection of sodium urate crystals. Clin. Res. **9**, 329 (1961)

Farber,S.J., Cohen,G.L., Castor,J.A.: The chemical and metabolic properties of acid mucopolysaccharides of renal papillae. Trans. Ass. Amer. Physcns. **75**, 154—159 (1962)

Frazier,P.D., Seegmiller,J.E.: Characterization of crystalline deposits in kidney tissue of patients with gout. Arthr. and Rheum. **9**, 504 (1966)

Garrod,A.B.: Treatise on gout and rheumatic gout (rheumatoid arthritis), 3rd Ed. London: Longmans, Green and Company, Inc. 1876

Howell,P.S.: Preliminary observations on local pH in gouty tophi and synovial fluid. Arthritis Rheum. **8**, 736—739 (1965)

Katz,W.A.: Deposition of urate crystals in gout. Altered connective tissue metabolism. Arthr. and Rheum. **19** (Suppl.), 275—285 (1975)

Katz,W.A., Ehrlich,G.E.: The solubility of monosodium urate in serum and connective tissue components (Abstr.), Arthr. and Rheum. **11**, 492 (1968)

Katz,W.A., Schubert,M.: The interaction of monosodium urate with connective tissue components. J. clin. Invest. **49**, 1783—1789 (1970)

Kerby,G.P.: The effect of inflammation on the hexuronate-containing polysaccharides of human plasma. J. clin. Invest. **37**, 962—965 (1958)

Klinenberg,J.R., Bluestone,R., Schlosstein,L., Waisman,J., Whitehouse,M.W.: Urate deposition disease. How is it regulated and how can it be modified? Ann. intern. Med. **78**, 99—111 (1973)

Klinenberg,J.R., Kippen,I.: The binding of urate to plasma proteins determined by means of equilibrium dialysis. J. Lab. clin. Med. **75**, 503—510 (1970)

Laurent,T.C.: Solubility of sodium urate in the presence of chondroitin-4-sulfate. Nature (Lond.) **202**, 1334—1335 (1964)

Loeb,J.N.: The influence of temperature on the solubility of monosodium urate. Arthr. and Rheum. **15**, 189—192 (1972)

McCarty,D.J.: The inflammatory reaction to microcrystalline sodium urate. Arthr. and Rheum. **8**, 726—734 (1965)

McCarty,D.J.: The gouty toe—A multifactorial condition. Ann. intern. Med. **86**, 234—236 (1977)

McCarty,D.J., Hollander,J.L.: Identification of urate crystals in gouty synovial fluid. Ann. intern. Med. **54**, 452—460 (1961)

Morris,J.E.: The transport of uric acid in serum. Amer. J. Med. Sci. **235**, 43—49 (1958)

Pal,S., Doganges,P.T., Schubert,M.: The separation of new forms of the proteinpolysaccharides of bovine nasal cartilage. J. biol. Chem. **241**, 4261—4266 (1966)

Peters,J.P., Van Slyke,D.D.: Quantitative clinical chemistry, Vol. 1. Baltimore: Williams and Wilkens 1946

Roberts,W.: The chemistry and therapeutics of uric acid gravel and gout. Brit. med. J. **1892 II**, 61—65

Rodnan,G.P.: Early theories concerning etiology and pathogenesis of the gout. Arthr. and Rheum. **8** (Suppl.), 599—609 (1965)

Sajdera,S.W., Hascall,V.C.: Proteinpolysaccharide complex from bovine nasal cartilage. J. biol. Chem. **244**, 77—87 (1969)

Schubert,M., Hamerman,D.: Metabolism of connective tissue. In: A primer of connective tissue biochemistry. Philadelphia: Lea and Febiger 1968

Seegmiller,J.E.: The acute attack of gouty arthritis. Arthr. and Rheum. **8**, 714—723 (1965)

Seegmiller,J.E., Howell,R.R., Malawista,S.E.: The inflammatory reaction to sodium urate. J. Amer. med. Ass. **180**, 469—475 (1962)

Shetlar,M.R., Shetlar,C.L., Richmond,V., Everett,M.R.: The polysaccharide content of serum fractions: carcinoma, arthritis, and infection. Cancer Res. **10**, 681—683 (1950)

Simkin,P.A.: Local concentration of urate in the pathogenesis of gout. Lancet **1973 II**, 1295—1298

Simkin,P.A.: The pathogenesis of podagra. Ann. intern. Med. **86**, 230—233 (1977)

Simkin,P.A., Pizzorno,J.E.: Transynovial exchange of small molecules in normal human subjects. J. appl. Physiol. **36**, 581—587 (1974)

Sokoloff,L.: The pathology of gout. Metabolism **6**, 230—243 (1957)

Spilberg,I., Tanphaichitr,K., Kantor,O.: Synovial fluid pH in acute gouty arthritis (Letter). Arthr. and Rheum. **20**, 142 (1977)

Thomas,L.L.: Reversible collapse of rabbit ears after intravenous papain and prevention of recovery by cortisone. J. exp. Med. **104**, 245—252 (1956)

Von Greiling,H., Herbertz,T.H., Schuler,B., Stuhlsatz,H.W.Z.: Biochemical studies on the cause of uric acid deposition in the connective tissue of gout. Z. Rheumaforsch. **21**, 50—55 (1962)

Yü,T.F., Gutman,A.B.: Ultrafilterability of plasma urate in men. Proc. Soc. exp. Biol. (N.Y.) **84**, 21—24 (1953)

CHAPTER 15

Role of the Leukocyte and Chemical Mediators of the Acute Gouty Attack

I. SPILBERG

A. Phagocytosis of Crystals

Experimental work in vivo (MCCARTY, 1970) has shown that the introduction of monosodium urate crystals into a joint cavity initiates an acute inflammatory response. Polymorphonuclear leukocytes are normally present in synovial fluid and phagocytosis of crystals by polymorphonuclear leukocytes occurs readily. Experimental work on animals has shown that the phagocytosis of crystals by polymorphonuclear leukocytes occurs independently of complement (SPILBERG and OSTERLAND, 1970). The crystals are taken into phagosomes which then merge with primary lysosomes to form phagolysosomes or secondary lysosomes. Electron microscopic studies indicate that after a crystal lies in contact with the membrane of the phagolysosome, dissolution of the membrane occurs and is followed by cell death (SCHUMACHER and PHELPS, 1968). Cell death, however, appears to be a slow process, since neutrophils which have previously ingested urate crystals in vitro have been reported to exhibit a normal phagocytic capacity for yeast (TURNER et al., 1973). WEISSMANN and RITA (1972) have postulated that lysis of the lysosomal membrane is due to the interaction of weakly anionic urate crystals with the membrane, forming cooperative hydrogen bonds with phosphate esters of membrane phospholipids. Not only do urate crystals disrupt lysosomal membranes, they also lyse red cells (WALLINGFORD and MCCARTY, 1971), the plasma membrane of polymorphonuclear leukocytes (SPILBERG et al., 1975), and liposomes (WEISSMAN and RITA, 1972), lamellar arrays of phospholipids containing cholesterol in their membranes. Incorporation of 17-estradiol into the liposome protects it from the lytic effect of the crystals, whereas testosterone does not. The protective effect of estradiol offers an explanation for the low incidence of gout, besides the lower levels of uric acid, among premenopausal women as compared to men. Studies by WEISSMANN and RITA, however, were performed using an artificial system, the liposome, with estradiol preincorporated at molar percentages 0.1–5.0 of the total lipid content. There are no data available on the concentration of estradiol in lysosome membranes of phagocytic cells.

The phagocytic process consists of particle ingestion, after which the particles are removed from the biologic system. The steps include adherence, phagosome formation, fusions of phagosomes with primary lysosomes, and the emptying of the lysosomal content into the formed secondary lysosome. Predictable changes in cell metabolism accompany these steps. Changes include increased glycogen breakdown, glucose utilization, phospholipid synthesis, and lactic acid formation (COHN and MORSE, 1960; ELSBACH, 1959; SBARRA and KARNOSKY, 1959). These increases are correlated in normal neutrophils with a concurrent increase in the activity of the hexosemonophosphate shunt (SBARRA and KARNOSKY, 1959). Indications that intact microtubules are necessary for the disposal of ingested material is supported both by the observation that colchicine and vinblastine, agents that prevent the normal polymerization of tubulin into microtubules (WILSON et al., 1974), interfere with degranulation and the formation of secondary lysosomes in the polymorphonuclear leukocyte (MALAWISTA, 1968) and by studies of cells from mice with Chediak-Higachi syndrome (OLIVER et al., 1974). Colchicine, however, does not interfere with phagocytosis per se of either bacteria (MALAWISTA and BODEL, 1967) or monosodium urate crystals (SPILBERG et al., 1974).

It has been postulated that following the initial phagocytosis of crystals, the release of lactic acid lowers the pH in the articular space, a change that would promote further crystallization of sodium urate. Incubation of polymorphonuclear leukocytes and monosodium urate crystals in isotonic saline, however, does not lead following phagocytosis to a decrease of the pH of the media below 7.2 (SPILBERG, 1975). Furthermore, the synovial fluid pH of 12 patients at the peak of an acute gouty attack has been found to be 7.43 ± 0.16 SD, and of 13 nongouty controls 7.5 ± 0.11 SD (SPILBERG et al., 1975). The amount of HCl required to bring the synovial fluid of an acute gouty joint from 7.5 to 7.0 has been found to be 36.5 mM (SPILBERG et al., 1977a). It appears, then, that the buffering capacity of synovial fluid is high enough to preclude major changes in pH. Moreover, changes in pH within physiological range have only minor effect on sodium urate solubility (KLINENBERG et al., 1973).

B. Mediators of the Inflammatory Response

Although the phlogistic effects of urate crystals are well documented, the mechanisms of the inflammatory reaction remain obscure. KELLERMEYER (1968) postulated that inflammation in acute gouty arthritis is initiated by Hageman factor. Anionic crystals activate Hageman factor (clotting factor XII), which enzymatically converts prekallikrein into kallikrein. Kallikrein acts upon plasma kininogen, releasing the active nonapeptide bradykinin and thus resulting in pain, vasodilation, and vascular permeability. The evidence indicates that catalytic amounts of kallikrein can activate precursor Hageman factor (COCHRANE et al., 1973), suggesting that Hageman factor and kallikrein became activated together in a positive feedback amplification loop. The neutral protease kallikrein has been shown to be chemotactic in vitro for polymorphonuclear leukocytes (GOETZL and AUSTEN, 1972) Leukocytes also possess neutral proteases capable of cleaving a vasoactive peptide from kininogen (GRENBAUM and KIN, 1967; MOVAT et al., 1976). Kinins have been found in the synovial effusions associated with arthritides of different etiologies (MELMON et al., 1967; EISEN, 1970). The concentration of these peptides, however, does not correlate well with the degree of inflammation (MELMON et al., 1967; EISEN, 1970) nor does the injection of kinin into the joints of animals produce synovial fluid leukocytosis or histological alterations of the synovium (MELMON et al., 1967), suggesting that kinins play a secondary role in the inflammatory response.

Other evidence has accumulated indicating that the Hageman factor-plasma kallikrein-kinin system may not play a primary role in initiating the inflammatory response. PHELPS et al. (1966) demonstrated that carboxypeptidase B, an enzyme cleaving the arginine residue at the carboxy terminal end of bradykinin, thereby converting it into an inactive octapeptide, has no effect upon the urate crystal-induced arthritis, either when injected simultaneously with urate crystals into the synovial space or when perfused into the artery supplying the affected joint. It also has been demonstrated that soybean trypsin inhibitor, an avid inhibitor of plasma kallikrein as well as of lysosomal kallikreinlike enzymes, has no effect upon the calcium pyrophosphate dihydrate inflammation induced in rabbit knees (SPILBERG, 1973). It is of further interest that acute urate arthritis has been produced in chickens (SPILBERG, 1974), an animal lacking Hageman factor (RATNOFF, 1966) and that no ornithokinin activity was detected in the synovial fluid of these birds despite the acute inflammation induced by the crystals. Spontaneous gouty arthritis has also been reported in chickens as well as in other fowl without Hageman factor (AUSTIC and COLE, 1972; SCHLUMBERGER, 1959; SCHOTTHAUER and BOLLMAN, 1934). The data obtained in animals and presented above may be different from the physiologic response to urate crystals in humans. The role of Hageman factor in human crystal-induced inflammation, therefore, requires clarification. It is of interest that rheumatoid arthritis has been shown to occur despite a severe deficiency of Hageman factor (DONALDSON et al., 1972).

Several components of complement have been implicated in the acute inflammatory response. The complement products $C3a$, $C5a$, and $C567$ have been shown to be chemotactic for polymorphonuclear leukocytes, and the complex $C1423$ is capable of inducing immune adherence and enhanced phagocytosis (RUDDY et al., 1972). NAFF and MYERS (1973) have reported that urate crystals can activate complement in vitro. They measured the complement components $C1$ to $C5$ after incubating the crystals in serum and found that $C2$, $C4$, $C3$, and $C5$ were depleted while $C1$ was only minimally reduced, suggesting a unique pathway of complement activation. Other components were not measured. This effect upon complement was lost by heating the urate crystals to $200°C$, as previously reported by PHELPS and McCARTY (1969). Levels of complement and its components in joints measured during acute attacks of gout, however, have been reported to be normal (FOSTIROPOULUS et al., 1965; BUNCH et al., 1974; PEKIN and ZVAIFLER, 1964; RYNES et al., 1974), and the phlogistic characteristics of the crystals are not abolished by subjecting them to high temperatures (SPILBERG and OSTERLAND, 1970; PHELPS and McCARTY, 1969). Furthermore, injection of *Naja-Naja* Cobra venom factor into rabbits (SPILBERG and OSTERLAND, 1970) and into a dog (PHELPS and McCARTY, 1969) did not diminish the leukocyte response to urate crystals in synovial fluid. This venom factor has been shown to deplete $C3$ and $C5$, (BRAI and OSTER, 1972) components of complement implicated in both chemotaxis and phagocytosis. It appears then that the inflammatory response to urate crystals does not depend on the presence of either complement or the Hageman factor-kallikrein-kinin system. It is not possible, however, to elicit a crystal-induced arthritis in animals rendered leukopenic by the use of either antipolymorphonuclear leukocyte sera (CHANG and GIALLA, 1968) or vinblastin (PHELPS and McCARTY, 1966; SPILBERG, 1973).

This accumulation of information has led investigators to focus attention on the polymorphonuclear leukocyte itself as the critical factor in the inflammatory response induced by urate crystals. Chemotactic activity for polymorphonuclear leukocytes has been reported to appear in the synovial fluid of canine joints injected

Table 1. Chemotactic response of WBC to urate-induced chemotactic factor

Cells	Chemotactic factors[a]	
	Human	Rabbit
Neutrophils		
Human peripheral blood	8.3 ± 0.2	8.5 ± 0.5
Rabbit peritoneal	7.7 ± 1.2	8.7 ± 0.6
Mononuclear cells		
Rabbit peritoneal	3.0 ± 0.4	3.9 ± 0.6
Macrophage		
Human alveolar	0	ND[b]
Lymphocytes		
Human peripheral blood	0	0
Eosinophiles		
Guinea-pig peritoneal	0	ND

[a] 6×10^{-6} M. Number represents the Chemotactic Index (Spilberg et. al., 1975) expressed as the Mean ± SD of three experiments.
[b] ND—"not done".

with urate crystals (Phelps, 1970b). In vitro studies have shown that, in the absence of complement, the phagocytosis of monosodium urate crystals by neutrophils (Phelps, 1970a; Spilberg et al., 1975) leads to the formation of a glycoprotein (mol. wt. 8400 daltons) chemotactic for other neutrophils and, to a lesser degree, for mononuclear cells (Spilberg et al., 1976) (Table 1). The appearance of chemotactic factor is abolished by preincubating the cells with protein synthesis inhibitors (Spilberg et al., 1974; Spilberg et al., 1977b), suggesting that chemotactic factor activity is produced by the induction of new protein synthesis, either of the factor itself or of a protein that modulates its activity, rather than by direct activation of a precursor protein. Colchicine, too, when incubated with cells and crystals at concentrations that are therapeutic for humans, inhibits the appearance of chemotactic factor activity (Phelps, 1970a; Spilberg et al., 1974) without affecting phagocytosis per se (Malawista and Bodel, 1967; Spilberg et al., 1974). This effect of colchicine offers an explanation to its known therapeutic value in gouty arthritis. It is not clear, however, whether the effect of colchicine is due to interference with microtubule assembly (Malawista, 1968) or to a direct effect upon the synthetic cell mechanism (Lohmander et al., 1976). The activity of the urate-induced chemotactic factor for neutrophils can be detected in vitro at a concentration of 1.8×10^{-7} M using the Boyden chamber technique. Comparison of the chemotactic activity of this cell-derived chemotactic factor with C5a suggests that the urate-induced factor is slightly less active on a molar basis. The concentration of the urate-induced factor that gives 50% maximal chemotactic activity has been calculated to be 1.5×10^{-6} M (Spilberg et al., 1976) and the amount of C5a required to give 50% activity 1.8×10^{-7} M (Gallin et al., 1975). Direct comparative studies, however, have not been performed. The intra-articular injection of urate-induced chemotactic factor obtained from rabbits into the joints of animals of other rabbits results in a massive accumulation of

Table 2. Characteristics of crystal-induced chemotactic factor

	Na urate	CPPD	Diamond
mol. wt.	8400	8400	8400
Glycoprotein	+	+	+
Equal migration from cathode on gel electrophoresis	+	+	+
Requirement of crystal phagocytosis	+	+	+
Heat sensitivity	+	+	+
Inhibition of appearance by protein synthesis inhibitors	+	+	ND
Inhibition of appearance by colchicine	+	+	ND
Deactivation	+	+	ND
Crossdeactivation	+	+	ND
Intracellular localization	Lysosomal fraction	Lysosomal fraction	Lysosomal fraction
Induction of arthritis in rabbits	+	ND [a]	ND
Inhibition of colchicine enhancement of capping in neutrophils	+	ND	ND

[a] ND—"not done".

polymorphonuclear leukocytes in the synovial fluid and of mononuclear cells and polymorphonuclear leukocytes in the synovial membrane, a picture that mimicks crystal-induced arthritis. The leukotactic effect of the factor is not accompanied by an increase in the vascular permeability. When histamine, a potent vasodilator, is injected intra-articularly into the joints of rabbits, an increment in vascular dilatation but no leukocytosis above that obtained with isotonic saline is observed (SPILBERG et al., 1977c). These experiments are in agreement with the postulate that the accumulation of leukocytes seen in the acute gouty joint is due to the chemotactic effect of the factor, vascular dilation playing a secondary role. Leukocytes contain enzymes that both produce and destroy kinins (GREENBAUM and KIN, 1967; MOVAT et al., 1976), mediators of vascular dilatation and pain; since vascular dilatation is seen in the inflammatory process induced by sodium urate crystals, it is likely that kinins and perhaps other unidentified substances play a supportive role in the development of the inflammatory process.

The sodium urate crystal is not unique in its ability to induce chemotactic factor activity from the neutrophil. A chemotactic factor with identical characteristics (Table 2) can be recovered from the granular fraction of human neutrophils that are allowed to phagocytose calcium pyrophosphate dihydrate crystals (SPILBERG et al., 1977b) and amorphous diamond crystals (SPILBERG et al., 1977d). Moreover, chemotactic activity for neutrophils has been reported in the media of neutrophils engulfing yeast (RYDGREN et al., 1976), or aggregated α-globulin in the absence of plasma (ZIGMOND and HIRSCH, 1973). Although additional studies are wanting, it is conceivable that the generation of a chemotactic factor may represent a uniform response of the neutrophil, and perhaps of other phagocytic cells, to the uptake process.

The mechanism by which polymorphonuclear leukocytes respond to a specific chemical gradient with directional migration has been investigated but not determined. ZIGMOND (1974) has shown that polymorphonuclear leukocytes are capable of recognizing a chemical gradient across their cell membranes. It has been postulated that chemotactic factors induce changes in the cellular membranes of polymorphonuclear leukocytes, thus making the cells more adhesive and thereby increasing their motility (CARTER, 1965), and that they affect the membrane potential of the cell by decreasing the negative surface charge (GALLIN et al., 1975). Using complement components as chemotactic factors, WARD and BECKER (1970) have shown that both potassium dependent ATPase and activation of a specific serine esterase are required for normal chemotaxis. A role for adenosine $3',5'$-cyclic monophosphate (cAMP) has not yet been clearly shown. It has been demonstrated that agents known to increase intracellular cAMP inhibit chemotaxis (TSE et al., 1972; RIVKIN et al., 1975). Prostaglandins E_1 and E_2 are known to increase intracellular cAMP (SCOTT, 1970; BUNCH et al., 1974; HORTON, 1969) and PGE_1 has been reported to act as a chemotactic factor (KALEY and WEINER, 1971). However, incubation of rabbit or human neutrophils with *E. coli*-derived factor or urate-induced chemotactic factor, procedures that render the cell inactive for future chemotactic response to the factors (WARD and BECKER, 1968; SPILBERG et al., 1976), produces no change in intracellular cAMP levels (RIVKIN, 1975) and only a minor elevation of cGMP (SPILBERG et al., unpublished observation).

BOUCEK and SNYDERMAN (1976) have shown that the incubation with complement-activated plasma is accompanied by an increase in the calcium content of the cell, suggesting a role of chemotactic factors in the regulation of intracellular Ca^{2+} necessary for the activation of actinomycinlike proteins, as is the case in the muscle. Another possible role for Ca^{2+} is in the control of microtubule assembly. Microtubule integrity is required for the chemotactic process (BANDMAN et al., 1974) and low calcium concentrations favor microtubule assembly (SCHLIWA, 1976). GOLDSTEIN et al. (1973) have shown that incubation of the chemotactic factor C5a with polymorphonuclear leukocytes leads to an increase in microtubule assembly. Furthermore, it has recently been shown that the disrupting effect of colchicine upon microtubules is inhibited by the urate-induced chemotactic factor (MANDELL et al., 1977). This protective effect of the factor is abolished by preincubating the cells with diisopropyl fluorophosphate (DFP), implicating a serine esterase in the process leading to microtubule assembly and chemotaxis (MANDELL and SPILBERG, 1977).

The preincubation of human polymorphonuclear leukocytes with complement-activated plasma or human urate-induced chemotactic factor has been shown to prevent the polymorphonuclear leukocytes from migrating towards a chemotactic gradient when, after washing, the cells were challenged with either of the factors in the Boyden chamber (SPILBERG et al., 1976). The chemotactic activity of complement-activated plasma has been shown to be due mainly to C5a and C567 (BECKER et al., 1974). The inhibition of the polymorphonuclear leukocyte chemotactic response by preincubation of the cells with the same chemotactic factor has been called "deactivation" by WARD and BECKER (1970). This property of chemotactic factor may be important in that it concentrates the polymorphonuclear leukocyte at the center of the inflammatory focus. Cross-deactivation between the chemotactic factors C5a and kallikrein (GOETZL and AUSTEN, 1974) and between different complement-derived chemotactic factors (BECKER et al., 1974) has been described. Cross-deactivation of polymorphonuclear leukocytes is consistent with the concept that chemotactic factors share one or more general recognition sites on the surface of the cell which can be saturated with chemotactic factor, thus preventing the recognition of a chemotactic gradient. Alternatively, different recognition sites may exist which, when bound to chemotactic factors, lead to the activation of a common pathway; once the pathway is fully activated, the cell is prohibited from responding with directional migration to another chemotactic factor, which it is, however, capable of recognizing. Support for the existence of a common pathway is found in the studies of BECKER and WARD (1967), WARD and BECKER (1968), GOETZEL and AUSTEN (1974) and studies from our laboratory (MANDELL and SPILBERG, 1977). These studies implicate an activated cell-bound serine esterase, susceptible to irreversible inhibition by DFP, in the polymorphonuclear chemotactic response to the complement-derived chemotactic factors, kallikrein and human urate-induced chemotactic factor. A second active serine esterase has also been described (BECKER and WARD, 1967). The role of the esterases, calcium, and other still undefined agents in the biochemical sequence of events leading to the directional stimulation of the contractile apparatus of the cell remains to be elucidated.

Recent studies have described the finding of IgM, IgG, fibrin, and C3 in the interstitium of tophi from two gouty patients (HASSELBACHER and SCHUMACHER, 1976). The ability of synthetic crystals to adsorb IgG and other proteins (KOZIN and MCCARTY, 1976a, 1976b) and the presence of IgM, IgG, IgA, fibrin, C3, and albumin on the surface of naturally occurring crystals have also been reported (HASSELBACH and SCHUMACHER, 1976). Little is known of the role that adsorbed proteins may play in the development of the crystal-induced inflammatory response. Preliminary reports suggest that the cytolytic properties of the crystal may be impaired (KOZIN et al., 1976; SKOSEY et al., 1976) and that the lysosomal enzyme release from polymorphonuclear leukocytic may be increased by crystals coated with IgG or Cohn fraction II.

The role of lysosomes in the mediation of the inflammatory reaction has been reviewed by WEISSMANN (1972). The intra-articular injection of lysosomal lysates from rabbit granulocytes leads to profound arthritis in rabbit knees (WEISSMANN et al., 1969). Since polymorphonuclear leukocyte lysosomes contain proteolytic enzymes as well as proteins with intrinsic phlogistic properties, it is important to emphasize the ability of the polymorphonuclear leukocyte to release its lysosomal contents concurrently with, as well as independently of, cell death. Various substances have been shown capable of inducing polymorphonuclear leukocyte lysosomal exocytosis (HENSON, 1976), including the complement subcomponent C5a and immune complexes. Of special relevance to the discussion here is the demonstrated ability of monosodium urate crystals to cause lysosomal enzyme release from cells. Monosodium urate crystals are able to induce release of the lysosomal contents of granulocytes during phagocytosis, following lysosomal membrane rupture due to the membranolytic properties of the crystal (WEISSMANN and RITA, 1973) (presumably after lysosomal digestion of the proteins coating the crystals), and by direct exocytosis (SPILBERG et al., 1975; HOFFSTEIN and WEISSMANN, 1975). Chemotactic factors are also capable of inducing lysosomal enzyme release (BECKER et al., 1974; GOLDSTEIN et al., 1975; SPILBERG et al., 1976) under certain conditions; however, the physiologic significance of these findings is still unclear. It has been proposed that cyclic nucleotide levels modulate the release of lysosomal enzymes via the cGMP/cAMP ratio; high values would tend to augment exocytosis while low values would be inhibitory (IGNARRO, 1975). Many parallels exist between the modulation of chemotaxis and

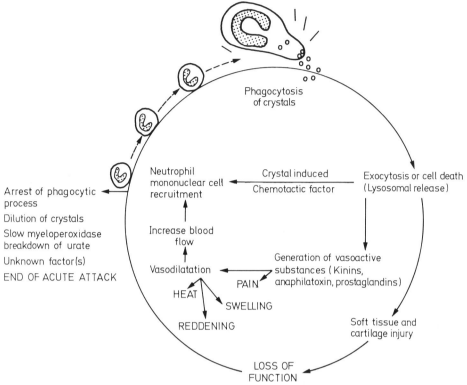

Fig. 1. Scheme of the acute gouty attack

lysosomal enzyme release, including the requirement for an activatable serine ester-ase (HENSON, 1976).

Prostaglandins (PG) have been shown to increase vascular permeability and modestly enhance leukocyte migration (KALEY and WEINER, 1971). There is evidence that clearly shows the ability of rabbit polymorphonuclear leukocytes (MCCALL and YOULTEN, 1973) and human platelets (SMITH and WILLIS, 1971) to generate prosta-glandins in vitro. However, the phlogistic action of these compounds is not com-pletely clear. While DENKO (1974) has suggested that PGE_1 is capable of enhancing the inflammation induced by monosodium urate crystals in the footpad of rats fed a diet deficient in essential fatty acids (precursors in the synthesis of prostaglandins), and GLATT et al. (1974) have shown an early intra-articular peak of PGE_2 in the avian model of crystal-induced arthritis, other reports have emphasized the anti-inflammatory properties of the same prostaglandins. DIPASQUALE et al. (1973) and ZURIER and QUAGLIATA (1971) have shown that PGE_1 and PGE_2 respectively can diminish adjuvant-induced arthritis and carrageenan-induced inflammation.

Perhaps the strongest argument implicating prostaglandins in the inflammatory reaction is the shared ability of aspirin, indomethacin, and other nonsteroidal anti-inflammatory agents to inhibit prostaglandin synthesis (VANE, 1971; SMITH and WILLIS, 1971). With specific reference to crystal-induced arthritis, it should be noted that aspirin has little if any therapeutic value in the management of the acute attack and that indomethacin has also been shown to exert a direct inhibitory effect on polymorphonuclear leukocyte phagocytosis of urate crystals (CHANG, 1972) in vitro.

Although the evidence is incomplete, available experimental work indicates that the only consistent requirement for crystal-induced arthritis is the presence of crystals and polymorphonuclear leukocytes in the joint cavity. Since few neutrophils are present in normal synovial fluid, the first encounter would depend solely on the concentration of crystals. The ensuing phagocytosis of crystals results in the formation of a factor chemotactically active for other neutrophils and leads to the disruption of their lysosomal membrane and to cell death. The release of lysosomal proteases by exocytosis (SPILBERG et al., 1975; HOFFSTEIN and WEISSMANN, 1975) and following cell death, into the joint cavity results in the destruction of cartilage proteoglycans (JANOFF et al., 1976) and in soft tissue injury (WEISSMANN et al., 1969). Leukocytes contain enzymes that both produce and destroy kinins (GRENBAUM and KIN, 1967; MOVAT et al., 1976). It is possible that kinins and other vasoactive substances play a role in later stages of the inflammatory process (Fig.1). This simplified concept of the inflammatory response to crystals is strengthened by the finding that the monosodium urate crystal-induced chemotactic factor obtained from rabbit neutrophils produces a marked inflammation when injected into joints of other rabbits (SPILBERG et al., 1977c).

C. Termination of the Acute Gouty Attack

The self-limited nature of the acute gouty attack is one of the most intriguing aspects of the acute inflammatory response. Several factors probably aid in terminating the attack: removal of sodium urate from the joint cavity by diffusion aided by increased blood flow, slow breakdown of urate to allantoin by lysosomal myeloperoxidase (CANELLAKIS et al., 1955), and release of corticosteroids from the adrenal cortex as a general stress response to the gouty attack.

Another clue to the understanding of the puzzling phenomena is provided by clinical experience; examination of synovial fluid in the later stages of the inflammatory response to crystals reveals that, although leukocytes and crystals are present, the latter are no longer intracellular, i.e., the phagocytic process has been arrested. The demonstration that phagocytosis of the crystals by the neutrophil is required for urate-induced chemotactic factor generation provides a possible explanation for the self-limited nature of the acute gouty attack since, in the absence of phagocytosis, the attraction of more cells to the site of inflammation would be curtailed. The mechanism by which phagocytosis is arrested, however, remains to be elucidated. Of relevance to this question is the recent finding of MUSSON and BECKER (1976) that some chemotactic factors can depress phagocytosis.

References

Austic, R. E., Cole, R. K.: Impaired renal clearance of uric acid in chickens having hyperuricemia and articular gout. Amer. J. Physiol. **223**, 525—530 (1972)

Bandmann, U., Rydgren, L., Norberg, B.: The difference between random movement and chemotaxis. Effects of antitubulins on neutrophil granulocyte locomotion. Exp. Cell Res. **88**, 63—73 (1974)

Becker, E. L., Sowell, H. J., Henson, P. M., Hsu, L. S.: The ability of chemotactic factors to induce lysosomal enzyme release. I. The characteristics of the release, the importance of surfaces and the relation of enzyme release to chemotactic responsiveness. J. Immunol. **112**, 2045—2054 (1974)

Boucek, M. M., Snyderman, R.: Calcium influx requirement for human neutrophil chemotaxis: inhibition by lanthanun chloride. Science **193**, 905—907 (1976)

Bourne, H. R. et al.: Cyclic adnosine-3', 5'-monophosphate and the regulation of human granulocyte function. J. clin. Invest. **49**, 11a Abstr. (1972)

Brai, M., Oster, A. G.: Studies on the C3 shunt activation in cobra venom induced lysis of unsensitized erythrocytes. Proc. Soc. exp. Biol. (Med.) **140**, 1116—1121 (1972)

Bunch, T. W., Hunder, G. G., McDuffie, F. C., O'Brien, P. C., Markowitz, H.: Synovial fluid complement determination as a diagnostic aid in inflammatory joint diseases. Mayo Clin. Proc. **49**, 715—720 (1974)

Canellakis, E. S., Tuttle, A. L., Cohen, P. P.: A comparative study of the end products of uric acid oxidation by peroxidases. J. biol. Chem. **213**, 397—404 (1955)

Carter, S. B.: Principle of cell motility: the direction of cell movement and cancer invasion. Nature (Lond.) **108**, 1183—1187 (1965)

Chang, Y.: Studies on phagocytosis. II. The effect of nonsteroidal anti-inflammatory drugs on phagocytosis and on urate crystal-induced canine joint inflammation. Pharm. exp. Ther. **183**, 235—244 (1972)

Chang, Y., Gialla, E. J.: Suppression of urate crystalinduced canine joints inflammation by heterologous antipolymorphonuclear leukocyte serum. Arthr. and Rheum. **11**, 145—150 (1968)

Cochrane, C. G., Revak, S. D., Aiken, B. S., Sitzer, S. S.: The structural characteristic and activation of Hageman factor in inflammation: mechanisms and control. In: Lepon, I. H., Ward, P. A. (Eds.). New York: Academic Press 1973

Cohn, A. Z., Morse, S. I.: Functional and metabolic properties of polymorphonuclear leukocytes. I. Observations in the requirements and consequences of particle ingestion. J. exp. Med. **111**, 667—687 (1960)

Denko, C. W.: A phlogistic function of prostaglandin E_1 in urate crystal inflammation. J. Rheum. **1**, 222—229 (1974)

Dipasquale, G., Rassaert, R., Welaj, P., Tripp, L.: Influence of prostaglandins (PG)E_2 and $F_{2\alpha}$ on the inflammatory process. Prostaglandins **3**, 741—757 (1973)

Donaldson, V. H., Gluek, H. I., Fleming, T.: Rheumatoid arthritis in a patient with Hageman trait. New Engl. J. Med. **286**, 528—530 (1972)

Eisen, V.: Plasma kinins in synovial exudates. Brit. J. exp. Path. **51**, 322—325 (1970)

Elsbach, P.: Composition and synthesis of lipids in resting and phagocyting leukocytes. J. exp. Med. **110**, 969—980 (1959)

Fostiropoulus, K., Austen, K. F., Bloch, K. J.: Total hemolytic complement and second component of complement activity in serum and synovial fluid. Arthr. and Rheum. **8**, 219—232 (1965)

Gallin, J. I., Durocher, J., Kaplan, A. P.: Interaction of leukocyte chemotactic factors with the cell surface. I. Chemotactic factor induced changes in human granulocyte surface charges. J. clin. Invest. **55**, 967—974 (1975)

Glatt, M., Peska, B., Brune, K.: Leukocytes and prostaglandins in acute inflammation. Experientia (Basel) **30**, 1257—1259 (1974)

Glatt, M., Peska, B., Brune, K.: Leukocytes and prostaglandins in acute inflammation. Experientia (Basel) **30**, 1257—1259 (1974)

Goetzl, E. J., Austen, K. F.: A method for assessing the in vitro chemotactic response of neutrophil utilizing CR51 labeled human leukocytes. Immunol. Commun. **1**, 421—430 (1972)

Goetzl, E. J., Austen, K. F.: Active site chemotactic factors and the regulation of the human neutrophil chemotactic response. Antibiot. Chemother. **19**, 218—232 (1974)

Goldfinger, S. E., Howell, R. R., Seegmiller, J. E.: Suppression of metabolic accompaniments of phagocytosis by colchicine. Arthr. and Rheum. **8**, 1112—1122 (1965)

Goldstein, I., Hoffstein, S., Gallin, J., Weissmann, G.: Mechanisms of lysosomal enzyme release from human leukocytes: Microtubule assembly and membrane fusion induced by a component of complement. Proc. nat. Acad. Sci. (Wash.) **70**, 2916—2920 (1973)

Goldstein, I., Hoffstein, S. T., Weissmann, G.: Influence of divalent cations upon complement-mediated enzyme release from human polymorphonuclear leukocytes. J. Immunol. **115**, 665—670 (1975)

Greenbaum, L. M., Kin, K. S.: The kinin forming and kinidase activities of rabbit polymorphonuclear leukocytes. Brit. J. pharm. Chemother. **29**, 238—247 (1967)

Hasselbacher, P., Schumacher, H. R. Jr.: Localization of immunoglobulin in gouty tophi by immunohistology, and on the surface of monosodium urate crystals (MSU) by immune agglutination. Arthr. and Rheum. **19**, 802 Abstr. (1976)

Henson, P. M.: Secretion of lysosomal enzymes induced by immune complexes and complement. In: Dingle, J. T., Dean, R. T. (Eds.): Lysosomes in Biology and Pathology, Vol. 5. New York: American Elsevier Publishers 1976

Hoffstein, S., Weissmann, G.: Mechanisms of lysosomal enzyme release from leukocytes. IV. Interaction of monosodium urate crystals with dogfish and human leukocytes. Arthr. and Rheum. **18**, 153—165 (1975)

Horton, E. W.: Hypothesis on physiological roles of prostaglandins. Physiol. Rev. **49**, 122—161 (1969)

Ignarro, L. J.: Regulation of lysosomal enzyme release by prostaglandins, autonomic neurohormones and cyclic nucleotides. In: Dingle, J. T., Dean, R. T. (Eds.): Lysosomes in Biology and Pathology, Vol. 4. New York: American Elsevier Publishers 1975

Janoff, A., Feinstein, G., Melemud, C., Elias, J. M.: Degradation of cartilage proteoglycan by human leukocyte granule neutral protease.—A model of joint injury. Penetration of enzyme into rabbit articular cartilage and release of $^{35}SO_4$-labeled material from the tissue. J. clin. Invest. **57**, 615—624 (1976)

Kaley, G., Weiner, R.: Prostaglandin E_1: A potential mediator of the inflammatory response. Ann. N.Y. Acad. Sci. **180**, 338—350 (1971)

Kellermeyer, R. W.: Hageman factor and acute gouty arthritis. Arthr. and Rheum. **11**, 452—459 (1968)

Klinenberg, J. R., Bluestone, R., Schlosstein, L., Waisman, J., Whitehouse, M. W.: Urate deposition disease. How it is regulated and how can it be modified? Ann. intern. Med. **78**, 99—111 (1973)

Kozin, F., McCarty, D. J.: Protein adsorption to monosodium urate, calcium pyrophosphate dihydrate, and silica crystals. Arthr. and Rheum. **19**, 433—438 (1976a)

Kozin, F., McCarty, D. J.: Adsorption of protein monosodium urate crystals: A possible mechanism of crystal-induced inflammation. Arthr. and Rheum. (Abstr.) **19**, 805 (1976b)

Kozin, F., Skosey, J. L., May, J., Chow, D. C.: Modification of responses of human neutrophils to monosodium urate crystals by coating of crystals with serum proteins. Clin. Res. (Abstr.) **24**, 331a (1976)

Lohmander, S., Moskalewski, S., Madsen, K., Thyberg, J., Friberg, V.: Influence of colchicine on the synthesis and secretion of proteoglycans and collagen by fetal guinea-pig chondrocytes. Exp. Cell Res. **99**, 333—345 (1976)

McCall, E., Youlten, L. J.: Proceedings: Prostaglandin E_1 synthesis by phagocytosing rabbit polymorphonuclear leukocytes: its inhibition by indomethacin and its role in chemotaxis. J. Physiol. (Lond.) **234**, 98—100 (1973)

McCarty, D. J., Jr.: On the crystal deposition diseases. Dis. Month. March (1970)

Malawista, S. E.: Colchicine: The common mechanism for its anti-inflammatory and anti-mytotic effects. Arthr. and Rheum. **11**, 191—197 (1968)

Malawista, S. E., Bodel, P. T.: The dissociation by colchicine of phagocytosis from increased oxygen consumption in human leukocytes. J. clin. Invest. **46**, 786—796 (1967)

Mandell, B., Spilberg, I.: Role of a chemotactic factor activated serine esterase in polymorphonuclear leukocytes capping. Clin. Res. **25**, (Abstr.) 363 A (1977)

Mandell, B., Spilberg, I., Lichman, J.: Inhibitions of polymorphonuclear leukocyte capping by a chemotactic factor. J. Immunol. **118**, 1375—1378 (1977)

Melmon, K. L., Webster, M. E., Goldfinger, S. E. et al.: The presence of a kinin in inflammatory synovial effusion from arthritides of varying etiologies. Arthr. and Rheum. **10**, 13—20 (1967)

Movat, H. Z., Habal, F. M., Macmorine, D. R. L.: Generation of a vasoactive peptide by a neutral protease of human neutrophil leukocytes. Agents Actions **6**, 183—190 (1976)

Musson, R., Becker, E. L.: The inhibitory effect of chemotactic factors on erythrophagocytosis by human neutrophils. J. Immunol. **117**, 433—439 (1976)

Naff, G. B., Myers, P. H.: Complement as a mediator of inflammation in acute gouty arthritis. I. Studies on the reaction between human serum complement and sodium urate crystals. J. Lab. clin. Med. **81**, 747—760 (1960)

Oliver, J. M., Zurier, R. B., Berlin, R. D.: Concanavalin-A cap formation on polymorphonuclear leukocytes of normal and beige (Chediak-Higashi) mice. Nature (Lond.) **253**, 471—473 (1974)

Pekin, T. J., Zvaifler, N. J.: Hemolytic complement in synovial fluid. J. clin. Invest. **43**, 1372—1382 (1964)

Phelps, P.: Polymorphonuclear leukocyte motility in vitro. IV. Colchicine inhibition of chemotactic activity formation after phagocytosis of urate-crystals. Arthr. and Rheum. **13**, 1—12 (1970a)

Phelps, P.: Appearance of chemotactic activity following intraarticular injection of monosodium urate crystals: effect of colchicine. J. Lab. clin. Med. **76**, 622—631 (1970b)

Phelps, P., McCarty, D. J., Jr.: Crystal induced inflammation in canine joints. II. Importance of polymorphonuclear leukocytes. J. exp. Med. **124**, 115—127 (1966)

Phelps, P., McCarty, D. J.: Crystal induced arthritis. Postgrad. med. **45**, 87—94 (1969)

Phelps, P., Prockop, D. J., McCarty, D. J.: Crystal induced inflammation in canine joints. III. Evidence against bradykinin as mediator of inflammation. J. Lab. clin. Med. **68**, 433—444 (1966a)

Ratnoff, O. D.: The biology and pathology of the initial stages of blood coagulation. Progr. Hematol. **5**, 204—245 (1966)

Rivkin, I., Rosenblat, J., Becker, E. L.: The role of cyclic AMP in the chemotactic responsiveness and expontaneous motility of rabbit peritoneal neutrophils. J. Immunol. **115**, 1126—1134 (1975)

Ruddy, S., Gigli, I., Austen, F.: The complement system in man. I. New Engl. J. Med. **287**, 489—495 (1972)

Rydgren, L., Simingskold, G., Bandman, V., Norberg, G.: The role of cytoplasmic microtubules in polymorphonuclear leukocyte chemotaxis. Exp. Cell Res. **99**, 207—220 (1976)

Rynes, R. I., Ruddy, S., Schur, P. H., Spragg, J., Austen, K. F.: Levels of complement components, properdin factors, and kininogen in patients with inflammatory arthritis. J. Rheum. **1**, 413—427 (1974)

Sbarra, A. J., Karnovsky, M. L.: The biochemical basis of phagocytosis. J. biol. Chem. **234**, 1355—1362 (1959)

Schliwa, M.: The role of divalent cations in the regulation of microtubule assembly. J. Cell Biol. **70**, 527—540 (1976)

Schotthauer, C. V., Bollman, J. I.: Spontaneous gout in turkeys. J. Amer. Vet. med. Ass. **85**, 98—103 (1934)

Schlumberger, H. G.: Synovial gout in the parakeet. Lab. Invest. **8**, 1304—1318 (1959)

Schumacher, H. R., Phelps, P.: Sequential changes in human polymorphonuclear leukocytes after urate crystal phagocytosis. An electron microscopy study. Arthr. and Rheum. **11**, 145—150 (1968)

Scott, R. E.: Effects of prostaglandins, epinephrine and NaF on human leukocyte, platelet and liver adrenyl cyclase. Blood **35**, 514—516 (1970)

Skosey, J. L., Kozin, F., Chow, D. C., May, J.: Differential responses of human neutrophils to monosodium urate crystals (MSU) and MSU coated with gamma globulin. Clin. Res. **24**, (Abstr.) 11a (1976)

Smith, J. B., Willis, A. L.: Aspirin selectively inhibits prostaglandin production in human platelets. Nature (Lond.) New Biol. **231**, 235—237 (1971)

Spilberg, I.: Studies on the mechanisms of inflammation induced by calcium pyrophosphate crystals. J. Lab. clin. Med. **82**, 86—91 (1973)

Spilberg, I.: Urate crystal arthritis in animals lacking Hageman factor. Arthr. and Rheum. **17**, 143—148 (1974)

Spilberg, I.: Current concepts of the mechanisms of acute inflammation in gouty arthritis. Arthr. and Rheum. **18**, 129—134 (1975)

Spilberg, I., Gallacher, A., Mandell, B.: Studies on crystal induced chemotactic factor. II. Role of phagocytosis. J. Lab. clin. Med. **85**, 631—636 (1975)

Spilberg, I., Gallacher, A., Mandell, B.: Calcium pyrophosphate dihydrate (CPPD) crystal induced chemotactic factor. Subcellular localization, role of protein synthesis and phagocytosis. J. Lab. clin. Med. **89**, 817—822 (1977b)

Spilberg, I., Gallacher, A., Mehta, J. M., Mandell, B.: Urate crystal induced chemotactic factor. Isolation and partial characterization. J. clin. Invest. **58**, 815—819 (1976)

Spilberg, I., Mandell, B., Wochner, R. D.: Studies on crystal induced chemotactic factor. I. Role of protein synthesis and neutral protease activity. J. Lab. clin. Med. **83**, 56—63 (1974)

Spilberg, I., Osterland, C. K.: Anti-inflammatory effect of the trypsin-kallikrein inhibitor in acute arthritis induced by urate crystals in rabbits. J. Lab. clin. Med. **76**, 472—479 (1970)

Spilberg, I., Rosenberg, D., Mandell, B.: Induction of arthritis by purified cell derived chemotactic factor. Role of chemotaxis and vascular permeability. J. clin. Invest. **59**, 582—585 (1977c)

Spilberg, I., Rosenberg, D., Mehta, J.: Induction of cell derived chemotactic factor and of arthritis by amorphous diamond crystals. Arthr. and Rheum. (Abstr.) **20**, 136 (1977d)

Spilberg, I., Tanphaichitr, K., Kantor, O.: Synovial fluid pH in acute gouty arthritis. Arthr. and Rheum. **20**, 142 (1977a)

Tse, R. L., Phelps, P., Urban, D.: Polymorphonuclear leukocyte motility in vitro. VI. Effect of purine and pyrimidine analogs: possible role of cyclic AMP. J. Lab. clin. Med. **80**, 264—274 (1972)

Turner, R. A., Schumacher, H. R., Myers, A. R.: Phagocytic function of polymorphonuclear leukocytes in rheumatic diseases. J. clin. Invest. **52**, 1632—1635 (1973)

Vane, J. R.: Inhibition of prostaglandin synthesis as a mechanism of action for aspirin-like drugs. Nature (Lond.) New Biol. **231**, 232—235 (1971)

Wallingford, W. R., McCarty, D. J.: Differential membranolytic effects of microcrystalline sodium urate and calcium pyrophosphate dihydrate. J. exp. Med. **133**, 100—112 (1971)

Ward, P. A.: Complement derived chemotactic factors and their interaction with neutrophilic granulocytes. Ingrahm proceedings of the international symposium on the biological activities of complement, pp. 108—116. Basel: Karger AG 1971

Ward, P. A., Becker, E. L.: The deactivation of rabbit neutrophils by chemotactic factor and the nature of the activatable esterase. J. exp. Med. **127**, 693—709 (1968)

Ward, P. A., Becker, E. L.: Biochemical demonstration of the activatable esterase of the rabbit neutrophil involved in the chemotactic response. J. Immunol. **105**, 1057—1067 (1970)

Weissmann, G.: Lysosomal mechanisms of tissue injury in arthritis. New Engl. J. Med. **286**, 141—147 (1972)

Weissmann, G., Rita, G. A.: Molecular basis of gouty inflammation: Interaction of monosodium urate crystals with lysosomes and lyposomes. Nature (Lond.) New Biol. **240**, 167—172 (1972)

Weissmann, G., Spilberg, I., Krakauer, K.: Arthritis induced in rabbits by lysates of granulocyte lysosomes. Arthr. and Rheum. **12**, 103—116 (1969)

Wilson, L., Banburg, J. R., Mizel, S. B. et al.: Interaction of drugs with microtubule proteins. Fed. Proc. **33**, 158—166 (1974)

Zigmond, S. H.: Mechanisms of sensing chemical gradients by polymorphonuclear leukocytes. Nature (Lond.) **249**, 450—452 (1974)

Zigmond, S. H., Hirsch, J. G.: Leukocyte locomotion and chemotaxis. New methods for evaluation, and demonstration of a cell-derived factor. J. exp. Med. **137**, 387—410 (1973)

Zurier, R. B., Quagliata, F.: Effect of prostaglandin E_1 on adjuvant arthritis. Nature (Lond.) **234**, 304—305 (1971)

CHAPTER 16

Role of Local Factors in the Precipitation of Urate Crystals

P. A. SIMKIN

A. Introduction

Over the past 15 years, the urate crystal has become accepted as the fundamental local factor in the pathogenesis of gout (McCARTY and HOLLANDER, 1961; McCARTY, 1977). In this concept, formation of crystals is the primary event underlying all gout, with acute arthritis or the growth of tophi invariably being secondary crystal-induced responses. Clearly, the conditions leading to urate precipitation are of paramount importance to an understanding of the syndrome of gout. Crystallization in vitro is a phenomenon well understood by physical chemists, who are thus able to determine precise solubility limits for any solute in a given solvent under defined conditions of temperature and pH. Formation of urate crystals in vivo, however, is not well understood by physicians, who have found that the incidence of gout correlates poorly with the concentration of urate in human serum, and that crystals, when present, are not randomly distributed but occur preferentially at well-recognized peripheral sites.

The careful epidemiologic studies in Framingham, Massachusetts provide the best data on the correlation between the serum concentration of urate and the incidence of gout (HALL et al., 1967). As a part of this work, serial observations were made on 2283 men over a period of 12 years. The highest serum urate level found in each of these men is listed in Table 1 and correlated with the observed incidence of gouty arthritis. If one conservatively considers 7 mg/100 ml as the borderline between normal and hyperuricemic concentrations of plasma urate, the poor correlation between hyperuricemia and gout is striking. In one-third (23) of the patients with gout, a serum urate as high as 7.0 mg/100 ml was never found. The largest group of gouty patients (27) had maximal urate concentrations between 7.0 and 7.9 mg/100 ml, yet only one in six subjects in this range developed gout over the entire 12 years of observation. For those in the next higher range, 8.0–8.9 mg/100 ml, the risk of developing gout remained low (25%). Each of these observations underscores the fact that serum urate concentration alone is a poor predictor of gouty arthritis. Additional factors must play a major role in determining when and where urate crystals form in human tissues.

"The extreme frequency of the affection first locating itself in the ball of the great toe, cannot be looked upon as a mere fortuitous circumstance, but is intimately connected with the pathology of the disease" (GARROD, 1859).

The distribution patterns characteristic both for acute gouty arthritis and for the formation of tophi clearly indicate the importance of local factors in determining sites of urate deposition. If all factors involved in urate crystallization were the same

Table 1. Prevalence of gouty arthritis in relation to serum urate level (HALL et al., 1967)

Highest serum urate (mg/100 ml)	Subjects examined (No.)	Subjects gouty (No.)
<6.0	1281	8
6.0–6.9	790	15
7.0–6.0	162	27
8.0–8.9	40	10
<9.0	10	9

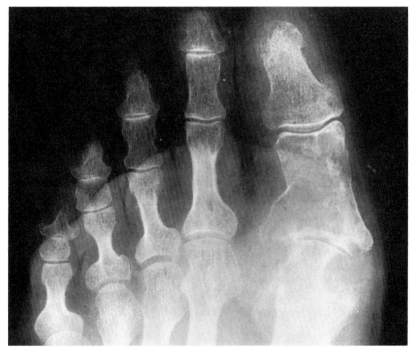

Fig. 1. Radiograph of a gouty foot. There are extensive tophaceous changes in the great toe, but the joints of all other toes are spared. (Courtesy of the Arthritis Foundation)

in all joints (as "systemic" factors would be), the incidence of gout would be the same in the hip as at the base of the big toe. Instead, there is a consistently uneven distribution of gouty involvement, with peripheral joints involved more than axial ones, the lower extremity involved more than the upper, and the base of the great toe invariably involved more often than any other joint (Fig. 1). The several series summarized in Table 2 are taken from Great Britain (GRAHAME and SCOTT, 1970), France (DE SÉZE et al., 1958), Denmark (BRØCHNER-MORTENSEN, 1941), and the United States (TALBOTT, 1964), and differ considerably in chronicity of the patients included, yet they share with each other and all other Western series the same pattern of involvement—a marked predilection for the bunion joint with the rest of

Table 2. Involved joints in patients with gout

Authors:	GRAHAME and SCOTT	DE SÉZE et al.	BRØCHNER-MORTENSEN	TALBOTT
Nationality:	England	France	Denmark	U.S.
Cases	354	100	100	
Units	%	#	#	Rank
Great toe	76	96	71	1
Ankle/foot	50	63/57	33	2
Knee	32	72	29	3
Finger	25	37	39	5
Elbow	10	45	14	6
Wrist	10	44	26	4
Tophi	21	59	33	—

the foot and the knee successively less involved, and the fingers, elbow, and wrist following behind. The remaining synovial joints are remarkably spared from the ravages of gouty arthritis.

The distribution of tophi is also characteristic; the classic site is over the pinnae of the ears (Fig. 2). Of the 59 tophaceous patients reported by DE SÉZE et al., 36 had such ear tophi, 32 had tophi in the hands, 27 had them on the feet, 24 over elbows, and 5 over knees. Once again, peripheral sites are primarily involved, although this pattern for tophi implies a reversal (also noted by GARROD) of the preference that acute gouty arthritis shows for the lower extremity. In either extremity, most tophi are found around joints, usually overlying extensor surfaces. Although tophi have occasionally been identified in such locations as the larynx and the valves of the heart, urate generally does not crystallize in skeletal muscle, in the lung, in the liver, in the spleen, in the nervous system, or in most other soft tissues.

Precipitation of sodium urate thus correlates poorly with its concentration in serum. Once crystallization occurs, however, it usually follows a highly characteristic pattern, with some sites involved with great regularity, while other sites are spared with equal consistency. This brief review will examine present knowledge of local factors that might determine this pattern.

B. Temperature

"To the disease, there is no great interval between the hands and the feet, both being of a similar nature, slender, devoid of flesh, and very near the external cold but very far from the internal heat." ARETAEUS, second century A.D., cited by GARROD (1859).

ARETAEUS was not alone in perceiving a relationship between the temperature of peripheral sites and the likelihood of their involvement by gout. To SCUDAMORE (1823), exposure of feet to the wet and to the cold was "by far the most frequent of the exciting causes" of acute gouty arthritis. Subsequent authors, including GARROD, have repeatedly reemphasized the importance of this association, which is now easily understood in terms of the central role of urate crystals in gout.

Everyone who has heated water to dissolve sugar is familiar with the effect of temperature on crystal solubility. Increasing the temperature will greatly increase the

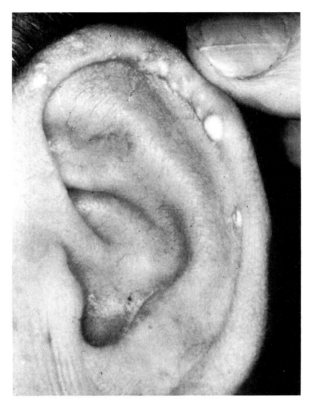

Fig. 2. Tophaceous deposits in an ear. This is the classic site for tophi. (Courtesy of the Arthritis Foundation)

Table 3. Solubility of urate as a function of temperature (in 150 mM NaCl) (LOEB, 1972)

Temperature (°C)	Maximal concentration of urate (mg/100 ml)
37	6.8
35	6.0
30	4.5
25	3.3
20	2.5
15	1.8
10	1.2

solubility of any solute and thus permit a higher concentration in aqueous solution. When the same solution is cooled, the solubility is reduced, rendering the solution supersaturated and leading to the precipitation of crystals. The calculations of LOEB (1972) (Table 3) suggest that temperature variations within the range expected in normal body tissues may profoundly affect urate solubility. In seven normal knees, HOLLANDER and HORVATH (1949) and HORVATH and HOLLANDER (1949) recorded a mean temperature of 32.3° C. Smaller, more peripheral joints have not been measured; however, it is reasonable to suppose that temperatures within such joints and within the ear are lower still. At such temperatures, even the serum urate concentration in normal males (5.3 mg/100 ml) would represent a supersaturated solution. It is, therefore, reasonable to postulate that low local temperatures are a major factor in the selection of peripheral locations for formation of tophi and involvement of joints by gout.

Temperature alone, however, is insufficient to explain the distribution of gouty involvement recorded in Table 2. There is every reason to believe that the interphalangeal joints of the toes, for instance, are subjected to temperatures at least as low as that at the base of the great toe. Involvement of the big toe, however, is many fold greater than that observed at other peripheral sites. Additional factors must be involved to explain this pattern.

It is also relevant to note that temperature changes work both ways on the solubility of urate. Whereas reduced temperature will promote crystallization of sodium urate, an increased temperature should promote its dissolution. Increased local temperature is one of the cardinal signs of inflammation and is classically present in acute gouty joints. This temperature response may play a major role in dissolving urate crystals, thus contributing to termination of acute gouty arthritis in many subjects.

C. pH

"It is probable that the fluids of these tissues (the ligaments and cartilages) are less alkaline than those of many others" (GARROD, 1859).

In recent years, more attention has focused on pH than on any other local factor affecting the solubility of sodium urate. This emphasis has resulted from the popularity of the cycle suggested by SEEGMILLER and HOWELL (1962) to explain the propagation of gouty episodes. Their thesis (Fig. 3) rests on the known chemotactic activity generated by urate crystals that lead to an influx of polymorphonuclear leukocytes to ingest offending crystals. The metabolic activity of these cells, however, leads to lactate release, with a resultant fall in intrasynovial pH. It was thought that this fall in pH would be sufficient to render the synovial fluid supersaturated for urate, with precipitation of additional crystals, thus starting the cycle anew. More recent findings, however, make it less likely that this theoretical cycle plays a major role in gout. Studies of synovial fluid from patients with a variety of disease states, including gout, have shown that it is extremely rare for the intrasynovial pH to fall below 7.0, even in the presence of severe synovitis (FALCHUK et al., 1970; TREUHAFT and McCARTY, 1971). As the pH of buffered saline is reduced from 7.4 to 7.0, the solubility of sodium urate does not fall at all but actually rises slightly (KIPPEN et al., 1974). These observations would appear to have closed the door on any role for local pH change in the precipitation of urate crystals.

The possibility was reopened, however, by WILCOX and KHALAF (1975), who reported that nucleation of urate crystals in supersaturated solutions was enhanced by a modest decrease in pH. The same authors also postulated that nucleation would be further enhanced by an increased concentration of ionic calcium at lower pH values. Since the body fluids of many hyperuricemic patients can be presumed to be

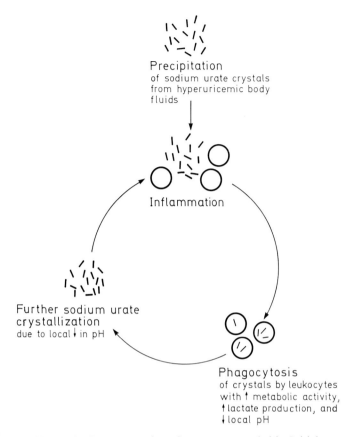

Fig. 3. The "Seegmiller cycle" for propagation of acute gouty arthritis. Initial urate crystals are chemotactic for polymorphonuclear leukocytes. The metabolic activity of these cells was thought to lower the intrasynovial pH, leading to precipitation of additional crystals. (SEEGMILLER and HOWELL, 1962)

supersaturated, it is appropriate to consider factors affecting nucleation rather than to retain a narrow focus on solubility alone. It may be, then, that a falling pH plays a role in promoting crystallization within the joint, even though the solubility of urate in synovial fluid does not fall. This may be especially true at the base of the big toe.

Determinations of pH have not been obtained during the classic acute attack of podagra. It is thought that the severe pain of these episodes is related to the high hydrostatic pressures accompanying the inflammation within this small joint. Under conditions of very high intraarticular pressure, the microvasculature in the toe might experience a much greater compromise than that observed in the larger joints, where most synovial fluid pH determinations have been recorded. Greater impairment of microvascular function would lead to more pronounced hypoxia and a larger fall in intrasynovial pH. Therefore, it remains possible that an exaggerated fall in pH may be an important factor contributing to the precipitation of urate crystals in the classic attack of podagra.

D. Cavitation

Agitation and stirring are well recognized as factors leading to precipitation of crystals from supersaturated solutions. Within joints, however, the synovial fluid exists primarily as a film over intra-articular structures and not as a large pool susceptible to easy mixing. It seem unlikely, therefore, that normal joint motion leads to major agitation or rapid mixing of the highly viscous intrasynovial fluid. It is possible, however, that rather than mixing, the related phenomenon of cavitation is important in the precipitation of urates within joints.

In his text on *Crystallization*, MULLIN (1972) reviews the evidence that nucleation of agitated solutions can be attributed to cavitation. It is cavitation that causes bubbles to form in the wake of a boat's propeller or behind a stirring bar in a laboratory beaker. It is now clear that the same process also occurs within joints and is, in fact, the cause of the noise produced by "cracking" ones knuckles (UNSWORTH et al., 1971). Presently, we have no data on the incidence of cavitation at the base of the big toe or at other favorite sites of urate precipitation. The process is important in nucleation of crystals in vitro (HUNT and JACKSON, 1966), however, and its possible role in vivo is an appropriate topic for clinical investigation.

E. Osteoarthritis

"I have very commonly found distinct evidence of injury on the surface of the cartilage (in nongouty first metatarsophalangeal joints) when these appearances were not present either in the corresponding joints of the other toes, or in any of the phalangeal articulations" (GARROD, 1859).

In his major review of the pathology of gout, SOKOLOFF (1957) introduced the term "dystrophic precipitation" of urate crystals and pointed out that European authorities have long favored such a concept. According to this idea, urate crystals may precipitate preferentially at sites that have abnormal connective tissues. SOKOLOFF pointed out that the most common sites for formation of tophi are exposed to frequent trauma and suggested that a local injury combined with a decreased blood supply might in some undefined way facilitate crystal formation. Strong support for this general idea is found in the predilection of gout for the base of the great toe. This joint has been shown to have more degenerative changes than any other weight bearing joint (KELLGREN and LAWRENCE, 1958). Conversely, the other metatarsophalangeal joints are rarely involved by osteoarthritis (MARTEL, 1970) and are almost always spared from acute attacks of gouty arthritis. It is reasonable to suggest that this preference of gout for the base of the big toe is a direct or an indirect result of the degenerative arthritic changes there. The predilection of acute gouty arthritis for older individuals supports the idea that the association is in some way causal (Fig. 4). Epidemiologic studies have clearly shown that mean serum urate concentrations do not progressively rise with advancing age in men (MIKKELSON et al., 1965). On the other hand, the mean age for the onset of gout is usually in the midforties. Thus, most gouty individuals probably attain their lifelong serum urate concentration at puberty but do not have their first attack of arthritis for another 25 years. Clearly, some factor other than serum concentration of urate must change to predispose the base of the big toe to acute attacks of podagra. The most likely change occurring with advancing age is the development of degenerative changes at this site.

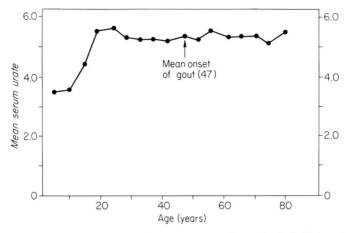

Fig.4. Age, serum urate, and the onset of gout. Men usually attain their lifelong level of serum urate around the time of puberty, yet most first attacks of gout occur in the forties. Some factor other than serum urate concentration must change in the intervening years to precipitate the onset of gout. (SIMKIN, 1977, modified from MIKKELSEN et al., 1965)

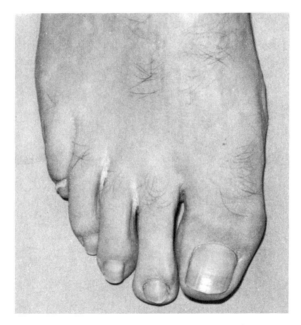

Fig.5. A gouty foot. This patient has no valgus angulation at the base of the great toe and has never had acute arthritis there. He does have significant angulation of the interphalangeal joint and has had repeated attacks of podagra at that site

Hallux valgus is such a common condition that physicians usually pay little attention to its presence in their patients. Valgus angulation at the base of the big toe is abnormal, however, and predisposes this joint to degenerative changes. Clinical experience suggests that hallux valgus and gout are also highly associated. This point may be illustrated anecdotally from the illustrations of an excellent recent textbook

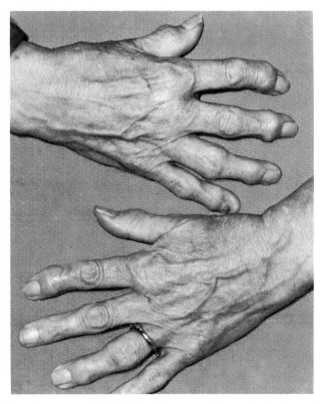

Fig. 6. Gout and erosive osteoarthritis. This older woman has typical osteoarthritic changes of the hand. The photograph was taken during the resolution of a superimposed acute gouty attack in the distal interphalangeal joint of the left index finger

on gout and uric acid metabolism (TALBOTT and YÜ, 1976). In this book hallux valgus is clear in each of five clinical photographs of gouty feet and in 14 or 15 radiographs used to illustrate gouty changes. This finding is not unique, but can readily be seen in illustrations from other textbooks of medicine, in collections of teaching slides, and in the feet of gouty patients in the clinic.

The association of degenerative changes with the presence of gouty involvement does not, in the author's experience, appear limited to the base of the big toe. The point may be illustrated in a gouty patient whose right foot is shown in Figure 5. This man's valgus deformity is in the middle rather than the base of the great toe. He has had repeated episodes of acute podagra over a 4-year period, with every one of these attacks clearly localized to the interphalangeal rather than the metatarsophalangeal joint. The same patient has had several serious injuries in his vocation as a prison guard and his avocation of motorcycle riding, with the most damage occurring in his right wrist, his right knee, and his left ankle. Each of these sites has been the focus of severe attacks of acute gouty arthritis, with no episodes in the contralateral wrist, knee, and ankle. Such a history of increased gouty prevalence at sites of old trauma is common in gouty patients and is best correlated with the degenerative changes induced by joint damage.

A different type of association between gout and degenerative joint disease is illustrated in the hands of another patient (Fig. 6). At the time of this photograph, the distal interphalangeal joint of the left index finger was recovering from an acute inflammatory episode. At the height of the inflammation, urate crystals were easily demonstrated in drainage from the inflamed site. It is clear, however, that the principal changes illustrated in the hands of this patient are those of "erosive osteoarthritis" (PETER et al., 1966). There is adduction of the thumbs, reflecting arthritis at the base of the first metacarpal, and Heberden's nodes are visible in the distal interphalangeal joints. It does not seem likely that this is a case of tophaceous gout simulating erosive osteoarthritis. Rather, this case is best interpreted as secondary urate precipitation in the degenerative changes of a distal interphalangeal joint affected primarily by erosive osteoarthritis. In their textbook, TALBOTT and YÜ comment that many patients with osteoarthritis of the hands have radiographic changes that are difficult to distinguish from those of gout. The case illustrated in Figure 6, as well as two similar patients seen at the University of Washington, suggests that gout may often be superimposed on osteoarthritis in the hands. In fact, some of the acute inflammatory episodes that characterize erosive osteoarthritis may represent unrecognized acute gout. Since most patients with erosive osteoarthritis are women, the possible superimposition of gout may not be considered. These patients are usually postmenopausal, however, and the higher urate concentrations of this age group may be sufficient to cause precipitation of crystals, with ensuing gouty arthritis.

F. Concentration

The concentration of serum urate is easily determined in good clinical laboratories, and the wide availability of the determination has led to over-dependence on this test in the diagnosis of gout. The concentration of urate within the joint space, however, has attracted little attention, since most physicians assume it to be equivalent to that found in plasma. This position, in fact, is supported by studies that have shown that the mean concentration of synovial fluid urate in groups of gouty patients closely approximates that found in serum (ROPES and BAUER, 1953; REEVES, 1965). It must be borne in mind, however, that any synovial fluid available for examination represents the inflammatory effusion of gouty arthritis. This fluid is not representative of the intraarticular fluid at the time that initial crystals first begin to induce the inflammatory response. Existing data, therefore, do not exclude the possibility that urate levels may be higher in synovial fluid than in plasma when crystallization first occurs.

A physiologic analysis of synovial effusions suggests that the urate concentration may, in fact, be much higher at some times than at others (SIMKIN, 1973 and 1977). This is particularly likely to be the case in joints with the degenerative changes discussed in the preceding section. It is a common clinical observation, confirmed by experimental studies in rabbits, that damaged joints develop effusions when used. Such effusions can be expected to develop during the course of activity and then to resolve at rest. If that activity is the classic long walk, excessive yard work, or hunting expedition so often preceding gouty arthritis (HENCH, 1933), the effusion may develop early in the day, remain present throughout continued utilization of the joint, and then resolve at night when the foot is elevated and at rest. Studies of normal human knees have shown that synovial permeability to small molecules is a function of molecular size (SIMKIN and PIZZORNO, 1974). In the case of water and urate, the

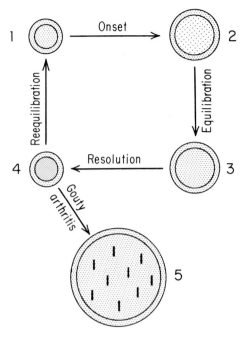

Fig. 7. Effect of synovial permeability on intrasynovial urate. Urate concentration in the plasma (outer ring) and in the joint (inner circle) is represented by intensity of shading. At rest (*1*), the concentrations are the same. During the onset of an effusion (*2*), water enters the joint space more rapidly than urate, thus transiently lowering the intrasynovial urate concentration. As the effusion persists (*3*), reequilibration of the two spaces will occur. During resolution of the effusion (*4*), water will leave more rapidly than urate and the intrasynovial concentration of urate will therefore exceed that of the plasma. At this point, crystals may precipitate and induce gouty arthritis (*5*) or reequilibration may occur with a return to the original conditions (*1*)

permeability of the normal synovium to urate was found to be $49 \pm 1\%$ of that found to water. This difference in permeability means that during the formation of a synovial effusion there will be more rapid ingress of water than of urate, and a transient decrease in the intrasynovial urate concentration will ensue. Once the effusion has reached its maximum volume, however, the continued influx of urate will lead to full equilibration of the urate concentration in the effusion with that found in plasma. When the effusion resolves, as would be expected with rest and elevation, water will again cross the synovium more rapidly than urate, leading to a transient increase in the intrasynovial urate concentration. It is at this point, during the resolution of an effusion, that the urate concentration of synovial fluid will exceed that of plasma, and it is at this time that the joint may be at special risk for the precipitation of urate crystals and the initiation of acute gouty arthritis (Fig. 7).

The process discussed above has been demonstrated experimentally with subcutaneous injections of Ringer's solution made equivalent in urate concentration to plasma and injected subcutaneously in human forearms (SIMKIN, 1973). In this model, the observed increase in tissue fluid urate concentration may be most analogous to the initiation of a tophus in an area of subcutaneous trauma. Unfortunately, there is as yet no model that might permit us to estimate the significance of this phenomenon at the base of the big toe, although the high prevalence of degenerative changes suggests that transient effusions would be especially likely there.

G. Shoes

"The pressure of too tight a shoe, and more especially if the patient walks much under such irritation, will occasionally induce gouty inflammation" (SCUDAMORE, 1823).

By the time of Aretaeus, new or tight shoes had already been implicated as important factors in the precipitation of acute gout, and their possible role is repeatedly mentioned in the older texts. In this context, the comment "there are no foot problems, only shoe problems" (ENGLAND cited by DAGNALL, 1963) seems relevant. In many patients, shoes play a major role in the induction of the hallux valgus deformity that appears to be associated with gout. Shoes may also be a factor in the absence of a fixed valgus deformation. In the foot illustrated in Figure 8, there was no obvious deformity, although this man had experienced three separate attacks of classic podagra at the base of his great toe. On comparing the configuration of his bare foot with that present in his shoe (shown in the middle frame), it was obvious, however, that this man experienced a functional hallux valgus whenever he was wearing these shoes. The flexors hallucis longus and brevis subject the base of the great toe to tremendous compressive forces during the pushoff phase of normal gait, and these forces cannot be evenly distributed across the articular cartilage when the

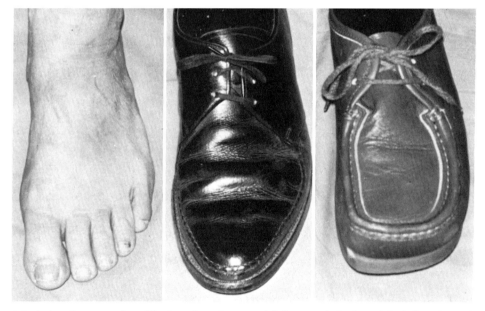

Fig. 8. Another gouty foot. The bare foot shown at left is normal. In the original shoe (center), however, the great toe is clearly forced into a valgus angulation. In more appropriate shoes (on the right) recurrent small effusions and acceleration of degenerative changes are less likely

toe is in a valgus position. This uneven distribution of forces seems likely then to accelerate degenerative changes, and the transient effusions that may lead to subsequent crystal formation and gouty arthritis at this joint. In the shoes shown on the right, the patient's feet were more comfortable and his gout readily controlled.

Physicians interested in the problem of gout are often asked what should be done for the patient with asymptomatic hyperuricemia. It may be that the most important advice one can offer such patients is to use shoes that do not cause hallux valgus deformities, which may secondarily precipitate gouty arthritis.

H. Crystal Deposits

The most obvious of the various factors that lead to precipitation of sodium urate is the presence of preexisting crystals at the same site. This factor is most apparent in the progressive growth of tophi, as illustrated in the patient shown in Figure 9. The tophus illustrated in the ring finger of this man began at the site of an old crush injury and grew progressively to the dimensions shown, without apparent tophi at any other location in the hands. Regardless of how or why the initial crystals formed at this site, it seems clear that it was the presence of an existing nidus of crystals that facilitated the precipitation of additional crystals from solution. The same process is presumably involved in the growth of any individual tophus. Similarly, the presence of a suspension of crystals may well lead to precipitation of additional crystals in synovial fluid during the onset of acute attacks of gouty arthritis.

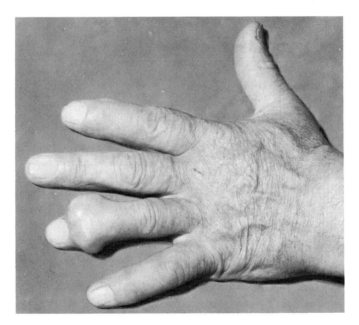

Fig. 9. Well-localized tophus over distal interphalangeal joint. Existing crystals at this site have formed the nidus on which additional crystals have successively formed. The end result is this large, solitary lesion

We should also consider the possibility that crystals other than those of sodium urate may serve as the nidus-potentiating nucleation of urate crystals from hyperuricemic solutions. Uric acid crystals in the urine accelerate precipitation of calcium oxalate as Dr. Coe discusses elsewhere in this volume. It could well be that calcium-containing crystals, such as hydroxyapatite, might in turn accelerate the precipitation of urate salts within joints. This becomes more likely, in view of the recent observation that apatite crystals may be present in the effusions of patients with osteoarthritis (DIEPPE et al., 1976). It is reasonable to suspect that this dystrophic effect may play a major role in the apparent association of osteoarthritis with gout. Similarly, several observers have been impressed by the frequency with which calcium pyrophosphate and sodium urate crystals are found within the same synovial fluid. In such an instance it is quite possible that the calcium crystals act as a nidus upon which urate crystals subsequently form. Since crystals of apatite are normally much smaller than those of urate and are not birefringent, there is unfortunately no present way that the clinician could recognize tiny apatite crystals in a gouty effusion.

"The rupture into a joint space of a previously formed urate deposit in the outer layer of cartilage precedes or precipitates an acute attack" (BROGSITTER, 1927).

A more obvious role of preexisting crystals in gout is that their "shedding" or release may well be responsible for precipitating episodes of acute arthritis. Up to this point, this discussion has focused on local factors that might enhance precipitation of urate crystals de novo. Many episodes of acute gouty arthritis, however, may result from the release of preformed crystals (as BENNETT et al., 1976 have suggested in pseudogout) rather than the precipitation of new ones. The best case in point is the acute gouty arthritis induced by rapid therapeutic lowering of the serum urate concentration. It also seems reasonable to suspect that some of the acute gouty episodes precipitated by surgery or other stress may reflect this phenomenon, as may local trauma to a synovium or articular cartilage, which is already loaded with preformed crystals. It is important to recognize, however, that although released crystals are themselves a local factor, there must have been other antecedent factors that led to their localization in the big toe and in other sites most likely to be attacked by gout.

By the time an individual has longstanding, severe gout with extensive tophaceous deposits, there may be nearly continuous inflammation as a result of repeated release of preformed crystals into the joint space. Figure 10 is a schematic diagram illustrating the life history of gout in such a patient. The figure reflects evolving concepts in the pathogenesis of gouty arthritis and is modified from an earlier figure of HENCH (1941). In phase 1 gout, acute episodes of arthritis are all related to new crystal formation and resolve entirely without continuation of deposits and, therefore, without the possibility of inducing gout by crystal release. The significant number of gouty patients who never become hyperuricemic probably all remain within phase 1 throughout their lives. In phase 2, however, there is the onset of a continuing precipitation of urate crystals from supersaturated extracellular fluids. This may occur on articular cartilage, within the synovium, or at other preferred sites of tophus formation. During this time, acute gouty episodes may occur from de novo precipitation of crystals, as in phase 1, but now may also be caused by the release of

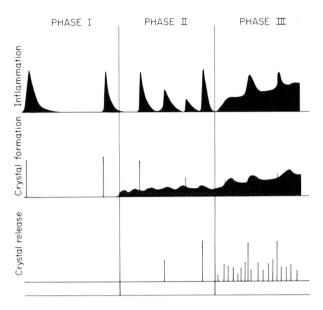

Fig. 10. Proposed course of tophaceous gout. Phase 1 gout begins with acute arthritis induced by precipitation of intraarticular crystals and proceeds on an intermittent basis, with each attack of gout produced by a new batch of crystals. In phase 2, formation and deposition of crystals are now essentially continuous, and acute arthritis may result either from newly formed or acutely released urate crystals. In phase 3, deposits are so extensive and the joint surfaces are sufficiently deformed that there is a near continuous release of crystals and a secondary chronic arthritis. (Modified from HENCH, 1941)

crystals from existing deposits. Patients with marked hyperuricemia may have a very short phase 1 or may, in fact, enter directly into phase 2 at puberty. Others, however, may have an extended phase 1 before beginning to have continuous crystal formation. In phase 3 there are now extensive crystal deposits, and most of the inflammation may be occurring from the release of preformed crystals. Fortunately, only a small minority of gouty patients who have extensive tophaceous gout would fall into this final phase.

J. Conclusion

If deposition of crystals underlies clinical gout, the disease will not be understood until the reasons for nucleation and growth of urate crystals in vivo have been fully worked out. Among the possible reasons for gout, research efforts have been appropriately focussed on mechanisms of hyperuricemia. It is now clear, however, that the serum urate concentration is an imperfect tool in both the diagnosis and the prediction of gout. Other factors must therefore be examined to determine what else may be involved in the crystallization process. The possible roles of serum proteins and of glycosaminoglycans are reviewed elsewhere in this volume. Such factors, however, are systemic and are presumably fairly constant. They cannot be expected to explain the typical nocturnal onset of acute gouty arthritis, the role of exercise and trauma, the onset of gout in middle age, and the predilection of the syndrome for the base of the big toe. Additional local factors must be involved in these phenomena. In the phrase of McCARTY (1965), "Not only do you need the seed (hyperuricemia), but you have to have the soil (local factors)."

In this chapter, a number of possible local factors have been considered. Temperature, pH, cavitation, osteoarthritis, intrasynovial urate concentration, badly fitting shoes, and preexisting crystal deposits are variables which may be logically considered as factors of importance in the deposition of urate crystals. For the most part, these possibilities are not new and were considered by GARROD and by other early workers. It is now an appropriate time, however, for a renewed interest in this problem. A more comprehensive understanding of all relevant factors, local as well as systemic, will be of immense value in the management and in the prophylaxis of gout and its sequelae.

References

Bennett, R. M., Lehr, J. R., McCarty, D. J.: Crystal shedding and acute pseudogout. Arthr. and Rheum. **19**, 93—97 (1976)

Brøchner-Mortensen, K.: One-hundred gouty patients. Acta med. scand. **106**, 81—107 (1941)

Brogsitter, A. M.: Histopathology of Gout. Leipzig: Vogel 1927

Dagnall, J. C.: Naming the profession. Brit. J. Chiropody **28**, 69—76 (1963)

De Séze, S., Ryckewaert, A., Levernieux, J., Marteau, R.: Physiopathology, clinical manifestations, and treatment of gout. Part 2. Clinical and therapeutic studies. Ann. rheum. Dis. **17**, 15—21 (1958)

Dieppe, P. A., Crocker, P., Huskisson, E. C., Willoughby, D. A.: Apatite deposition disease: A new arthropathy. Lancet **1976 I**, 266—269

Falchuk, K. H., Goetzl, E. J., Kulka, J. P.: Respiratory gasses of synovial fluids. An approach to synovial tissue circulatory-metabolic imbalance in rheumatoid arthritis. Amer. J. Med. **49**, 223—231 (1970)

Garrod, A. B.: The Nature and Treatment of Gout and Rheumatic Gout. London: Walton and Maberly 1859

Grahame, R., Scott, J. T.: Clinical survey of 354 patients with gout. Ann. rheum. Dis. **29**, 461—468 (1970)

Hall, A. P., Barry, P. E., Dawber, T. R., McNamara, P. M.: Epidemiologie of gout and hyperuricemia. A long-term population study. Amer. J. Med. **42**, 27—37 (1967)

Hench, P. S.: Diagnosis and treatment of gout and gouty arthritis. J. Amer. med. Ass. **116**, 453—459 (1941)

Hench, P. S., Darnall, C. M.: A clinic on acute, old-fashioned gout; with special reference to its inciting factors. Med. Clin. N. Amer. **16**, 1371—1393 (1933)

Hollander, J. L., Horvath, S. M.: The influence of physical therapy procedures on the intra-articular temperature of normal and arthritis subjects. Amer. J. med. Sci. **218**, 543—548 (1949)

Horvath, S. M., Hollander, J. L.: Intra-articular temperature as a measure of joint reaction. J. clin. Invest. **28**, 469—473 (1949)

Hunt, J. D., Jackson, K. A.: Nucleation of solid in an undercooled liquid by cavitation. J. appl. Physiol. **37**, 254 (1966)

Kellgren, J. H., Lawrence, J. S.: Osteo-arthrosis and disc degeneration in an urban population. Ann. rheum. Dis. **17**, 388—397 (1958)

Kippen, I., Klinenberg, J. R., Weinberger, A., Wilcox, W. R.: Factors affecting urate solubility in vitro. Ann. rheum. Dis. **33**, 313—317 (1974)

Loeb, J. N.: The influence of temperature on the solubility of monosodium urate. Arthr. and Rheum. **15**, 189—192 (1972)

Martel, W.: Acute and chronic arthritis of the foot. Semin. Roentgenol. **5**, 391—406 (1970)

McCarty, D. J., Jr.: The inflammatory reaction to microcrystalline sodium urate. Arthr. and Rheum. **8**, 726—735 (1965)

McCarty, D. J.: The gouty toe—a multifactorial condition. Ann. intern. Med. **86**, 234—236 (1977)

McCarty, D. J., Hollander, J. L.: Identification of urate crystals in gouty synovial fluid. Ann. intern. Med. **54**, 452—460 (1961)

Mikkelsen, W. M., Dodge, H. J., Valkenburg, H.: The distribution of serum uric acid values in a population unselected as to gout or hyperuricemia. Tecumseh, Michigan 1959—1960. Amer. J. Med. **39**, 242—251 (1965)

Mullin, J. W.: Crystallisation, 2nd Ed. London-Cleveland: Butterworth 1972

Peter, J. B., Pearson, C. M., Marmor, L.: Erosive osteoarthritis of the hands. Arthr. and Rheum. **9**, 365—388 (1966)

Reeves, B.: Significance of joint fluid uric acid levels in gout. Ann. rheum. Dis. **24**, 569—571 (1965)

Ropes, M. W., Bauer, W.: Synovial Fluid Changes in Joint Disease. Cambridge: Harvard University Press 1953

Scudamore, C.: A Treatise of the Nature and Course of Gout, 4th Ed. London: Mallett 1823

Seegmiller, J. E., Howell, R. R.: The old and new concepts of acute gouty arthritis. Arthr. and Rheum. **5**, 616—623 (1962)

Simkin, P. A.: Local concentration of urate in the pathogenesis of gout. Lancet **1973 II**, 1295—1298

Simkin, P. A.: The pathogenesis of podagra. Ann. Intern. Med. **86**, 230—233 (1977)

Simkin, P. A., Pizzorno, J. E.: Transynovial exchange of small molecules in normal human subjects. J. appl. Phys. **36**, 581—587 (1974)

Sokoloff, L.: The pathology of gout. Metabolism **6**, 230—243 (1957)

Talbott, J. H.: Gout. New York-London: Grune & Stratton 1964

Talbott, J. H., Yü, T.-F.: Gout and Uric Acid Metabolism. New York: Stratton Intercontinental Medical 1976

Treuhaft, P. S., McCarty, D. J.: Synovial fluid pH, lactate, oxygen, and carbon dioxide partial pressure in various joint diseases. Arthr. and Rheum. **14**, 475—484 (1971)

Unsworth, A., Dowson, D., Wright, V.: Cracking joints. A bioengineering study of cavitation in the metacarpophalangeal joint. Ann. rheum. Dis. **30**, 348—358 (1971)

Wilcox, W. R., Khalaf, A. A.: Nucleation of monosodium urate crystals. Ann. rheum. Dis. **34**, 332—339 (1975)

Wynngaarden, J. B., Kelley, W. N.: Gout and Hyperuricemia. New York-San Francisco-London: Grune & Stratton 1976

CHAPTER 17

Uric Acid Nephrolithiasis

Ts'ai-Fan Yü

A. Introduction

Urinary tract stones were known in prehistoric times. The oldest stone was unearthed in upper Egypt, dated approximately 4800 B.C. (SHATTOCK, 1905). Stones have been discovered from Egyptian mummies of different dynasties (MILLER, 1929; WESSON, 1935; GUTHRIE, 1946; SIGERIST, 1951; BUTT, 1956). WILLIAMS recorded one from North Arizona, estimated to be 3000 years old (WILLIAMS, 1926). Stone disease has been described from China and India (THOMSON, 1921; McCARRISON, 1931). Lithotomy was mentioned in ancient India in the first century B.C. (GUTHRIE, 1946). Stones were then almost exclusively found in the bladder, kidney stones being rare. For some unknown reason, the prevalence of bladder stones has decreased steadily from western countries since the turn of the century (SALLINEN, 1959).

B. Prevalence of Uric Acid Nephrolithiasis (Table 1)

Kidney stones in adults in modern industrialized countries consist predominantly of calcium oxalate and calcium phosphate. Stones composed chiefly of uric acid constitute only a small fraction of total renal calculi. From Australia, WARDLAW reported that 5.6% of 196 upper urinary tract stones were composed of "urate" (WARDLAW, 1952). They are likewise infrequent in England and the Scandinavian countries. Uric acid as the chief constituent was reported in only a relatively small proportion of 856 stones from Great Britain and Northern Ireland, uric acid in 2.3%, uric acid dihydrate in 1.3%, ammonium acid urate 2.6%, and sodium acid urate 0.4% (SUTOR et al., 1974). An incidence of uric acid stones varying from 3% to 6% has been reported from the Scandinavian countries (HELLSTROM, 1938; JENSEN, 1941; LAGERGREN, 1956). In Spain, 17% of 1200 cases of renal lithiasis were uric acid stones. Of the 280 cases in this series with uric acid stones, 204 had normouricemia and 76 had hyperuricemia (CIFUENTES DELATTE et al., 1972). In the Federal Republic of Germany, uric acid stones have been estimated to constitute 13% of all stones (EBBINGHAUS and PRIEBER, 1960), though there has been a constant rise of uric acid stone formation in the last 10 years (MAY and SCHINDLER, 1972). In MAY and SCHINDLER's series, 25% of patients with urolithiasis had uric acid stones, and 25% of uric acid stone patients had hyperuricemia. The average occurrence of urolithiasis in Czechosolovakia has been reported to be 1 per 1000 population; uric acid stones constitute 15% of these (KRIZEK, 1957). Of 179 cases of urolithiasis reported from France, 23% were uric acid stones (COTTET and WEBER, 1959). Urolithiasis is quite common in Israel; and 39.5% of 544 patients with urolithiasis has been found to have uric acid stones (ATSMON et al., 1963).

Table 1. Prevalence of uric acid stones in patients with nephrolithiasis from different areas of the world

Location	Patients or stones No.	Uric acid stones %	Author	(Year)
Sydney, Australia	196	5.6	WARDLAW	(1952)
Great Britain, N Ireland	856	6.6	SUTOR et al.	(1974)
Sweden	100	5	HELLSTRÖM	(1938)
Sweden	77	3.6	LAGERGREN	(1956)
Denmark	111	6	JENSEN	(1941)
Czechoslovakia	—	14.8	KRIZEK	(1957)
Spain	1200	17	CIFUENTES, DELATTE et al.	(1972)
Germany	94	12.8	EBBINGHAUS and PRIEBER	(1960)
Germany	—	25	MAY and SCHINDLER	(1972)
France	179	23	COTTETT and WEBER	(1959)
Israel	544	39.5	ATSMON et al.	(1963)
USA and Canada				
1. Winston-Salem	500	3.4	BOYCE et al.	(1955)
2. Durham	287	1.8	HUGHES et al.	(1960)
3. Pensacola	772	4.3	LEONARD	(1961)
4. Houston	2500	3.6	NICHOLAS	(1961)
5. Boston	207	9.7	MELICK and HENNEMAN	(1958)
6. Chicago	300	17	VERMEULEN and FRIED	(1965)
7. Various Areas	10000	9.4	HERRING	(1962)
8. Various Areas	24000	8	PRIEN	(1963)
9. Toronto, Ontario	439	5	YENDT	(1970)

The prevalence of uric acid stones in the United States, likewise, is different in different localities. They are less frequent in the stone belt of the southern states, where uric acid occurs in about 4% of all stones examined (BOYCE et al., 1955; HUGHES, 1960; LEONARD, 1961; NICHOLAS, 1961). From Chicago, it was reported as 17% (VERMEULEN et al., 1965). Approximately 10% of all stones reported from all over the United States were uric acid stones (MELICK and HENNEMAN, 1958; HERRING, 1962; PRIEN, 1963). YENDT found 5% of 439 stones to be composed of uric acid from Toronto General Hospital in a period of 13 years (YENDT, 1970). About 0.1% of the adult population entering hospitals every year is diagnosed as having renal stone (BOYCE et al., 1956), and if 10% of these calculi are composed of uric acid, one would expect the prevalence of uric acid stones to be 0.01% in the general population.

C. Chemistry of Uric Acid

Using various isotopically labeled compounds, the purine ring of uric acid has been shown to be assembled from molecules of glycine, carbon dioxide, formate, and ammonia by way of aspartate and glutamine, all of which are common metabolites within the cell (Fig. 1) (BUCHANAN, 1958). Uric acid is a trioxypurine, with oxygen at positions 2, 6, and 8 of the purine ring. It is a weak acid, which ionized at the N-9

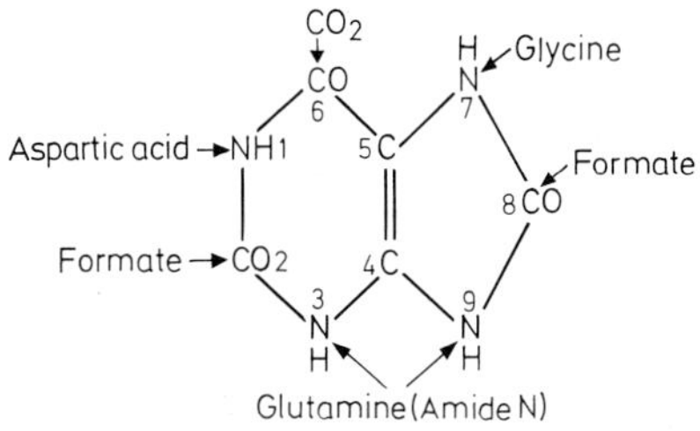

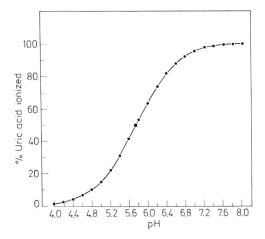

Fig. 1. Uric acid, indicating numbering of purine ring and source of each atom in *de novo* purine biosynthesis (reproduced with permission of Am. J. Med.).

Fig. 2. Dissociation of uric acid in relation to pH, calculated from the Henderson-Hasselbach equation and a pK_A of 5.75 for uric acid (reproduced with permission of Am. J. Med.)

position, with a pK_A at pH 5.75 (BERGMANN and DIKSTEIN, 1955). The degree of ionization of uric acid in relation to pH, calculated from the HENDERSON-HASSEL-BALCH equation, is shown in Figure 2. At pH 7.4, uric acid is virtually completely ionized as urate, the form in which it exists in plasma. The relative amounts of ionized and un-ionized uric acid in urine depend largely upon the urine acidity. In distinctly acid urine with pH less than 5, uric acid exists largely un-ionized as free acid to the extent of more than 90%; at pH 5.4, the un-ionized form is decreased to about 70%. The relative amounts of the ionized and the un-ionized forms are equal at pH 5.75. The ionized moiety rapidly increases beyond its pK_A at 5.75. Given a urinary uric acid excretion of 1000 mg at pH 6.0 (un-ionized = 36%), the calculated amount of free acid would be 360 mg; but a lesser excretion of 500 mg at pH 5.0 (un-ionized = 85%) will provide more free acid, 425 mg, due to the lesser ionization at lower pH (Fig. 2). The significance of the amount of ionized and un-ionized lies in the fact that the un-ionized form, the free uric acid, is less soluble than the ionized form.

D. Structure and Formation of Uric Acid Stones

Uric acid precipitates in acid urine in either anhydrous or its dihydrate form (Lonsdale and Mason, 1966). Pure uric acid stones are generally round or ellipsoid
(Fig. 3). They generally absorb urochromes, which appear yellow, orange, or yellow-
ish brown. The pigment is suggested by Pinto and his coworkers to consist of two
pyrollic rings of low molecular weight (Pinto et al., 1976).

The ultrastructure of uric acid stones obtained from patients were studied
(Meyer et al., 1971). Each stone appeared to be a pure polycrystalline aggregate of
orthorhombic uric acid by X-ray diffraction. Ultrastructure of uric acid stone by
transmission electronmicroscopy of thin-sectioned material reveals at least three
distinctive features (Fig. 4): (1) The uric acid blocks are laid down in approximately
parallel rows. The blocks butt into each other, and appear to fuse across broad
interfaces. They join from row to row with narrow bridges; (2) the interiors are
usually inhomogeneous; (3) a serpiginous interconnected network of uric acid is
another common feature of uric acid stones. These blocks usually range from 1000–
5000 Å in size and tend to be randomly arranged. Many blocks have a two-phase
labyrinth interior. Apparently, the wall of the block is formed first, then the interior
fills in. Uric acid in urine tends to hover near the saturation point. With the concentration fluctuating above and below saturation, sintering can be expected to occur in
the region of highest concentration gradient between those uric acid blocks.

Crystal nucleating and growth by epitaxy consists of the growth of one crystal on a
substrate of another, with a near geometric fit between the respective networks that
are in contact. According to Lonsdale (1968), epitaxy may be of considerable importance in stone growth, once a suitable seed is deposited. Without such a seed, the
urine can attain a very high degree of supersaturation of certain relatively insoluble
components without precipitation. Precipitation from a saturated or supersaturated
solution of a stone-forming compound will occur at once on a suitable seed or
substrate, provided there is an epitaxial relationship. A variety of excellent fits are
possible for epitaxial growth on a nucleus of uric acid or calcium oxalates. By using
crystallographic techniques, Lonsdale demonstrated that urate and uric acid may
prompt epitaxial growth of calcium oxalate crystals because of certain interatomic or
intramolecular interaction (Lonsdale, 1968). Finlayson, on the other hand, considered that the uric acid blocks could have nucleated independently at random positions, aggregated, and finally become sintered (Finlayson and Meyer, 1972).

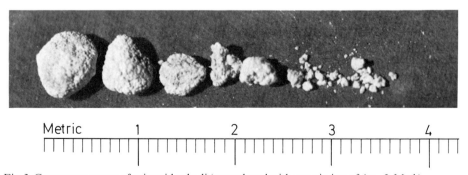

Fig. 3. Gross appearance of uric acid calculi (reproduced with permission of Am. J. Med.)

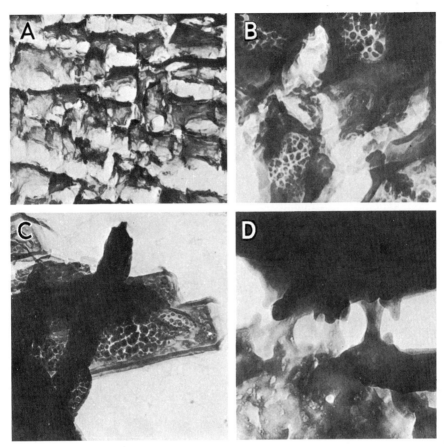

Fig. 4. Ultrastructure of uric acid calculi through transmission electron micrographs. (A) Blocks of uric acid are arranged in roughly parallel rows, joined together by interblock bridges (× 33 600). (B) The uric acid blocks are irregular in shape and position. The interiors of the blocks are labyrinths with various degrees of densification (× 41 600). (C) Blocks of uric acid grown in vitro from human urine, showing some regular walls and labyrinth interiors (× 43 200). (D) Interblock bridging in uric acid stones. Several bridges are well formed, and two bridges appear to be forming (× 50 000) (reproduced with permission from Dr. B. Finlayson)

E. Association of Other Crystalline Constituents in Uric Acid Stones

Determination of the composition of 164 calculi from the GUTMAN and YÜ Gout Research Clinic showed that pure uric acid occurred in only 132 (or 80%), a prevalence not different from that reported several years previously (YÜ and GUTMAN, 1967). Nineteen (12%) contained calcium oxalate only. Mixed stones of uric acid with calcium oxalate occurred in three, with calcium phosphate in six, with magnesium ammonium phosphate in two, and with cystine in two, totalling 8%.

Calcium oxalate is the most common constituent of all stones in the general population (MELICK and HENNEMAN, 1958). It may appear as calcium oxalate monohydrate or calcium oxalate dihydrate. Both hydrates may be found in the same stone. The presence and concentrations of other urinary constituents may influence the state of hydration of calcium oxalate (SUTOR, 1969). Further, both calcium oxalate and uric acid are equally insoluble in acid urine, although calcium oxalate is also insoluble at higher urine pH as well. It is probably not a pure coincidence that uric acid and calcium oxalate are present in the same patient, or even in the same stone (YÜ and GUTMAN, 1967; PRIEN and PRIEN, 1968).

Uric acid may often be the nucleus or exist in a distinct layer of mixed calculi in association with calcium oxalate, or less frequently, with apatite. Alteration of light and dark layers in a calculus composed of a single substance occurs commonly in both calcium oxalate monohydrate and uric acid stones (PRIEN and PRIEN, 1968).

Some interesting studies have been made on the sequence of deposition of the various components in laminated calculi (MEYER, 1929). Calcium oxalate, uric acid, and cystine precipitate in acid urine; magnesium ammonium phosphate deposits in alkaline urine. Calcium phosphate will precipitate from a solution at a pH above 6, becoming increasingly insoluble as the pH rises. As a stone grows, the composition of the outer layers may change with change in urine reaction. When urine becomes infected, magnesium ammonium phosphate and calcium phosphate are deposited; if renal function is adequate, they are supersaturated; and when renal insufficiency is present, the stone may stop growing. Calcium oxalate, calcium phosphate, and uric acid may be deposited in alternate layers as a stone is built up. But once magnesium ammonium phosphate appears in a stone, there will be no further change and it appears as its outermost layer.

Hyperuricosuria and hypercalciuria were frequently found to coexist in patients with calcium stones (SMITH et al., 1969; DENT and SUTOR, 1971; COE and KAVALACH, 1974). According to SMITH and his co-workers, most of their 394 patients with calcium stones have hyperuricemia. They suggested that if a patient has hyperuricemia and hypercalciuria, he will form calcium stones, whereas if he has hyperuricosuria and hypocalciuria, uric acid stones will result. DENT and SUTOR remarked that hyperuricemia occurs very commonly in the chronic stone formers both in those with and without hypercalciuria. COE and KAVALACH found 12% of 230 patients with calcium stones to have hyperuricosuria and hypercalciuria. HODGKINSON on the other hand did not find any significant differences in the daily excretion of uric acid by the control subjects and stone formers, nor any significant relationship between uric acid and calcium excretion (HODGKINSON, 1976). It is assumed that this inconsistency is related to the differences in the consumption of purine-rich foods.

Calcium stones may be formed by patients with hyperuricosuria, who present no abnormal calcium metabolism (PAK and ARNOLD, 1975). PAK and ARNOLD showed that seeds of monosodium urate may initiate heterogeneous nucleation of calcium oxalate and calcium phosphate. Crystals of uric acid or monosodium urate were seeded in Ca oxalate solution, containing tracer ^{14}C-oxalate. Aliquots of the suspension were filtered through a Millipore filter at different time intervals. Radioactive ^{14}C was assayed in a liquid scintillation counter, oxalate was determined, and Ca assayed by atomic absorption spectrometry. At pH 6.7, seeds of monosodium urate over a concentration range of 0.5–5.0 mg/ml, caused a rapid decline in ^{14}C-oxalate of the filtrate, indicating crystallization of calcium oxalate. At lower concentration of urate, there was a lag of 3 h before a decrease of ^{14}C radioactivity appeared. At a more acidic pH of 5.7, the radioactivity disappeared at a slower rate. In contrast, seeds of free uric acid as high as 5 mg/ml failed to cause crystallization of calcium oxalate at either pH. The heterogeneous nucleation of calcium phosphate by seeding of monosodium urate or uric acid was similar.

Unlike uric acid stone formers, urine pH of patients with hyperuricosuria and calcium stones usually exceeds 5.7. Their urine samples are usually supersaturated with respect to monosodium urate. Despite the normal calcium content, the urine samples from patients with hyperuricosuria and calcium stones are often metastably supersaturated with respect to calcium oxalate and calcium phosphate. This accounts for the formation of calcium stones with hyperuricosuria and normocalciuria.

In cystinuria, increased urinary excretion of cystine is associated with increased excretion of lysine, ornithine, and arginine. Cystine is the least soluble amino acid, while the other three amino acids are relatively soluble. Cystine stones are uncommon, unlike calcium oxalate stones. They are usually multiple and tend to recur, predisposing to urinary tract obstruction and secondary infection.

Hyperuricemia in coexistence with cystinuria has been reported (KING and WAINER, 1967; MELONI and CANARY, 1967; VERGIS and WALKER, 1970; KRIZEK, 1972). Cystine stone and uric acid stone may be present in the same patient. In the series of SMITH et al., 12 of the 17 cystine stone patients had a history of uric acid calculi (SMITH et al., 1969). In our series of 10 patients with cystine stones, there were two patients with a plasma uric acid abnormally high above 9 mg/100 ml; one had frequent gouty arthritis and extensive tophaceous deposits, and another had a family history of gout. Three had mild hyperuricemia only, and in two patients, uric acid stones and cystine stones coexisted. It is not possible to determine whether hyperuricemia in cystinuria is related to renal damage, or whether the two metabolic abnormalities are causally related.

F. Pathogenesis of Uric Acid Nephrolithiasis

I. Hyperuricosuria and Hyperuricemia

The lower forms of animal possess a full complement of enzymes necessary for complete degradation of purines. The capacity for metabolizing purines becomes more deficient as life ascends the phylogenetic scale (CAMPBELL, 1973). Thus, some invertebrates degrade purines via uric acid, allantoin, allantoic acid, and urea, finally to ammonia and CO_2. The end products of purine metabolism among animals vary, depending on the loss of particular sequential purine metabolizing enzymes (Table 2). In most mammals, the end product of purine is allantoin, and most of the nitrogen waste is urea. Man and higher primates, like other mammals, excrete urea in large quantities. Uric acid represents the end product of purine metabolism in man, since he lacks uricase. The kidney efficently reabsorbs the uric acid filtered at the glomerulus, and urinary uric acid is secreted by the renal tubules (GUTMAN and YÜ, 1961). As much as one-third of the uric acid is eliminated extrarenally (SORENSEN, 1960). The major extrarenal route of uric acid disposal is via the intestinal tract, where uricolysis takes place due to the intestinal flora. A small amount of uric acid is excreted through the skin (ATSMON et al., 1963), the saliva (SORENSEN, 1960), and the

Table 2. Biologic degradation of purine bases

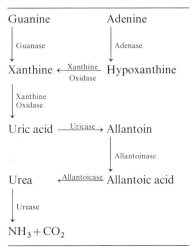

hair and nails (Bollinger and Gross, 1953). Extrarenal elimination is increased as a compensatory measure when impairment of renal function is present.

With a normal renal glomerular filtration rate of 100–120 ml/min and a daily excretion of 500–600 mg of uric acid in urine, man usually maintains a plasma urate of 5–6 mg/100 ml. In primary gout, hyperuricemia is the rule and hyperuricosuria is frequent. Uric acid nephrolithiasis occurs in approximately 20% of gouty subjects. Its presence is estimated to be 1000 times greater than in the nongouty population (Yü and Gutman, 1967).

By giving ^{15}N-glycine, it was found that overexcretors of uric acid incorported more of the isotope into uric acid (Benedict et al., 1952, 1953). When dietary protein was increased, there was further increase in the rate of incorporation into uric acid (Bien et al., 1953; Bowering et al., 1970). Thus, the overexcretion of uric acid is indeed due to overproduction of uric acid; the overproduction is enhanced with increased dietary protein.

Urinary uric acid excretion depends largely upon the total amount of purine and protein ingested. Hence, a person with a protein intake of 100 g, which yields 16 gm nitrogen, will excrete approximately 14.4 g nitrogen in the urine, calculated on the basis of about 90% elimination via the kidney, and 10% via the intestine. If uric acid nitrogen is approximately 1.5% of the total nitrogen in the urine, 216 mg uric acid nitrogen or 648 mg uric acid will be found in urine. When the protein intake is increased by 30%, 130 g protein will yield 20.8 g total nitrogen, and 18.7 g nitrogen will appear in urine. Assuming the same proportion of uric acid nitrogen to total nitrogen in urine, 280 mg uric acid nitrogen, or 840 mg uric acid, an excess of about 200 mg uric acid, will be excreted.

A disproportionate amount of uric acid nitrogen is excreted by gouty patients, whereas in the normal patient the uric acid nitrogen-to-total nitrogen ratio averages 1.5±0.3% (Talbott and Yü, 1976). It frequently exceeds 1.8% in gouty patients,

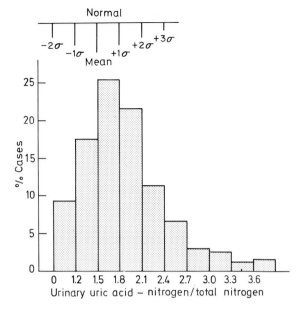

Fig. 5. Distribution of urinary uric acid nitrogen to total nitrogen ratios in patients with uric acid nephrolithiasis compared with nongouty subjects

Table 3. Relation of plasma urate concentrations to prevalence of nephrolithiasis in primary gout

Plasma uric acid mg/100 ml	Primary gout: total patients		Patients with nephrolithiasis	
	No.	%	No.	%
5.1– 7.0	83	7	16	20
7.1– 9.0	472	38	126	27
9.1–11.0	491	40	181	37
11.1–13.0	144	12	66	46
13.1–16.0	38	3	19	50

particularly in those with uric acid lithiasis (Fig. 5). About 22% of gouty patients have urinary uric acid nitrogen-to-total nitrogen ratios exceeding 1.8% (+1 S.D. of the nongouty mean); 11% of them exceed 2.1% (+2 S.D.), and another 15% of patients have a ratio above 2.4% (+3 S.D.). In 9% of gouty nephrolithiasis patients, the uric acid nitrogen is actually less than 1.2% (−1 S.D. of the nongouty mean), due to renal damage. When renal damage is present, hyperuricemia becomes more striking. Thus, the degree of hyperuricosuria does not necessarily correspond to that of hyperuricemia.

Uric acid nephrolithiasis is more frequent in gouty subjects with extreme hyperuricemia and hyperuricosuria (Tables 3 and 4). Lithiasis occurs in less than 30% of gouty patients when plasma urate is less than 9 mg/100 ml; and it occurs in approximately 50% when plasma urate concentrations exceed 11 mg/100 ml. Similarly, the

Table 4. Relation of urinary uric acid excretion to prevalence of nephrolithiasis in primary gout

Urinary uric acid	Primary gout: total patients		Patients with nephrolithiasis	
mg/day	No.	%	No.	%
< 400	152	12	32	24
400– 599	482	36	113	24
600– 799	397	30	127	32
800– 999	208	16	64	31
1000–1600	80	6	38	49

prevalence of nephrolithiasis is less than 30% in gouty patients when urinary excretion of uric acid is less than 600 mg a day; it increased to 50% when the urinary uric acid exceeded 1 g a day.

II. Undue Urinary Acidity and Subnormal Ammonium Excretion

Secretion of hydrogen ions into tubular fluid occurs largely in the proximal tubule, but it is in the distal tubule and the collecting duct where a distinctly acidic urine is formed. Normally the urine is distinctly more acid at night and in the early morning hours. There is a circadian rhythm with a postprandial alkaline tide (ELLIOT et al., 1959). The type of diet, the degree of hydration, and one's physical activity may influence the urine acidity significantly.

In the case of the gouty patient, particularly those with uric acid lithiasis, there is undue acidity of urine (Yü and GUTMAN, 1967), as studied by determining the early-morning urine pH after an overnight fast (Table 5). In almost half the subjects with uric acid nephrolithiasis this was found to be less than 5.1. It was between 5.1 and 5.3 in 29% and 5.4–5.6 in 17%. In normal subjects, only 15% had urine pH less than 5.1; 59% had urine pH between 5.1 and 5.6; urine pH was more than 5.6 in 26%. The circadian rhythm is absent in many gouty patients. There is no indication of abnormal metabolic generation of hydrogen ions, nor any evidence of abnormal tubular secretion of hydrogen ions. The persistently acidic urine is thought to be due to some alteration in the excretion of ammonium or titratable acidity. Cumulative data from the GUTMAN and Yü series showed that there was a distinct deficit of ammonium in

Table 5. Urine pH in primary gout with uric acid stones, compared with primary gout without stones and normal subjects

Urine	Primary gout with Stones		Primary gout without stones		Normal subjects	
pH	No.	%	No.	%	No.	%
4.8–5.0	87	47	82	28	12	15
5.1–5.3	54	29	108	37	27	34
5.4–5.6	32	17	76	26	20	25
5.7–5.9	11	6	17	6	10	13
>5.9	2	1	12	4	11	13

Table 6. Urinary excretion of ammonium and titratable acid in 2-h morning urine samples after overnight fast in patients with uric acid nephrolithiasis and normal subjects according to urine pH

Urine pH	Subjects	No.	NH_4^+ mEq/min	TA^a mEq/min	NH_4^+/TA^a	$C_{Creatinine}$ ml/min
4.8–5.0	Normal	11	31.2 ± 5.1	25.8 ± 4.0	1.27 ± 0.25	104 ± 18
	lithiasis	31	24.0 ± 6.9 ($p=0.001$)	29.9 ± 7.1 ($p=0.05$)	0.80 ± 0.21 ($p=0.001$)	117 ± 18 (ns)
5.1–5.3	Normal	25	33.2 ± 8.2	26.1 ± 5.7	1.27 ± 0.44	107 ± 19
	lithiasis	24	23.6 ± 6.6 ($p=0.001$)	26.1 ± 7.0 ($p=$ ns)	0.40 ± 0.29 ($p=0.001$)	109 ± 12 (ns)
5.4–5.6	Normal	18	32.5 ± 7.5	23.5 ± 9.0	1.53 ± 0.16	121 ± 18
	lithiasis	10	19.4 ± 3.8 ($p=0.02$–0.01)	21.7 ± 3.7 ($p=$ ns)	0.89 ± 0.17 ($p=0.001$)	103 ± 17 (ns)
5.7–5.9	Normal	8	25.5 ± 5.9	17.9 ± 2.3	1.45 ± 0.42	112 ± 16
	lithiasis	7	18.5 ± 9.3 ($p=$ ns)	16.6 ± 3.9 ($p=$ ns)	1.11 ± 0.40 ($p=$ ns)	100 ± 12 (ns)

[a] TA, titratable acid

p = probability. ns = not significant when p is greater than 0.05.

Table 7. Urinary ammonium excretion in nephrolithiasis, age matched with normal subjects

Age (yrs.)		No.	Urinary NH_4^+ (m Eq./min)
40 or less	Normal	44	32.5 ± 7.1
	lithiasis	48	26.8 ± 6.2
41–60	Normal	10	35.2 ± 7.6
	lithiasis	72	26.7 ± 8.0

a majority of the gouty patients. The deficit was more prevalent in the gouty with lithiasis, compared at similar ranges of urine pH, matched age groups, and all with normal renal functions (Tables 6 and 7). Titratable acidity was found to be essentially the same in both groups. The ratio of ammonium to titratable acid is 1.25 to 1.45 in normal subjects. This ratio is barely 1 or less than 1 in patients with lithiasis. No significant differences were seen when urine pH was higher than 5.6. The persistently acidic urine in gouty patients is assumed by some to be due to a subnormal ammonium excretion at a given acid load or urine pH (HENNEMAN et al., 1962; GUTMAN and YÜ, 1965; RAPOPORT et al., 1967; PLANTE et al., 1968; FALLS, 1972) and by others to be due to high values of titratable acidity (DELBARRE et al., 1964; FRANK et al., 1960; BARZEL et al., 1964; METCALFE-GIBSON et al., 1965).

Since glutamine is the major source of ammonia produced by the kidney, the decreased excretion of ammonia may be interpreted to be the result of deficient extraction of glutamine at the peritubular border of the renal tubular cells or of a defect in renal enzymatic release of ammonia from glutamine. The deficient ammonia excretion is associated with overexcretion of uric acid.

III. Organic Matrix and Crystallization

The usual components of urinary calculi have one property in common; they are all relatively insoluble substances. Uric acid in urine is invariably supersaturated if the urine pH is below 5.5. The degree of supersaturation of the urine in respect to uric acid may sometimes be quite remarkable. It was suggested that urinary mucoprotein, such as the TAMM-HORSFALL mucoprotein, might act as solubilizer for uric acid to maintain uric acid in a supersaturated state (SPERLING et al., 1965). However, no differences in the capacity for saturation were found between idiopathic uric acid stone formers and normal subjects.

It has recently been shown that some nondialyzable substances on crystallization rates and supersaturation levels were present in both the stone formers and the normal subjects; there were appreciable differences between the two groups of subjects (GILL and ROMA, 1976).

Additional studies are needed to determine more precisely the physico-chemical nature of the nondialyzable material. Perhaps a number of other constituents in urine may influence the properties of this solubilizer. It is also possible that uric acid stones may respond differently than other types of stones.

G. Natural History of Uric Acid Nephrolithiasis

I. Primary Gout and Hyperuricemia Without Gout

Approximately 22% (421) of 1900 patients with primary gout from the GUTMAN and YÜ Gout Research Clinic gave a history of nephrolithiasis. This is somewhat higher than that of other reported series (DE SÉZE and RYCKEWAERT, 1960; WEISS and SEGALOFF, 1959); perhaps the difference is the result of the prolonged period of follow-up in the GUTMAN and YÜ study, in many cases up to 25 years. More than 90% of the cases with renal calculi were men, reflecting the preponderance of males among gouty patients. The mean age of onset of lithiasis was not much different from that of gout. However, lithiasis developed first, and gout supervened at a much more advanced age in 40% of the patients (Table 8). Renal calculi preceded gouty arthritis more frequently in younger age groups; but after 50 years of age more calculous patients gave history of gout preceding lithiasis. The attacks of renal colic are recurrent in about half the patients. The intervals between the recurrences are quite unpredictable; the frequency may vary from several attacks in a year to none in 10–20 years. Surgical intervention has been necessary in about 10% of the cases. In the preantibiotic era, recurrent calculi with infected urine frequently required repeated surgical intervention, even nephrectomy. In those patients without clinically recognizable evidence of renal damage, the urine is unduly acidic, and many have hyperuricosuria. Tophi occur in 40% of calculous patients, the same incidence as in gout without lithiasis.

Of 98 female gouty patients, 14 had a history of renal calculi (YÜ, 1977). The mean age of onset of stone in these females was 53 years, corresponding to the relatively late age of onset of gout as compared to males. Of the 14 females with calculi, 9 were also tophaceous. Of the 14, 8 had recurrent lithiasis, 7 prior to onset of gout. The hyperuricosuria was not evident in most cases possibly because of the

Table 8. Years intervening between onset of lithiasis and arthritis in primary gout

Years intervening	Lithiasis preceded gouty arthritis		Gouty arthritis preceded lithiasis	
	No.	%	No.	%
Same year	21	5	19	5
1– 2	28	7	26	6
3– 5	14	3	52	12
6–10	43	10	55	13
11–15	29	7	50	12
16–20	22	5	23	5
21–40	11	3	28	7
Total	168	40	253	60

frequent use of diuretics for coexisting hypertension or obesity. Accurate urine pH could not be determined in a few because of urinary infection or the use of drugs for coexisting medical problems.

One hundred fifty cases of uric acid nephrolithiasis without gout have been studied. The course of lithiasis proves to be equally unpredictable in this group as in primary gout. Many of these patients have remained asymptomatic without developing gout.

II. Uric Acid Lithiasis in Secondary Gout, Associated with Blood Dyscrasia

Hyperuricemia, with excessive excretion of uric acid, has long been recognized in polycythemia, myeloid metaplasia, and certain types of leukemia. Despite the frequent hyperuricemia, the incidence of secondary gout is only about 5–10% (LYNCH, 1962; GRAHAME and SCOTT, 1970; TALBOTT, 1959). Isotope study has shown relatively low incorporation of uric acid from ^{15}N-glycine in the first few days; instead, there is a progressive increase in incorporation, reaching a maximum by the end of 2 weeks (LASTER and MULLER, 1953; YÜ et al., 1953; YÜ et al., 1956). Hyperuricemia and increased uric acid excretion are frequent in myelocytic leukemia (NUGENT et al., 1962; SANDBERG et al., 1956; RIESELBACH et al., 1964; KRAKOFF, 1965). When gout occurs in leukemia, it is usually in patients with chronic myelocytic leukemia in the terminal blastic phase (YÜ, 1965). Lymphatic leukemia seldom gives rise to hyperuricemia and excessive uricosuria (KRAKOFF, 1965). When cytolytic agents and/or other therapeutic measures are instituted, the turnover rate of nucleic acids is accelerated and the degree of hyperuricemia greater, as is the extent of excessive uricosuria.

Prevalence of nephrolithiasis in secondary gout is twice as frequent as in primary gout (YÜ et al., 1976). It occurred in 25 of 63 patients with secondary gout associated with chronic myeloproliferative diseases. It is particularly frequent in "spending" polycythemia vera or meyloid metaplasia. According to a recent prospective study of polycythemia vera, the sex incidence is almost equal (WASSERMAN, 1975). However, secondary gout is still male preponderant (M:F, 6:1), as is renal lithiasis in blood dyscrasias (M:F, 5:1).

Calculi were recurrent in a majority of the cases, depending to a large extent on the activity of the hemopoietic system. Lithiasis preceded gouty arthritis in 12 of the 25 calculus cases (40%), which is the same as that seen in primary gout. The intervening years between lithiasis and gout may be as many as 15 or more; but eight patients had both conditions within a year. Interestingly enough, the onset of lithiasis in three patients actually led to the discovery of the underlying blood disease. The mean age at onset of the blood disease was 52 ± 9 years old; the age at onset of lithiasis was 57 ± 10, and that of gouty arthritis was 58 ± 9 years old. Fifteen of the 25 calculous cases (60%) were found to be tophaceous, a much higher incidence than in primary gout. Some patients developed tophi before the onset of gouty arthritis or lithiasis. In 9 cases, uric acid aggregates resulted in acute ureteral obstruction and bacterial infection. Nephrectomy had to be resorted to in one patient, and death from uremia occurred in three. The natural course of renal lithiasis in blood dyscrasias is less favorable than that of renal lithiasis in primary gout, largely because of the prognosis of the underlying disease.

III. Hypoxanthine Guanine Pyrophosphoribosyl Transferase (HPRT) Deficiency and Other Enzyme Abnormalities

The most fulminant form of renal lithiasis occurs in patients with HPRT deficiency, or in those with excessive PRPP synthetase activity. Accelerated purine biosynthesis de novo using ^{14}C-glycine is demonstrated in Lesch-Nyhan syndrome. The isotope is rapidly incorporated into uric acid, and the cumulative incorporation over a 7-day period may be as much as 20 times the normal (LESCH and NYHAN, 1964; NYHAN et al., 1965). In partial HPRT deviciency there is likewise an increased rate of de novo biosynthesis of uric acid (KELLEY et al., 1967). The uric acid turnover rate is exceedingly rapid, as a reflection of increased production and excretion. The serum urate of such patients is as a rule over 10 mg/100 ml. The urinary excretion of uric acid is frequently more than 1 g a day. The urinary uric acid to creatinine ratio in adults is normally 0.3 to 0.5. In HPRT deficient children, uric acid/creatinine ratio frequently exceeds 1, reaches as high as 3 or 5 (KAUFMAN et al.,1968). The urinary uric acid nitrogen to total nitrogen ratios in HPRT deficiency subjects goes as high as 3%, the normal being $1.5 \pm 0.3\%$. The high urinary uric acid excretion is often reflected in the frequent occurrence of renal calculi. Of 18 patients with HPRT deficiency 13 gave a history of calculi (KELLEY et al., 1969). In 8 of the patients, the first clinical symptoms were related to passage of renal stones. Of the 13 patients, 10 passed the first stones before the age of 20 and 6 at less than 8 years of age. A group of eight cases of partial HPRT deficiency in three generations was found in one Italian family (YÜ et al., 1972). Five had recurrent renal lithiasis with repeated ureteral obstructions and anuria.

Several families are now known to have increased activity of phosphoribosyl pyrophosphate synthetase activity as the explanation for purine overproduction, with gouty arthritis or renal lithiasis (BECKER, 1972; SPERLING et al., 1972; YÜ et al., 1975). As in HPRT deficiency, the renal lithiasis tends to be recurrent.

Renal lithiasis may appear in type I glycogen storage disease, associated with hyperuricemia and gouty symptoms. The hyperlacticacidemia and the increased availability of PRPP for uric acid biosynthesis contribute to hyperuricemia, and in turn renal calculi (HOLLING, 1963; KELLEY et al., 1968).

IV. Chronic Renal Disease

Chronic renal disease is a frequent cause of hyperuricemia, but incidence of gouty arthritis in renal insufficiency is rather low (SARRE and MERTZ, 1965; RICHET et al., 1965). We have recorded 253 patients with varying degrees of renal involvement in 1700 primary gout patients, and 76 had primary intrinsic renal disease (YÜ and BERGER, 1975). The causes of the renal disease in the 76 were chronic glomerular nephritis, chronic pyelonephritis, congenital cystic disease of the kidneys, and proteinuria of undertermined etiology. In renal insufficiency, the uric acid excretion is usually reduced, since the amount filtered is diminished and tubular transport is impaired. Thus, only 10 of the 76 had renal lithiasis, mainly among those with less renal damage. In these 10, urinary uric acid excretion was 656 ± 207 mg/day (not excessive), and the serum uric acid was 10.1 ± 1.2 mg/100 ml. Four of the 10 patients had recurrent calculi. A persistently acidic urine may play an important role in producing renal calculi, despite the absence of marked hyperuricosuria in such patients.

EMMERSON found no renal stones in his series of 34 cases of saturnine gout (EMMERSON, 1968). This is not surprising, since uric acid excretion is rather low in lead nephropathy. Furthermore, no evidence of urate overproduction from ^{14}C-glycine was found in saturnine gout (BALL and SORENSEN, 1969).

V. Chronic Ulcerative Colitis and Regional Ileitis

Uric acid lithiasis is fairly common in patients with ulcerative colitis and regional ileitis (DEREN et al., 1962; MARATKA and NEDBAL, 1964; GROSSMAN and NUGENT, 1967). DEREN et al. reported 28 cases of nephrolithiasis among 583 patients with ulcerative colitis and regional ileitis admitted to the Mt. Sinai Hospital in New York City during a 10-year period from 1950 to 1960. Uric acid stone occurred in 13 patients, calcium stone in nine, and the composition of stone was not determined in the remaining six. Pyelonephritis was found in more than half the subjects. MARATKA and NEDBAL reported 512 patients with ulcerative colitis, of whom 438 were treated medically and 74 surgically. Renal stone developed in 10; nine of the 10 patients were in the surgically treated group. GROSSMAN and NUGENT reviewed 1100 cases of ulcerative colitis and regional ileitis. Excisional surgery of small or large intestine was done in 827 of the 1100 cases. Renal stones occurred in 35 patients; 31 occurred in the surgically treated group. It is generally observed that uric acid lithiasis is relatively more common in ileostomy patients (BENNETT and JEPSON, 1966; CLARKE and MCKENZIE, 1969; GIGAX and LEACH, 1971).

In patients who have developed uric acid stones after ileostomy or colostomy, uric acid excretion is usually within normal limits (MELICK and HENNEMAN, 1958). These patients, as a rule, excrete rather acidic urine, produce small urine volume, and are prone to urinary infections. The excessive loss of intestinal bicarbonate is partly compensated by bicarbonate reabsorption by the kidney. In addition, the intestinal sodium loss leads to increased renal sodium reabsorption, which takes place partially in exchange for hydrogen ion. If hypokalemia coexists, hydrogen ion secretion is further facilitated, leading to an even more acidic urine. Further, with loss of fluid by the intestinal tract, either transiently during an exacerbation of the condition or chronically due to a diminished absorptive surface, a diminution of urine volume may result (GALLAGHER et al., 1962; WILMORE and GOTS, 1969; REISNER et al., 1973).

VI. Idiopathic Uric Acid Lithiasis

A hereditary form of idiopathic uric acid nephrolithiasis, without hyperuricemia or hyperuricosuria, has been described (DE VRIES et al., 1962; ATSMON et al., 1963). It affects females almost as frequently as males and is more common among Jews and Italians than other ethnic groups. It is transmitted as an autosomal dominant trait and is characterized by early onset with recurrent attacks. Many of the patients have urinary tract infection and renal damage. A majority of the patients die in uremia. The characteristic findings are low urine pH and absence of postprandial alkaline tides.

HENNEMAN and co-workers reported two cases of idiopathic uric acid nephrolithiasis with reduced ammonium excretion (HENNEMAN et al., 1962). WOEBER and co-workers confirmed the low ammonia formation in a case of uric acid nephrolithiasis (WOEBER et al., 1962). RAPOPORT reported on 16 cases with uric acid calculi, compared to 16 cases with calcium oxalate calculi, and 11 normal subjects. The mean ammonium-to-titratable acidity ratios were significantly lower in the uric acid calculi cases. Each of the 16 patients with uric acid calculi had hyperuricemia (RAPOPORT et al., 1967). On the other hand, the uric acid lithiasis cases reported by WRONG did not reveal any abnormally low urinary ammonium excretion (METCALFE-GIBSON et al., 1965). It is possible that the so-called "idiopathic uric acid lithiasis" may include uric acid lithiasis of various unknown causes, some with renal damage.

H. Detection of the Chemical Nature of the Stone

Information on the chemical nature of any stone is important in view of the satisfactory therapeutic measures for different types of stones. The stones may be recurrent, and the nature of the stone may be changed in some patients. A uric acid calculus may be mixed with calcium oxalate, calcium phosphate, or magnesium ammonium phosphate. A uric acid calculus usually becomes radiopaque when there is change in its chemical nature.

Whenever a calculus is obtained, bits of material should be scraped from different parts of the calculus for routine chemical analysis and polarizing-light microscopy. A uric acid stone is usually deeply pigmented. A tiny piece may be dissolved in lithium carbonate and its differential optical densities determined on a UV spectrophotometer at 292 nm, using uricase. A cystine stone appears flaky and light colored. A nitroprusside test for cystine is simple enough to perform; or an amino acid chromatogram of the urine may be done. For detection of calcium, oxalate, phosphate, or magnesium chemical and/or optical methods may be used. For more exact and accurate analysis, X-ray diffraction, electron microscopy and other optical methods may be done, although not so easily carried out routinely. The essence is to know the nature of the stone for more precise treatment.

J. Management of Uric Acid Naphrolithiasis

General principles involved in the management of uric acid lithiasis include correction of undue urine acidity and control of hyperuricosuria, elminination of urinary tract infection, and treatment of underlying disease if present.

I. Correction of Undue Urine Acidity

According to the estimates of PETERS and VAN SLYKE, the free uric acid concentration in a saturated solution of uric acid in urine would be approximately 60 mg/liter at pH 5.0 and 37° C. The solubility is greatly increased to 220 mg/l at pH 6.0, and to 1580 mg/l at pH 7.0 (PETERS and VAN SLYKE, 1946). In order to promote the solubility of uric acid in urine, one must have adequate hydration to produce satisfactory urine volume, a sensible diet to lessen urinary uric acid excretion, and induce a reasonable urine pH.

1. Adequate Hydration

It is a long-established routine to encourage adequate hydration in renal lithiasis. This seems to be simple and yet not always easy to accomplish, particularly if a liberal amount of liquid intake is to be maintained uniformly throughout day and night. In order to be able to produce a satisfactory urine volume of 2 l/day (approximately 1.5 ml/min), an amount of liquid equal to urine loss, plus an additional liter of fluid, should be ingested daily. Whenever there is excessive loss of body water through the skin and the intestinal tract due to hot environment, exercise, febrile disease, or diarrheal state, it is extremely important to make up the loss with extra intake of liquid. When a copious urine flow is maintained, the urine acidity usually diminishes. Fruit juices help dilute and alkalinize the urine.

2. Sensible Diet

A sensible diet with a low purine content and a moderate amount of proteins is important. A sensible diet does not imply a restricted diet, since the average American diet tends to be too generous, particularly in proteins and calories. A protein intake of 1 gm/kg body weight should be more than adequate for maintaining nutrition. With moderate reduction in protein intake, hyperuricosuria in many may be partially or completely corrected. It has been repeatedly indicated that uric acid excretion becomes much lower with less total nitrogen output in urine, which in turn depends on protein intake (BOWERING, 1970; GUTMAN and YÜ, 1952, 1963). It has been recognized for many years that a high-protein diet is uricosuric (BODANSKY, 1938). A low-protein diet has been advocated in the management of uric acid stones (BOGASH and DOWBEN, 1954). In replacing high-purine and high-protein foods, one should include more fresh vegetables to have a relatively more alkaline ash diet. This in turn produces a less acid urine.

3. Alkalinizing Agents

Despite vigilance in maintaining an adequate fluid and low-purine and protein intake, the urine acidity in many calculous patients may still be excessive. Since uric acid is highly dissociated beyond pH 6.0 to form urate, which is more soluble than free uric acid (Fig. 2), the urine pH should be maintained between 6.0 and 6.5. It is not necessary to achieve a urine pH approaching or beyond 7. Over alkalinization favors the precipitation of calcium phosphate or carbonate. The most convenient means of alkalinizing the urine is to employ sodium bicarbonate, 0.6–1.2 g three or four times/ 24 h. Appropriate dosage for use can be adjusted by determination of the acidity of freshly voided urine by the patient himself using the pH paper.

In patients with coexisting hypertension or cardiac insufficiency, use of a sodium salt should be kept at a minimum; alkaline potassium salts are preferred instead. Diuretics in general may produce some favorable effect on patients with increased uricosuria, since they promote urine flow and diminish uric acid output. Acetazolamide, a potent carbonic acid anhydrase inhibitor, favorably produces an alkaline urine and decreases uric acid excretion. But it may also increase the incidence of calcium stone by reducing citrate excretion, thus complicating uric acid lithiasis (Davis, 1959).

II. Control of Infection

In former years it was not infrequent for patients with recurrent calculi to require cysto- or pyelo-lithotomy. In some, surgical intervention had to be repeated and nephrectomy became necessary. A pure uric acid calculus may become infected, leading to magnesium ammonium phosphate stones due to urea-splitting organisms. Urine pH becomes alkaline with bacterial infection. When urine contains many WBC or RBC, it is important to culture the urine, to determine bacterial sensitivity to antibiotics if the culture is positive and to employ an appropriate antibiotic. In recent years recurrent nephrolithiasis with accompanying bacterial infection is less frequent. This is in part due to the availability of more potent antibiotics and in part due to the use of allopurinol.

III. Control of Hyperuricosuria—Allopurinol

The final steps in the synthesis of uric acid involve the conversion of hypoxanthine to xanthine and xanthine to uric acid in the presence of xanthine oxidase (Fig. 6). Allopurinol, an analog of hypoxanthine, is a potent inhibitior of xanthine oxidase (Feigelson et al., 1957). Its administration reduces the serum and urinary uric acid (Rundles et al., 1963; Yü and Gutman, 1964). Thus, it is useful in patients with uric acid lithiasis who have hyperuricosuria, especially when it is difficult to alkalinize the urine due to coexisting conditions.

Allopurinol has a rather short plasma half-life of only 1–3 h. Its metabolite, oxipurinol, has a much longer half-life, ranging from 17–48 h (Elion et al., 1966). Allopurinol has a rapid renal clearance, approximating the glomerular filtration rate; but oxipurinol, extensively reabsorbed, has a renal clearance only about three times the uric acid clearance (Elion et al., 1968). Whereas allopurinol is an analog of hypoxanthine, oxipurinol is an analog of xanthine (Fig. 6). Allopurinol, like hypoxan-

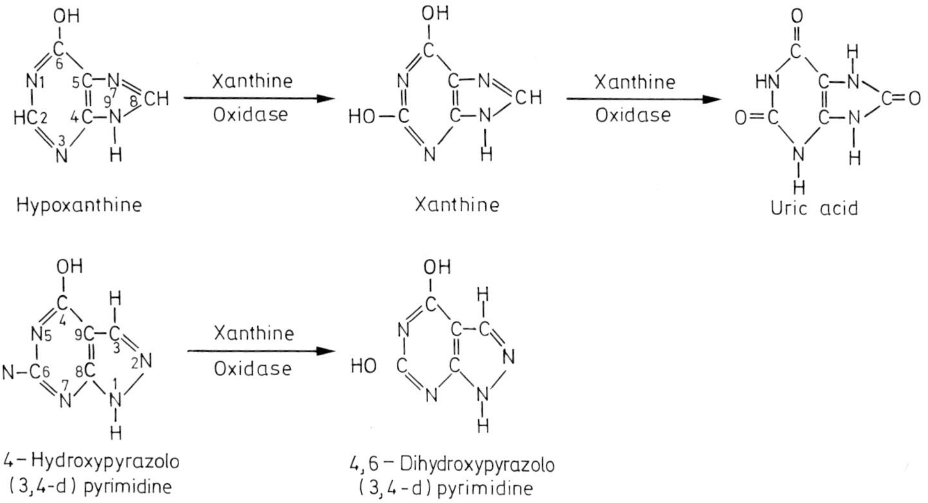

Hypoxanthine   Xanthine   Uric acid

4-Hydroxypyrazolo
(3,4-d) pyrimidine

4,6-Dihydroxypyrazolo
(3,4-d) pyrimidine

Fig. 6. Conversion of hypoxanthine to xanthine and to uric acid; conversion of 4-hydroxypyrazolo (3,4-d) pyrimidine (allopurinol) to 4,6-dihydroxypyrazolo (3,4-d) pyrimidine (oxipurinol) and their respective structural relationship to hypoxanthine and xanthine

Table 9. Solubilities of purine bases in serum and urine

	pH	Uric acid mg/100 ml	Xanthine mg/100 ml	Hypoxanthine mg/100 ml
Serum	7.4	7	10	115
Urine	5.0	15	5	140
Urine	7.0	200	13	150

thine, is relatively soluble in aqueous medium, but oxipurinol shares the insolubility of xanthine. KLINENBERG and co-workers studied the solubilities of the purine at 37° C for up to 24 h (KLINENBERG et al., 1965). After removing the crystals by Millipore filtration, the purine concentrations in the filtrate were determined. The solubility in serum of monosodium urate expressed as uric acid is about 7 mg/100 ml, that of xanthine 10 mg/100 ml. The solubility of uric acid is increased more than 10-fold at pH 7 as compared to pH 5, but no such striking difference is seen for xanthine. Hypoxanthine in both serum and urine at both pH levels is quite soluble (Table 9).

Following allopurinol administration, hypoxanthine and xanthine excretion is greatly increased with minimal accumulation in the blood, since hypoxanthine and xanthine are rapidly cleared by the kidneys at the rate of glomerular filtration (GOLDFINGER et al., 1965). The distribution of hypoxanthine and xanthine in urine is usually in favor of the latter. Since xanthine is as insoluble as uric acid, a potential hazard in the use of allopurinol is the formation of xanthine stones. However, xanthine stones have not been observed in patients without specific enzyme deficiencies, because the decrease in uric acid excretion is not followed by a stoichiometric increase in excretion of hypoxanthine and xanthine after allopurinol. However, the stoichiometric relationship between the decrease in uric acid and the increase in oxypurines after allopurinol exists in HPRT deficiency patients. Hence, xanthine stones following allopurinol in patients with Lesch-Nyhan syndrome have been reported (GREENE et al., 1969). Xanthine nephropathy has also been observed in patients with lymphoma or lymphosarcoma treated with allopurinol (BAND et al., 1970; ABLIN et al., 1972). Apparently, the initial hyperuricemia and hyperuricosuria in such patients may be excessive, and the increased xanthine output is markedly enhanced following a combination of chemotherapy and allopurinol.

Oxipurinol stones have been reported in a patient who had some neurologic disorder but with no HPRT deficiency (LANDGREBE et al., 1975). The patient developed hematuria and stones, leading to acute urinary tract obstruction after large doses of oxipurinol and allopurinol. The stone was identified as oxipurinol on infrared spectrum analysis. In patients receiving allopurinol, about 50% of the drug may be oxidized to oxipurinol. When large amounts of oxipurinol together with allopurinol are given, oxipurinol excretion may increase significantly to exceed its solubility in urine.

In general, allopurinol is well tolerated with a low order of toxicity (RUNDLES et al., 1963; YÜ and GUTMAN, 1964; KLINENBERG et al., 1965; KUZELL, 1966). Nevertheless, drug fever, skin rash, granulocytopenia, hepatitis, vasculitis, and epidermal necrolysis have been reported (MILLS, 1971; STRATIGOS, 1972; LIDSKY and SHARP, 1967; SIMONS et al., 1972; GREENBERG and ZAMBRANO, 1972; JARZOBSKI et al., 1970). Asymptomatic elevations of serum glutamic pyruvate transaminase and serum glutamic oxaloacetic transaminase have been observed (YÜ, 1974). Most of the reactions are allergic in nature. Some effects are toxic and are dose related.

Since many patients with renal calculi suffer single attacks without recurrences for a number of years, and in many the chemical nature of the stone has never been ascertained, allopurinol may not be indicated in such cases. But in recurrent uric acid nephrolithiasis, allopurinol is essential and highly effective.

Allopurinol is indicated in hyperuricosuria despite careful diet, as well as in those with difficulty in alkalinizing urine and with coexisting complicated medical conditions. Allopurinol should be started before cytolytic therapy for blood dyscrasias to avoid extreme hyperuricemia and/or hyperuricosuria. In stone formers with HPRT deficiency, or with other enzyme abnormalities, allopurinol can be life saving. The use of allopurinol does not preclude the proper treatment of coexisting medical conditions.

The required dosage of allopurinol in uncomplicated uric acid nephrolithiasis is usually 200–300 mg/day. Up to 600 mg/day may be required occasionally for a short period of time. Patients' compliance with the general measures of treatment and the concomitant treatment for underlying disorders are important considerations in planning dose schedules. A poor renal function status may require less allopurinol, since the rate of drug excretion will be more sluggish (ELION et al., 1968). In patients receiving cytotoxic drugs, allopurinol dosage must be maintained at a minimum, since cyclophosphamide toxicity is enhanced in presence of allopurinol (Boston Collaborative Study, 1974). Allopurinol slows the metabolism of Coumadin by reducing the activity of the hepatic microsomal drug metabolizing enzyme systems (VESELL et al., 1970). Hence, a patient taking coumadin should be kept on a minimal amount of allopurinol.

To obtain more satisfactory responses in preventing recurrent nephrolithiasis, it is most important to make patients understand the problem for better cooperation. Serum and urine for uric acid, urine pH, and urine volumes, as well as renal function status and coexisting conditions, should be periodically reassessed so that allopurinol dosage may be adjusted appropriately.

Observations on allopurinol for uric acid nephrolithiasis have been expanded to 150 from 108 patients reported previously (GUTMAN and YÜ, 1968). Altogether, 16 patients had recurrence of symptoms. Five had large "mixed" uric acid calculi and persistent infection. Four had recurrence of gravel in the first year of allopurinol treatment. Repeated attacks of renal colic were apparently related to calcium oxalate stones that had been present prior to allopurinol therapy in two patients. Another patient with severe dehydration developed a single attack of renal colic and a calcium stone on a hot day. In one patient with myeloid metaplasia, allopurinol dosage became insufficient when repeated blood transfusions and large doses of androgen were given. In two others, one with HPRT deficiency and another one with excessive activity of PRPP synthetase, uric acid gravel recurred following the omission of allopurinol for a few days only. It is apparent that success of allopurinol treatment of uric acid nephrolithiasis depends in part on the eradication of infection, control of coexisting conditions, as well as appropriate allopurinol dosage, and knowing the nature of the calculi. And lastly, not all flank pains are renal colic; a nonrenal pain can develop in patients with renal lithiasis.

K. Conclusion

Uric acid nephrolithiasis constitutes about 10% of all calculi in the population at large. The prevalence of renal calculi in patients with primary gout is approximately 20%, and that in secondary gout associated with myeloproliferative disorders is twice as great. Renal calculi occur frequently in hyperuricemic and hyperuricosuric conditions associated with HPRT deficiency or other purine metabolizing enzyme abnormalities. Persistent undue acidity of the urine and increased concentration of uric acid in the urine are critical predisposing factors in the formation of uric acid calculi. Increased concentrations of uric acid occur when there is hyperuricosuria resulting from increased biosynthesis of uric acid and/or contraction of urine volume. Persistent undue acidity of the urine in uric acid stone formers is attributable to deficient urinary ammonium excretion.

Uric acid nephrolithiasis is infrequent in chronic renal disease, but it occurs fairly commonly in chronic diarrheal syndromes, particularly in ileostomy patients. The infrequent occurrence of renal calculi in chronic renal insufficiency is at least in part related to diminished urinary excretion of uric acid. In chronic diarrheal syndromes, there is no hyperuricosuria. The predisposing factors here are undue urine acidity and small urine volume due to excessive loss of intestinal water and electrolytes.

Idiopathic uric acid nephrolithiasis is frequent among certain races in certain localities. There is no hyperuricemia nor hyperuricosuria, but persistent undue acidity of urine is present.

Management of uric acid nephrolithiasis should include correction of urine hyperacidity, control of hyperuricosuria, elimination of urinary tract infection, and treatment of associated disease if present. Adequate hydration, moderation in dietary intake of purines and proteins, and appropriate use of alkali may avoid recurrence of renal calculi in most patients. Allopurinol should be recommended in patients known to have excessive production and excretion of uric acid, in those with difficulty in alkalinizing urine, and in those with coexisting medical complications. Allopurinol is particularly useful in patients with HPRT deficiency or other purine metabolizing enzyme abnormalities and in patients with myeloproliferative diseases prior to cytotoxic therapy. Appropriate dosage is essential for prevention of recurrent nephrolithiasis without causing drug toxicity.

References

Ablin, A., Stephens, B.G., Hirata, T., Wilson, H.K., Williams, H.E.: Nephropathy, xanthinuria and orotic aciduria, complicating Burkitt's lymphoma treated with chemotherapy and allopurinol. Metabolism **21**, 771—778 (1972)

Atsmon, A., Vries, A. de, Frank, M.: Uric Acid Lithiasis. Amsterdam: Elsevier 1963

Ball, G.V., Sorensen, L.B.: Pathogenesis of hyperuricemia in saturnine gout. New Engl. J. Med. **280**, 1199—1202 (1969)

Band, P.R., Silverberg, D.S., Henderson, J.F., Ulan, A.A., Wensel, R.H., Banerjee, T.K., Little, A.S.: Xanthine nephropathy in a patient with lymphosarcoma treated with allopurinol. New Engl. J. Med. **283**, 354—357 (1970)

Barzel, U.S., Sperling, O., Frank, M., Vries, A. de: Renal ammonium excretion and urinary pH in idiopathic uric acid lithiasis. J. Urol. **92**, 1—5 (1964)

Becker, M.A., Meyer, L.J., Wood, A.W., Seegmiller, J.E.: Gout associated with increased PRPP synthetase activity. Arthr. and Rheum. **15**, 430 (1972)

Benedict, J.D., Roche, M., Yü, T.F., Bien, E.J., Gutman, A.B., Stetten, W. de: The incorporation of glycine nitrogen in uric acid in normal and gouty man. Metabolism **1**, 3—12 (1952a)

Benedict, J.D., Yü, T.F., Bien, E.J., Gutman, A.B., Stetten, W de: A further study of the utilization of dietary glycine nitrogen for uric acid synthesis in gout. J. Clin. Invest. **32**, 775—777 (1953b)

Bennett, R.C., Jepson, R.P.: Uric acid stone formation following ileostomy. Aust. N.Z.J.Surg. **36**, 153—158 (1966)

Bergmann, F., Dikstein, S.: Relationship between spectral shifts and structural changes in uric acids and related compounds. J. Amer. Chem. Soc. **77**, 691—696 (1955)

Bien, E.J., Yü, T.F., Benedict, J.D., Gutman, A.B., Stetten, W. de: The relation of dietary nitrogen consumption to the rate of uric acid synthesis in normal and gouty man. J. Clin. Invest. **32**, 778—780 (1953)

Bodansky, M.: Introduction to Physiological Chemistry, 4th Ed. New York: John Wiley and Sons 1938

Bogash, M., Dowben, R.M.: Low protein diet in the management of uric acid stones. J. Urol. **72**, 1057—1060 (1954)

Bollinger, A., Gross, R.: Ammonia, urea and uric acid content of toe nails in renal insufficiency and gout. Aust. exp. Biol. med. Sci. **31**, 385—390 (1953)

Boston Collaborative Drug Surveillance Program: Allopurinol and cytotoxic drugs interaction in relation to bone marrow depression. J. Amer. med. Ass. **227**, 1036—1040 (1974)

Bowering, J., Calloway, D.H., Margen, S., Kaufman, N.A.: Dietary protein level and uric acid metabolism in normal man. J. nutr. **100**, 249—261 (1970)

Boyce, W.H., Garvey, F.K., Strawcutter, H.E.: Incidence of urinary calculi among patients in general hospitals, 1948—1952. J. Amer. med. Ass. **161**, 1437—1442 (1956)

Boyce, W.H., Garvey, F.K., Norfleet Jr., C.M.: The metal chelate compounds of urine. Their relation to the initiation and growth of calculi. Amer. J. Med. **19**, 87—95 (1955)

Buchanan, J.M.: The enzymatic synthesis of the purine nucleotides. Harvey Lect. **54**, 104—130 (1958/1959)

Butt, A.J. (Ed.): Etiological Factors in Renal Lithiasis. Springfield (Ill.): Ch. C. Thomas 1956

Campbell, J.W.: Nitrogen excretion Ch 7. In: Prosser, C.L. (Ed.): Comparative Animal Physiology, pp. 279—316. Philadelphia: W.B. Saunders 1973

Cifuentes, Delatte, L., Rapado, A., Abehsera, A., Traba, M. L., Cortes, M.: Uric acid lithiasis and gout in urinary calculi. Int. Symp. Renal Stones Res., Madrid, 1972, pp. 115—118

Clarke, A. M., McKenzie, R. G.: Ileostomy and the risk of urinary uric stones. Lancet **II**, 395—397 (1969)

Coe, F. L., Kavalach, A. G.: Hypercalciuria and hyperuricosuria in patients with nephrolithiasis. New Engl. J. Med. **291**, 1344—1350 (1974)

Cottet, J., Weber, A.: Intér pratique de l'analyse clinique des calculs urinaire. Pathol. Biol. Sem. Hôp. **7**, 1975—1978 (1959)

Davis, D. W.: Acetazolamide therapy with renal complication. Brit. med. J. **I**, 214—215 (1959)

Delbarre, F., Auscher, C., Lac, Y du: Documents pour l'étude du rein goutteux IV. Documents sur le pH-urinaire et ses variations. Rein Foie **6**, 53—62 (1964)

Dent, C. E., Sutor, D. J.: Presence or absence of inhibitor of calcium oxalate crystal growth in urine of normal and of stone formers. Lancet **1971 II**, 775—778 (1971)

Deren, J. J., Porush, J. G., Levitt, M. F., Khilnani, M. T.: Nephrolithiasis as a complication of ulcerative colitis and regional ileitis. Ann. Intern. Med. **56**, 843—853 (1962)

Ebbinghaus, K. D., Prieber, S.: Die Behandlung hoher Harnleiterstein. Dtsch. med. Wschr. **85**, 1045—1048 (1960)

Elion, G. B., Kovensky, A., Hitchings, G. H., Metz, E., Rundles, R. W.: Metabolic studies of allopurinol, an inhibitor of xanthine oxidase. Biochem. Pharmacol. **15**, 863—880 (1966a)

Elion, G. B., Yü, T. F., Gutman, A. B., Hitchings, G. H.: Renal clearance of oxipurinol, the chief metabolite of allopurinol. Amer. J. Med. **45**, 69—77 (1968)

Elliot, J. S., Sharp, R. F., Lewis, L.: Urinary pH. J. Urol. **81**, 339—343 (1959)

Emmerson, B. T.: The clinical differentiation of lead gout from primary gout. Arthr. and Rheum. **11**, 623—634 (1968)

Falls W. F., Jr.: Comparison of urinary acidification and ammonium excretion in normal and gouty subjects. Metabolism **21**, 433—445 (1972)

Feigelson, P., Davidson, J. D., Robins, R. K.: Pyrozolopyrimidines as inhibitors and substrates of xanthine oxidase. J. Biol. Chem. **226**, 993—1000 (1957)

Finlayson, B., Meyers, A. S.: In: Finlayson, B., Hench, L. L., Smith, L. H. (Eds.): Stone Ultrastructure in Urolithiasis Physical Aspects, pp. 115—128. Washington, D.C.: National Academy of Sciences 1972

Frank, M., Vries, A. de, Atsmon, A., Kochwa, S.: Urinary pH, ammonia and calcium excretion in renal uric acid stone patients. Israel Med. J. **19**, 299—301 (1960)

Gallagher, N. D., Harrison, D. D., Skyring, A. P.: Fluid and electrolyte disturbances in patients with long-established ileostomies. Gut **3**, 219—223 (1962)

Gigax, J. H., Leach, J. R.: Uric acid calculi associated with ileostomy for ulcerative colitis. J. Urol. **105**, 797—799 (1971)

Gill, W. B., Roma, M. J.: Determinants of supersaturation levels and crystallization rates of calcium oxalate from urine of normal humans and stone formers: Effects of nondialyzable materials. J. Surg. Res. **21**, 45—49 (1976)

Goldfinger, S., Klinenberg, J. R., Seegmiller, J. E.: The renal excretion of oxypurines. J. Clin. Invest. **44**, 623—628 (1965)

Grahame, R., Scott, J. T.: Clinical survey of 354 patients with gout. Ann. Rheum. Dis. **29**, 461—468 (1970)

Greenberg, M. S., Zambrano, S. S.: Aplastic agranulocytosis after allopurinol therapy. Arthr. and Rheum. **15**, 413—416 (1972)

Greene, M. L., Fujimoto, W. Y., Seegmiller, J. E.: Urinary xanthine stones: a rare complication of allopurinol therapy. New Engl. J. Med. **280**, 426—427 (1969)

Grossman, M. S., Nugent, F. W.: Urolithiasis as a complication of chronic diarrheal disease. Amer. J. Dig. Dis. **12**, 491—497 (1967)

Guthrie, D.: History of Medicine. Philadelphia: J. B. Lippincott 1946

Gutman, A. B., Yü, T. F.: Gout, a derangement of purine metabolism. Advanc. Intern. Med. **5**, 227—302 (1952a)

Gutman, A. B., Yü, T. F.: A three-component system for regulation of renal excretion of uric acid in man. Trans. Ass. Amer. Physcns **74**, 353—365 (1961b)

Gutman, A. B., Yü, T. F.: Urinary ammonium excretion in primary gout. J. Clin. Invest. **44**, 1474—1481 (1965c)

Gutman, A. B., Yü, T. F.: Uric acid nephrolithiasis. Amer. J. Med. **45**, 756—779 (1968d)

Hellstrom, J.: The significance of staphylococci in the development and treatment of renal and ureteral stones. Brit. J. Urol. **10**, 348—372 (1938)

Henneman, P. A., Wallach, S., Dempsey, E. F.: The metabolic defect responsible for uric acid stone formation. J. Clin. Invest. **41**, 537—542 (1962)

Herring, L. C.: Observations on the analysis of 10000 urinary calculi. J. Urol. **88**, 545—562 (1962)

Hodgkinson, A.: Uric acid disorders in patients with calcium stones. Brit. J. Urol. **48**, 1—5 (1976)

Holling, H. E.: Gout and glycogen storage disease. Ann. Intern. Med. **58**, 654—663 (1963)

Hughes, J., Coppridge, W. M., Roberts, L. C., Mann, V. I.: Oxalate urinary tract stones. J. Amer. med. Ass. **172**, 774—776 (1960)

Jarzobski, J., Ferrey, J., Wombolt, D., Fitch, D. M., Egan, J. D.: Vascultis with allopurinol therapy. Amer. Heart J. **79**, 116—121 (1970)

Jensen, A. T.: On concrements from the urinary tract. III. Acta Chir. Scand. **85**, 473—500 (1941)

Kaufman, J. M., Greene, M. L., Seegmiller, J. E.: Urinary uric acid/creatinine ratio—a screening test for inherited disorders of purine metabolism. J. Pediat. **73**, 583—592 (1968)

Kelley, W. M., Greene, M. L., Rosenbloom, F. M., Henderson, J. F., Seegmiller, J. E.: Hypoxan-thine-guanine phosphoribosyltransferase deficiency in gout. Ann. Intern. Med. **70**, 155—206 (1969c)

Kelley, W. M., Rosenbloom, F. M., Henderson, J. F., Seegmiller, J. E.: A specific enzyme defect in gout associated with overproduction of uric acid. Proc. Nat. Acad. Sci. (Wash.) **57**, 1735—1739 (1967a)

Kelley, W. M., Rosenbloom, F. M., Seegmiller, J. E., Howell, R. D.: Excessive production of uric acid in type I glycogen storage disease. J. Pediat. **72**, 488—496 (1968b)

King, J. S., Wainer, A.: Cystinuria with hyperuricemia and methioninuria. Amer. J. Med. **43**, 125—130 (1967)

Klinenberg, J. R., Goldfinger, S. F., Seegmiller, J. E.: The effectiveness of xanthine oxiase inhibitor allopurinol in the treatment of gout. Ann. Intern. Med. **62**, 639—647 (1965)

Krakoff, I. H.: Studies of uric acid biosynthesis in the chronic leukemia. Arthr. and Rheum. **8**, 772—779 (1965)

Krizek, V.: Anthropologische Merkmale und Nierensteinkrankheit. Dtsch. Z. Verdau.-Stoffwech-selkr. **17**, 133—139 (1957)

Krizek, V.: Uricemia in cystinuria. Horm. Metab. Res. **4**, 51—53 (1972)

Kuzell, W. B., Seebach, L. M., Glover, R. P., Jackman, A. E.: Treatment of gout with allopurinol and sulfinpyrazone in combination and with allopurinol alone. Ann. Rheum. Dis. **25**, 634—642 (1966)

Lagergren, C.: Biophysical investigation of urinary calculi. An X-ray crystallographic and micro-radiographic study. Acta Radiol. [Suppl.] **133**, 1—71 (1956)

Landgrebe, A. R., Nyhan, W. L., Coleman, M.: Urinary tract stones resulting from the excretion of oxypurinol. New Engl. J. Med. **292**, 626—627 (1975)

Laster, L., Muller, A. F.: Uric acid production in a case of myeloid metaplasia associated with gouty arthritis, studied with ^{15}N-labeled glycine. Amer. J. Med. **15**, 857—861 (1953)

Leonard, R. H.: Quantitative composition of kidney stones. Clin. Chem. **7**, 546—551 (1961)

Lesch, M., Nyhan, W. L.: A familiar disorder of uric acid metabolism and central nervous system function. Amer. J. Med. **36**, 561—570 (1964)

Lidsky, M. D., Sharp, J. P.: Jaundice with the use of 4-hydroxypyrazolo (3,4-d)-pyrimidine (4-HPP). Arthr. and Rheum. **10**, 294 (1967)

Lonsdale, K.: Epitaxy as a growth factor in urinary calculi and gall stones. Nature (Lond.) **217**, 56—58 (1968)

Lonsdale, K., Mason, P.: Uric acid, uric acid dihydrate and urates in urinary calculi, ancient, and modern. Science **152**, 1511—1512 (1966)

Lynch, E. C.: Uric acid metabolism in proliferative diseases of the marrow. Arch. Intern. Med. **109**, 639—653 (1962)

McCarrison, R.: A lecture on the causation of stone in India. Brit. Med. J. **I**, 1009—1015 (1931)

Maratka, Z., Nedbal, J.: Urolithiasis as a complication of the surgical treatment of ulcerative colitis. Gut **5**, 214—217 (1964)

May, P., Schindler, E.: Methods and results of conservative treatment of uric acid stones. In: Urinary Calculi. Int. Symp. Renal Stone Res., Madrid, 1972, pp. 111—114

Melick, R. A., Henneman, P. H.: Clinical and laboratory studies of 207 consecutive patients in a kidney stone clinic. New Engl. J. Med. **259**, 307—314 (1958)

Meloni, C. R., Canary, J. J.: Cystinuria with hyperuricemia. J. Amer. med. Ass. **200**, 169—171 (1967)

Metcalfe-Gibson, A., McCallum, F. M., Morrison, R. B. I., Wrong, O.: Urinary excretion of hydrogen ion in patients with uric acid calculi. Clin. Sci. **28**, 325—342 (1965)

Meyer, A. S., Finlayson, B., Dubois, L.: Direct observation of urinary stone ultrastructure. Brit. J. Urol. **43**, 154—163 (1971)

Meyer, J.: Über die Ausfällung von Sedimenten und die Bildung von Konkrementen in den Harnwegen. Z. klin. Med. **111**, 613—687 (1929)

Miller, J. L.: Some diseases of ancient man. Ann. med. Hist. **1**, 394—402 (1929)

Mills, Jr., R. M.: Severe hypersensitivity reactions associated with allopurinol. J. Amer. med. Ass. **216**, 799—802 (1971)

Nicholas, H. O.: Urinary calculi. III. Further observations on calculi from patients in the southeast Texas area. Clin. Chem. **7**, 175—177 (1961)

Nugent, C. A., MacDiarmid, W. D., Tyler, F. H.: Renal excretion of uric acid in leukemia and gout. Arch. intern. Med. **109**, 540—544 (1962)

Nyhan, W. L., Oliver, W. J., Lesch, M.: A familiar disorder of uric acid metabolism and central nervous system function. II. J. Pediat. **67**, 257—263 (1965)

Pak, C. Y. C., Arnold, L. H.: Heterogeneous nucleation of calcium oxalate by seeds of monosodium urate. Proc. Soc. Exp. Biol. Med. (N.Y.) **149**, 930—932 (1975)

Peters, J. P., Van Slyke, D. D.: Quantitative clinical chemistry, 2nd Ed., Vol. I. Baltimore: Williams and Wilkins 1946

Pinto, B., Rocha, E., Ruiz-Marcellán, F. J.: Isolation and characterization of uricine from uric acid stones. Kidney Int. **10**, 437—443 (1976)

Plante, G. E., Durivage, J., Lemieux, G.: Renal excretion of hydrogen in primary gout. Metabolism **17**, 377—385 (1968)

Prien, E. L.: Crystallographic analysis of urinary calculi; a 25 year survey study. J. Urol. **89**, 917—924 (1963)

Prien, E. L., Prien Jr., E. L.: Composition and structure of urinary stone. Amer. J. Med. **45**, 654—672 (1968)

Rapoport, A., Crassweller, P. O., Husdan, H., From, G. L. A., Zweig, M., Johnson, M. D.: The renal excretion of hydrogen ion in uric acid stone formers. Metabolism **16**, 176—188 (1967)

Reisner, G. S., Wilansky, D. L., Schneiderman, S.: Uric acid lithiasis in the ileostomy patient. Brit. J. Urol. **45**, 340—343 (1973)

Richet, G., Mignon, F., Ardaillou, R.: Goutte secondaire de nephropathies chroniques, Presse Méd. **73**, 633—638 (1965)

Rieselbach, R. E., Bentzel, C. J., Cotlove, E., Erei, E. III., Freireich, E. J.: Uric acid excretion and renal function in the acute hyperuricemia of leukemia Pathogenesis and therapy of uric acid nephropathy. Amer. J. Med. **37**, 872—884 (1964)

Rundles, R. W., Wyngaarden, J. B., Hitchings, G., Elion, G. B., Silberman, H. R.: Effects of xanthine oxidase inhibitor on thiopurine metabolism, hyperuricemia and gout. Trans. Ass. Amer. Physcns **76**, 126—140 (1963)

Sallinen, H.: Some aspects of urolithiasis in Finland. Acta Chir. Scand. **118**, 479—487 (1959)

Sandberg, A. A., Cartwright, G. E., Wintrobe, M. M.: Studies of leukemia: I uric acid excretion. Blood **11**, 154—166 (1956)

Sarre, H., Mertz, D. P.: Sekundäre Gicht bei Niereninsuffizienz. Klin. Wschr. **43**, 1134—1140 (1965)

Seze, S. de, Ryckewaert, A.: La Goutte. Paris: Expansion Scientifique Francaise 1960

Shattock, S. G.: A prehistoric or predynastic Egyptian calculus. Trans. Path. Soc. (Lond.) **56**, 275—291 (1905)

Sigerist, H. E.: A History of Medicine. New York: Oxford Univ. Pr. 1951

Simons, F., Feldman, B., Gerety, D.: Granulomatous hepatitis in a patient receiving allopurinol. Gastroenterology **62**, 101—104 (1972)

Smith, M. J., Hunt, L. D., King Jr., J. S., Boyce, W. H.: Uricemia and urolithiasis. J. Urol. **101**, 637—642 (1969)

Sorensen, L. B.: Role of the intestinal tract in the elemination of uric acid. Arthr. and Rheum. **8**, 694—706 (1965)

Sperling, O., Persky-Brosh, S., Boer, P., Vries, A. de: Uric acid lithiasis associated with excessive purine production due to mutant PRPP synthetase. In: Urinary Calculi. Int. Symp. Renal Stone Res., Madrid, 1972, pp. 96—104

Sperling, O., Vries, A. de, Kedem, O.: Studies on the etiology of uric acid lithiasis. IV. Urinary non-dialyzable substances in idiopathic uric acid lithiasis. J. Urol. **94**, 286—292 (1965)

Stratigos, J. D., Bartsokas, S. K., Capetanakis, J.: Further experiences of toxic epidermal necrolysis incriminating allopurinol pyrazolone and derivatives. Brit. J. Derm. **86**, 564—567 (1972)

Sutor, D. J.: Growth studies of calcium oxalate in presence of various ions and compounds. Brit. J. Urol. **41**, 171—178 (1969)

Sutor, D. J.: In: Finlayson, B., Hench, L., Smith, L. H. (Eds.): The Nature of Urinary Stones in Urolithiasis; Physical Aspects, pp. 43—46. Washington, D.C.: Nat. Acad. Sci. 1972

Sutor, D. J., Wooley, S. E., Illingsworth, J. J.: Some aspects of the adult urinary stone problem in Great Britain and Northern Ireland. Br. J. Urol. **46**, 275—288 (1974)

Talbott, J. H.: Gout and blood dyscrasias. Medicine **38**, 173—205 (1959)

Talbott, J. H., Yü, T. F.: Gout and Uric Acid Metabolism. New York: Stratton Inter. med. Book Co. 1976

Thomson, J. O.: Urinary calculus at the Canton Hospital, Canton, China. Surg. Gynec. Obstet. **32**, 44—55 (1921)

Vergis, J. G., Walker, B. R.: Cystinuria, hyperuricemia and uric acid nephrolithiasis. Nephron **7**, 577—579 (1970)

Vermeulen, C. W., Fried, F. A.: Observations on dissolution of uric acid calculi. J. Urol. **94**, 293—296 (1965)

Vermeulen, C. W., Lyon, E. S.: Mechanisms of genesis and growth of calculi. Amer. J. Med. **45**, 684—692 (1968)

Vesell, E. S., Passananti, G. T., Greene, F. E.: Impairment of drug metabolism in man by allopurinol and nortriptyline. New Engl. J. Med. **283**, 1484—1488 (1970)

Vries, A. de, Frank, M., Atsmon, A.: Inherited uric acid lithiasis. Amer. J. Med. **33**, 880—892 (1962)

Wardlaw, H. S. H.: Observation on the incidence and composition of urinary calculi. Med. J. Aust. **1**, 180—186 (1952)

Wasserman, L. R.: Polycythemia vera study group, sponsored by National Cancer Institute, USPHS. Personal communication, 1975

Weiss, T. E., Segaloff, A.: Gouty Arthritis and Gout. Springfield (Ill.): Charles C. Thomas 1959

Wesson, M. B.: Renal calculi; etiology and prophylaxis. J. Urol. **34**, 289—295 (1935)

Williams, G. D.: An ancient bladder stone. J. Amer. med. Ass. **87**, 941 (1926)

Wilmore, D. W., Gots, R. E.: The etiology of uric acid urolithiasis following ileostomy. Arch. Surg. **99**, 421—423 (1969)

Woeber, K. A., Ricca, L., Hills, A. G.: Pathogenesis of uric acid urolithiasis. Clin. Res. **10**, 45 (1962)

Yendt, E. R.: Renal calculi. Canad. MA J. **102**, 479—489 (1970)

Yü, T. F.: Secondary gout associated with myeloproliferative diseases. Arthr. and Rheum. **8**, 765—771 (1965)

Yü, T. F.: Milestones in the treatment of gout. Am. J. Med. **56**, 676—685 (1974)

Yü, T. F.: Some unusual features of gout in females. Semin. Arthritis Rheum. **6**, 247—255 (1977)

Yü, T. F., Balis, M. E., Krenitsky, T. A., Dancis, J., Silvers, D. N., Elion, G. B., Gutman, A. B.: Rarity of X-linked partial hypoxanthine guanine phosphoribosyltransferase deficiency in a large gouty population. Ann. Intern. Med. **76**, 255—264 (1972)

Yü, T. F., Balis, M. E., Yip, L.: Overproduction of uric acid in primary gout. Arthr. and Rheum. [Suppl.] **18**, 695—698 (1975)

Yü, T. F., Berger, L.: Renal disease in primary gout; a study of 253 gouty patients with proteinuria. Semin. Arthritis Rheum. **4**, 293—305 (1975)

Yü, T. F., Gutman, A. B.: Effect of allopurinol (4-hydroxypyrazolo(3,4-d)-pyrimidine) on serum and urinary uric acid in primary and secondary gout. Amer. J. Med. **37**, 885—898 (1964)

Yü, T. F., Gutman, A. B.: Uric acid nephrolithiasis in gout predisposing factors. Ann. intern. Med. **67**, 1133—1148 (1967)

Yü, T. F., Wasserman, L. R., Benedict, J. D., Bien, E. J., Gutman, A. B., Stetten, W., de: A simultaneous study of glycine-^{15}N incorporation into uric acid and heme and of ^{59}Fe utilization, in a case of gout associated with polycythemia secondary to congenital heart disease. Amer. J. Med. **15**, 845—856 (1953)

Yü, T. F., Weinreb, N., Wittman, R., Wasserman, L. R.: Secondary gout associated with chronic myeloproliferative disorders. Semin. Arthritis Rheum. **5**, 247—256 (1976)

Yü, T. F., Weissmann, B., Sharney, L., Kupfer, S., Gutman, A. B.: On the biosynthesis of uric acid from glycine-^{15}N in primary and secondary polycythemia. Amer. J. Med. **21**, 901—917 (1956)

CHAPTER 18

Association of Calcium Nephrolithiasis with Disorders of Uric Acid Metabolism

F. L. COE

A. Introduction

The observation that calcium stones of renal origin may be associated with uric acid disorders has been made on many occasions. PRIEN and PRIEN (1968) noted that patients with gout, who also suffered from stones, frequently passed stones which contained, or were composed of, calcium oxalate. GUTMAN (1968) also mentioned the surprisingly high frequency of calcium oxalate stones in gout patients and called attention to crystallographic studies of LONSDALE (1968a, b) showing a significant enough structural correspondence between crystals of uric acid, sodium hydrogen urate, and calcium oxalate to allow one to grow upon the surface of another or to act for one another as heterogeneous seed nuclei. DENT and SUTOR (1971), in a study examining inhibitors of calcium oxalate crystal growth in urine from normal people and patients with recurrent calcium oxalate renal stones, found that stone formers were more often hyperuricemic than normals, even though none of the patients had clinical gout. SMITH and his colleagues (1969) have made similar observations and have suggested that calcium stone formers with uric acid disorders represent a significant metabolic subgroup of calcium stone disease.

Our own observation, that hyperuricosuria was very frequent among patients with calcium oxalate nephrolithiasis (COE and RAÎSEN, 1973; COE and KAVALICH, 1974) was consonant with what had come before and provided evidence for an abnormality of urine chemistry that could link uric acid disorders to the formation of calcium stones in the kidney or upper urinary tract. Subsequent research has centered mainly on the hyperuricosuric calcium oxalate stone former, probably because patients with gout or asymptomatic hyperuricemia but without hyperuricosuria lack an apparent, decisive urine chemistry abnormality and offer less immediate research opportunities. Study of such patients has provided four kinds of evidence, in addition to statistical association, linking hyperuricosuria to calcium stone formation and setting hyperuricosuric patients apart from other calcium stone formers. These include an atypical natural history of stone disease, in vitro evidence for heterogeneous nucleation of calcium oxalate crystallization by seed crystal of sodium hydrogen urate or uric acid, a reduction by urate or uric acid of the inhibiting effect that urine normally has upon the growth of calcium oxalate crystals, and an apparently dramatic effect of allopurinol to reduce new stone formations. Taken altogether, the weight of evidence supports the existence of a distinct syndrome of hyperuricosuric calcium oxalate nephrolithiasis.

B. Frequency of Hyperuricosuria in Calcium Stone Formers

Before describing later and more specific research, it seems worthwhile to review the basic statistical association that, in large measure, initiated subsequent investigation. A recent survey of 460 calcium oxalate stone formers illustrates the very large fraction of patients who excreted above 800 mg (men) or 750 mg (women) of uric acid in at least one of two 24 h urine samples collected for the purpose of making such measurements (Table 1). Of the 121 hyperuricosuric patients, 40 men (39%) and four women (22%) were hyperuricemic by usual definition. Normal men and women, who had no history of stone disease, excreted such large amounts of uric acid only infrequently (Table 2). If higher limits are used, stone formers depart more drastically from normals, who rarely contributed values above 900 mg/24 h (men) or 800 mg/24 h (women).

There is a natural difficulty in defining upper limits of normal for uric acid excretion, because there is no obvious bimodality to the distribution of excretion rates among stone patients or normal people, but only a tendency—quite marked— for higher values to occur in patients (Table 2). GUTMAN (1968), facing the same problem, suggested limits of 800 and 750 mg for men and women, respectively, which we have also used to define hyperuricosuria. A point 2 standard deviations above the mean values of uric acid excretion by our normals of each sex could replace these arbitrary limits, because only 5% of the normal points depart so widely from the mean. But such limits might not offer a diagnostically useful advance. The extent of urine saturation with uric acid, sodium hydrogen urate, or both, determined mainly by the urine concentrations of the substances, not the amount excreted daily, is the property that can influence crystallization in the urine. The normal range should be defined in terms of concentration, something that has not yet been accomplished. In

Table 1. Metabolic and clinical disorders in 460 consecutive calcium stone formers

	Number of patients	%
Idiopathic hypercalciuria	95	20.7
Marginal hypercalciuria[a]	53	11.5
Hyperuricosuria	67	14.6
Hypercalciuria and hyperuricosuria[b]	54	11.7
Hyperuricemia alone	26	5.7
Primary hyperparathyroidism	24	5.2
Renal tubular acidosis[c]	17	3.7
Inflammatory bowel disease[d]	21	4.6
Medullary sponge kidney	7	1.5
Sarcoidosis	3	0.7
No disorder found	93	20.2
Total	460	

[a] Urine calcium and 140 mg/gm creatinine.
[b] Marginal hypercalciuria not included.
[c] Distal, hereditary form.
[d] Regional enteritis, ulcerative colitis, granulomatous ileocolitis.

Table 2. Frequency of various uric acid excretion rates among calcium oxalates stone formers (P) and normal subjects (N)

Urine uric acid (mg/24 h)	Men[a]		Women	
	N (128)	P (1046)	N (77)	P (302)
< 200	0	0	0	0
200– 400	2	1	36	25
400– 600	38	17	54	53
600– 800	48	50	9	8
800– 900	6	14	0	6
900–1000	4	11	—	5
> 1000	2	7	—	3

[a] Numbers are the percentage of 24-h urine samples containing the amounts of urate indicated. Total number of urine samples in each group is shown in parentheses.

the meantime, given the indirect relationship that exists between excretion rate and concentration, the lower limits of GUTMAN may be just as useful in predicting oversaturation as higher limits and have also proven reasonably effective in selecting patients for treatment.

C. Mechanisms of Hyperuricosuria

Excessive dietary purine intake is a natural mechanism to explain so widespread a tendency to large uric acid excretion rates. The other likely basis, perhaps acting in concert, is uric acid overproduction from endogenous purine metabolism. A tubule defect of urate reabsorption is an unattractive hypothesis in view of the absence of hypouricemia. The issue is unsettled, but purine overingestion and urate overproduction both seem to occur and contribute to hyperuricosuria.

I. Role of Diet

The first essential question, whether hyperuricosuric stone formers habitually consume more purine than normal people, has been approached by estimating purine and calorie intake by 10 men who were normouricemic, hyperuricosuric calcium oxalate stone formers age and weight and 5 matched normals drawn from a comparable social and economic class. For 18 days, each person kept a detailed diary of all foods consumed. With standard listings of purine and calorie contents of foods and beverages, a nutritionist computed daily intakes of both (BRIDGES and MATTICE, 1942). The final conclusion, summarized in Table 3, was that patients invested a higher proportion of their dietary intake in purine rich foods (KAVALICH et al., 1976). By chance, the average caloric intakes of patients and controls were virtually identical, a fact that greatly simplifies comparison of their purine intakes. The specific diet abnormality in patients was preferential consumption of meat, fish, and poultry at the expense of breads, grains, and starches (Fig. 1). This dietary pattern may well

Table 3. Purine and caloric intake by patients and normal subjects

	Purine intake (mg/24 h)	Caloric intake (cal/24 h)
Patients (10)	259 ± 29 [a]	2109 ± 161
Normal men (5)	155 ± 21	2104 ± 147

[a] $F = 9.16$ $p < 0.01$, for patients vs. normal men.
Values are means ± 1 SEM.

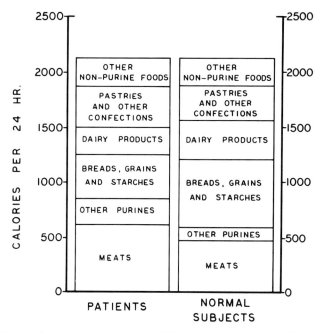

Fig. 1. Diets of hyperuricosuric and normal men. Dietary calories consumed in the form of meat, fish, and poultry were greater in hyperuricosuric men, almost entirely at the expense of reduced bread, grains, and starches

reflect a not uncommon tendency of men to eat their meat and leave bread and potatoes aside; it is uncertain whether such a diet pattern is actually wide spread, even among the majority of hyperuricosuric calcium oxalate stone formers, since our sample was very small.

A useful byproduct of the study is the regression line relating uric acid excretion to dietary purine intake in normal men (Fig. 2). The intercept of the equation—5.53 mg/kg/24 h, the predicted daily excretion of uric acid given no exogenous purine—corresponds well with the actual average value for uric acid excretion measured for these normal men after 7 days of a purine-free diet—5.6 mg/kg/24 h (Kavalich et al., 1976). This correspondence supports the validity of the diet diary method for estimating purine intake.

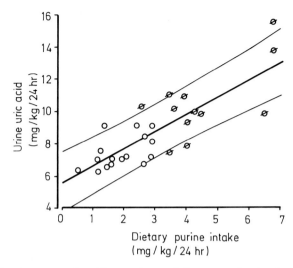

Fig. 2. Correlation between uric acid excretion and dietary purine intake in normal subjects. Values obtained on ambient diet (O) and during deliberate increase in meat intake (⊖). The linear regression relating excretion (Y) to intake (×) has slope 1.07 and intercept 5.53 mg/kg/24 h (KAVALICH et al., 1976)

II. Role of Over-Production

In addition to consuming excessive purine, some of the 10 patients we studied appeared to overproduce uric acid. The 95% confidence band relating normal urine uric acid excretion to dietary purine intake, derived from the regression shown in Figure 2, is shown as a cross-hatched area in Figure 3. Of the 10 patients we studied, three excreted more uric acid than would normal subjects eating the same amount of purine. After 7 days of a purine-free diet, these three patients continued to excrete more uric acid than normal subjects usually do and certainly more than the five normal subjects we studied, shown by open circles. Presumably, the surplus uric acid they excreted on their own high-purine diet or a purine-free diet reflected over-production of uric acid during the course of endogenous purine metabolism.

III. Possible Renal Tubular Disturbance

All 10 patients we studied were normouricemic, in common with a majority of hyperuricosuric calcium oxalate stone formers. But the absence of hyperuricemia is itself surprising. Excess dietary purine tends to increase serum urate levels in normal people to abnormal or nearly abnormal levels (STEELE and RIESELBACH, 1967), so one would expect hyperuricemia to be more the rule than the exception. Figure 4 compares serum urate levels to urine uric acid excretion for our 10 patients; the 95% confidence interval derived from the five normal people is cross-hatched. The normal subjects had each deliberately increased their purine intake for 3 days so that hyperuricosuria would be present on some occasions, allowing construction of the confidence band. Serum urate levels in normals exceeded those in patients. After

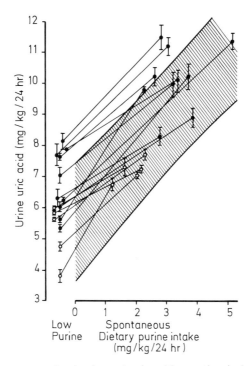

Fig. 3. Relationship between purine intake and uric acid excretion in hyperuricosuric patients compared to normals. The 95% confidence band for the normal regression is cross-hatched. Data from three of the ten patients (*closed circles*) exceeded the upper limit of the band, indicating an abnormal rate of uric acid excretion for the corresponding purine intake. After 7 days of a purine-free diet, these three patients continued to excrete an abnormal amount of uric acid compared to the five normal subjects (*open circles*). All values are means (± 1 SEM) of three separate determinations (Coe and Kavalich, 1974)

7 days of a purine free diet, serum and urine urate values were within the normal range (open circles).

The abnormal relationship between serum urate concentration and urine urate excretion rate in the patients could reflect an inherent tubule disturbance, such as enhanced secretion or reduced post secretory reabsorption. It could also reflect an alteration acquired because of the chronicity of purine loading; our normal subjects were loaded for only a few days. So far, no studies of chronic purine loading in normals that have extended over many months have documented whether or not a gradual fall in serum urate level occurs. Such a study would be profitable, as renal adaptation might occur.

D. Natural History of Stone Disease

Idiopathic hypercalciuria of marginal or severe degree occurred alone in 32.2% of calcium stone formers and in association with hyperuricosuria in 11.7%. Another 20.2% of patients had no discernable metabolic defect, and 14.6% had only hyper-

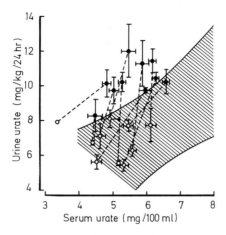

Fig. 4. Relationship between serum urate level and urine uric acid excretion in patients and normal subjects. The 95% confidence band derived from five subjects is cross-hatched. In order to obtain hyperuricosuric data from the normals, each was briefly purine loaded by increased meat intake for 5 days, and three 24-h urine collections were obtained—on days 3, 4, and 5 of loading. On their own diets, patients had lower serum urate levels for their degree of hyperuricosuria than did the normals (*closed circles*). After 7 days of a purine-free diet (*open circles*), their values were in the normal zone. Each point is the mean (± 1 SEM) of three determinations

uricosuria (Table 1). Because of their numbers, it is possible to draw reasonably clear conclusions about the natural history of stones in patients within these metabolic subgroups. All of the remaining diseases that cause calcium stones, including primary hyperparathyroidism, renal tubular acidosis, hyperoxaluric states, and other rarer entities, are represented by too few patients for reliable measurement of stone formation rates.

Hyperuricosuric patients formed the majority of their stones at a later average age than other types of patients (Fig. 5). This was not simply due to a later age of stone onset (Table 4) but mainly to a more prolonged course of disease. The severity of stone disease was also greater for hyperuricosuric patients (Table 4); stone formation rates were higher, and rates of cystoscopy and surgical procedures were also higher, partly because of the greater number of stones formed and partly because of a higher rate of complications for each 100 stones formed. The lateness and the severity of their stone disease support the notion that hyperuricosuric calcium oxalate stone formers constitute a separate metabolic subclass of renal stone disease. They also suggest that treatment may be a more urgent matter in hyperuricosuric than in other calcium oxalate stone formers, because their disease is likely to be more severe and more protracted.

E. Urate-Oxalate Epitaxis

Epitaxis is the oriented overgrowth of crystalline material upon the surface of another crystal of different chemical composition but similar structure (LONSDALE,

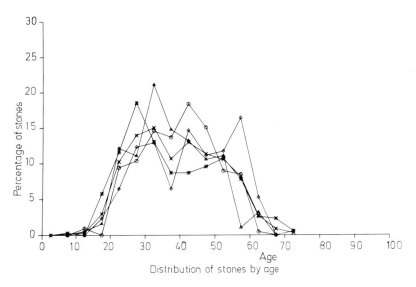

Fig. 5. Occurrence of calcium stones at various ages. Each point shows the fraction of all stones formed by the population of patients in each metabolic subgroup in each 5-year age interval. Symbols: ○, hyperuricosuria; ×, hyperuricosuria and hypercalciuria; △, hypercalciuria; ◇ marginal hypercalciuria; × ×, no metabolic defect. Average age at stone onset shown in Table 4 for each subgroup. Peak stone occurrance in hyperuricosuric patients occurred in the interval of 40–45 years; the other groups had peak ages of 25–30, no defect; 30–35, hypercalciuria and admixed hypercalciuria and hyperuricosuria; marginally hypercalciuric patients had three peaks of stone formation, at 30–55, 40–45, and 55–60

Table 4. Characteristics of stone disease in patients with hyperuricosuria, hypercalciuria, or no discernable disorder

	HU[a]	HU+IH	IH	MIH	Neither
Number of patients	51	43	81	45	64
Percent men	81	90.5	71.5	67.6	69.5
Mean age at stone onset (year)	35.6	33	33.3	35.2	36.3
Stones/pt	4.17	4.6	4.8	4.24	3.59
Stones/100 pt/year	64.9	53.1	41	37.7	42.8
Hospitalizations/100 stones	33.8	16.1	17.1	27.7	21.7
Cystoscopies/100 stones	20.5	19.8	9.8	11.7	16.5
Surgical procedures/100 stones	16.8	14.1	13.4	17.3	13.4

[a] Abbreviations: HU, hyperuricosuria; IH, idiopathic hypercalciuria; MIH, marginal hypercalciuria.

1968 a, b). The importance of epitaxis is related to the process of nucleation, the initiating event in the creation of a solid phase in an oversaturated solution. As the concentrations of materials like calcium and oxalate rise in solution, seed nuclei of calcium oxalate will tend to form. Their formation is favored by the magnitude of the free ion activity product (UHLMAN, 1972), their dissolution by the natural tendency

Table 5. Geometrical correspondences between naturally occuring faces of uric acid and calcium oxalate crystals

	Face	Dimensions (Å)
Uric acid	100	6.21×7.40
Uric acid $\cdot 2H_2O$	100	6.35×7.40
$CaO_x \cdot H_2O$ [a]	001	6.28×14.57
$CaO_x \cdot H_2O$ [b]	101	12.30×14.32

[a] Whewellite, calcium oxalate monohydrate.
[b] Weddellite, calcium oxalate dihydrate.

of molecules to break away from crystal nuclei and reenter the solution. Above an activity product that is characteristic for each salt, called the formation product, nuclei will form, reach a size large enough to be stable, and then grow, a phenomenon called homogenous nucleation. The activity product in a solution in equilibrium with a mass of solid phase that is neither growing nor decreasing in size is called the thermodynamic equilibrium product or solubility product. In simple salt solutions, the formation product for calcium oxalate is approximately 8.5 times above the equilibrium product (PAK and HOLT, 1976). The zone between solubility and formation products is called the metastable zone.

If preformed nuclei are added to a metastable solution, nucleation is bypassed; all that is necessary to increase the mass of the solid phase is growth of the preformed nuclei, which can occur at any activity product within the metastable range. In other words, heterogeneous seed nuclei can facilitate the formation of a solid phase of calcium oxalate from a metastable urine by obviating the thermodynamically costly process of homogenous nucleation, provided the heterogeneous nuclei possess sufficient structural similarities to calcium oxalate to permit epitaxial growth. Crystallographic evidence and heterogeneous seeding experiments both suggest that sodium hydrogen urate uric acid and calcium oxalate crystals share sufficient structural similarities to allow epitaxis.

I. Crystallographic Evidence

LONSDALE (1968a, b) has summarized the most critical data concerning structural similarities between uric acid and calcium oxalate crystals. Anhydrous uric acid crystals, commonly found as a constituent of human stones (LONSDALE, 1968b), have network dimensions for their 100-face that are very close to those of the 001-face of calcium oxalate monohydrate or the single face, 101, of calcium oxalate dihydrate crystals (Table 5). For epitaxy to occur, the dimensions must match within a few percent either directly or as integral multiples of one another. The percentage misfits for the corresponding dimensions of the 001-face of whewellite and the 100-face of uric acid dihydrate, for example, are 1.1% and 1.6%, if one divides the 14.57 Å dimension of whewellite by two to obtain the closest integral result, 7.285. Both forms of uric acid and of calcium oxalate are well-enough matched to allow epitaxis

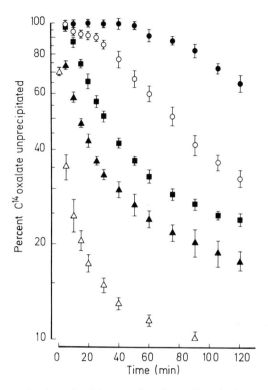

Fig. 6. Heterogenous nucleation of calcium oxalate by sodium hydrogen urate seed crystals. A saturated solution containing calcium 5 mM and ^{14}C-labeled sodium oxalate 200 μM, pH 5.7, 5 mM barbitol-acetate buffer, KCl 150 mM, was shaken at 24° C. At intervals, aliquots were filtered through 5 μ pore diameter filters and the radioactivity of the filtrate determined. In the absence of seed crystal (●), precipitation began after 40 min. 0.1 mM of sodium acid urate crystals (○) greatly accelerated precipitation; 2.5 mM (■) was more effective. Equivalent amounts of calcium oxalate monohydrate seed crystals (▲ and △) were far more effective, especially during the first few minutes. All points are means (±1 SEM) of three determinations. (From COE et al., 1975)

in any order among them. Sodium hydrogen urate is not listed in the table, because its unit cell dimensions are not yet determined.

II. Heterogeneous Nucleation

Direct evidence for nucleation of calcium oxalate solutions by uric acid and its salt has been presented by (PAK (PAK and ARNOLD, 1975) and ourselves (COE et al., 1975). In our experiment, a metastable calcium oxalate solution, buffered at pH 5.7 in 5 mM acetate barbital, was labeled with ^{14}C-oxalate. Incubated with shaking, the solution lost none of its labeled oxalate to the solid phase over a 30-min period (Fig. 6), as judged by determining the ^{14}C-radioactivity level of aliquots passed through a 5-μ-pore-diameter millipore filter, which would retain crystal nuclei. Addition of even small amounts of preformed sodium hydrogen urate crystals caused a rapid loss of

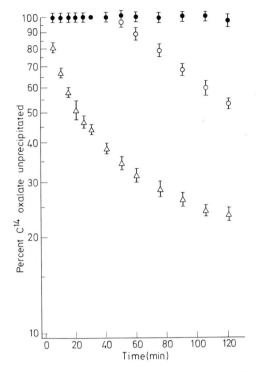

Fig. 7. Nucleation of calcium oxalate by seed crystals of uric acid. The system described in Figure 6 was altered to pH 4.4. Unseeded (●), no precipitation of oxalate occurred during 2 h. 2.5 mM of uric acid crystals (○) promoted precipitation but less than did the same amount of calcium oxalate monohydrate crystals (△). All values are means (±1 SEM) of three experiments

counts, reflecting the accretion of oxalate to the solid phase. Crystal growth, not adsorption of radio-labeled oxalate to a urate surface, was occuring as shown by the absence of a fall in radioactivity when calcium was omitted and, in separate experiments, by simultaneous equimolar loss of oxalate and calcium from the filtrate.

Uric acid seed crystals were also able to initiate calcium oxalate crystal growth, although a lag phase was present (Fig. 7) and initial growth appeared to be slower. With time, crystal growth rose toward the level seen with sodium hydrogen urate. These experiments were performed at pH 4.4 rather than at pH 5.7, to prevent conversion of uric acid to urate. Unseeded, the system remained stable for a longer period than at the higher pH values used for the urate experiments, and growth of added preformed calcium oxalate crystals was also slower. The difference in growth rates with both seed crystals makes it difficult to compare the effects of urate uric acid directly.

To facilitate comparison, the rate of oxalate precipitation onto urate or uric acid seed nuclei was compared at each time interval to the rate of oxalate precipitation onto preformed calcium oxalate seed nuclei incubated under the same conditions. This calculation expresses the relative empirical efficiency of either heterogeneous

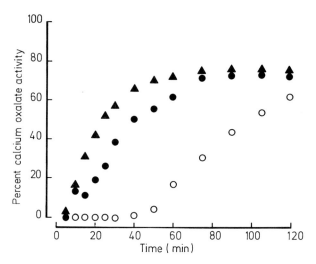

Fig. 8. Comparison of urate and uric acid seed nuclei to seeds of calcium oxalate. The increment of oxalate precipitated in each of the time intervals shown in Figure 6 with urate seeds of 0.1 mM (○) and 2.5 mM △ is shown divided by the increment of oxalate precipitated in the same period with an equivalent solid-to-liquid ratio of calcium oxalate monohydrate seed crystals. Effects of uric acid and calcium oxalate seeds, 2.5 mM each (○), shown in Figure 7, are also compared. The effectiveness of either heterogenous nucleus rises towards that of calcium oxalate with time

nucleus to calcium oxalate monohydrate itself. At early time periods, urate seed crystals were very inefficient compared to calcium oxalate seed crystals (Fig. 8), but with time the differences decreased. This may reflect the gradual coating of urate seed nuclei with calcium oxalate crystals, which by their growth then accelerated the transfer of oxalate from the solution to the solid phase. The response was similar for low and high solid-to-liquid ratios of seed crystals, provided that comparable concentrations of urate and calcium oxalate crystals were compared. Uric acid crystals, because of their lag phase, were inert for the first 30 min (Fig. 8). Thereafter, they became more efficient heterogeneous nuclei, gradually rising to equal urate in effect. Presumably, the lag phase reflects the relatively slow growth of calcium oxalate crystals on the surface of the uric acid seeds, whereas the later onset of detectable oxalate precipitation reflects growth of the calcium oxalate surface. Inspection of Figure 6 reveals that a lag phase was also present when sodium acid urate seed crystals were used. Even at a very high concentration, urate nuclei did not produce appreciable oxalate precipitation at 5 min, whereas large amounts of oxalate were deposited in 5 min on preformed calcium oxalate nuclei.

The role of heterogeneous nucleation in vivo is uncertain. Sodium hydrogen urate crystals are not seen in fresh warm human urine, raising a natural barrier to the direct extension of the present in vitro studies to human stone disease. Furthermore, ROBERTSON et al. (1976) have shown that urine from stone formers and normal subjects often appears to be undersaturated or metastable with respect to urate or uric acid, and that in the few cases where uric acid levels were above the formation, product calcium oxalate activity products were high enough that crystallization could have occured without a need for heterogenous nucleation. Furthermore, by their calculations, urine would remain below the urate formation product even if 2000 mg urate were excreted at pH 6.3 in 1 liter of urine.

PAK, on the other hand (PAK, 1977), has provided evidence that urine is more saturated with respect to urate and uric acid, enough so that spontaneous crystallization of either one would be common, especially in hyperuricosuric patients. His methods differ from those of ROBERTSON. Whereas ROBERTSON computes the activity product of sodium hydrogen urate from the properties of a given urine and compares it to solubility and formation products observed in equivalent salt solutions, PAK seeds urine with preformed nuclei of urate or uric acid, observes to what extent the concentrations of uric acid or the product of urate and sodium concentrations decline, and compares the extent of oversaturation thus measured to the corresponding formation product rates in that urine sample. Given this difference of methodology and conclusions, the role of calcium oxalate heterogeneous nucleation by urate or uric acid in urine is unsettled.

In addition, the urine is itself an uncertain locale for stone development. Nascent nuclei will tend to wash away within a few minutes, as their dimensions, even when unusually large, are less than 1 mm, compared to urinary structures many millimeters in diameter. If mere growth and aggregation of newly formed nuclei caused stones to form in the urine, the bladder would be the site of most stones, whereas it is in the kidneys themselves, in the calyces, and on the renal papillae that most calcium stones are formed. In order to develop there, stones must grow on anchored nuclei. Nuclei could lodge in the niches of calyces or infundibula; an even more attractive site is upon the open ends of collecting ducts plugged with crystals, which form a permanent surface of anchored seed nuclei. The dimensions of terminal collecting ducts, about 200–300 μ in diameter, could permit plugging by masses of calcium oxalate crystals, which are commonly above 12 μ in diameter in stone-forming urine (ROBERTSON, 1976) or by uric acid crystals, which can occlude even the ureter under extreme conditions and certainly do occlude renal collecting ducts in some hyperuricosuric patients (EMERSON and GRAHAM-ROW, 1975).

Much remains uncertain. Obstructing intraluminal deposites of uric acid are well known (EMERSON and GRAHAM-ROW, 1975), but urate crystals are usually found in the renal interstitium, not plugging renal tubules. It may be that detailed study of renal tissue from stone formers will reveal intratubular or calyceal masses of urate that have been hitherto overlooked, or that future studies of filtered urine sediments will reveal that sodium urate crystalluria is not rare. Alternatively, it may be that uric acid itself, which surely does plug tubules and may produce copious crystalluria, is an important source of heterogeneous nuclei that compensate for their inefficiency by being widely distributed.

The potential importance of heterogeneous nuclei for calcium oxalate is much greater in urine than it would be in simple salt solution, because urine contains potent inhibitors of nucleation and crystal growth that raise the formation product and slow the growth of calcium oxalate nuclei, retarding the development of an appreciable crystal mass (ROBERTSON et al., 1976). One of these inhibitors is inorganic pyrophosphate (FLEISCH and BISAZ, 1962); the other(s), one or more larger molecules (MEYER and SMITH, 1975), are of uncertain composition. These inhibitors do not affect uric acid or sodium hydrogen urate, which crystallize in urine at the same rate as in a similarly constructed salt solution.

F. Reduced Urine Inhibitors

ROBERTSON (1976) has recently presented evidence for the intriguing idea that sodium acid urate may promote calcium oxalate stone disease by interfering with naturally occuring urine inhibitors of calcium oxalate crystal growth, inhibitors that he believes may be acid mucopolysaccarides (amps) (ROBERTSON et al., 1976). His method for measuring inhibitors is to observe the effects of 1% urine on the rate at which seed crystals of calcium oxalate grow and aggregate in a metastable calcium oxalate solution. He observed that urines containing more urate have less inhibitory effect per milligram of amps than urines with lower urate concentrations, a rather indirect fact whose interpretation depends upon the unproven assumption that amps is the major inhibitor present and not merely one of many inhibitors. A more direct demonstration that he presented is that urate added to urine in vitro reduces, and removal of urate restores, inhibitory activity (ROBERTSON, 1976; ROBERTSON et al., 1976), but as yet this has not been documented in detail, only described in an overall review fashion.

The observations may be of extreme importance. If generally correct, they could explain the syndrome of hyperuricosuric calcium oxalate stones without a need to invoke massive urate or uric acid crystalluria, neither of which are especially common in the urine of calcium oxalate stone formers. The problem of anchored nuclei is also lessened as, uninhibited by the usual properties of urine, calcium oxalate crystal nuclei could readily grow and aggregate sufficiently to occlude collecting ducts in the renal papillae or lodge in calyces. Reduced inhibition could also explain the critical, and as yet unpublished observations, by PAK (PAK, 1976) that induction of hyperuricosuria in normal people leads to their producing a urine in which the formation product for calcium oxalate, usually very elevated in urine compared to simple salt solutions, presumably because of the inhibitors urine contains, is reduced towards levels seen in simple media. Heterogeneous nucleation could cause such a reduction of formation product, but so could a reduction of inhibitory activity. Finally, the impressive therapeutic effects of allopurinol would be simply explained.

G. Allopurinol Treatment

Perhaps the most dramatic evidence linking hyperuricosuria to calcium oxalate stones is the seeming ability of allopurinol to reduce new stone formation far below pretreatment rates. Thus far we have observed 48 patients with recurrent calcium stones who had hyperuricosuria as a sole detected metabolic disorder and were treated with allopurinol for at least 1 year. Before treatment, these patients formed 67.9 stones/100 pt/yr (Table 6) and would therefore be expected to form 124.8 stones during the 186 pt years of treatment, if the pretreatment stone production rate continued to apply. In fact, they formed only eight stones (Fig. 9), $X^2 = 109.3$, $p < 0.001$, indicating that stone production rate had altered greatly.

Table 6. Effects of allopurinol treatment in patients with hyperuricosuric calcium oxalate stones[a]

	HU[b]	IH+HU	Untreated patients
Number of patients	48	42	34
Pretreatment interval (pt. yr.)	298	357	292
Pretreatment stones	200	188	123
Stones/pt	4.17	4.48	3.62
Years/pt	6.21	8.5	8.6
Stones/100 pt/yr	67.1	52.7	42.2
Treatment interval (pt. yr.)	186	119	109
Years/pt	3.88	2.83	3.21
New stones formed	8	6	29
Predicted new stones	124.8	62.7	46.2
New stones/predicted (%)	6.4	9.6	62.8
X^2, pred. vs. obs.	109.3	51.3	6.4
P	< 0.001	< 0.001	< 0.05

[a] These patients are the subset of those shown in Tables 1 and 4 for whom detailed follow-up data were available.

[b] Abbreviations: HU, hyperuricosuria; IH, idiopathic hypercalciuria.

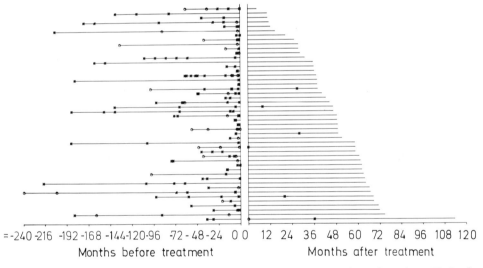

= -240 -216 -192 -168 -144-120-96 -72 - 48 -24   0 0   12 24   36 48 60   72   84 96 108 120

Months before treatment   Months after treatment

Fig. 9. The effect of allopurinol upon new stone production in hyperuricosuric patients. Each of 48 patients is indicated by a horizontal line. Single (×) and multiple (○) events are shown. New stone production was greatly reduced during treatment. The statistical details are shown in Table 6. Allopurinol was given 100 mg twice daily except in three subjects who required 300 mg/day to reduce hyperuricosuria

The interpretation of these results is not completely straightforward. Thus far, there has been no prospective control population with the same characterisics left untreated; factors other than allopurinol may have produced the fall in stone production. Some estimates of the likely effects of nonspecific factors, such as diet, better attention to fluid intake, avoidance of dehydration and continued contact with the

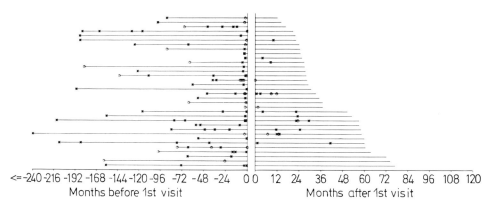

<=-240-216 -192 -168 -144 -120 -96 -72 -48 -24   0 0 12 24   36 48 60 72   84 96 108 120
Months before 1st visit   Months after 1st visit

Fig. 10. The course of calcium oxalate stone disease in untreated patients. Symbols as in Figure 9; statistics are shown in Table 6. Despite contact with the stone clinic and advice concerning diet and hydration, new stone production was reduced by only 37.2% compared to the nearly ten fold reduction observed in the allopurinol treated patients

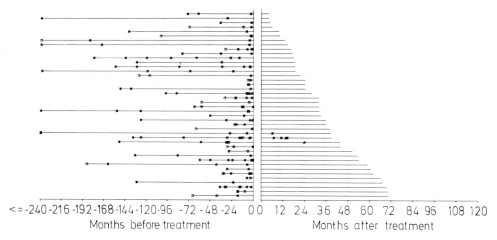

< =-240 -216 -192 -168 -144 -120 -96 -72 -48 -24   0 0 12 24 36 48 60 72 84 96   108 120
Months before treatment   Months after treatment

Fig. 11. Effects of combined allopurinol and thiazide treatment of patients with hyperuricosuria and hypercalciuria. Symbols as in Figures 9 and 10; statistics are in Table 6. Combined treatment lowered stone reccurrence dramatically. The thiazide used was trichlormethiazide, 2 mg twice daily; allopurinol was given 100 mg twice daily

stone clinic, can be derived from the response of a separate group of calcium stone formers, who had no detectable metabolic disorders and were, therefore, given no specific form of treatment.

This group of 34 patients had a less active form of stone disease before entering the program (Table 6), a fact mentioned previously. During the follow-up interval, new stone formation declined, so that only 62.8% of the stones that would have been predicted actually occurred (Fig. 10). These observations suggest that nonspecific factors related to our follow-up program probably do foster a moderate decline in stone formation. But even though these patients were relatively less active before

Table 7. Effects of allopurinol on new stone production by recurrent calcium oxalate stone formers with serum urate levels above 6 mg-% [a]

Year of follow-up	Allopurinol treated patients—new stones			Placebo-treated patients—new stones			X^{2} [c]	p
	Yes	No	All [b]	Yes	No	All		
0.5	21	28	49	30	13	43	6.57	<0.01
1	11	27	38	24	3	27	20.70	<0.001
2	10	20	30	19	1	20	16.84	<0.001
3	6	17	23	12	1	13	14.54	<0.001
4	4	15	19	11	1	12	14.73	<0.001
5	2	10	12	4	1	5	5.97	<0.02

[a] Adapted from (SMITH, 1977), Table 2. Numbers are patients who have or have not formed new stones at each follow-up interval.
[b] Includes patients remaining in the study; some were lost due to failure of treatment compliance, personal decisions to leave the study or drug intolerance. Patients entered the study at different times and therefore had varying lengths of total follow-up.
[c] Calculated X^{2} for placebo vs. allopurinol treated patients; p values are for 1° of freedom.

entering the program, compared to hyperuricosuric patients, they formed nearly 10 times more stones per 100 patients per year during the follow-up interval, suggesting that allopurinol treatment may well have contributed to stone prevention in hyperuricosuric patients.

Because it is a common disorder, hyperuricosuria was often found to coexist with idiopathic hypercalciuria in some individuals. Their coexistence was almost precisely what would be expected by change alone, given their independent rates of occurance. In this group of patients, the only treatment data available are based upon combined use of thiazide, an agent that has an established effect to lower urine calcium excretion (EDWARDS et al., 1973), and allopurinol. These combined treatment data, which show a marked fall in stone production (Table 6, Fig. 11), are mainly confirmatory; either agent alone may well have been sufficient, and only a failure of treatment, which would be unexpected, could have any major impact upon the hypothesis that hyperuricosuria may contribute to calcium stone production.

In addition to these prospective, uncontrolled treatment data derived from metabolically well-defined patients, there has been a controlled, randomized prospective study based upon the treatment with allopurinol of patients who formed calcium oxalate calculi and had serum urate levels above 6 mg/% with or without hyperuricosuria (SMITH, 1977). Apparently, hypercalciuric patients were excluded. The principle data from the study are summarized in Table 7. The number of stone-free, placebo-treated patients fell rapidly, from 13 at 6 months to one at 1 year; among the allopurinol treated patients, the fraction of stone free remained significantly more elevated throughout the study. The difference in occurrance of stone-free patients for each of the 5 years, tested by X^{2}, was significant at each interval. SMITH divided the patients who continued to form new stones into those improved, by which was meant a reduced rate of new stone production, and those unchanged. These two categories, which were distinguished on subjective grounds and on the basis of the number of stone events in single subjects, a small and highly variable index that is notoriously capricious for stone disease, are lumped together in Table 7 under the heading of new stones formed.

These treatment results are quantitatively different from our own but nevertheless lead to the same basic conclusion. In each year, 20–35% of Smith's treated patients formed new stones, whereas overall recurrence was below 10% in our 48 treated patients with hyperuricosuric calcium oxalate stones; still, the Smith data demonstrate an impressive allopurinol treatment effect. Quantitative differences in the magnitude of the effect could easily have arisen from the different patient populations studied. Our patients all were hyperuricosuric; some were hyperuricemic and some were not. In the Smith (1977) study, the selection criterion, serum urate level above 6 mg/%, could have included many patients whom we would have classified as idiopathic stone formers.

The problem of selection is far from trivial. Both proposed mechanisms of stone production, heterogeneous nucleation and reduction of inhibitor activity, depend upon abnormally elevated urine urate or uric acid concentrations. However, patients with normal urine urate levels could conceivably benefit from allopurinol by virtue of a reduction in the background effects, which even normal amounts of urate may produce. The magnitude of the therapeutic response in such patients would predictably be reduced to the extent that factors other than the effects of urate were responsible for stones. Given this mechanism for potential degradation of allopurinol effect, the significant fall in new stone production from allopurinol that Smith observed supports the notion that this drug, probably because of its effects upon urine urate level, is an efficient therapeutic agent in certain forms of calcium oxalate stone disease.

H. Conclusion

A variety of observations support the existence of a new, gradually evolving syndrome that may be called hyperuricosuric calcium oxalate nephrolithiasis. It consists of calcium oxalate stones, hyperuricosuria, and the absence of any of the well-defined causes of calcium oxalate stones, such as hypercalciuric states, primary hyperparathyroidism, hyperoxaluria from any cause, and medullary sponge kidney disease. It seems to affect mainly men and is caused by a combination of dietary purine excess and, in some cases, endogenous uric acid over-production. Stone disease is maximal during the fourth and fifth decades of life and is often of unusual severity. Allopurinol therapy appears to be an effective form of treatment, although this has not yet been established by a controlled, prospective study but only by prospective observation of treated patients. The mechanism linking hyperuricosuria to calcium oxalate stone production is not known. Heterogeneous nucleation of calcium oxalate by crystals of sodium hydrogen urate or uric acid, in the urine, calyceal niches, or at the open ends of plugged renal collecting ducts is one attractive hypothesis that is supported by some in vitro evidence. Attenuation of urine crystal growth inhibitors by an excess of urine urate, perhaps existing in the form of a gel, is another.

The true prevalence, clinical importance, and cohesiveness of the syndrome are all uncertain. Our data suggest a prevalence of about 20%–30%, either alone or associated with idiopathic hypercalciuria. Prevalence will generally reflect diet, so the affluent may well suffer more frequently from hyperuricosuria and its presumed consequences than will the poor. The syndrome may also vary in importance with time, depending upon cultural patterns of diet in this country and elsewhere. The clinical importance of the syndrome is supported mainly by the apparent success of allopurinol treatment. If this can be reproduced during a fully controlled study, confidence in the value of long-term treatment will be much increased. Dietary measures have never been evaluated as a treatment measure. They may be as effective as allopurinol and offer the obvious advantage of simplicity and avoidance of a drug.

References

Bridges, M. A., Mattice, M. R.: Food and Beverage Analyses. Philadelphia: Lea and Febiger 1942

Coe, F. L., Kavalich, A. G.: Hypercalciuria and hyperuricosuria in patients with calcium nephrolithiasis. New Engl. J. Med. **291**, 1344—1350 (1974)

Coe, F. L., Lawton, R. L., Goldstein, R. B., Tembe, V.: Sodium urate accelerates precipitation of calcium oxalate in vitro. Proc. Soc. exp. Biol. (N.Y.) **149**, 926—929 (1975)

Coe, F. L., Raisen, L.: Allopurinol treatment of uric-acid disorders in calcium-stone formers. Lancet **1973 I**, 129—131

Dent, E. D., Sutor, D. J.: Presence or absence of inhibitor of calciumoxalate crystal growth in urine of normals and of stone formers. Lancet **1971 I**, 776—778

Edwards, B. R., Baer, P. G., Sutton, R. A. L., Dirks, J. H.: Micropuncture study of diuretic effects on sodium and calcium reabsorption in the dog nephron. J. clin. Invest. **52**, 2418—2427 (1973)

Emerson, B. T., Graham-Row, P.: Pathogenesis of the gouty kidney. Kidney Int. **8**, 65—71 (1975)

Fleisch, H., Bisaz, S.: Isolation from urine of pyrophosphate, a calcification inhibitor. Amer. J. Physiol. **203**, 671—675 (1962)

Gutman, A. B.: Uric acid nephrolithiasis. Amer. J. Med. **45**, 756—779 (1968)

Gutman, A. B., Yü, T. F.: Renal function in gout, with a commentary on the renal regulation of urate excretion, and the role of the kidneys in the pathogenesis of gout. Amer. J. Med. **23**, 600—625 (1957)

Kavalich, A. G., Moran, E., Coe, F. L.: Dietary purine consumption by hyperuricosuric calcium oxalate kidney stone formers and normal subjects. J. chron. Dis. **29**, 745—760 (1976)

Lonsdale, K.: Human stones. Science **159**, 1159—1207 (1968 a)

Lonsdale, K.: Epitaxy as a growth factor in urinary calculi and gallstones. Nature (Lond.) **217**, 56—58 (1968 b)

Meyer, J. L., Smith, L. H.: Growth of calcium oxalate crystals. Inhibition by natural crystal growth inhibitors. Invest. Urol. **13**, 36—39 (1975)

Pak, C. Y. C.: Personal communication 1976

Pak, C. Y. C., Arnold, L. H.: Heterogeneous nucleation of calcium oxalate by seeds of monosodium urate. Proc. Soc. exp. Biol. (N.Y.) **149**, 930—932 (1975)

Pak, C. Y. C., Holt, K.: Nucleation and growth of brushite and calcium oxalate in urine of stone formers. Metabolism **25**, 665—673 (1976)

Pak, C. Y. C., Waters, O., Ornold, L., Holt, K., Cox, C., Barilla, D.: Mechanism for calcium urolithiasis among patients with hyperuricosuria: supersaturation of urine with respect to monosodium urate. J. clin. Invest. (1977) (in press)

Prien, E. L., Prien, E. L., Jr.: Composition and structure of urinary stone. Amer. J. Med. **45**, 654—672 (1968)

Robertson, W. G.: Physical chemical aspects of calcium stone formation in the urinary tract. In: Fleisch, H., Robertson, W. G., Smith, L. H., Vahlensieck, W. (Eds.): Urolithiasis Research, pp. 25—40. London: Plenum Press 1976

Robertson, W. G., Knowles, F., Peacock, M.: Urinary acid mucopolysaccharide inhibitors of calcium oxalate crystallization. In: Fleisch, H., Robertson, W. G., Smith, L. H., Vahlensieck, W. (Eds.): Urolithiasis Research, pp. 331—334. London: Plenum Press 1976

Robertson, W. G., Marshall, R. W., Peacock, M., Knowles, F.: The saturation of urine in recurrent, idiopathic calcium stone formers. In: Fleisch, H., Robertson, W. G., Smith, L. H., Vahlen-sieck, W. (Eds.): Urolithiasis Research, pp. 335—338. London: Plenum Press 1976

Smith, M. J. V.: Placebo vs. Allopurinol for renal calculi. J. Urol. (1977) (in press)

Smith, M. J. V., Hunt, L. D., King, J. S., Jr., Boyce, W. H.: Uricemia and urolithiasis. J. Urol. **101**, 637—642 (1969)

Steele, T. H., Rieselbach, R. E.: The renal mechanism for urate homeostasis in normal man. Amer. J. Med. **43**, 868—875 (1967)

Uhlman, D. R.: Crystal growth from solutions. Interface structure and interface kinetics. In: Finlayson, B. et al. (Ed.): Urolithiasis-Physical Aspects, pp. 169—176. Washington, D.C.: Nat. Acad. Sci. 1972

CHAPTER 19

Pathology of Urate Nephropathy

J. H. TALBOTT

A. Introduction

Although urate nephropathy frequently is assumed to be synonymous with gouty kidney, there are certain objections to either term in this context. In the former the onus is placed solely upon the uric acid moiety for the nephropathy. Proof is lacking that this is always the fact. An objection to the implications of gouty kidney is its restricted sense, since in this discussion selected features beyond the kidney in patients with gout will be included. Furthermore, urates may not be demonstrated in the parenchyma of the kidney of many patients with gout, and the functioning units of the kidney may show alterations or changes not usually attributed to reactions either initiated or augmented by uric acid deposition. The focus of this discussion, however, will concern the kidney in gout, but other aspects including selected features of the transport of uric acid through the kidney will be considered briefly.

The kidney is altered structurally or functionally in most patients whose natural history of primary gout extends over a period of years. The dysfunction may be minor or major when carefully investigated. Since hyperuricemia is the sine qua non of gouty arthritis and urate crystals can usually be demonstrated in synovia or synovial fluid of affected joints as early as the first articular attack, it is reasonable to believe, although by no means proven, that the hyperuricemia has been relatively long standing and any reaction by the kidney, usually occult and minimal, to hyperuricemia was probably present at that time.

On the other hand, the development of irreversible kidney dysfunction as the primary cause of death occurs in approximately 10% of patients with gout (TALBOTT and TERPLAN, 1960). The incidence has been found in smaller series to be as high as 25% (GUDZENT, 1928; MAYNE, 1955).

B. Gross Examination

Early in the clinical course of gouty arthritis in most patients the kidneys may be normal grossly whether under adequate or inadequate control of the articular distress by antigout drugs. This normal appearance may persist for years or throughout the natural history of the disease. In other patients, even though renal function tests may be essentially normal, section of the kidneys at postmortem examination may show urate deposits in the parenchyma. If multiple deposits are seen they tend to aggregate in the medullary portion or in the papillae (Fig. 1). Late in the course of the disease of those with well-developed or severe renal insufficiency, the kidneys may be small and symmetrically or asymmetrically atrophic and shrunken to a small per-

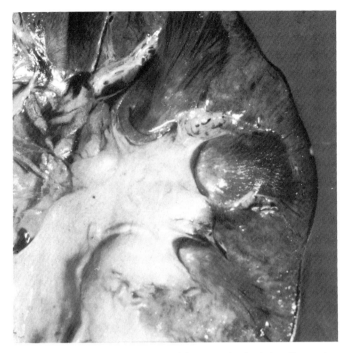

Fig. 1. Sagittal section of a kidney of a patient with gout who had the disease for more than 20 years. He died during his second myocardial infarction at the age of 76. The parenchyma looks very healthy except for small white urate deposits throughout the parenchyma

centage of their previous size (HEPTINSTALL, 1966) (Fig. 2). Further examination shows that the capsule may strip easily or it may be adherent. The exposed surface may show marked fibrotic scarring and, on section, marked reduction in volume of cortex as well as medulla, with loss of most normal parenchymal identity. Uric acid stones, large or small, sometimes are found in the calyces or pelvis if the kidney is contracted.

Congenital lesions of the kidney have been reported in patients with typical primary gouty arthritis (YÜ, 1975). Furthermore, if articular gout appears in the clinical course of the disease of patients with polycystic kidneys with well-developed renal insufficiency, it usually is late. On the other hand, chronic renal disease such as acquired chronic glomerulonephritis, even late in the course with advanced renal insufficiency, is not usually associated with clinical gouty arthritis (TALBOTT and YÜ, 1976). One explanation for this low incidence of gouty arthritis and chronic glomeru- lonephritis is the relatively short period of persistent hyperuricemia.

Be this as it may, a few patients with gout, less than 5% of any large series and usually those with chronic tophaceous deposits—severe in degree—will have ad- vanced degenerative changes of the kidney not clearly distinguishable from the late structural changes of chronic glomerulonephritis except for the possible presence of urate tophi (TALBOTT and TERPLAN, 1960). One example of this low association is the study by RICHET et al. (1975) of 166 uremic patients. They found only 17 examples of

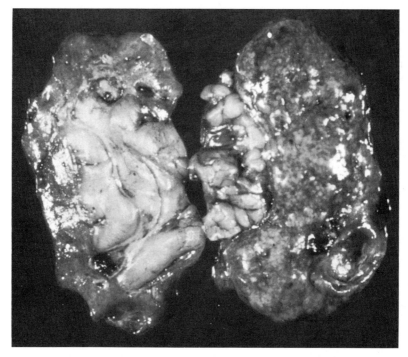

Fig. 2. Marked contraction of the kidney of a 52-year-old white male with a clinical history of gout and severe hypertension that extended over a decade. He died in renal failure. The other kidney was similarly contracted

overt gouty arthritis. Furthermore, it would be my suspicion that most of these patients were probably suffering initially from primary articular gout and hyperuricemia, followed by secondary renal disease than from articular gout secondary to chronic glomerulonephritis.

C. Acute Obstructive Uric Acid Nephropathy in Blood Dyscrasias and Neoplasms

In the natural history of some solid tumors and a number of blood diseases, an increased turnover of nucleoproteins may lead to a persistent hyperuricemia and, in some, acute attacks of gouty arthritis identified as secondary gout appear. Secondary gout accounts for approximately 10% of all patients with clinical gout in any large series (TALBOTT, 1959; YÜ et al., 1976).

Frequently, a more critical reversible phenomenon appears in patients with acute leukemia undergoing radiation or leukemic patients given cytotoxic drugs in management. The breakdown of nucleoproteins and the progressive increase in the concentration of uric acid in blood and body fluids is so rapid and of such a magnitude that the overproduction of uric acid may greatly exceed the capacity of the kidneys to excrete this excess. This sequence rapidly leads to acute oliguric renal failure with massive un-ionized uric acid deposition in the renal tubules. In addition the patients may be seriously ill, anorexic, dehydrated, and acidotic from the primary disease. The presence of a highly concentrated urine of low pH may result in a three- or four-fold increase in amount of uric acid in body fluids before the seriousness is appreciated. The subsequent precipitation of massive amounts of uric acid into tubules, renal pelvis, and lower urinary tract may be fatal. Currently, with adequate hydration, administration of alkalinizing agents, and use of allopurinol to depress uric acid formation, many of the acute problems of the past may be avoided.

FREI et al. (1963) discussed uric acid nephropathy as a function of treatment of a selected group of patients with cancer at the National Cancer Institute. Six among a total of 57 patients developed uric acid nephropathy while undergoing antitumor therapy for acute leukemia. No mention was made of articular gout in this small series nor in the discussion of uric acid nephropathy generally. It was reiterated, however, that the clearance of inulin and PAH rapidly improved—even returned to normal—with aggressive management. The reversibility was consistent with the relief of mechanical obstruction and was not compatible with permanent parenchymal damage of sufficient severity to depress the glomerular filtration rate.

DEGER and WAGONER (1972) discussed peritoneal dialysis in acute uric acid nephropathy in a 23-year-old female with acute lymphoblastic leukemia. During antileukemic therapy, the blood urea rose to 312 mg/100 ml and the serum urate to 79 mg/100 ml. Following dialysis, the serum uric acid decreased to 10.1 mg/100 ml. A total of 19 gm uric acid were recovered in the dialysate in slightly less than 3 days. Six months later the patient died. Leukemic infiltrations of the kidneys and other organs were noted at autopsy. Microscopically, the renal histology showed normal-appearing glomeruli, tubules, and interstitium. The exception was the finding of scattered dense infiltrations of immature lymphocytes in the interstitium related to the primary disease. One can conclude from this single case report that in an oliguric patient, excreting only 120 ml urine/24 h, associated with an excessively elevated serum uric acid concentration, that acute uric acid nephropathy may be a reversible phenomenon.

In contrast to a reversible phenomenon in acute uric acid nephropathy, either with adequate specific or nonspecific therapy, any long-term beneficial action of antigout drugs on well-developed renal lesions in chronic gouty arthritis has not been demonstrated. There are reports of a favorable action of allopurinol in preventing further deterioration of renal parenchyma, and urate tophi in the renal parenchyma may be mobilized (RUNDLES, 1963), but controlled studies of a permanent beneficial effect of antihyperuricemic drugs on renal disease in gout have not been recorded. It has seemed empirically, abundantly clear to me for some time that once a patient has been placed on long-term prophylactic medication, no further clinical evidence of renal deterioration may be expected (TALBOTT, 1967).

D. Experimental Production of Acute Uric Acid Nephropathy

KLINENBERG et al. (1973) have designed an experimental model in rats of urate nephropathy. The animals were given a prepared died containing uric acid and oxonate, the latter an inhibitor of uricase. The experiments were associated with levels of serum urate of five to eight times normal within 3 weeks. Another group of subacute experiments using RNA as the uric acid precursor were then performed. Serum urate values only twice normal were achieved in these experiments.

The principle changes in the experimental animals reflected proximal tubular dilatation from precipitation of un-ionized uric acid in the collecting ducts with secondary blockage of the tubules. The tubular cells contained mitotic figures and other nuclear changes compatible with degeneration. There were also collections of inflammatory cells and crystal deposits in and around the dilated tubules. Some of the dilated collecting tubules contained masses of inflammatory cells, amorphous material, and neutrophils in the interstitium. In contrast to glomerular changes sometimes seen in gouty patients, the glomeruli in the experimental rats were unaffected and were similar to those of the control animals.

E. Structural Alterations in the Gouty Kidney

The kidneys of patients with primary as well as secondary gout in many instances are associated with considerable variation in structural changes, frequently related to severity and duration of articular disease. If the gout is secondary to drug ingestion or a blood dyscrasia, structural changes of the primary disease unrelated to hyperuricemia may also be present. Uric acid passing through the kidney in higher-than-normal concentration is probably the number-one initiating agent. Firm proof is lacking that hyperuricemia per se, without precipitation of uric acid, can produce renal disease; frequently, neither crystals of uric acid nor monosodium urate monohydrate can be demonstrated either on renal biopsy or at postmortem study. One of the largest studies of renal function in patients with gout was by BERGER and YÜ (1975). They found that hyperuricemia alone had no deleterious effect on renal function over a decade or more of observation.

In other gouty patients, irrespective of the stage of the articular disease, urate deposits in the kidney are evident. Any reaction to hyperuricemia is probably confined initially, and possibly before the first attack of gouty arthritis, to mechanical damage to the epithelium of the loop of the Henle from precipitated uric acid or the salts of urates.

With precipitation of uric acid in the tubule, it is conceivable that an accumulation of inflammatory cells, as in experimental nephropathy, may be observed (KLINENBERG et al., 1973).

At this stage, no associated changes in the glomerulus, the walls of the blood vessels, or development of an extensive inflammatory reaction in the interstitial spaces characteristic of or associated with deposits of sodium urate, may be present. On the other hand, with the deposition of crystals in the tubules and subsequently in the interstitium of the medulla or pyramids, a urate tophus surrounded by multinucleated giant cells will result. Later in the pathogenesis, vascular changes may be prominent, associated or unassociated with an inflammatory reaction.

The incidence of demonstrable urate deposits in the gouty kidney varies greatly. By renal biopsy the incidence may be less than 10% (GONICK, 1965). At postmortem examination, MAYNE (1955) found urate deposits in 63% of a total of 27 patients. TALBOTT and TERPLAN (1960) identified needle crystals, thought to be urate or uric acid crystals in 93% of 191 kidney specimens of cases examined postmortem.

Sokoloff (1957) studied the histologic appearance of tophi in the renal parenchyma and considered them to be identical with nonrenal tophi, either in the subcutaneous spaces or in and about joints. Monosodium urate monohydrate crystalline deposits were present, as well as a variable inflammatory reaction. Seegmiller and Frazier (1966) examined by X-ray diffraction crystals deposited in renal tissue obtained at autopsy from gouty patients and from patients with acute leukemia. The crystalline patterns were identical to those of monosodium urate monohydrate crystals in four patients with gouty arthritis and identical to calcium oxalate monohydrate crystals in the remaining two. The diffraction patterns, identical to those of uric acid, were obtained in five of 12 patients suffering from acute leukemia.

The uric acid crystals were found only within the lumen of renal tubules of the patients with leukemia and were assumed to be in equilibrium with the urine components flowing through the tubules. The opposite situation was found in gouty patients. None of the monosodium urate monohydrate crystals were found within the tubular lumen but rather in the parenchymal tissue and in the renal pyramids. Here they were surrounded by collagen with varying degrees of an inflammatory reaction, similar to that found in a gouty tophus. No evidence was found of any basement membrane surrounding the deposits in the tubular lumen. The deposition of urates in the kidney was thought to be a direct effect of the naturally occurring purine degradation products present in excessive amounts in tubular urine in a supersaturated state, although immunologic phenomena or possibly a chemical variant of urates to account for the structural damage had not been excluded.

There are notable differences between the solubility of uric acid and the solubility of sodium salts of urates in simulated body fluids. The solubility in physiologic salt concentrations at body temperature and at the physiologic pH is about 8.8 mg/ 100 ml. This is considerably lower than the maximum solubility of uric acid in vivo, which has been observed to be as high as 100 mg/100 ml in patients. Changes in pH within the physiologic range have a minor effect on sodium urate solubility, while uric acid solubility is highly dependent on pH in the same range. The fact that the monosodium urate monohydrate crystals found in gouty kidney are similar to those found in gouty tophi supports the conclusion that these deposits are in equilibrium with vascular fluids with a high sodium content in a relative alkaline media, while the tubular deposits are composed of uric acid crystals and are in equilibrium with tubular urine, a relatively acid medium.

The parenchymal deposition of sodium urate has a preferential location for the renal medulla between the tubules and the vasa recta in the interstitial spaces. This medullary concentration of urate crystals has been assumed to be a result of a countercurrent multiplication, as a consequence of resorption beyond the proximal tubules, or a countercurrent exchange by the vasa recta after the passage followed by absorption in the collecting ducts.

The precipitated uric acid in the tubules may be crystalline and may be present without any associated particulate matter or it may be mixed with proteinaceous material. Tubular atrophy, diminution in size of the epithelial cells, and pycnotic nuclei may eventually appear. The atrophic changes may be particularly evident in the tubules in the medulla, where there may be an increase in the parenchymal stroma and fibrosis. From renal biopsy studies, Greenbaum (1961) assumed that the initial structural change with urate precipitation probably takes place within the

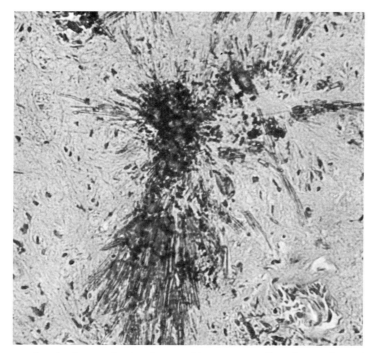

Fig. 3. Urate tophus in the renal parenchyma without surrounding giant cells (H & E, × 285)

lumen of the tubules and deposits later appear in the interstitial spaces. Other changes include an increase of liprochrome pigment in the epithelium of Henle's loop and the collecting tubules.

The deposits of crystalline uric acid or urate salts may vary in size and shape. They may lie free in the parenchyma without evidence of a foreign body reaction (Fig. 3), or they may attract foreign body giant cells and form a typical urate tophus (Fig. 4). Proper fixation and staining will retain the structural appearance of the urate deposits. If the tissue has been fixed in an aqueous media, however, the crystals may dissolve and lose the characteristic crystalline shape (Fig. 5). The crystalline pattern should be retained if absolute alcohol is the fixative and if special stains for uric acid are used. The needle crystals with such a protected procedure are clearly evident. Amorphous deposits may be seen in some sections side-by-side with crystalline deposits.

Following the deposition of urates in and around the tubules, three additional histopathologic changes may be observed. These are vascular lesions, inflammatory changes, and, rarely, amyloid deposition. Lacking precise information, it seems reasonable to assume that the changes in the walls of the blood vessels of the renal parenchyma or the glomerular capillary bed with hypertrophy of the intima and frequently of the media probably occur at approximately the same time as the urate deposits. There is no experimental evidence that one phenomenon precedes the other. Primarily, on the basis of incidence, it is assumed that the inflammatory changes and amyloid deposition develop later, if at all.

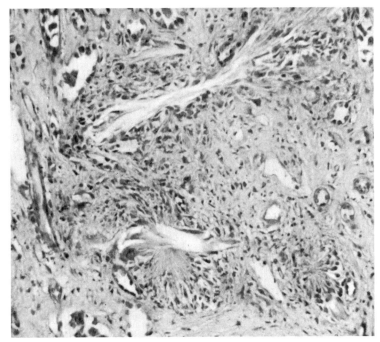

Fig.4. Sheaves of uric acid crystals surrounded by multinucleated foreign body giant cells (H & E, × 330)

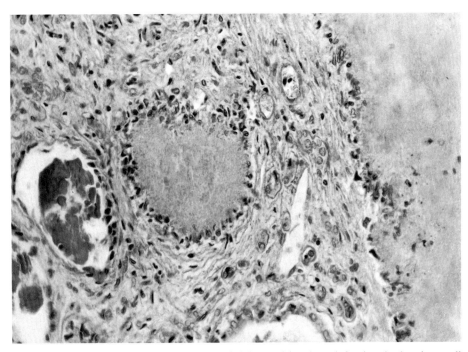

Fig.5. Amorphous deposit of urate surrounded by multinucleated foreign body giant cells (H & E, × 312)

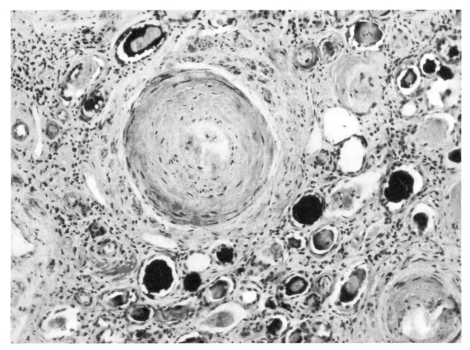

Fig. 6. Marked intimal thickening and hyalinization in an interlobular artery. The tubules are lined with atrophic flattended epithelium, and the lumen contains homogeneous casts (H & E, × 164)

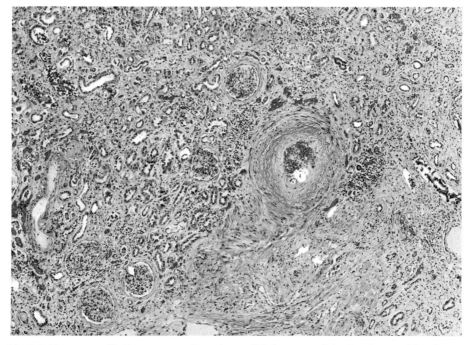

Fig. 7. Diffuse areas of inflammatory cells and vasculitis in an arteriole plus degenerative changes in tubules and glomeruli (H & E, × 108)

Table 1. Clinical and pathologic data from 191 postmortem protocols of cases of gout (Talbott and Terplan, 1960)

Pathologic findings	Clinical evaluation of gouty arthritis	
	Mild	Moderate
Well-developed pyelonephritic scarring	20	9
Minimal chronic changes of gout usually combined with minimal cortical-pyelonephritic scarring	13	2
Distinct vascular changes with severe structural alterations associated with urate deposits	3	15
Distinct vascular changes, pyelonephritic scarring and well-developed changes of urate deposits	12	12
Minimal evidence of urate deposits combined with distinct vascular changes	11	7
Evidence of severe pyelonephritis and changes associated with urate deposits	2	12

The changes in the vessels, both arteries and arterioles, and in the glomeruli vary greatly in degree and may be indistinguishable from similar structural changes in nongouty patients with benign hypertension. Since about 40% of gouty patients have hypertension (Talbott, 1967), an elevation of blood pressure that usually follows a benign course, vascular changes are not unanticipated. Only a few cases of gouty arthritis have sufficient clinical and laboratory evidence to warrant a diagnosis of malignant renal hypertension, with marked proliferation of the arteriolar walls and hyalinization. Vessels may show homogeneous casts within their lumen and increased basophilia and degenerative changes out of proportion to parenchymal damage. An example of an interlobular artery with almost complete obliteration of the lumen is shown in Figure 6.

The glomeruli may show changes similar to glomerulonephritis with fibrillar thickening of capillary basement membrane and partial or complete obliteration. However, Barlow and Beilin (1968) failed to discover any significant difference in the incidence of glomerular atrophy and nephrosclerosis between hypertensive and nonhypertensive gouty patients and assumed that the development of renal insufficiency was more close related to increasing age than to the gouty process, per se. On the other hand, Gonick et al. (1965) found changes characteristic of glomerulosclerosis in patients with gouty arthritis and, contrary to the majority who have speculated on the pathogenesis of the gouty kidney, believed that the primary lesion was in the glomerulus rather than in the tubules.

Another relatively common structural change in the gouty kidney is attributed to chronic inflammation (Fig. 7), usually unassociated with urinary tract infection. Mention has already been made of scattered inflammatory cells around the tubules, believed to represent a nonspecific, noninfectious reaction to deposition of uric acid crystals in the tubular lumen. In contrast, some patients with extensive areas of inflammation have had a clinical history of chronic pyelonephritis or atypical findings of ascending pyelonephritis. The interstitial tissue may show fibrosis and collec-

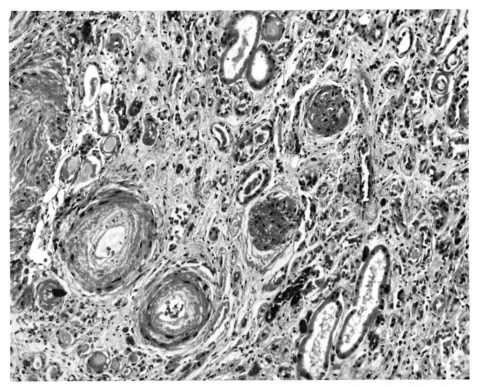

Fig. 8. Diffuse deposits of amyloid-staining material in the glomerulus of a patient with a history of tophaceous gout for many years (Congo Red, × 135)

tion of lymphocytes, plasma cells, and macrophages, characteristic of pyelonephritis unrelated to urate deposits. However, the presence of extensive inflammatory changes in the kidneys in the microscopic study by TALBOTT and TERPLAN (1960) of 191 postmortem kidneys (Table 1) was surprisingly high. The majority were suffering from primary gout. The usual special stains failed to show bacteria, even in cases of chronic pyelonephritis and obvious infection. SOKOLOFF (1965) assumed that the appearance of scar tissue in the gouty kidney was a mixture of chronic pyelonephritis and arteriolar nephrosclerosis.

The final structural change in the kidney is amorphous material in the glomeruli, which stains with an amyloid dye (Congo Red). This is an infrequent phenomenon in patients with gout. The amyloid-like deposits may be focal or the entire glomerulus may be involved (Fig. 8). I have observed this phenomenon only in patients with a chronic urate ulcer or a sinus draining urate sludge, usually unrelated or some distance removed from a gouty joint. There are two other possibilities for the development of amyloid disease in gouty patients. Amyloid or amyloid-like material may appear in the kidney of any long-standing chronic disease, such as in chronic deforming rheumatoid arthritis or indolent tuberculosis. These deposits may be related also to chronic pyelonephritis, a complication sometimes observed in patients with recurring small urate stones or large staghorn calculi.

None of the patients with gout showing amyloid deposits in the kidney that I have seen had evidence of amyloid in other parts of the body at postmortem examination. Nor was amyloid found in any patients in our series with uncomplicated mild primary gout or gout secondary to a blood dyscrasia with but one exception. This was a patient with amyloid deposits associated with multiple myeloma that developed a decade after the onset of clinical gouty arthritis.

F. Miscellaneous Observations

In the development of degenerative vascular disease of the kidney, the observations by TRAUT et al. (1954) that urates may aggregate in vessel walls has not been confirmed. It was suggested that this aggregation may reflect coexisting disturbances of other metabolic systems as well as those of urates.

TALBOTT and YÜ (1976) discussed in their monograph the correlation between tophaceous gout, graded 0–3 in severity, with proteinuria and hypertension. There was a progressive increase in the percentage of cases with hypertension as a function of tophaceous deposits. Similar findings were reported regarding the severity of tophaceous deposits and the incidence of proteinuria. Less than 10% of patients with nontophaceous gout in the GUTMAN and YÜ series had proteinuria. This incidence increased to 82% for those with tophi. When age was plotted as a function of tophi, there was progressive increase in incidence in the severity of tophaceous deposits up to the age of 50. Thereafter, the incidence for the next two decades remained essentially stationary. In the eighth decade of life the incidence of tophi of all degrees was slightly greater than in the preceding decade. It seems reasonable to believe, and probably unrelated to therapy, that as the gouty patient grows older, tophaceous deposits increase in incidence and severity correlated with the increasing incidence of proteinuria and hypertension.

No consistent correlation has been found between renal insufficiency and attacks of gouty arthritis (YÜ and BERGER, 1975). Even in those gouty patients whose joint symptoms had been present for several years, attacks of acute gout were less frequent in spite of severe renal insufficiency. In addition to proteinuria, a significant number of patients with well-developed gouty arthritis will show an inability to concentrate urine maximally, as well as various types of casts in the urinary sediment.

Saturnine gout (BALL and MORGAN, 1968) has many features in common with primary gout except for the history and clinical findings of lead intoxication. Also, the pathologic changes in the kidney are similar to primary gout, except for a paucity of inflammatory cells. However, EMMERSON (1968, 1971) has shown that in saturnine gout the hyperuricemia may be mediated by excessive tubular reabsorption of urate. LILIS et al. (1968) studied renal function in 102 patients with lead poisoning who had suffered for a decade or more with lead intoxication. It was specifically noted that not one of the patients had suffered an attack of clinical gout.

G. Selected Laboratory Procedures

I. Roentgenography

KRÖPELIN and MERTZ (1972), using various roentgenographic procedures for the diagnosis of changes in the kidney that included tomography and intravenous pyelography, reported the findings on 18 males and 4 females with primary gout. The average age was 52 years. The sclerotic form of papillary necrosis in the gouty kidney could be differentiated radiologically from the infectious-toxic form, which occurs in chronic pyelonephritis or diabetes mellitus. In spite of the above findings, however, it was concluded that the radiologic changes of the gouty kidney are not necessarily specific.

II. Renal Biopsy

GREENBAUM et al. (1961) described the histologic findings at renal biopsy in 12 patients with clinical gouty arthritis. The ages ranged from 4 to 69 years. Only two of the patients, one aged 55 who had suffered from gout for 38 years and another aged 40 who had suffered for only 6 years, each with a family history of gout but no gouty tophi, showed normal renal function and normal histologic features. The first case, however, had proteinuria 1 +. At the other end of the spectrum were two patients in renal failure who showed atrophic glomerular lesions, tubular atrophy, an increase in interstitial fibrosis, and arteriolar hypertrophy. No urate deposits were seen in any of the sections examined. No significant specific contributions were made concerning the pathogenesis of the histopathology from the renal biopsy material in these 12 patients when compared to the postmortem study of a larger number of cases.

BARLOW and BEILIN (1968) made a study of renal disease in 53 gouty patients. Slightly less than half of the number were subjected to renal biopsy. Two of the patients had diabetes mellitus and showed severe arteriolar lesions that were different from the sections studied in gouty patients without diabetes mellitus. The most prominent features in the biopsy of the nondiabetic gouty patient were glomerular and tubular atrophy. The incidence and severity of these lesions was twice that found in a comparable autopsy study of renal histology in 100 nongouty cases matched for age.

In the absence of inflammatory changes, atrophy of the nephron was attributed to ischemia. The degree of arteriosclerosis was not correlated with the severity of nephrosclerosis in these patients. Although there was a strong association between hypertension and nephrosclerosis in the nongouty subjects, this association was not apparent in the gouty patient. The overall severity of nephrosclerosis was no greater in the hypertensive group than in the normotensive group. The investigation emphasized the importance of vascular nephrosclerosis as a cause of renal damage at an early stage in the gouty patient.

The development of severe nephrosclerosis was considered in relation to the relatively high incidence of hypertension and other occlusive arterial diseases as an associated phenomenon in gouty patients. They emphasized what was discussed in detail sometime later by TALBOTT and YÜ (1976). To wit, the gouty patient with atherosclerosis and diabetes mellitus or the gouty patient with hypertension shares many of the clinical problems seen in nongouty patients with these diseases. These include the sequelae of disorders of purine, lipid, and carbohydrate metabolism. They also found what had been mentioned a generation ago (TALBOTT, 1943), that some degree of renal dysfunction is observed in approximately 40% of gouty patients, even after consideration of the natural decline and development of degenerative changes in the kidney as a function of age. However, the renal impairment is mild in most patients. The exceptions observed by BARLOW and BEILIN were two patients with coincident diabetic glomerulosclerosis. Nor was there any indication of any disparity between loss of glomerular function and loss of tubular function. The development of renal insufficiency was assumed to be related to increasing age rather than to the gouty process. Enzyme histochemical techniques provided no evidence of tubular damage in an earlier stage than was detectable by routine histologic techniques.

PARDO et al. (1968) examined with the electron microscope sections from renal biopsies of 13 patients with primary gout for comparison with 11 nongouty patients with essential hypertension. There were no distinct renal lesions as seen by electron microscopy in the gouty kidneys not observed in the nongouty except for large and small electron-opaque interstitial deposits in the gouty cases. Comparable mesangial, vascular, cortical, medullary, and tubular lesions were observed in biopsy specimens from either group. Cells in the loops of Henle and in the collecting tubules in either condition showed increased lipofuscin pigment. Indifferent as well as obsolete tubular elements were frequent. An associated thickening of the lamina densa with hypertension was observed in both groups, which alteration was thought to depend upon the severity and duration of the hypertension and did not appear to be directly related to the hyperuricemia.

The vascular lesions were quantitatively indistinguishable in the gouty and nongouty cases regardless of the presence or absence of hypertension. However, the degree of vascular involvement was more severe in the gouty patients with renal insufficiency. PARDO et al. (1968) also reported the findings from adolescent normotensives with juvenile onset diabetes mellitus. Well-developed arteriolar hyalinosis was found, which suggested that diabetes mellitus favors the development of such vascular lesions. These findings were believed to support the possibility that the metabolic defect recognized as primary gout may, as is noted with diabetes mellitus and hypertension, accentuate the vascular lesions generally attributed to aging, although the mechanism(s) are unknown.

In another phase of the study, lithium monourate was injected intravenously into rabbits in acute experiments and the animals sacrificed. No glomerular changes were seen in the sections studied. This finding was interpreted as further evidence that the glomerulus is not affected by excessive urate transport and that the glomerular changes noted in gouty patients are probably related to hypertension or to arteriosclerosis rather than hyperuricemia.

GONICK et al. (1965) investigated the evolutionary progression of the renal lesion in gout with material from 28 percutaneous biopsies and 42 autopsies. Most of the patients were in the middle-to-late decades of life and had carried a diagnosis of gout for a number of years. The majority displayed hypertension and proteinuria. The primary objective of the study was to identify and give priority if possible to the structural changes in the glomeruli, tubules, interstitial tissue, and blood vessels. A uniform fibrillar thickening of the glomerular capillary basement membrane was present, with an increased number of nuclei in the capillary loops. Both endothelial and epithelial cells had more abundant cytoplasm than anticipated. Any glomerulosclerosis was not associated with a stiffened or wilted appearance of the glomeruli nor with hyaline basement membrane thickening as seen in diffuse glomerulosclerosis of diabetes mellitus. There were no characteristic abnormalities of the proximal convoluted tubules. The loops of Henle, however, tended to show consistent early alterations with atrophy, dilatation, regeneration, and sometimes brown pigment deposition in the epithelium.

Distinctive architectural changes in the macula densa and distal convolutions were lacking. Collecting tubular abnormalities consisted of hyperplastic epithelial cells palisaded to a significant degree. When urate tophi were present, chronic inflammation and scarring was seen in the peripheral medulla and overlying cortex. In kidneys without urate tophi, the distribution of inflammatory changes was unusual, and the lesions appeared to develop in an area proximal to the loop of Henle. Unlike the ordinary pyelonephritis process, the lesions tended to avoid the medulla and juxtamedullary cortex. Both arteries and arterioles showed degenerative changes out of proportion to the changes in the parenchyma, which included exaggerated hyalinization of the intima. Unusual basophilia of the degenerated intima, media, or the entire vessel wall, including the adventitia, was common.

They concluded that the renal abnormalities began early in the course of clinical gouty arthritis (associated with hyperuricemia) and rejected the possibility that gouty nephropathy is initiated by deposition of urates in the collecting tubules. The absence of proximal tubular dilatation argued against a major obstructive component; rather, atrophy, and pigment deposition in Henle's loop were found as consistent early alterations. Vascular changes both in the glomerular capillary bed and in larger blood vessels were also frequent. The histochemical findings suggested that the pathogenesis of gouty nephropathy was not an obstructive phenomenon but more likely a reaction of the kidney to an increased filtered load of uric acid from identified urate precursors.

H. Conclusion

Neither studies of renal function nor histopathologic studies by the light or electron microscope provide definitive evidence of a specific lesion or lesions that can adequately be identified as the specific feature in the kidneys of patients with gout. Hyperuricemic glomerular filtrate, with or without the demonstration of uric acid deposits in the tubules, is probably primary to the pathogenesis. A significant number of patients will show transient or persistent proteinuria as an associated phenomenon. In most patients and usually 1 or more years after the onset of articular distress—in the natural history of gout—deposits of monosodium urate monohydrate crystals may appear in the interstitium together with fibrosis and vascular changes, frequently associated with hypertension. Inflammatory changes may be minimal and associated with deposition of uric acid crystals in the tubules or as multinucleated giant cells surrounding parenchymal urate deposits or as massive accumulation of inflammatory cells associated with pyelonephritis. A few patients will show amyloid or amyloid-staining deposits in the glomeruli or interstitium.

Acknowledgement: Several of the illustrations have been reproduced from TALBOTT and YÜ (1976) with permission.

References

Ball, G. V., Morgan, J. M.: Chronic lead ingestion and gout. South Med. J. **61**, 21—24 (1968)

Barlow, K. A., Beilin, L. J.: Renal disease in primary gout. Quart. J. Med. **37**, 79—96 (1968)

Berger, L., Yü, T. F.: Renal function in gout. IV. An analysis of 524 gouty subjects including long term follow up studies. Amer. J. Med. **59**, 605 (1975)

Deger, G. E., Wagoner, R. D.: Peritoneal dialysis in acute uric acid nephropathy. Mayo Clin. Proc. **47**, 189—192 (1972)

Emmerson, B. T.: The clinical differentiation of lead gout from primary gout. Arthritis Rheum. **11**, 623—634 (1968)

Emmerson, B. T., Mirosch, W., Douglas, J. B.: The relative contributions of tubular reabsorption and secretion to urate excretion in lead nephropathy. Aust. N.Z. J. Med. **4**, 353—362 (1971)

Frei, E. III, Bentzel, C. J., Rieselbach, R., Block, J. B.: Renal complications of neoplastic disease. J. chron. Dis. **16**, 757—776 (1963)

Gonick, H. C., Rubini, M. E., Gleason, I. O., Sommers, S. C.: The renal lesion in gout. Ann. intern. Med. **62**, 667—674 (1965)

Greenbaum, D., Ross, J. H., Steinberg, V. L.: Renal biopsy in gout. Brit. med. J. **1961 I**, 1502—1504

Gudzent, F.: Gicht und Rheumatismus. Berlin: Springer 1928

Heptinstall, R. H.: Pathology of the Kidney, pp. 495—506, 2nd Ed. Boston: Little Brown 1966

Kjellstrand, C. M., Campbell, D. C., von Hartitzsch, B., Buselmeier, T. J.: Hyperuricemia acute renal failure. Arch. intern. Med. **133**, 349—359 (1974)

Klinenberg, J. R., Bluestone, R., Schlosstein, L., Waisman, J., Whitehouse, M. W.: Urate deposition disease: how is it regulated and how can it be modified? Ann. intern. Med. **78**, 99—111 (1973)

Kröpelin, T., Mertz, D. P.: Zur Röntgendiagnostik der Gichtniere. Dtsch. med. Wschr. **97**, 71—75 (1972)

Lesch, M., Nyhan, W. L.: A familial disorder of uric acid metabolism and central nervous system function. Amer. J. Med. **36**, 561—570 (1964)

Lilis, R., Gavrilescu, N., Nestorescu, B., Dumitriu, C., Roventa, A.: Nephropathy in chronic lead poisoning. Brit. J. industr. Med. **25**, 196—202 (1968)

Mayne, J. G.: Pathological study of the renal lesion found in 27 patients with gout. Ann. rheum. Dis. **15**, 61—62 (1955)

Pardo, V., Perez-Stable, E., Fisher, E. R.: Ultrastructural studies in hypertension. III. Gouty nephropathy. Lab. Invest. **18**, 143—150 (1968)

Richet, P., Mignon, G. F., Ardaillou, R.: Gout secondary to chronic kidney disease (Fre). Presse med. **73**, 633—638 (1975)

Rieselbach, R. E., Bentzel, C. J., Cotlove, E., Frei, E., Frereich, E. J.: Uric acid excretion and renal function in the acute hyperuricemia of leukemia: pathogenesis and therapy of uric acid nephropathy. Amer. J. Med. **37**, 872—884 (1964)

Rundles, R. W., Wyngaarden, J. B., Hitchings, G. H., Elion, G. B., Silberman, H. R.: Effects of xanthine oxidase inhibitor on thiopurine metabolism, hyperuricemia, and gout. Trans. Ass. Amer. Physicians **76**, 126—140 (1963)

Schultz, A.: Zur Frage der Beziehungen zwischen Leukämie und Gicht. Zugleich Mitteilung histologischer Darstellungsmethoden der Harnsäure und der Urate. Virchows Arch. path. Anat. **280**, 519—533 (1931)

Seegmiller, J. E., Frazier, P. D.: Biochemical considerations of the renal damage of gout. Ann. rheum. Dis. (Suppl.) **25**, 668—672 (1966)

Sokoloff, L.: The pathology of gout. Metabolism **6**, 230—243 (1957)

Sokoloff, L.: Pathology of gout. Arthritis Rheum. **8**, 707—713 (1965)

Sorensen, L. B.: The pathogenesis of gout. Arch. intern. Med. **109**, 379—390 (1962)

Talbott, J. H.: Gout. New York: Oxford Univ. Pr. 1943

Talbott, J. H.: Gout and blood dyscrasias. Medicine (Baltimore) **38**, 173—205 (1959)

Talbott, J. H.: Gout, 3rd Ed. New York: Grune and Stratton 1967

Talbott, J. H., Terplan, K. L.: The kidney in gout. Medicine (Baltimore) **39**, 405—462 (1960)

Talbott, J. H., Yü, T. F.: Gout and Uric Acid Metabolism. New York: Stratton Intercon 1976

Traut, E. F., Knight, A. A., Szanto, P. M., Passerelli, E. W.: Specific vascular changes in gout. J. Amer. med. Ass. **156**, 591—593 (1954)

Yü, T. F., Berger, L.: Renal disease in primary gout; a study of 253 gout patients with proteinuria. Semin. Arthritis Rheum. **4**, 293—307 (1975)

Yü, T. F., Weinreb, N., Wittman, R., Wasserman, L. R.: Secondary gout associated with chronic myeloproliferative disorders. Semin. Arthritis Rheum. **5**, 247—257 (1976)

CHAPTER 20

Uricosuric Drugs

H. S. DIAMOND

A. Introduction

Renal transport of urate is influenced by many endogenous metabolites and drugs. Any drug whose net effect on renal tubular transport of urate results in increased urate clearance can be considered a uricosuric agent. By this definition, uricosuric drugs include a large number of compounds with diverse chemical structures and pharmacologic properties. Only a few of these drugs have been widely employed clinically as uricosuric agents.

The clinically important uricosuric agents have a number of characteristics in common that are important to an understanding of their clinical pharmacology and mechanisms of interactions with transport of other drugs and compounds including urate. Thus, it is useful to outline the general characteristics of this group of drugs and the postulates derived from them before discussing the pharmacology of specific drugs.

B. Tubular Transport of Uricosuric Drugs

In common with many other drugs (KOCH-WESER and SELLARS, 1976) most uricosuric drugs are extensively bound to serum albumin and are therefore not completely filtered at the glomerulus; they enter the urine largely by tubular secretion. Secretion of these compounds occurs in the proximal tubule, including the pars recta, via the secretory system for weak organic acids (WEINER, 1973). Most of these drugs appear to compete with p-aminohippuric acid (PAH) and with each other for secretion (WEINER et al., 1960; WEINER et al., 1964; PEREL et al., 1969). There appear to be at least two transport systems for secretion of organic acids in the proximal tubule. Recent evidence suggests that in man and the chimpanzee urate is secreted by a carrier system different from the system responsible for secretion of PAH and most uricosuric drugs (BONER and STEELE, 1973; FANELLI et al., 1971a; MEISEL and DIAMOND, 1977). Secretion is required for expression of the uricosuric effect of most uricosuric drugs (YÜ et al., 1963; DANTZLER, 1973). Inhibition of secretion of uricosuric drugs by co-administration of PAH impairs the uricosuric effect of these drugs without directly altering urate secretion (FANELLI et al., 1973a; MEISEL and DIAMOND, 1977). This effect is attributed to a decrease in the concentration of the drug at the luminal membrane of the renal tubule (Fig. 1). This and other evidence support the concept that uricosuria is induced by interaction between uricosuric drugs and a reabsorptive carrier for urate at the luminal membrane (GUTMAN, 1966). Direct measurement of drug concentrations at the luminal membrane in man are unavail-

PAH-PROBENECID ORGANIC ACID
SECRETORY CARRIER TRANSPORT

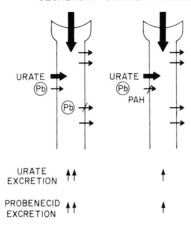

Fig. 1. PAH competitively inhibits the tubular secretion of probenecid, reducing its concentration at the luminal membrane and thereby impairing its uricosuric effect. Probenecid secretion in the absence of PAH permits intraluminal probenecid to inhibit urate reabsorption. PAH inhibits both probenecid secretion and probenecid-induced uricosuria

able. However, several additional indirect observations support this concept. Alkalinization, which increases excretion of some uricosuric drugs, increases uricosuric potency (Yü et al., 1959). In two series of drugs, phenylbutazone analogues and probenecid analogues, there is a relationship between potency as uricosuric agents and extent of drug excretion in the urine (GUTMAN et al., 1960; BLANCHARD et al., 1972). Maximal uricosuric potency in these series correlated with pK_a. In many of the studies cited, urine concentration of uricosuric drugs is a better correlate of uricosuric activity than is serum concentration of the drugs.

Under physiologic conditions and in an acid urine the net renal clearance of many anionic uricosuric drugs is quite low. Low clearance appears to be accounted for by passive non-ionic reabsorption of organic acids (WEINER et al., 1964). Increases in urinary pH result in marked increases in excretion of many uricosuric drugs (GUTMAN et al., 1955; WEINER et al., 1959, 1964). In some cases the increment in excretion is sufficient to demonstrate net secretion of the drug. Excretion is also directly correlated with the rate of urine flow and is dependent (in an inverse manner) upon lipid solubility. Thus, in a series of phenylbutazone analogs of similar lipid solubility but varying pK_a, renal excretion varied inversely with pK_a. The greater excretion rates of compounds with low pK_a were attributed both to increased secretion by an active process and lesser or absent reabsorption by passive non-ionic diffusion.

There is no direct evidence for active reabsorption of any uricosuric drug in man or mammals. Nonetheless, this possibility cannot be discounted. The concept of competitive inhibition of active urate reabsorption by uricosuric drugs, which are themselves not actively reabsorbed and are therefore "refractory substrates," is similar to concepts advanced to explain competitive inhibition or organic acid secretion

Table 1. Effect of some drugs which alter urate excretion in man on urate excretion in other species

	Cebus monkey	Mongrel dog	Dalmation dog	Rat	Rabbit	Fowl	Man
Probencid	+ +	0	– –	+ +	–	– –	+ +
Sulfinpyrazone	+	?	?	0	?	– –	+ +
Benzbromerone or Benziodarone	+ +	?	?	+ +	?	±	+ +
Tienilic Acid	?	+ +	+ +	+ +	– –	– –	+ +
Pyrazinoate	– –	0	0	–	+	0	– –
PAH	–	–	–	–	?	– –	+
Zoxazolamine	0	0	0	?	?	–	+ +

Data represents standard clearance studies where available or micropuncture if no other data available. Uricosuria = +; urate retention = –; single symbol, mild effect; double symbol, pronounced effect; 0 = no change; ? = unknown (MUDGE et al., 1973; LEMIEUX et al., 1973; WEINER and FANELLI, 1975; WEINER, 1976; LEMIEUX, et al., 1977; MEISEL and DIAMOND, 1977).

by some of these drugs prior to the recognition of passive reabsorption. There are several examples of active bidirectional transport of organic acids other than urate and uricosuric drugs in mammalian species (CHO and CAFRUNY, 1970; MAY and WEINER, 1970).

Many uricosuric drugs have been observed to inhibit urate excretion at low doses. While this paradoxical effect on urate excretion could result from any one of many possible mechanisms, inhibition of urate secretion by low doses of uricosuric drugs has been the mechanism most often proposed. In man, this mechanism has been invoked to account for decreased urate excretion following low doses of salicylate (YÜ and GUTMAN, 1959), probenecid, and phenylbutazone (YÜ and GUTMAN, 1955). However, net tubular secretion of urate in man can be demonstrated by administration of sulfinpyrazone during osmotic diuresis and urate loading (GUTMAN et al., 1959). This is accounted for with difficulty by the hypothesis that the paradoxical affect on urate excretion of these drugs represents inhibition of secretion at low drug doses and both secretion and reabsorption at high drug doses, and suggests a more complex interaction. These observations can easily be accounted for by the concept of at least two organic acid secretory carriers in the proximal tubule with differing affinities for urate and uricosuric drugs. Inhibition of the component of urate secretion derived from a carrier with low affinity for urate but high affinity for the uricosuric agent, could account for modest degrees of urate retention at low doses of the uricosuric drug without affecting the major urate secretory carrier. Some of the marked species variability in response to uricosuric drugs might be accounted for if there were more than one secretory carrier for organic acids (including urate) with species variation in the relative affinity of each carrier (Table 1). In general, drugs that are uricosuric in man tend to cause urate retention in species normally showing net secretion of urate such as the chicken (BERGER et al., 1960; NECHAY and NECHAY, 1959), but are uricosuric in species showing net urate reabsorption such as the chimpanzee (FANELLI et al., 1971 a, b) and Cebus monkey (FANELLI et al., 1970). The effects of these drugs in other species are striking because of the range of variation among species. Species variability in response to uricosuric drugs limits the usefulness of animal studies for analysis of mechanism and site of action.

Most uricosuric drugs are organic acids. These drugs are generally thought to exert their uricosuric effects by interacting with a reabsorptive system for urate that is sensitive to certain organic acids. There are several exceptions. The organic base chlorprothixene is uricosuric in man (HEALEY et al., 1965). However, recent studies with this agent suggest that this drug may be a nonspecific proximal tubule toxin since uricosuria is associated with inhibition of tubular transport of many other substances transported in the proximal tubule (WEINSHILBOUM et al., 1975). A similar explanation appears to account for uricosuria associated with "outdated" tetracycline (FULOP and DRABKIN, 1965). Zoxazolamine is a weak organic base with potent and selective uricosuric properties (BURNS et al., 1958). Zoxazolamine does not appear to be transported by the PAH-sensitive organic acid secretory system and would not be anticipated to interact with an organic acid reabsorptive carrier. Its mechanism of action is uncertain. There is no evidence that its uricosuria is due to an organic acid metabolite although this possibility has not been completely excluded. The major known metabolite is a phenolic glucuronide, an organic acid that has no uricosuric activity. However, not all metabolites of this drug have been identified. The anticholinergic agent glycopyrolate is another organic base found to be uricosuric in some hyperuricemic patients (POSTHLETHWAITE et al., 1974). Drug metabolism or anticholinergic effects may account for uricosuria associated with this agent.

C. Drug Metabolism

Since most uricosuric drugs are weak organic acids that are reabsorbed extensively by passive non-ionic diffusion, elimination of the drugs is largely dependent on metabolism. The well-characterized metabolites are generally stronger organic acids than the parent compounds, which are, therefore, more rapidly eliminated in the urine. Many of these metabolites are themselves secreted by the organic acid secretory systems and thus, may potentially compete with the parent compound, urate, and/or each other for secretion. Some of these metabolites are also uricosuric and in some cases may account for a significant proportion of the uricosuric activity of the parent compound. The metabolism of most uricosuric drugs is incompletely characterized. Moreover, few metabolites have been carefully studied for their interactions with organic acid transport systems in the kidney. The potential interactions among drug, metabolite, and urate are obviously complex and could account for many poorly understood drug effects.

Drug metabolism occurs largely in the liver and requires hepatic uptake of the drugs. Hepatic uptake is not passive but is carried out by organic acid transport systems that appear to be closely analogous to those in the kidney. For example, PAH and many uricosuric drugs compete for binding with ligandin and related hepatic binding proteins (KIRSCH et al., 1975). Ligandin is also found in the proximal renal tubule with highest concentration in the pars recta (ARIAS et al., 1976). Probenecid is known to impair the hepatic uptake of many compounds. These effects do not appear to be accounted for by competition for binding to ligandin and may be secondary to competition for uptake at the plasma membrane (KENWRIGHT and

LEVI, 1973). In animals some uricosuric drugs might alter urate metabolism by inhibition of hepatic uptake. Further complex drug interactions can result from saturable metabolic pathways or hepatic uptake, which may result in the relative proportions in the circulation of parent compound and metabolites varying with administered dose of drug. Inhibition of hepatic uptake of drug by drug metabolites may add to the potential interactions. This entire area has been incompletely studied. Interactions of these types may account for many drug effects on urate transport that are at present either unexplained or explained in other ways.

D. Mechanisms of Uricosuria

Present evidence suggests that the clinically important uricosuric drugs inhibit renal tubular reabsorption of urate by interacting at the luminal membrane of the renal tubule with a reabsorptive system for urate. The discussion of the mechanism of action of uricosuric drugs that follows is based upon postulates as to the mechanism of renal handling of uric acid in man. According to these postulates, uric acid is freely or very nearly freely filtered at the glomerulus. Additional urate enters the tubule by secretion. The magnitude of urate secretion is large, perhaps equal to the filtered load of urate. The organic acid carrier accounting for most urate secretion is distinct from the organic acid carrier responsible for secretion of PAH and most uricosuric drugs. Both filtered and secreted urate are extensively reabsorbed in the renal tubule. However, reabsorption of filtered urate is more nearly complete so that most excreted urate is derived from secretion. These concepts and the evidence supporting them have been presented in an earlier chapter and reviewed elsewhere (RIESELBACH and STEELE, 1974; DIAMOND et al., 1976-7).

The postulates are consistent with several mechanisms for uricosuria. Increase in the filtered load of urate could theoretically result in increased urate clearance. At 4° C and in an albumin solution of 4 g/dL concentration in dilute buffer approximately 30% of the urate is bound to albumin (KLINENBERG and KIPPEN, 1970; CAMPION et al., 1973). Uricosuric drugs displace albumin-bound urate under these conditions (KIPPEN et al., 1974).

Uricosuria could result from increased urate secretion or diminished reabsorption of filtered and/or secreted urate. Differentiation among these possibilities have proved difficult. Studies in man have relied upon analysis of effects of inhibitors of urate transport on drug-induced uricosuria. The complexity of interactions involved has rendered interpretation of results difficult and less than definitive. Micropuncture and perfusion studies in animals have provided more nearly definitive results. However, in view of the marked species variability in response to uricosuric drugs (Table 1), the applicability of this data to man is uncertain. Several factors initially suggested that uricosuric drugs acted to inhibit urate reabsorption. In normal man, urate excretion is approximately 8% of the filtered load (GUTMAN and YÜ, 1975a). Even a minor decrease in the reabsorptive flux for urate could result in substantial uricosuria. Thus, the increase in urate clearance that followed administration of uricosuric drugs was more easily accounted for by inhibition of reabsorption than by enhanced secretion. Probenecid and other uricosuric drugs were known to inhibit tubular secretion of many organic acids (BEYER et al., 1951; WEINER et al., 1960).

Moreover, many uricosuric drugs including probenecid and phenylbutazone (YÜ and GUTMAN, 1955) and salicylate (YÜ and GUTMAN, 1959) were urate retaining when administered in small doses. Urate retention was attributed to inhibition of urate secretion. This made increased urate secretion an unlikely mechanism for uricosuria induced by these drugs (GUTMAN et al., 1959; GUTMAN and YÜ, 1961).

The uricosuric effect of many drugs in man is largely or completely abolished following administration of pyrazinamide (STEELE and BONER, 1973; DIAMOND and PAOLINO, 1973). Pyrazinamide is a potent inhibitor of urate secretion (STEELE and RIESELBACH, 1967; WEINER and TINKER, 1972). Pyrazinamide suppression of uricosuria induced by several uricosuric drugs, including benzbromarone (LEMIEUX et al., 1973) and radiocontrast agents (POSTLETHWAITE and KELLEY, 1971), was initially attributed to stimulation of urate secretion by these drugs. The recognition of reabsorption of secreted urate made this interpretation unnecessary.

Micropuncture and microperfusion studies have supported the concept of inhibition of urate reabsorption by uricosuric drugs and tended to localize these effects to the proximal tubule (WEINMAN et al., 1976; FRANKFORT and WEINMAN, 1977; KRAMP and LENOIR, 1975). Because of species differences in responsiveness to uricosuric drugs and in urate metabolism, localization of the site of inhibition of urate reabsorption by uricosuric drugs in man remains uncertain. Most uricosuric drugs are more effective inhibitors of reabsorption of the component of urate excretion that is pyrazinamide suppressible than of the postpyrazinamide component of urate excretion (STEELE and BONER, 1973), which is consistent with the suggestion that they may be better inhibitors of reabsorption of secreted than of filtered urate. However, alternate interpretations of this data are possible as noted by STEELE and RIESELBACH (1975). Secretion of uricosuric drugs is required for expression of their uricosuric effect. Most uricosuric drugs compete for secretion with PAH, and PAH secretion probably occurs to a substantial extent in the late proximal tubule including the pars recta. Thus, concentrations of uricosuric drugs may be low at the luminal membrane in the earliest segment of the proximal tubule. Uricosuric drugs may be less effective inhibitors of urate reabsorption in this segment of the proximal nephron where intraluminal urate might be largely derived from filtration. They might be more effective inhibitors of urate reabsorption in more distal segments of the nephron where a larger fraction of intraluminal urate is derived from secretion.

From the preceding discussion, it should be obvious that several different mechanisms could account for paradoxical urate retention by uricosuric drugs. Many diuretics that are uricosuric when given intravenously produce urate retention when given for longer periods (HEALEY et al., 1959). Urate retention appears to be secondary to extracellular fluid volume depletion and can be prevented by volume replacement (STEELE and OPPENHEIMER, 1969; WEINMAN and EKNOYAN, 1975).

The paradoxical effects of most other uricosuric agents are probably related to competetive inhibition of transport carriers by drugs. However, this interaction may be more complex than has generally been appreciated. For example, the paradoxical effect of salicylate on urate excretion has been attributed to inhibition of urate secretion at low blood salicylate levels and of both urate secretion and reabsorption at higher blood levels (YÜ and GUTMAN, 1959). This interpretation fails to consider the metabolic sequence in which ingested salicylate is conjugated, and the complex renal interactions by which salicylate metabolites as well as free salicylate are se-

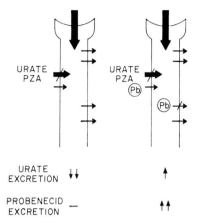

Fig. 2. Pyrazinamide inhibits urate secretion but does not affect tubular secretion of probenecid. Inhibition of urate secretion impairs the uricosuric response to probenecid by reducing the urate concentration in the tubule of the urate reabsorptive site inhibited by probenecid

creted by the renal tubule and may compete with each other for secretion, with salicylate conjugates accounting for more than 80% of normal excretion (Schacter and Manis, 1958; Weiner et al., 1959). The interactions of salicylate and metabolites with putative urate secretory and reabsorptive carriers have not been studied. Although it is possible that free salicylate interacts with both the PAH and urate secretory carriers, the alternative possibility that salicylate metabolites account in part for the "paradoxical" effects of salicylate on urate excretion has not been excluded. Saturation of metabolic pathways for salicylate results in dose-dependent differences in proportions of salicylate and its metabolites in plasma, which might account for differences in the degree of inhibition of secretory and reabsorptive transport carriers at different salicylate blood levels.

The uricosuric response to probenecid in man is intact or enhanced when uricosuria is induced by urate loading or volume expansion (Diamond and Meisel, 1977) and in patients with hyperuricemia and endogenous urate overproduction (Diamond et al., 1975). The uricosuric response to probenecid is attenuated following administration of low doses of uricosuric drugs (Diamond and Meisel, 1977), or of other drugs that compete with probenecid for secretion (Meisel and Diamond, 1977).

Pyrazinamide markedly reduces urate excretion in man during probenecid-induced uricosuria (Steele and Boner, 1973; Diamond and Paolino, 1973). This appears to be due to inhibition of urate secretion by pyrazinamide without a direct effect on probenecid action, but the interrelationships are complex (Meisel and Diamond, 1977) (Fig. 2). The urate-retaining effect of pyrazinamide is due to a metabolite, pyrazinoic acid, which in the chimpanzee has a biphasic effect on urate excretion (Fanelli and Weiner, 1973; Weiner and Tinker, 1972). Urate retention occurs at low pyrazinoic acid blood levels, approximating those attained in man following oral pyrazinamide. Uricosuria occurs at much higher blood levels. Pyrazinoate does not alter PAH secretion or probenecid excretion (FANELLI and WEINER, 1973; MEISEL and DIAMOND, 1977) but does prolong probenecid half-life (YÜ et al., 1977), possibly by inhibition of hepatic uptake. Thus probenecid may alter pyrazinamide metabolism and pyrazinoate concentration. Pyrazinoate is both actively secreted and reabsorbed in the proximal tubule in dogs (WEINER and TINKER, 1972). Thus, in addition to its effects on urate secretion, pyrazinamide might interact with probenecid through effects on metabolism of both drugs, renal transport of both drugs, and even at a putative urate reabsorptive site.

From the preceding discussion, it should be obvious that the complexity of possible interactions with urate transport occurring when uricosuric drugs are administered simultaneously is beyond the capacity for rational analysis at our present level of understanding. For most combinations of uricosuric drugs, drug combinations show additive uricosuria up to the maximum uricosuria attainable with the more potent of the agents (GUTMAN, 1966; DIAMOND and MEISEL, 1977). No uricosuric drug or drug combination has produced net secretion of urate in normal man in the absence of urate loading and osmotic diuresis. Mutual suppression of uricosuria is observed when salicylate is administered together with many other uricosuric drugs including probenecid, sulfinpyrazone (YÜ et al., 1963), phenylbutazone (OYER et al., 1965), zoxazolamine (BURNS et al., 1958), and benzbromarone (SINCLAIR and FOX, 1975). This effect is probably not accounted for by competition for drug secretion since probenecid and sulfinpyrazone compete for secretion without suppressing each others uricosuric action (PEREL et al., 1969). Inhibition of urate secretion by salicylate or its metabolites may account for suppression of uricosuria by salicylate (STEELE and BONER, 1973; MEISEL and DIAMOND, 1977).

E. Clinical Pharmacology and Use

The primary goal of uricosuric drug therapy is reduction of increased serum uric acid to the normal range. There is no universally accepted agreement among experienced physicians as to indications for the use of uric acid-lowering drugs. Treatment with uric acid-lowering agents is not warranted for most hyperuricemic patients. With infrequent exceptions, patients with asymptomatic hyperuricemia do not require antihyperuricemic therapy. Not all patients who have had one or more attacks of gouty arthritis require therapy to lower serum uric acid. Patients with infrequent and mild attacks of gout and modest elevation of serum uric acid may be treated successfully with colchicine prophylaxis or treated only for acute attacks. Lowering serum uric acid is not effective or useful treatment of acute gouty arthritis. Acute gout is treated with colchicine or potent nonspecific anti-inflammatory drugs.

Indications for uric acid-lowering treatment similar to those recommended by WYNGAARDEN and KELLEY (1976) are employed by many physicians. These authors propose four general indications for use of either uricosuric drugs or allopurinol:

1. Tophi visibile on physical examination. If the nature of the lesion is uncertain its tophaceous character should be verified by aspiration and by identification of urate crystals in the aspirate.

2. Roentgenographic lesions consistent with tophi in a patient with proven gout.

3. A proven attack of gout in a patient with a serum urate concentration persistently above 8–8.5 mg/dL by a phosphotungstic acid method or two severe attacks of

proven gout within 1–2 years in a patient with a lower serum urate level. The appropriate level of serum uric acid must be adjusted for the method used and for the normal range in an individual laboratory. In general, equivalent limits for "autoanalyzer" methods are 10–20% higher than the concentrations indicated here for phosphotungstic acid methods.

4. Asymptomatic hyperuricemia without a secondary cause with urate levels persistently 9.0 mg/dL or greater by a phosphotungstic acid method (10–20% greater than this by some "autoanalyzer" methods).

With initiation of effective uricosuric therapy in man there is a prompt rise in urate clearance resulting in a decrease in the body pool of urate accompanied by an initial sharp rise in urinary uric acid. This rise persists until the body urate pool is reduced sufficiently to lower serum uric acid to a concentration at which a steady-state balance between urate production and excretion is again achieved despite persistence of increased urate clearance (GUTMAN, 1966). At this point the uric acid content in 24-h urine collections will be approximately the same as that prior to uricosuric therapy. A persistent, slight increase in uric acid excretion per 24 h is often observed. Since gastrointestinal elimination of urate is directly correlated with serum urate concentration, elimination of urate in the gastrointestinal tract is decreased at the lower serum urate concentrations found during uricosuric therapy (SORENSON, 1965). In normal man the total body urate pool is less than twice the daily urate elimination, and the increase in urinary uric acid usually abates after one or two days. The body urate pool is increased in patients with hyperuricemia and may be enormously increased in patients with extensive tophaceous gout. In these patients urinary uric acid may remain persistently elevated for weeks or months after initiation of uricosuric therapy.

Once the urate pool is reduced, 24-h excretion of uric acid will be determined by the rate of urate production. When patients are not on a purine-restricted diet, dietary purines will also alter urinary uric acid. Thus urinary excretion of uric acid will remain persistently elevated during uricosuric therapy in patients with uric acid overproduction but will generally fall to the normal range once the expanded body pool of urate is reduced in patients whose hyperuricemia was secondary to urate underexcretion.

The increase in renal excretion of urate that accompanies uricosuric therapy makes these drugs less desirable in patients with renal complications of gout. In patients with a history of renal stones, hyperuricosuria, or gouty nephropathy, allopurinol, which lowers both serum and urine uric acid, is to be preferred to uricosuric drugs. Successful uricosuric therapy requires reduction of serum uric acid to the normal range (GUTMAN, 1966), preferably to 1–2 mg/dL below the concentration at which plasma is saturated with urate. This satisfactory response cannot be achieved in all patients. In general, patients with significantly impaired renal function respond poorly, if at all, to uricosuric drugs (YÜ, 1974).

The sharp rise in urate excretion which accompanies initiation of uricosuric therapy is the time of greatest risk for renal stone formation or tubular deposition of urate. This risk is minimized by introduction of uricosuric therapy at low doses, with gradual increments until optimum control of serum uric acid is achieved. Patients are instructed to drink large amounts of fluid to maintain a large urine volume. Alkalinization of the urine can be employed to increase urate solubility but is not routinely required. Chronic alcohol ingestion may render uricosuric therapy ineffective. Inhibition of urate secretion ablates the response to uricosuric agents (Meisel and Diamond, 1977). Alcohol is metabolized to lactate in concentrations sufficient to inhibit urate secretion and the uricosuric response (Lieber et al., 1962; Yü et al., 1957).

Acute gout may develop during the initial reduction of the uric acid pool size toward normal. Prophylactic oral colchicine is generally administered along with uricosuric drugs to reduce the frequency of acute attacks of gout during the first several months of therapy or until all tophi have resolved.

F. Clinically Important Uricosuric Drugs

Probenecid was the first generally acceptable uricosuric agent (Taibott et al., 1951; Gutman and Yü, 1951) and remains the most widely used. Sulfinpyrazone, developed as an analog of phenylbutazone (Burns et al., 1957), is also available throughout the world. Zoxazolamine (Burns et al., 1958), a potent uricosuric agent, has largely been withdrawn from use because of hepatic and bone marrow toxicity. A newer potent uricosuric agent, benzbromarone, has been used for several years in Europe (Zollner et al., 1970; Sinclair and Fox, 1975) and is in clinical trials in the United States (Yü, 1976; Sorenson and Levinson, 1976). Ticrynafen is one of only a few diuretic agents with potent uricosuric properties (Reese and Steele, 1976).

I. Probenecid

1. Chemistry, Methods of Assay, and Pharmakokinetics

It is appropriate to begin the discussion of uricosuric drugs with probenecid, the first practical therapeutic uricosuric agent.

Probenecid was developed as part of a planned pharmacologic attempt to develop an organic acid inhibitor of renal tubular secretion of penicillin (Beyer, 1950). Carinamide was the first drug to be tried clinically as a result of this search. Its weak uricosuric properties were noted by Wolfson et al. (1948) while investigating its metabolism. Its rapid excretion and, therefore, short duration of action made it an impractical drug, and it was superceded by the introduction of probenecid (Beyer et al., 1951). Probenecid was synthesized as part of a systematic program to find an analog of carinamide that was a longer acting and more potent inhibitor of penicillin secretion.

In these studies probenecid was selected after it was found that dialkylsulfamyl benzoic acids were more potent than monoalkylsulfamyl benzoic acids and that these in turn were more potent than alkylsulfamilobenzoic acids of similar structure (Beyer et al., 1951). Among dialkylsulfamyl benzoic acids increasing length of the N-alkyl substitution is associated with decreasing clearance. Excretion of the dipropyl analog approaches zero (Weiner et al., 1960). Decreasing clearance in this series is related to increasing lipid solubility with increasing length of the N-alkyl substitution, which permits more complete reabsorption by passive non-ionic back diffusion in acid urine (Weiner et al., 1960).

Probenecid, p-(di-n-propylsulfamyl) benzoic acid (Fig. 3), is a white, odorless, crystalline powder that is practically insoluble in water and dilute acid but is soluble

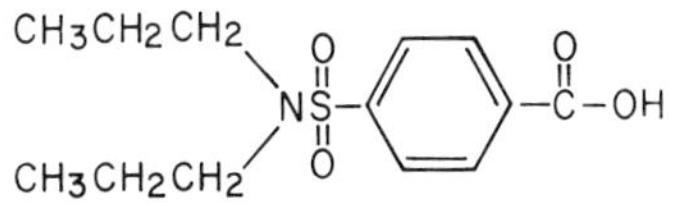

CH₃CH₂CH₂ ... Probenecid structure ... –C–OH

Fig. 3. Structure of probenecid

in alcohol, chloroform, acetone, and dilute alkali. The pK of probenecid is 3.4, which is high enough to permit almost complete reabsorption by passive non-ionic diffusion and along with its lipid solubility accounts for its low excretion rate and relatively long biologic half-life (WEINER et al., 1964). The 2-nitro, 2-hydroxyl, and 2-chloro analogs, which are all stronger acids, are about ten times as potent as probenecid on a weight basis as uricosuric agents (BLANCHARD et al., 1972). There is no correlation between ability to inhibit PAH excretion or renal excretion of these drugs and uricosuric potency. The basis for this difference in uricosuric potency is uncertain. Uricosuric activity might correlate with drug concentration in the proximal tubule as proposed by GUTMAN et al. (1960) but this has not been established.

Probenecid concentration in biologic fluids has most often been measured by spectrophotometric methods (DAYTON et al., 1963). These methods lack specificity, are only moderately sensitive and reproducible, and may detect some probenecid metabolites. Gas chromatography using the n-dibutyl analog of probenecid as an internal standard provides a more specific and sensitive assay (ZACCHEI and WEIDNER, 1973). The internal standard is prepared by mixing for 10 min 1 ml of plasma or 3 ml of urine containing 15 µg internal standard (in 1 ml phosphate buffer pH 7.0) with 2 N HCl (1 ml) and 25 ml of benzene. At least 20 ml of the organic phase is removed after centrifugation and mixed weth 2 ml of 0.1 N NaOH. The organic phase is discarded and free acids are extracted from the aqueous phase into methylene chloride (5 ml) after adjustment of the pH to 1. The methylene chloride phase is then treated with 0.1 ml of an ethereal solution of diazomethane and evaporated in a warm water bath under nitrogen. The residue is dissolved in ethyl acetate and aliquots are injected into the gas chromatograph. Standard curves are constructed by plotting peak height ratios (probenecid/dibutyl analog) versus weight ratios. The amount of probenecid in unknown samples is then determined from peak heights when standard and unknown samples are run simultaneously.

Probenecid is rapidly absorbed following oral administration in man (DAYTON and PEREL, 1971). Peak serum concentrations are obtained in 2–3 h following 1 g oral dose. The plasma half-life is variable and dose dependent, ranging from 4–12 h, probably due to saturation of metabolic pathways or hepatic uptake (DAYTON et al., 1963; DAYTON and PEREL, 1971). Considerable differences in half-life in individual subjects are also noted. Probenecid is almost completely reabsorbed by non-ionic diffusion in acid urine so that elimination is largely by metabolism. Only 4–13% of administered probenecid is excreted unchanged (MELETHIL and CONWAY, 1976). The major metabolic product excreted in the urine is probenecid monoacyl glucuronide (34–47%). Other excreted products include the mono N-propyl, secondary alcohol, and carboxylic metabolites. Some of the metabolites have uricosuric activity in animals (ISRAILI et al., 1972). Probenecid and its conjugated metabolites are excreted in the bile and may undergo enterohepatic circulation (SABIH et al., 1971). At concentrations in the

Table. 2. Inhibition of organic acid transport by probenecid

1. Inhibition of tubular secretion of organic acids	
Penicillin	(BEYER et al., 1951)
p-Aminosalicylic acid	(BOGER and PITTS, 1950)
p-Aminohippuric acid	(BEYER et al., 1951)
Phenolsulfonphthalein	(BEYER, 1950)
Androsterone	(GARDNER et al., 1951)
Salicylate and its acyl and phenolic glucuronides	(GUTMAN et al., 1955; SCHACTER and MANIS 1958; WEINER et al., 1959)
Pantothenic acid	(BOGER et al., 1953)
Phlorizon and its glucuronide	(BRAUN et al., 1957)
Acetazolamide	(WEINER et al., 1959)
Corticotropin	(BONAR and PERKINS, 1962)
Ampicillin	(KLEIN and FINLAND, 1963)
Dapsone	(GOODWIN and SPARELL, 1969)
Indomethacin	(SKEITH et al., 1968)
Sulfinpyrazone	(PEREL et al., 1969)
Cephradine	(MISCHLER et al., 1974)
Methrotrexate	(BOURKE et al., 1975)
2. Inhibition of hepatic uptake	
Bromsulfonphthalein	(GOETZEE et al., 1960)
Indocyanine Green	(VOGIN et al., 1960)
Rifamycin	(KENWRIGHT and LEVI, 1973)
Methrotrexate	(KATES et al., 1976)
3. Inhibition of cerebrospinal fluid transport	
Biogenic amines	(TAMARKIN et al., 1970)
Penicillin	(SPECTOR and LORENZO, 1974)

therapeutic range, probenecid is extensively bound to plasma proteins (89–94%) and its volume of distribution is limited largely to extracellular fluid (DAYTON and PEREL, 1971). Probenecid crosses both the cerebrospinal fluid and placental barriers. Renal excretion of probenecid is greatly increased when passive non-ionic reabsorption is inhibited in alkaline urine, and net tubular secretion can then be demonstrated (WEINER et al., 1964). This increased excretion is associated with an increase in uricosuric effect (YÜ et al., 1977).

2. Biologic Effects

Most biologic effects of probenecid (Table 2) appear to result from inhibition of transport of organic acids across membrane barriers. Probenecid is a competitive inhibitor of renal tubular secretion and thereby of excretion of many organic acids including PAH and penicillin (BEYER, 1951; GUTMAN and YÜ, 1957a; WEINER et al., 1959). Probenecid is also known to inhibit the hepatic uptake and biliary excretion of several drugs including bromsulfthalein (GOETZEE et al., 1960), iodocyanine green (VOGIN et al., 1966), rifamycin (KENWRIGHT and LEVI, 1973), and methotrexate (KATES et al., 1976). Competition for hepatic uptake has not been well studied, and some drug interactions may be explained in part by this mechanism. For example, pyrazinamide administration increases probenecid blood levels, perhaps by impairing the hepatic uptake and metabolism or biliary excretion of probenecid (YÜ et al.,

Table 3. Comparison of some clinically useful uricosuric drugs

	Probenecid	Sulfinpyrazone	Benzbromarone	Tienilic acid
After oral dose:				
Time of:				
Peak blood level	2— 3 h	1 h	2— 4 h	3— 4 h
Peak uricosuric	2— 3 h	1— 3 h	6—12 h	3— 5 h
Duration of uricosuria	4—12 h	6—10 h	48 h	12—24 h
Starting dose per day	500 mg	200 mg	20—40 mg	125 mg
Maximum dose per day	2 g	800 mg	80 mg	500 mg
Effect of PZA on uricosuric response	Marked inhibition	Marked inhibition	Partial inhibition	Partial inhibition
Specific toxicity in man	G.I.	G.I. marrow (rare)	diarrhea, other G.I.	hypokalemia, azotemia

G.I. = gastrointestinal; PZA = pyrazinamide

1977). Changes in volume of distribution of penicillin group drugs (GIBALDI and SCHWARTZ, 1968) may also reflect impaired hepatic uptake. Inhibition of hepatic uptake of drugs and normal metabolites might lead to a variety of unanticipated biologic effects. This area has not been extensively studied. Probenecid increases the concentration of biogenic amines in cerebrospinal fluid (TAMERKIN et al., 1970; PEREL et al., 1974) and inhibits the transport of penicillin and p-aminosalicylic acid into the choroid plexus and out of cerebrospinal fluid (SPECTOR and LORENZO, 1974). Drugs may affect the uricosuric response to probenecid by inhibition of probenecid secretion (YÜ et al., 1963; MEISEL and DIAMOND, 1977), inhibition of urate secretion (STEELE and BONER, 1973; MEISEL and DIAMOND, 1977), or inhibition of non-ionic reabsorption of probenecid (YÜ et al., 1977). Other possible mechanisms of interaction including changes in probenecid metabolism (YÜ et al., 1977) and inhibition of binding to the urate reabsorption carrier are possible but have not been demonstrated.

The uricosuric response to probenecid appears promptly after intravenous administration and is evident within 30–40 min after oral administration. Following a 2-g oral dose of probenecid, urate excretion increases approximately fourfold with peak excretion usually occurring 1–2 h after the oral dose (SIROTA et al., 1952). In one large series of patients with gout, serum urate was satisfactorily controlled on 1 g or less of probenecid in approximately 50% of patients and on 2 g or less in 85% of patients (GUTMAN and YÜ, 1957b). When used for the treatment of gout, the initial dose is 250 mg twice daily (one-half of a 500-mg tablet). The uricosuric response and serum urate levels are then observed, and the dose is increased at weekly intervals (by 500 mg/day in divided doses) until a satisfactory therapeutic response is achieved (Table 3).

3. Toxicology

Acute toxicity from overdosage both in animals and man is primarily related to the central nervous system. Clinical features include vomiting, muscle twitching, hyperactive deep tendon reflexes, coma, and seizures (RIZZUTO, V.J., et al., 1965). As much as 47.5 g has been ingested with survival.

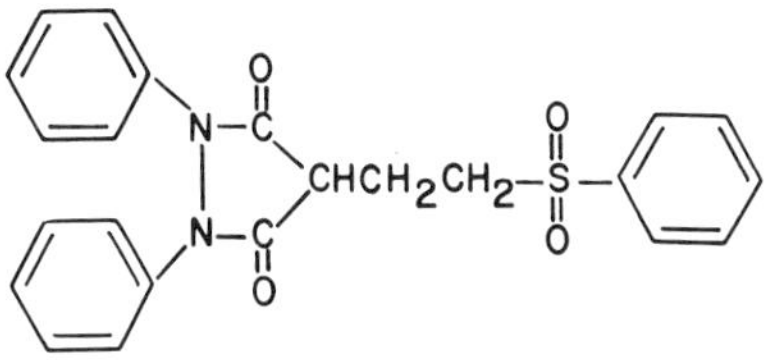

Sulfinpyrazone

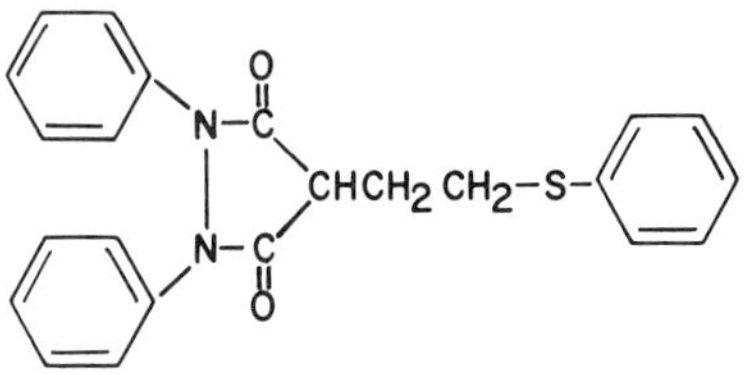

G-25671

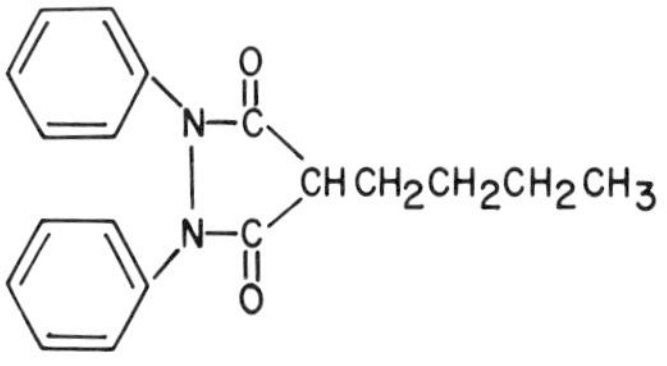

Phenylbutazone

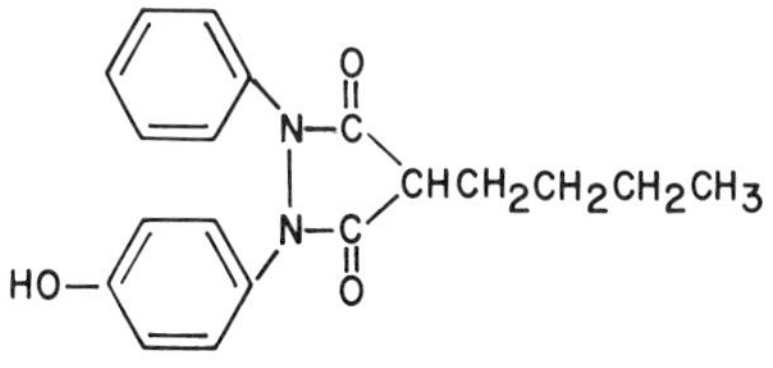

Oxyphenbutazone

Fig. 4. Structure of sulfinpyrazone and related pyrazolidinedrones

Probenecid is well tolerated in long-term use. In the large series reported by GUTMAN and YÜ (1957b) gastrointestinal side effects were noted in 80% of patients and rash or other hypersensitivity reaction in 5%. Other complications of probenecid therapy are precipitation of acute attacks of gout, seen in 10% of patients treated by GUTMAN and YÜ (1957b) and urolithiasis, observed in 9% of patients in this series. Both these complications are common to all uricosuric drugs and are largely preventable. The incidence of acute gout following uricosuric therapy can be greatly reduced by concommitant low-dose colchicine prophylaxis. The incidence of renal stones can be reduced by gradual introduction of uricosuric therapy, maintenance of a large urine volume, and alkalinization of the urine when necessary.

II. Sulfinpyrazone and Related Pyrazolidinediones

Sulfinpyrazone (1,2-diphenyl-4-(2′-phenylsulfinethyl)-3,5-pyrazolidinedione) was first isolated from urine (BURNS et al., 1957) as the sulfoxide metabolite of the phenylbutazone analogue G-25671 (Fig. 4). Identification of sulfinpyrazone was the end point of studies of properties of more than 80 pyrazolidinediones beginning with phenylbutazone. Structure activity relationships of this group of drugs have been reviewed in detail by GUTMAN (1966). Uricosuric potency varies inversely with pK_a—analogs with $pK_a < 4$ are potent uricosuric agents (GUTMAN et al., 1960). Maximum uricosuria is attained at a pK_a of approximately 3 (pK_a of sulfinpyrazone is 2.8) with no further increment in uricosuric activity with more acidic analogs. The rate of excretion of these compounds also varies inversely with pK_a indicating that reabsorption is attributable to non-ionic back diffusion. Uricosuric potency correlates directly with excretion rate and thus with concentration in the renal tubule. There is no correlation among the pyrazolidinediones between uricosuric potency and lipid solubility, plasma protein binding, or plasma half-life (GUTMAN, 1966). Sulfinpyrazone lacks the potent anti-inflammatory activity of phenylbutazone and oxyphenbutazone.

1. Method of Assay

Assay of sulfinpyrazone and its analogs has generally been performed by an ultraviolet spectrophotometric method (DAYTON et al., 1961), with limited specificity. Recently, a more specific method employing liquid chromatography with ^{14}C sulfinpyrazone as an internal standard has been reported (INABA et al., 1975).

In this method, 0.5-ml serum aliquots are mixed with 0.5 ml 1 N HCl, 2 ml 1-chlorobutane, and ^{14}C sulfinpyrazone as an internal standard. Aliquots (1 ml) are evaporated to dryness, the residue is dissolved in 100 μl methanol, and 8 μl is injected into a Varian Model 4010-01 liquid chromatograph equipped with a Micro-Pak S 1-10 column (silicon gel 10-μm particle; Varian 25 cm, 2.2 mn internal diameter). A dioxane-methanol solvent (65:35) is delivered at a flow of 0.7 ml/min. Samples are read at 254 nm in an ultraviolet detector, and the peak area is read against a standard curve after subtraction of blanks and correction for recovery of radioactive internal standard.

2. Pharmacokinetics

Pharmacokinetics have been studied following administration of ^{14}C-labeled sulfinpyrazone (DIETERLE et al., 1975). Absorption of sulfinpyrazone from the gastrointestinal tract is rapid and complete in normal man, the plasma concentration reaching a peak of approximately 20 μg/ml after 1 h. The half-life after an oral dose is approximately 2–3 h. Tissue distribution of sulfinpyrazone is largely limited to extracellular fluid. In man, approximately 98% of plasma sulfinpyrazone is bound to plasma proteins. Renal excretion, therefore, is by tubular secretion. More than 85% of an administered dose was recovered from the urine within four days. Approximately 30% of excreted material is unaltered sulfinpyrazone. Even in acid urine, sulfinpyrazone with a pK_a of 2.8 is largely ionized and therefore little is reabsorbed by nonionic diffusion. The major urinary metabolite is the glucuronide of sulfinpyrazone. Approximately 8% is excreted as the para-hydroxyl metabolite. This metabolite is known to be a potent uricosuric agent itself and may contribute to the uricosuric activity of the parent compound (DAYTON et al., 1961). Sulfinpyrazone competes for secretion with PAH, probenecid, and salicylate (BURNS et al., 1957; YÜ et al., 1963; PEREL et al., 1969).

3. Biologic Effects

Sulfinpyrazone is a potent uricosuric agent with activity on a molar or weight basis two to six times that of probenecid (BURNS et al., 1957; EMMERSON, R., 1963). A 35-mg intravenous dose has a uricosuric effect compared to a minimum 100-mg dose of probenecid (BURNS et al., 1957). In chronic use, 400 mg per day produces uricosuria equivalent to 1.5 g to 2 g per day of probenecid. Maximum uricosuric response is about seven times control and increases urate excretion to approximately 50% of the

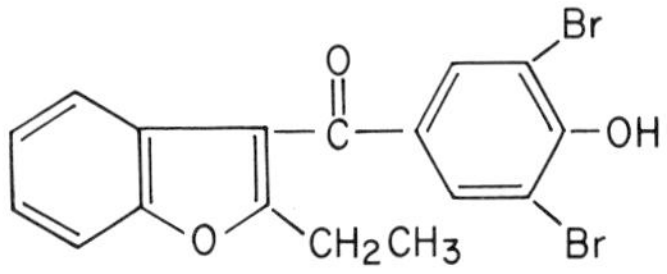

Benzbromarone

Fig. 5. Structure of benzbromarone

estimated filtered load. Net urate secretion can be demonstrated in man by administration of sulfinpyrazone after urate loading and mannitol infusion (GUTMAN et al., 1959). A paradoxical effect on urate excretion in man has not been unequivocally demonstrated. The uricosuric effect is attenuated by salicylate (YÜ et al., 1963) and by pyrazinamide (DIAMOND and PAOLINO, 1973).

Sulfinpyrazone impairs platelet aggregation and prolongs platelet survival (SMYTHE et al., 1965). Thus, its use has been advocated for prevention of venous thrombosis and formation of thrombi on prostheses (WEILY and GENTON, 1970; STEELE et al., 1973).

In the treatment of gout, the initial dose is 50 mg twice daily. The dose is then increased in 100 mg/day increments weekly until serum uric acid is in the normal range. Hyperuricemia can be controlled in most patients on 200–400 mg per day divided between two doses. Precautions to prevent tubular deposition of urate and stone are the same as for probenecid.

4. Toxicology

Gastrointestinal toxicity is found in 10–15% of patients, rash in less than 3% (EMMERSON, 1963; GUTMAN, 1966). Bone marrow depression is infrequent but has been reported (GUTMAN, 1966). Sulfinpyrazone may potentiate the activity of sulfa drugs and oral hypoglycemic agents.

III. Benzbromarone and Related Drugs

The benzofuran derivative benzbromarone (3-(3,5 dibromo-4 hydroxybenzoyl)-2 ethylbenzofuran) (Fig. 5) is a potent uricosuric agent that has been used extensively in Europe and is presently undergoing clinical trials in North America. The closely related compound benzioderone, which differs only in substitution of iodine for bromine atoms, was developed first and is also a potent uricosuric agent but was withdrawn because of toxicity related to the iodine content.

1. Pharmacokinetics and Assay

Benzbromarone is essentially insoluble in water and only slightly soluble in $1N$ sodium hydroxide. Absorption following oral administration in man is variable, with micronized preparations employed in recent studies in North America giving significantly better absorption than the nonmicronized preparations used in earlier studies in Europe. Following absorption the drug is rapidly dehalogenated to the monobromine, bromobenzarone, and then the dehalogenated compound, benzarone, so that beyond 2–4 h after administration of a single dose most drug in plasma appears as metabolites, notably benzarone (BROEKHUYSEN et al., 1972; YÜ, 1976). Some of the metabolites are conjugated with glucuronic acid. Renal excretion is slow with biliary excretion, primarily of benzarone, being the major route of elimination and accounting for approximately 60% of benzarone excretion. After a single oral dose of benzbromarone, peak serum levels are found at 2–4 h and decline rapidly therafter. Peak levels of the metabolites occur at 4–6 h or later and decline more slowly with a half-life in excess of 12 h. Time of peak uricosuric response varies widely among different subjects but does not correlate with benzbromarone blood levels. The dehalogenated metabolite benzarone is uricosuric (DELBARRE et al., 1967), and uricosuric activity correlates better with plasma concentration of metabolites than with concentration of benzbromarone.

Benzbromarone and its principle metabolites can be assayed by gas-liquid chromatography after extraction from acidified urine with cyclohexane and acetylation with acetic anhydride (YÜ et al., 1976).

In rats, a species showing a uricosuric response to benzbromarone comparable to that of man, microinjection studies indicate that benzbromarone decreases urate reabsorption in the proximal tubule (KRAMP and LENOIR, 1975). In common with other uricosuric drugs, benzbromarone inhibits tubular secretion of other organic acids. On a weight basis benzbromarone is about twice as potent as sulfinpyrazone in prolonging the disappearance from plasma of intravenously injected phenol red. However, benzbromarone does not interfere with the urinary excretion of penicillin. Benzbromarone has no clinically significant anti-inflammatory or platelet aggregation-inhibiting properties.

2. Biologic Effects

Benzbromarone is one of the most potent of the known uricosuric agents with 100 mg per day of micronized benzbromarone giving a uricosuric response approximately equivalent to that obtained with 1 g per day of probenecid (JAIN et al., 1974). Uricosuric response increases gradually to a maximum at 8–12 h and persists for 48 h after a single oral dose (ZOLLNER et al., 1970; JAIN et al., 1974).

Benzbromarone inhibits xanthine oxidase in vitro, but this effect is probably not clinically important since concentrations necessary to inhibit the enzyme are in excess of those achieved by recommended oral doses in man (SINCLAIR and FOX, 1975). There is no increase in urinary oxypurines following benzbromarone administration, suggesting that xanthine oxidase is not inhibited in vivo (SORENSON and LEVINSON, 1976).

Benzbromarone is administered in single daily doses with maximum recommended doses varying with the form (micronized 80 mg/day; nonmicronized 100 mg/day). Adjustment of dose and precautions to prevent acute attack of gout, tubular deposition of urate, and stone formation are the same as for other uricosuric drugs. In common with other uricosuric drugs, the uricosuric effect of benzbromarone is antagonized by salicylate (SORENSON and LEVINSON, 1976; SINCLAIR and FOX, 1975). However, benzbromarone retains significant uricosuric activity during salicylate administration. Pyrazinamide also antagonizes the uricosuric effect (SORENSON and LEVINSON, 1976).

3. Toxicology

In most published reports benzbromarone appears to have been well tolerated. Gastrointestinal side effects, including diarrhea, are the most commonly reported side effects in clinical use (YÜ, 1976). Rash and hypersensitivity reactions have been reported but appear to be infrequent. There is little data on drug interactions other than as they relate to urate excretion.

IV. Tienilic Acid (Ticrynafen) and Other Uricosuric Diuretics

Most diuretic agents cause renal retention of uric acid probably due to extracellular fluid volume depletion (WEINMAN et al., 1975; STEELE and OPPENHEIMER, 1969), although thiazide diuretics are uricosuric when given intravenously (HEALEY et al., 1959; DEMARTINI et al., 1962). Net secretion of urate can be readily demonstrated in the chimpanzee by the administration of the organomercurial mersalyl (FANELLI et al., 1973b). Intravenous mersalyl is also a potent uricosuric agent in man although net secretion of urate in man is not demonstrated after mersalyl (FANELLI and HITZENBERGER, 1974). FANELLI and co-workers (1977a, b) have reported on the pharmacology and uricosuric properties in the chimpanzee of a new uricosuric and diuretic agent with the chemical structure (6,7-dichloro-2-methyl-1-oxo-2-phenyl-5-indenyloxy)acetic acid. This agent appears to inhibit both urate secretion and reabsorption and may, therefore, be a less effective uricosuric agent in man than in the chimpanzee.

Tienilic acid,2,3-dichloro-4-(2-thienylcarbonyl)phenoxy acetic acid (Ticrynafen) is a diuretic, chemically related to ethacrynic acid (Fig. 6) but lacking the alpha-beta unsaturated side chain which confers sulfhydryl reactivity on the latter compound (STOTE et al., 1976). Its saluretic action is more nearly like that of a thiazide diuretic than ethacrynic acid. However, unlike thiazide diuretics it is a potent uricosuric agent in man following oral administration (MASBERNARD and GIUDICELLI, 1974; REESE and STEELE, 1976; STOTE et al., 1976). It also has been used in the management of arterial hypertension (MASBERNARD and GIUDICELLI, 1974). Tienilic acid is presently in clinical trial in Europe (ANP-3624, Anphar Laboratories) and in the United States (SKF-62698, Smith, Kline, and French Laboratories; generic name in the United States, Ticrynafen) for use as a diuretic, antihypertensive, and uricosuric agent.

Tienilic acid is the most potent uricosuric agent yet reported in the mongrel dog (LEMIEUX et al., 1977), a species where most urate transport is thought to occur in the proximal tubule (ZINS and WEINER, 1968). This and stop-flow studies in the dog (LEMIEUX et al., 1977) suggest a proximal tubule site of action for the uricosuric effect. As a diuretic, the drug is thought to act on the cortical diluting segment (STOTE et al., 1976). Tienilic acid competes with PAH for secretion and would probably interact with other drugs secreted by the PAH-sensitive organic acid carrier system (LEMIEUX et al., 1977; REESE and STEELE, 1976). Tienilic acid is also uricosuric in the rat but is urate retaining in the rabbit, Dalmation dog, guinea pig, and chicken (LEMIEUX et al., 1977). Diuretic activity can also be demonstrated in many animal species. A paradoxical effect on urate excretion has not been found with doses of 10–50 mg (STOTE et al., 1976).

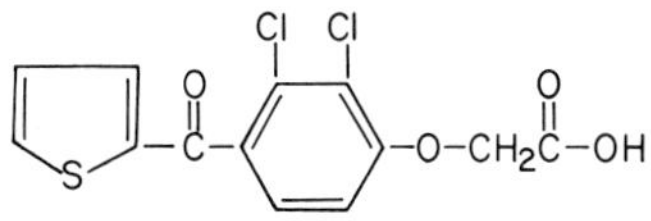

Tienilic Acid

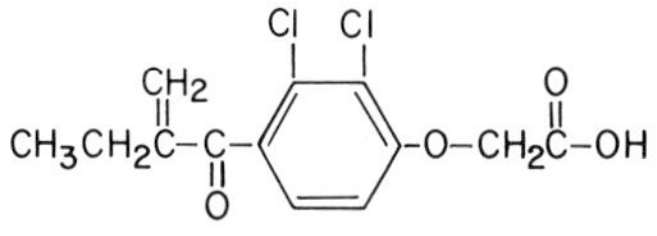

Ethacrynic Acid

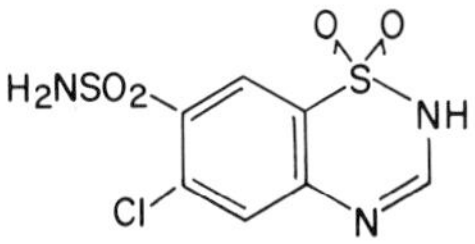

Chlorothiazide

Fig. 6. Structure of tienilic acid (Ticrynafen), ethacrynic acid, and chlorothiazide

1. Pharmacokinetics and Assays

A gas-chromatographic method for assay of tienilic acid in biologic material has recently been developed and used for improved assay of the pharmacokinetics of the drug (HWANG et al., 1978). This method employs methylation of carboxylic acid groups and transmethylsilyation of the hydroxyl group of one metabolite. Earlier methods did not separate the parent drug from one of its metabolites. Urine, plasma, and serum samples (1 ml) are diluted with 2 ml of $1N$ HCl, mixed for 45 min with 10 ml of diethyl ether and centrifuged. Seven ml of the organic layer is mixed with 0.5 ml of diazomethane solution at ice bath temperature for 1 h, then evaporated at 40° C under nitrogen, washed with methanol, and dried by evaporation. One ml of a mixture of acetonitrile containing an internal standard (the methyl ester of ethacrynic acid), pyridene, and silylating agent (bis-trimethylsilyl-trifluro-acetamide plus 10% trimethylchlorosilane) (75:10:15), is added and 3 h allowed before injection of the sample into the gas chromatograph for analysis.

Tienilic acid is extensively bound to plasma proteins in all mammals studied (DORMARD et al., 1976). Tienilic acid is metabolized to two major metabolites, one formed by reduction of the ketone, the other by oxidation of the thienyl carbonyl moiety to an acid (DORMARD et al., 1976). Glycine conjugates of these metabolites probably also appear in some mammals. Not all of the urinary metabolites of tienilic acid have been identified. Plasma levels of tienilic acid and its metabolites reach a peak value 3–4 h after administration in man (HWANG et al., 1978). Conjugated metabolites of the drug are found in bile in some species. Pharmacokinetic studies in man are incomplete. The major metabolites have not been studied for uricosuric activity in man. Half-life in man appears to be 6–12 h or less.

2. Biologic Effects

In recent studies, the uricosuric activity of tienilic acid is comparable to other established uricosuric drugs, a single 1-g dose producing a three- to fivefold increase in urate excretion (STOTE et al., 1976). In chronic use, uricosuric effects may be somewhat less striking, perhaps because of volume depletion induced by the drug's diuretic effect.

The uricosuric response to tienilic acid is reduced but not eliminated following administration of pyrazinamide (STOTE et al., 1976; REESE and STEELE, 1976; PRASAD et al., 1977). Tienilic acid does not alter pyrazinamide metabolism or net excretion (PRASAD et al., 1977). These results have been interpreted as suggesting that tienilic acid inhibits reabsorption of both filtered and secreted urate. Differences in degree of suppression of uricosuric response by pyrazinamide in reported studies can be accounted for by differences in the timing of administration of the two drugs and in the dose of tienilic acid. Following oral administration in man pyrazinamide is metabolized slowly to pyrazinoic acid, the actual inhibitor of urate secretion (WEINER and TINKER, 1972). Maximum suppression of urate secretion does not appear for at least 90 min after oral administration but then is stable for several hours. Thus for accurate studies of pyrazinamide-induced suppression of uricosuria, pyrazinamide should be administered 90 min prior to administration of the uricosuric drug and uricosuric response compared to that obtained when the uricosuric drug is administered alone.

Diuretic and antihypertensive effects appear comparable to those of commonly used thiazide diuretics except that there may be an increased propensity to hypokalemia (REESE and STEELE, 1976; STOTE et al., 1976). In common with some thiazide diuretics, tienilic acid may potentiate prothrombin antagonist anticoagulants and may impair glucose tolerance. Recommended doses for chronic clinical use of tienilic acid have not been established.

3. Toxicology

Known toxicity of tienilic acid relates to its uricosuric and diuretic properties. Risk of tubular deposition of urate or renal stone formation is similar to that with other uricosuric agents and similar precautions are indicated although the concomitant diuretic effect of tienilic acid may provide some protection. Substantial increases in serum uric acid, which may occur upon discontinuation of medication, can be accounted for by diuretic-induced volume depletion.

Hyponatremia, hypokalemia, hypochloremic alkalosis, and elevations in blood urea nitrogen and serum creatinine can occur and are secondary to its diuretic properties.

The clinical importance of tienilic acid and other uricosuric diuretics is uncertain. Hypertension is a frequent clinical finding in patients with gout (CANNON et al., 1966) and hyperuricemia, most often asymptomatic, is a frequent complication of diuretic management (DOLLERY et al., 1960). Both hyperuricosuria (EMMERSON and Row, 1975) and hyperuricemia (MURRAY and GOLDBERG, 1975) have been suggested as risk factors for nephropathy. Uricosuric diuretics would reduce hyperuricemia at the expense of at least intermittant hyperuricosuria. Indications for use of these drugs remain to be established.

References

Arias, I. R., Fleischner, G., Kirsch, R., Mishkin, S., Gatmaiten, Z.: On the structure, regulation, and function of ligandin. In: Arias, I. M., Jakoby, W. B. (Eds.): Glutathione: Metabolism and Function. New York: Raven Press 1976

Berger, L., Yü, T. F., Gutman, A. B.: Effect of drugs that alter uric acid excretion in man on uric acid clearance in the chicken. Amer. J. Physiol. **198**, 575—580 (1960)

Beyer, K. H.: Functional characteristics of renal transport mechanisms. Pharmacol. Rev. **2**, 227—280 (1950)

Beyer, K. H.: Factors basic to the development of useful inhibitors of renal transport mechanisms. Arch. int. Pharmacodyn. **98**, 97—117 (1954)

Beyer, K. H., Russo, H. F., Tillson, E. K., Miller, A. K., Verwey, W. F., Gass, S. R.: "Benemid," p-(di-N-propyl-sulfamyl)-benzoic acid: its renal affinity and elimination. Amer. J. Physiol. **166**, 625—640 (1951)

Blanchard, K. C., Maroske, D., May, D. G., Weiner, I. M.: Uricosuric potency of 2-substituted analogs of probenecid. J. Pharmacol. exp. Ther. **180**, 397—410 (1972)

Bluestone, R. I., Kippen, I., Klinenberg, J. R., Whitehouse, M. W.: Effect of some uricosuric and antiinflammatory drugs on the binding of uric acid to human serum albumen. J. Lab. clin. Med. **76**, 85—91 (1970)

Boger, W. P., Bayne, G. M., Gylfe, J., Wright, L. D.: Renal clearance of pantothenic acid in man: inhibition by probenecid ("Benemid"). Proc. Soc. exp. Biol. (N.Y.) **82**, 604—608 (1953)

Boger, W. P., Pitts, F. W.: Plasma concentrations of p—Amino Salicylic acid (PAS) increased by p(Di-n-propylsulfamyl)benzoic acid. Science **112**, 149—153 (1950)

Bonar, J. A., Perkins, W. H.: Inhibition of urinary excretion of iodine[131]-labeled corticotropin by probenecid. J. clin. Endocr. **22**, 38—42 (1962)

Boner, G., Steele, T. H.: Relationship of urate and p-aminohippurate secretion in man. Amer. J. Physiol. **225**, 100—104 (1973)

Bourke, R. S., Chheda, G., Bremer, A., Watanabe, O., Tower, D. B.: Inhibition of renal tubular transport of methotrexat by probenecid. Cancer Res. 35, 110—116 (1975)

Braun, W., Whittaker, V. P., Lotspeich, W. F.: Renal excretion of phlorizon and phlorizon glucuronide. Amer. J. Physiol. **190**, 563—567 (1957)

Broekhuysen, J., Pacco, M., Sion, R., Demeulen, L., Vanhee, M.: Metabolism of benzbromarone in man. Europ. J. clin. Pharmacol. **4**, 125—130 (1972)

Burns, J. J., Yü, T. F., Berger, L., Gutman, A. B.: Zoxazolamine. Physiological disposition, uricosuric properties. Amer. J. Med. **25**, 401—408 (1958)

Burns, J. J., Yü, T. F., Ritterand, A., Perel, J. M., Gutman, A. B., Brodie, B. B.: A potent new uricosuric agent, the sulfoxide metabolite of the phenylbutazone analogue, G-25671. J. Pharmacol. exp. Ther. **119**, 418—426 (1957)

Campion, D. S., Bluestone, R., Klinenberg, J. R.: Uric acid: characterization of its interaction with human serum albumen. J. clin. Invest. **52**, 2383—2387 (1973)

Cannon, P. J., Stason, W. B., DeMartini, F. E., Sommers, S. C., Laragh, J. H.: Hyperuricemia in primary and renal hypertension. New Engl. J. Med. **275**, 457—464 (1966)

Cho, K. C., Cafruny, E. J.: Renal tubular reabsorption of p-aminohippuric acid (PAH) in the dog. J. Pharmacol. exp. Ther. **173**, 1—12 (1970)

Dantzler, W. H.: Characteristics of urate transport by isolated perfused snake tubules. Amer. J. Physiol. **224**, 445—453 (1973)

Dayton, P. G., Perel, J. M.: The metabolism of probenecid in man. Ann. N.Y. Acad. Sci. **179**, 399—402 (1971)

Dayton, P. G., Perel, J. M., Snell, M. M., Yü, T. F., Gutman, A. B.: The physiological disposition of probenecid including renal clearance in man; studies by an improved method for its estimation in biologic material. J. Pharmacol. exp. Ther. **140**, 278—286 (1963)

Dayton, P. G., Sicam, L. E., Landrau, M., Burns, J. J.: Metabolism of sulfinpyrazone (anturiane) and other thio analogues of phenylbutazone in man. J. Pharmacol. exp. Ther. **132**, 287—290 (1961)

Delbarre, F., Auscher, C., Oliver, J., Rose, A.: Traitement des hyperuricemics et de la goutte par des derives du benzofuranne. Sem. Hôp. Paris **43**, 1127—1133 (1967)

Demartini, F. E., Wheaton, E. A., Healey, L. A., Laragh, J. H.: Effect of chlorothiazide on the renal excretion of uric acid. Amer. J. Med. **32**, 572—577 (1962)

Diamond, H. S., Meisel, A. D.: Effect of pharmacological inhibitors on urate transport during induced uricosuria. Clin. Sci. Mol. Med. **53**, 133—139 (1977)

Diamond, H. S., Meisel, A. D., Kaplan, D.: Renal tubular transport of urate in man. Bull. rheum. Dis. **27**, 876—881 (1976-7)

Diamond, H. S., Meisel, A., Sharon, E., Holden, D., Cacatian, A.: Hyperuricosuria and increased tubular secretion of urate in sickle cell anemia. Amer. J. Med. **59**, 796—802 (1975)

Diamond, H. S., Paolino, J. S.: Evidence for a post secretory reabsorptive site for uric acid in man. J. clin. Invest. **52**, 503—510 (1973)

Dieterle, W., Faigle, J. W., Richter, W. J., Theobald, W.: Biotransformation and pharmacokinetics of sulfinpyrazone (Anturan) in man. Eur. J. clin. Pharmacol. **9**, 135—145 (1975)

Dollery, C. T., Duncan, H., Schumer, B.: Hyperuricemia related to treatment of hypertension. Brit. med. J. **1960 II**, 832—835

Dormard, Y., Levron, J. C., Adnot, P., Lebedeff, T., Ejaubault, G.: Pharmacokinetic study of 2,-3dichloro4-(2-thienyl keto ^{14}C)phenoxyacetic acid (Tienilic acid) in mammals. Europ. J. Drug. Metab. Pharmac. **1**, 41—49 (1976)

Emmerson, B. T.: A comparison of uricosuric agents in gout with special reference to sulfinpyrazone. Med. J. Aust. **1**, 839—844 (1963)

Emmerson, B. T., Row, P. G.: An evaluation of the pathogenesis of the gouty kidney. Kidney Int. **8**, 65—71 (1975)

Fanelli, G. M., Bohn, D., Reilly, S.: Renal urate transport in the chimpanzee. Amer. J. Physiol. **220**, 613—620 (1971 a)

Fanelli, G. M., Bohn, D. L., Reilly, S. S.: Renal effects of uricosuric agents in the chimpanzee. J. Pharmacol. exp. Ther. **177**, 591—599 (1971 b)

Fanelli, G. M., Bohn, D. L., Reilly, S. S.: Effects of merurial diuretics on renal transport of urate and p-aminohippurate in the cebus monkey. Amer. J. Physiol. **224**, 993—996 (1973 a)

Fanelli, G. M., Bohn, D. L., Reilly, S. S., Weiner, I. M.: Effects of mercurial diuretics on renal transport of urate in the chimpanzee. Amer. J. Physiol. **224**, 985—992 (1973 b)

Fanelli, G. M., Bohn, D. L., Scriabine, A., Beyer, K. H.: Saluretic and uricosuric effects of (6,7-dichloro-2-methyl-1-oxo-2-phenyl-5-indanyloxy)acetic acid (Mk-196) in the chimpanzee. J. Pharmacol. exp. Ther. **200**, 402—412 (1977 a)

Fanelli, G. M., Bohn, D. L., Stafford, S.: Functional characteristics of renal urate transport in the cebus monkey. Amer. J. Physiol. **218**, 627—636 (1970)

Fanelli, G. M., Bohn, D. L., Zacchei, A. G.: Renal excretion of a saluretic-uricosuric agent (Mk-196) and interaction with a urate-retaining drug, pyrazinoate, in the chimpanzee. J. Pharmacol. exp. Ther. **200**, 413—419 (1977 b)

Fanelli, G. M., Hitzenberger, G.: Uricosuric activity of intravenous mersalyl in man. Medikon. **3**, 12—13 (1974)

Fanelli, G. M., Weiner, I. M.: Pyrazinoate excretion in the chimpanzee; relation to urate disposition and the actions of uricosuric drugs. J. clin. Invest. **52**, 1946—1957 (1973)

Farrel, P. C.: Protein binding of urate ions in vitro and in vivo. Progr. Biochem. Pharmacol. **9**, 153—162 (1972)

Fulop, M., Drabkin, A.: Potassium depletion syndrome secondary to nephropathy apparently caused by "outdated" tetracycline. New Engl. J. Med. **272**, 986—989 (1965)

Frankfort, S. J., Weinman, E. J.: The effect of probenecid on urate transport in the rat kidney. Proc. Soc. exp. Biol. (N.Y.) **155**, 554—557 (1977)

Gardner, L. I., Crigler, J. R., Migeon, C. J.: Inhibition of urinary 17-ketosteroid excretion produced by benemid. Proc. Soc. exp. Biol. (N.Y.) **78**, 460—463 (1951)

Gibaldi, M., Schwartz, M. A.: Apparent effect of probenecid on distribution of penicillin in man. Clin. Pharmacol. Ther. **9**, 345—349 (1968)

Goetzee, A. E., Richards, T. G., Tindall, V. R.: Experimental changes in liver function induced by probenecid. Clin. Sci. **19**, 63—78 (1960)

Goodwin, C. S., Sparell, G.: Inhibition of dapsone excretion by probenecid. Lancet **1969 II**, 884—885

Gutman, A. B.: Uricosuric drugs, with special reference to probenecid and sulfinpyrazone. Advanc. Pharmacol. **4**, 91—142 (1966)

Gutman,A.B., Dayton,P.G., Yü,T.F., Berger,L., Chen,W., Sicam,I.E., Burns,J.J.: A study of the inverse relationship between pK and rate of renal excretion of phenylbutazone analogs in man and dog. Amer. J. Med. **29**, 1017—1033 (1960)

Gutman,A.B., Yü,T.F.: Benemid(p-(di-N-propylsulyfamyl)-benzoic acid) as a uricosuric agent in chronic gouty arthritis. Trans. Ass. Amer. Phycns **64**, 279—288 (1951)

Gutman,A.B., Yü,T.F.: Renal function in gout. With a commentary on the renal regulation of urate excretion and the role of the kidney in the pathogenesis of gout. Amer. J. Med. **23**, 600—622 (1957a)

Gutman,A.B., Yü,T.F.: Protracted uricosuric therapy in tophaceous gout. Lancet **1957IIb**, 1258—1260

Gutman,A.B., Yü,T.F.: A three-component system for regulation of renal excretion of uric acid in man. Trans. Ass. Amer. Phycns. **74**, 353—365 (1961)

Gutman,A.B., Yü,T.F., Berger,L.: Tubular secretion of urate in man. J. clin. Invest. **38**, 1778—1781 (1959)

Gutman,A.B., Yü,T.F., Sirota,J.H.: A study by simultaneous clearance techniques, of salicylate excretion in man. Effect of alkalinization of the urine by bicarbonate administration; effect of probenecid. J. clin. Invest. **34**, 711—721 (1955)

Healey,L.A., Harrison,M., Decker,J.L.: Uricosuric effect of chlorprothixene. New Engl. J. Med. **272**, 526—527 (1965)

Healey,L.A., Magid,G.J., Decker,J.L.: Uric acid retention due to hydrochlorthiazide. New Engl. J. Med. **261**, 1358—1362 (1959)

Hwang,B., Konicki,G., Dewey,R., Miao,C.: Gas chromatograpgic determination of ticrynafen (tienilic acid) and its metabolites in urine, serum, and plasma of man and animals. J. Pharm. Sci. In press

Inaba,T., Besley,M.I., Chow,E.J.: Determination of sulfinpyrazone in serum by high-performance liquid chromatography. J. Chromatogr. **104**, 165—169 (1975)

Israili,Z.H., Perel,J.M., Cunningham,R.F., Dayton,P.G., Yü,T.F., Gutman,A.B., Long,K.R., Long,R.C.: Metabolites of probenecid. Chemical physical and pharmacological studies. J. med. Chem. **15**, 709—713 (1972)

Jain,A.K., Ryan,J.R., McMahan,F.G., Noveck,R.J.: Effect of single oral doses of benzbromarone on serum and urinary uric acid. Arthr. and Rheum. **17**, 149—157 (1974)

Jenkins,P., Rieselbach,R.E.: Unique characteristics of the mechanism for reabsorption of filtered versus secreted urate. Proc. Amer. Soc. clin. Invest. (Abst.) p.36a (1974)

Kates,R.E., Tozer,T.N., Sorby,D.L.: Increased methotrexate toxicity due to concurrent probenecid administration. Biochem. Pharmacol. **25**, 1485—1488 (1976)

Kenwright,S., Levi,A.J.: Impairment of hepatic uptake of rifamycin antibiotics by probenecid and its therapeutic implications. Lancet **1973II**, 1401—1404

Kippen,I., Whitehouse,M.W., Klinenberg,J.R.: Pharmacology of uricosuric drugs. Ann. rheum. Dis. **33**, 391—396 (1974)

Kirsch,R., Kamisaka,K., Fleischner,G., Arias,I.M.: Structure and functional studies of ligandin, a major renal organic anion binding protein. J. clin. Invest. **55**, 1009—1019 (1975)

Klein,J.O., Finland,M.: Ampicillin activity in vitro and absorption and excretion in normal young men. Amer. J. med. Sci. **245**, 544—555 (1963)

Klinenberg,J.R., Kippen,I.: The binding of urate to plasma protein determined by means of equilibrium dialysis. J. Lab. clin. Med. **75**, 503—510 (1970)

Koch-Weser,J., Sellars,E.M.: Binding of drugs to serum albumin. New Engl. J. Med. **294**, 311—316 (1976)

Kovarsky,J., Holmes,E., Kelley,W.N.: Absence of significant urate binding to human serum proteins. Clin. Res. **24**, 21A (1976)

Kramp,R., Lenoir,R.: Distal permeability to urate and effects of benzofuran derrivatives in the rat kidney. Amer. J. Physiol. **228**, 875—883 (1975)

Lemieux,G., Kiss,A., Vinay,P., Gougoux,A.: Nature of the uricosuric effect of tienilic acid, a new diuretic. Kidney Int. **12**, 104—114 (1977)

Lemieux,G., Vinay,P., Gougoux,A., Michaud,G.: Nature of the uricosuric action of benziodarone. Amer. J. Physiol. **224**, 1440—1449 (1973)

Lieber,C.S., Jones,D.P., Lasowsky,M.S., Davidson,C.S.: Interrelation of uric acid and ethanol metabolism in man. J. clin. Invest. **41**, 1863—1870 (1962)

Masbernard, A., Giudicelli, C. P.: Etude clinique de l'action antihypertensive de l'acide chloro-2,3(tienil-2-ceto)-phenoxyacetique en administration prolongee. Lyon Med. **232**, 165—174 (1974)

May, D. G., Weiner, I. M.: Bidirectional active transport of n-hydroxy-benzoate in proximal tubules of dogs. Amer. J. Physiol. **218**, 430—436 (1970)

Meisel, A. D., Diamond, H. S.: Inhibition of probenecid uricosuria by pyrazinamide and para-aminohippurate. Amer. J. Physiol. **232**, F 222—F 226 (1977)

Melethil, S., Conway, W. D.: Urinary excretion of probenecid and its metabolites in humans as a function of dose. J. Pharm. Sci. **65**, 861—865 (1976)

Mischler, T. W., Sugerman, A. A., Willard, D. A., Brannick, L. J., Neiss, E. S.: Influence of probenecid and food on the bioavailability of cephardine in normal subjects. J. clin. Pharmacol. **14**, 604—611 (1974)

Mudge, G. H., Berndt, W. O., Valtin, H.: Tubular transport of urea, glucose, phosphate, uric acid, sulfate, and thiosulfate. In: Orloff, J., Berliner, R. W. (Eds.): Handbook of Physiology, Section 8, Renal Physiology, pp. 587—652. Washington, D.C.: American Physiological Society 1973

Murray, T., Goldberg, M.: Chronic interstitial nephritis: Etiologic factors. Ann. Intern. Med. **82**, 453—459 (1975)

Nechay, B. R., Nechay, L.: Effects of probenecid, sodium salicylate, 2,4-dinitrophenol and pyrazinamide on renal secretion of uric acid in chickens. J. Pharm. exp. Ther. **126**, 291—295 (1959)

Oyer, J. H., Wagner, S. L., Schmid, F. R.: Suppression of salicylate-induced uricosuria by phenylbutazone. Amer. J. Med. Sci. **251**, 39—45 (1965)

Perel, J. M., Dayton, P. G., Snell, M. M., Yü, T. F., Gutman, A. B.: Studies of interactions among drugs in man at the renal level: Probenecid and sulfinpyrazone. Clin. Pharmacol. Ther. **10**, 834—840 (1969)

Perel, J. M., Levitt, M., Dunner, D. L.: Plasma and cerebrospinal fluid probenecid concentration as related to accumulation of acidic biogenic amine metabolites in man. Psychopharmacology **35**, 83—90 (1974)

Postlethwaite, A. E., Kelley, W. N.: Uricosuric effect of radiocontrast agents: A study in man of four commonly used preparations. Ann. intern. Med. **74**, 845—852 (1971)

Postlethwaite, A. E., Ramsdell, C. M., Kelley, W. N.: Uricosuric effect of an anticholinergic agent in hyperuricemic subjects. Arch. int. Med. **134**, 270—276 (1974)

Prasad, D. R., Weiner, I. M., Steele, T. H.: Diuretic-induced uricosuria: interaction with pyrazinoate transport in man. J. Pharm. exp. Ther. **200**, 58—64 (1977)

Reese, O. G., Steele, T. H.: Renal transport of urate during diuretic-induced hypouricemia. Amer. J. Med. **60**, 973—979 (1976)

Rieselbach, R. E., Steele, T. H.: Influence of the kidney upon urate homeostasis in health and disease. Amer. J. Med. **56**, 666—675 (1974)

Rizzuto, V. J., Inglesby, T. V., Grace, W. J.: Probenecid (Benemid) intoxication with status epilepticus. Amer. J. Med. **38**, 646—648 (1965)

Sabih, K., Klaassen, C. D., Sabih, K.: Combined GC and high resolution mass spectrometric determination of probenecid. J. Pharm. Sci. **60**, 745—751 (1971)

Schacter, D., Manis, J. G.: Salicylate and salicyl conjugates: Fluorometric estimation, biosynthesis and renal excretion in man. J. clin. Invest. **37**, 800—807 (1958)

Sinclair, D. S., Fox, I. H.: The pharmacology of hyperuricemic effect of benzbromarone. J. Rheumatol. **19**, 183—190 (1975)

Sirota, J. H., Yü, T. F., Gutman, A. B.: Effect of benemid on urate clearance and discrete renal functions in gouty subjects. J. clin. Invest. **31**, 692—701 (1952)

Skeith, M. D., Simkin, P. A., Healey, L. A.: Renal excretion of indomethacin and its inhibition by probenecid. Clin. Pharmacol. Ther. **9**, 89—93 (1968)

Smythe, H. A., Ogryzlo, M. A., Murphy, E. A., Mustard, J. F.: The effect of sulfinpyrazone (Anturan) on platelet economy and blood coagulation in man. Can. med. Ass. J. **92**, 818—821 (1965)

Sorenson, L. B.: Role of the intestinal tract in the elimination of uric acid. Arthr. and Rheum. **8**, 694—703 (1965)

Sorenson, L. B., Levinson, D. J.: Clinical evaluation of benzbromarone; a new uricosuric drug. Arthr. and Rheum. **19**, 183—190 (1976)

Spector, R., Lorenzo, A. V.: The effects of salicylate and probenecid on the cerebrospinal fluid transport of penicillin, aminosalicylic acid and iodide. J. Pharmacol. exp. Ther. **188**, 55—65 (1974)

Steele, T. H., Boner, G.: Origin of the uricosuric response. J. clin. Invest. **52**, 1368—1375 (1973)

Steele, T. H., Oppenheimer, S.: Factors affecting urate excretion following diuretic administration in man. Amer. J. Med. **47**, 464—574 (1969)

Steele, T. H., Rieselbach, R. E.: The renal mechanism for urate in normal man. Amer. J. Med. **43**, 868—875 (1967)

Steele, T. H., Rieselbach, R. E.: Renal urate excretion in normal man. Nephron **14**, 21—32 (1975)

Steele, P. P., Weily, H. S., Genton, E.: Platelet survival and adhesiveness in recurrent venous thrombosis. New Engl. J. Med. **288**, 1148—1152 (1973)

Stote, R. M., Maass, A. R., Cherrill, D. A., Mirza, M. A., Beg, M. D., Alexander, F.: Tienilic acid: A potent diuretic-uricosuric agent. J. Pharmacol. Clin. Special Issue, 19—27 (1976)

Talbott, J. H., Norcross, B. M., Lockie, L. M.: The clinical and metabolic effects of Benemid in patients with gout. Trans. Amer. Ass. Phycns **14**, 372—377 (1951)

Tamarkin, N. R., Goodwin, F. K., Axelrod, J.: Rapid elevation of biogenic amine metabolites in human CSF following probenecid. Life Sci. **9**, 1397—1408 (1970)

Vogin, E. E., Scott, W., Boyd, J., Bear, W. T., Mattis, P. A.: Effect of probenecid on indocyanine green clearance. J. Pharmacol. exp. Ther. **152**, 509—515 (1966)

Weily, H. S., Genton, E.: Altered platelet function in patients with prosthetic mitral valves: Effects of sulfinpyrazone therapy. Circulation **42**, 967—972 (1970)

Weiner, I. M.: Transport of weak acids and bases. In: Orloff, J., Berliner, R. W. (Eds.): Handbook of Physiology, Section 81, Renal Physiology, pp. 521—554. Washington, D.C.: American Physiological Society, 1973

Weiner, I. M.: Comparative pharmacology of uricosuric drugs. Gen. Pharmacol. **7**, 1—4 (1976)

Weiner, I. M., Blanchard, K. C., Mudge, G. H.: Factors influencing renal excretion of foreign organic acids. Amer. J. Physiol. **207**, 953—963 (1964)

Weiner, I. M., Fanelli, G. M.: Renal urate excretion in animal models. Nephron. **14**, 33—47 (1975)

Weiner, I. M., Tinker, J. P.: Pharmacology of pyrazinamide: metabolic and renal function studies related to the mechanism of drug induced urate retention. J. Pharm. exp. Ther. **180**, 411—434 (1972)

Weiner, I. M., Washington, J. A., Mudge, G. H.: Studies on the renal excretion of salicylate in the dog. Bull. Johns Hopkins Hosp. **105**, 284—297 (1959)

Weiner, I. M., Washington, J. A., Mudge, G. H.: On the mechanism of action of probenecid on renal tubular secretion. Bull. Johns Hopkins Hosp. **106**, 336—346 (1960)

Weinman, E. J., Eknoyan, G.: Chronic affects of chlorothiazide on reabsorption by the proximal tubule of the rat. Clin. Sci. Mol. Med. **49**, 107—113 (1975)

Weinman, E. J., Eknoyan, G., Suki, W. N.: The influence of extracellular fluid volume on the tubular reabsorption of uric acid. J. clin. Invest. **55**, 283—291 (1975)

Weinman, E. J., Knight, T. F., McKenzie, R., Eknoyan, G.: Dissociation of urate from sodium transport in the rat proximal tubule. Kidney Int. **10**, 295—300 (1976)

Weinshilboum, R. M., Geldstein, J. L., Kelley, W. N.: Prolonged hypouricemia associated with acute chlorprothixene ingestion. Arthr. and Rheum. **18**, 739—741 (1975)

Wolfson, W. Q., Cohn, C., Levine, R., Huddlestun, B.: Transport and excretion of uric acid in man. III. Physiological significance of the uricosuric effect of caronamide in man. Amer. J. Med. **4**, 774 (1948)

Wyngaarden, J. B., Kelley, W. N.: Gout and Hyperuricemia. New York-San Francisco-London: Grune and Stratton 1976

Yü, T. F.: Milestones in the treatment of gout. Amer. J. Med. **56**, 676—685 (1974)

Yü, T. F.: Pharmacokinetic and clinical studies of a new uricosuric agent, benzbromarone. J. Rheumatol. **3**, 305—312 (1976)

Yü, T. F., Burns, J. J., Gutman, A. B.: Results of a clinical trial of G-28 315 a sulfoxide analog of phenylbutazone, as a uricosuric agent in gouty subjects. Arthr. and Rheum. **1**, 532—543 (1958)

Yü, T. F., Dayton, P. G., Gutman, A. B.: Mutual suppression of the uricosuric effects of sulfinpyrazone and salicylate: a study of interactions between drugs. J. clin. Invest. **42**, 1330—1339 (1963)

Yü, T.F., Gutman, A.B.: Paradoxical retention of uric acid by uricosuric drugs in low dosage. Proc. Soc. exp. Biol. (N.Y.) **90**, 542—547 (1955)

Yü, T.F., Gutman, A.B.: Study of the paradoxical effects of salicylate in low, intermediate and high dosage on the renal mechanisms for excretion of urate in men. J. clin. Invest. **38**, 1298—1315 (1959)

Yü, T.F., Perel, J., Berger, L., Roboz, J., Israili, Z.H., Dayton, P.G.: The effect of interaction of pyrazinamide and probenecid on urinary uric acid excretion in man. Amer. J. Med. **63**, 723—728 (1977)

Yü, T.F., Sirota, J.H., Berger, L., Halpern, M., Gutman, A.B.: Effect of sodium lactate infusion on urate clearance in man. Proc. Soc. exp. Biol. (N.Y.) **96**, 809—813 (1957)

Zacchei, A.G., Weidner, L.: GLC determination of probenecid in biological fluids. J. Pharm. Sci. **62**, 1972—1974 (1973)

Zins, G.R., Weiner, I.M.: Bidirectional urate transport limited to the proximal tubule in dogs. Amer. J. Physiol. **215**, 411—422 (1968)

Zollner, N., Griebsch, A., Fink, J.K.: On the effect of benzbomarone on serum uric acid levels and uric acid excretion in patients with gout. Dtsch. med. Wschr. **95**, 2405—2412 (1970)

Allopurinol and Other Inhibitors of Urate Synthesis

GERTRUDE B. ELION

A. Introduction

The ideal drug for the treatment of hyperuricemia would be one which reduces uric acid synthesis without interfering with important anabolic pathways or normal regulatory functions. In theory, uric acid production may be inhibited at a number of different enzymatic steps, either those involved in the de novo pathway of purine biosynthesis or those concerned with the final stages of purine catabolism. Compounds such as azaserine and diazo-oxo-norleucine which block the early steps of purine biosynthesis reduce uric acid synthesis but also interfere with nucleic acid synthesis and are therefore cytotoxic (GRAYZEL et al., 1960; ZUCKERMAN et al., 1959). Inhibition of xanthine oxidase, on the other hand, has proven to be a clinically safe and effective method of reducing uric acid formation.

Although xanthine oxidase has long been known to oxidize hypoxanthine and xanthine to uric acid, it has not always been apparent that the bulk of uric acid production in man involves this enzyme. Indeed, the discovery that inosinate was the first purine synthesized de novo (BUCHANAN et al., 1957) suggested the possibility that the conversion of hypoxanthine to xanthine to uric acid might occur at the ribonucleoside or ribonucleotide level (GREENBERG, 1957). The finding that patients with congenital xanthinuria lacked xanthine oxidase (WATTS et al., 1964), although they apparently could convert inosinate to xanthylate via the enzyme inosinate dehydrogenase, focused attention on the importance of xanthine oxidase in uric acid production. It was open to question, however, whether or not xanthine oxidase inhibition could be achieved in vivo. WESTERFELD et al. (1959) had succeeded in inhibiting xanthine oxidase in rats only with toxic levels of carbonyl reagents. Moreover, a pteridine which was a potent xanthine oxidase inhibitor in vitro failed to give any inhibition in vivo (BYERS, 1952).

Allopurinol (4-hydroxypyrazolo(3,4-d)pyrimidine) was chosen for in vivo studies of xanthine oxidase inhibition because it was a potent inhibitor of the enzyme in vitro, was relatively nontoxic, and did not appear to interfere with anabolic processes within the cell, as judged by its lack of inhibition of the growth of bacteria or tumors (ELION et al., 1963). In this chapter allopurinol and its oxidation product, oxipurinol, will be discussed together for reasons which will be apparent. Other xanthine oxidase inhibitors will be discussed as well.

B. Inhibition of Xanthine Oxidase In Vitro

Allopurinol, a structural analog of hypoxanthine (Fig. 1), is both a substrate for and a potent inhibitor of xanthine oxidase in vitro. The binding of allopurinol to xanthine

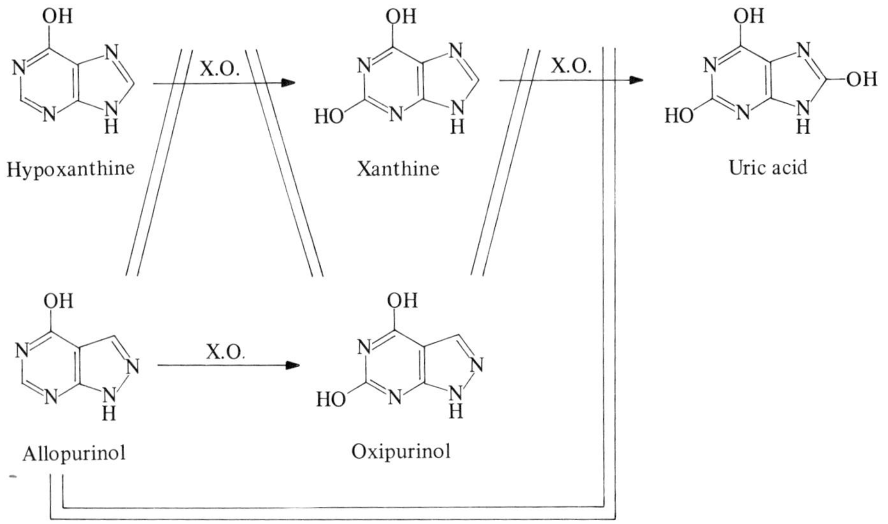

Fig. 1. Structural formulas of oxypurines, uric acid, allopurinol, and oxipurinol

oxidase is about ten- to fortyfold greater than the binding of xanthine to the enzyme and the inhibition appears to be competitive when initial reaction kinetics are considered (ELION, 1966). The K_i of allopurinol depends on the source of xanthine oxidase and the pH at which the kinetics are measured. For the bovine cream enzyme the $K_i = 7 \times 10^{-7}$ M at pH 7.4 (ELION, 1966), for the human liver enzyme it is 1.9×10^{-7} M at pH 7.4 (ELION, 1966), and for the human small intestinal enzyme it has been reported to be $K_i = 7.6 \times 10^{-9}$ M (WATTS et al., 1965). However, it was recognized in early studies that the enzyme kinetics of allopurinol were not simple and that preincubation of the enzyme for several minutes with allopurinol led to inactivation of the enzyme (ELION, 1966).

The product of the enzymatic oxidation of allopurinol is the xanthine analog oxipurinol (Fig. 1) (4,6-dihydroxypyrazolo(3,4-d)pyrimidine; alloxanthine; oxoallopurinol; DHPP). Although the apparent K_i of this compound initially appeared to be higher than that of allopurinol (ELION, 1966), rapid inactivation of the enzyme occurred in the presence of a substrate, e.g. xanthine. Preincubation of the enzyme with oxipurinol alone did not inactivate the enzyme.

The explanation for these observations was soon forthcoming from experiments performed anaerobically (MASSEY et al., 1970; EDMONDSON et al., 1972) or in the presence of a chemical reductant (SPECTOR and JOHNS, 1970). Oxipurinol complexes very tightly ($K_i = 5 \times 10^{-10}$ M) with partially reduced xanthine oxidase in which the molybdenum is in the Mo(IV) state (MASSEY et al., 1970, 1970a; SPECTOR and JOHNS, 1970, 1970a). This binding is stoichiometric, mole for mole, to functional enzyme, i.e., only to enzyme which is turning over. The binding is not covalent, and oxipurinol can be removed by prolonged dialysis or by oxidation of the enzyme, the latter either on prolonged standing in air or by electron acceptors such as ferricyanide or 2,6-dichlorophenolindophenol. The halftime for reactivation of the oxipurinol-xanthine-oxidase complex under aerobic conditions is about 5 h (MASSEY et al., 1970). These studies on the enzyme inhibition have been recently reviewed (SPECTOR, 1977).

The success of allopurinol as a xanthine oxidase inhibitor in vivo is undoubtedly due in large measure to the properties of oxipurinol as an enzyme inhibitor and to its persistence in body fluids (cf. Section IV).

C. Inhibition of Xanthine Oxidase In Vivo

I. Exogenous Purines

The first evidence that allopurinol was an inhibitor of xanthine oxidase in vivo was its ability to prevent the oxidation of 6-mercaptopurine (6-MP) to 6-thiouric acid (TU) in mice (ELION et al., 1962; ELION et al., 1963). The conversion of 6-MP to TU is mediated by xanthine oxidase (ELION et al., 1954; ELION et al., 1959) and is a major catabolic pathway in the metabolism of 6-MP in man as well as in lower animals (ELION et al., 1954, 1959, 1963, 1963a; HAMILTON and ELION, 1954). The inhibition of the oxidation of 6-MP by allopurinol in mice is accompanied by an equivalent potentiation of the antitumor and immunosuppressive properties of 6-MP and with some (unproportional) increase in toxicity (ELION et al., 1963). The biological activities of other 6-substituted purines, e.g. 6-chloropurine, 6-methylthiopurine, and 6-propylthiopurine, all of which are substrates for xanthine oxidase, are potentiated by allopurinol in a similar manner.

In man the oxidation of 6-MP to TU is inhibited by relatively low doses of allopurinol, as evidenced by the reduction in urinary thiouric acid and the increase in the excretion of 6-MP (ELION et al., 1963, 1963a; RUNDLES et al., 1963; VOGLER et al., 1966). The antileukemic activity of 6-MP is also potentiated (RUNDLES et al., 1963; VOGLER et al., 1966). The more efficient utilization of 6-MP for the synthesis of thiopurine nucleotides when conversion to thiouric acid is blocked undoubtedly accounts for this potentiation (ELION, 1975).

II. Inhibition of Uric Acid Production

The ability of allopurinol to inhibit the oxidation of endogenous purines by xanthine oxidase results in a reduction of uric acid levels in both serum and urine and in an increase in the urinary excretion of hypoxanthine and xanthine (RUNDLES et al., 1963, 1966; HITCHINGS, 1966; YÜ and GUTMAN, 1964). This has made the drug an extremely useful therapeutic agent for the treatment of the primary hyperuricemia of gout (RUNDLES et al., 1963, 1966, 1966a, 1969; YÜ and GUTMAN, 1964; KLINENBERG et al., 1965; SCOTT, 1966) as well as for the secondary hyperuricemias associated with malignancies (KRAKOFF and MEYER, 1965; KRAKOFF and MURPHY, 1968; RUNDLES et al., 1963, 1969; SCOTT, 1966). The decrease in uric acid production is dose-related, and serum urate levels can be regulated to the desired level by dose adjustment (HITCHINGS, 1966; RUNDLES et al., 1966) unless there is serious impairment of renal function (LEVIN and ABRAHAMS, 1966). When serum urate levels are maintained below the saturation level of sodium urate, crystalline deposits of urate dissolve and tophi decrease in size. The rate of disappearance of such deposits is dependent on the level of serum urate maintained. Some acute attacks of gout have been reported to occur at the beginning of therapy, as they do with uricosuric agents, probably as the result of the mobilization of urate deposits. With the maintenance of serum urate levels below the saturation point, destructive arthritis improves, acute attacks become less frequent and severe, and gouty nephropathy appear to halt in most patients (SCOTT, 1966; RUNDLES et al., 1969).

In lower mammals which oxidize uric acid to allantoin via uricase, the effect of allopurinol is to reduce allantoin production and increase oxypurine excretion (HITCHINGS, 1966; ELION et al., 1968). Longterm animal studies have shown that the degree of inhibition of xanthine oxidase remains constant at a constant dose of allopurinol, indicating that no induction of enzyme occurs as a consequence of prolonged inhibition (HITCHINGS, 1966). This is also true in man. Gout patients do not require increased amounts of allopurinol after years of treatment; indeed, the dose may often be reduced once tophi have disappeared.

Because allopurinol reduces urinary uric acid as well as serum urate, it is used to prevent the hyperuricosuria, uric acid crystals, urinary stone formation, and urinary tract obstruction that often result from the rapid lysis of cells in patients with malignancies who are undergoing intensive chemotherapy or radiation (RUNDLES et al., 1969). It is similarly possible to prevent the overproduction of uric acid in patients with chronic myeloproliferative diseases, e.g. polycythemia vera, multiple myeloma, and myeloid metaplasia. In individuals who are chronic uric acid stone-formers, allopurinol therapy has been able to prevent urinary stone formation (DE - VRIES et al., 1966; DE VRIES and FRANK, 1967; RUNDLES et al., 1969).

III. Oxypurines

The oxypurines hypoxanthine and xanthine are the immediate precursors of uric acid, whether the purines are derived from food, biosynthesis, or nucleic acid degradation. They might be expected to accumulate when xanthine oxidase is inhibited. A factor which mitigates against this is the rapid clearance by the kidney of hypoxanthine and xanthine. Unlike uric acid, the oxypurines are cleared at a rate close to the glomerular filtration rate (GOLDFINGER et al., 1965). Consequently, serum oxypurine levels rise minimally during allopurinol therapy, in most cases remaining below 0.5 mg/100 ml (YÜ and GUTMAN, 1964; ELION et al., 1968; GOLDFINGER et al., 1965; HITCHINGS, 1969), well below the solubilities of hypoxanthine and xanthine. The oxypurine crystals reported in the muscle of some allopurinol-treated gout patients (WATTS et al., 1971) are probably artifacts of the method of preparation (HITCHINGS, 1971).

Elevated levels of oxypurines appear in the urine during allopurinol therapy. In most patients, however, the increase in oxypurine excretion is not as great as the decrease in uric acid excretion (HITCHINGS, 1966; RUNDLES et al., 1963, 1966), i.e., the total amount of purine endproduct decreases. A similar decrease in purine endproduct is seen in rats and dogs (HITCHINGS, 1966). One reason for this is the ability of hypoxanthine and xanthine to be reutilized for nucleic acid synthesis when their oxidation to uric acid is inhibited. This has been demonstrated both in mice (PO-MALES et al., 1963, 1965) and in man (RUNDLES et al., 1963, 1966). This reutilization has the effect of reducing the amount of oxypurine excreted and of providing the nucleotides, adenylic acid and guanylic acid, which act as feedback inhibitors of the

first enzyme of purine biosynthesis, glutamine phosphoribosylpyrophosphate amidotransferase. The reutilization of the oxypurines provides by the "salvage" pathway
the nucleotides which would ordinarily be synthesized de novo. The fact that the
total amount of nucleic acid synthesized is not affected is evidenced by the lack of
either inhibition (SKIPPER et al., 1957) or stimulation of tumor growth (ALEXANDER et
al., 1966) when allopurinol is given.

Another explanation which has been advanced for the decreased de novo purine
synthesis seen in the majority of patients is the formation of allopurinol ribonucleotide which acts as a pseudofeedback inhibitor of the amidotransferase (MCCOLLIS-
TER et al., 1964). While this is theoretically a possibility, the quantitative aspects of
nucleotide formation from allopurinol (v.i. Sections V and VI) make it unlikely in a
clinical situation.

The enzyme hypoxanthine-guanine phosphoribosyltransferase (HGPRTase) is
essential to both the reutilization of oxypurines and the formation of allopurinol
ribonucleotide. Consequently, in children with the Lesch-Nyhan syndrome and in
the small percentage of gout patients (estimated at 1%–2% (YÜ et al., 1972)) who are
deficient in this enzyme, the amount of oxypurine excreted in the urine exactly
parallels the decrease in uric acid production caused by allopurinol (BALIS et al.,
1967; ROSENBLOOM et al., 1967). Thus, although such patients can still be relieved of
hyperuricemia and hyperuricosuria by allopurinol, their de novo synthesis of purines
is not decreased.

While variable, the ratio of xanthine to hypoxanthine appearing in the urine as a
result of xanthine oxidase inhibition is generally about 2:1. Although hypoxanthine
is a very watersoluble compound, xanthine and uric acid have approximately the
same low solubility in urine (KRAKOFF and MEYER, 1965; LEVIN and ABRAMS, 1966).
There is, therefore, the possibility that excessive xanthine excretion might result in
crystalluria or xanthine stone formation. Renal xanthine deposits can be produced in
animals by chronic administration of allopurinol (HITCHINGS, 1966). The smaller the
animal, the greater the amount of purine endproduct excreted in relation to its water
flux. Thus, in rats and mice, which ordinarily excrete the highly soluble endproduct
allantoin, the substitution of xanthine as endproduct and the relatively small volume
of urine can lead to urinary xanthine concentrations of as high as 1.7 mg/ml, well
above the saturation level. The limiting toxicity in these animals is the formation of
renal calculi. Xanthine calculi have not, except in rare circumstances, been seen in
patients treated with allopurinol. Even with aggressive therapy, urate production is
rarely decreased more than 50%, and the total amount of xanthine excreted is
generally below 150 mg/day. In a urine volume of 1500 ml, this would give a xanthine
concentration of only 0.1 mg/ml, and where reutilization of xanthine for nucleic acids
can occur, xanthine excretion is often less. However, in children with the Lesch-
Nyhan syndrome, children who are tremendous overproducers of uric acid and who
lack HGPRTase, aggressive therapy with allopurinol (e.g. 9 mg/kg) has produced
xanthine precipitates in the urine (SORENSEN, 1968). Xanthine crystalluria has also
been reported in two cases of Burkitt's lymphoma and lymphosarcoma treated with
aggressive chemotherapy and allopurinol (GREENE et al., 1969; BAND et al., 1970;
ALBIN et al., 1972). The natural occurrence of xanthine stones in man is not unknown, but the number reported in the literature is small (RUNDLES et al., 1969). In
xanthuric patients who have a congenital lack of xanthine oxidase and whose purine

endproduct is almost totally xanthine, xanthine stones are rare even at levels of xanthine excretion considerably higher than those reached under allopurinol therapy. The maintenance of a high water flux is nevertheless recommended as a precautionary measure.

D. Pharmacokinetics and Clearance

Allopurinol has a solubility in water of 0.44 mg/ml at 25° C and 0.75 mg/ml at 37° C (ELION, unpublished). Its $pK_a = 9.34$ (KRENITSKY et al., 1967), similar to that of hypoxanthine ($pK_a = 8.9$). The monosodium salt is soluble to the extent of 13.6 mg/ml and can be used for intravenous (i.v.) infusion.

Oxipurinol is less watersoluble than allopurinol. Its solubility in water is 0.35 mg/ml at 37° C. Its $pK_a = 7.74$ (KRENITSKY et al., 1967), close to that of xanthine ($pK_a = 7.4$), and its solubility in urine is much greater at pH 8 (700 mg/l) than at pH 5 (20 mg/l) (LEVIN and ABRAHAMS, 1966).

Allopurinol is rapidly well absorbed from the gastrointestinal tract. Peak plasma levels in man generally occur at 0.5–1 h after ingestion (ELION et al., 1966; NELSON, unpublished). An oral dose of 300 mg produces a maximum plasma level of allopurinol of about 2 μg/ml (NELSON, unpublished). Approximately 20% of the ingested drug has been found to be excreted in the feces (ELION et al., 1966). Because of its rapid oxidation to oxipurinol and a renal clearance rate approximating that of glomerular filtration, allopurinol has a plasma halflife in man of about 2 h at the usual therapeutic doses (3–6 mg/kg) (ELION et al., 1966). However, oxipurinol has a very long plasma halflife (18 h–30 h), and effective xanthine oxidase inhibition can thus be maintained at a steady state with even a single daily dose of allopurinol (RODNAN et al., 1975).

Because of the oxidation of allopurinol, the ratio of allopurinol to oxipurinol in the plasma changes rapidly (Table 1). At high intravenous doses of allopurinol (50–100 mg/kg), the degree of xanthine oxidase inhibition is so great that the oxidation of allopurinol itself is inhibited and its plasma halflife then approaches the glomerular filtration rate, e.g. 100 mg/kg i.v. in a dog (Table 1).

The long plasma halflife of oxipurinol is not due to either plasma protein binding or concentration in tissues. Both allopurinol and oxipurinol show no binding to plasma proteins, are freely diffusable, and are distributed in total body water. However, levels in the brain are only about $1/3$ of those in other tissues (ELION et al., 1966).

Whereas allopurinol is cleared essentially by glomerular filtration, oxipurinol is reabsorbed in the kidney tubules in a manner similar to the reabsorption of uric acid (ELION et al., 1968). The clearance rate of oxipurinol in a man with normal renal function is approximately 15 ml/min, or 3 times the rate of urate clearance. Tubular reabsorption of oxipurinol is inhibited by uricosuric agents, e.g., probenecid, in the same way as is the reabsorption of uric acid (ELION et al., 1966, 1968). Consequently, combined treatment with allopurinol and a uricosuric agent will lead to a lower plasma concentration of oxipurinol and to less xanthine oxidase inhibition than when allopurinol alone is given.

As oxipurinol is itself a potent xanthine oxidase inhibitor and produces a prolonged duration of enzyme inhibition, it can be used as an alternative drug in the

Table 1. Ratios of allopurinol to oxipurinol in plasma following allopurinol administration

Species	Dose mg/kg	Time h	Allopurinol/ Oxipurinol	Ref.
Man	4.5, p.o.	1	0.5	NELSON, unpublished
		2	0.17	
		6	0.02	
Dog	4, i.v.	1	2.0	ELION et al., 1966
		2	0.35	
	100 i.v.	1	35	ELION, unpublished
		6	11	
Rat	50 , i.v.	1	3.1	NELSON et al., 1973
		6	0.3	

treatment of hyperuricemia (RUNDLES, 1966a; CHALMERS et al., 1968). However, because of its relatively poor solubility and absorption, oxipurinol must be given in doses twice as high as allopurinol to achieve the same degree of xanthine oxidase inhibition (CHALMERS et al., 1968; ELION et al., 1968; SIMMONDS, 1969; ELION, unpublished). It therefore appears to offer no therapeutic advantage over allopurinol.

Patients with impaired renal function poorly clear both uric acid and oxipurinol. Lower than normal doses of allopurinol are required for individuals with gouty nephropathy to maintain a plasma concentration of oxipurinol adequate for xanthine oxidase inhibition. The relationship of steady-state plasma levels of oxipurinol to clearance of oxipurinol (or urate) at various doses of allopurinol can be approximated by a nomogram (ELION et al., 1968). The theoretical values based on the assumption that 70% of the daily dose is excreted as oxipurinol agree well with the experimentally determined plasma concentrations (ELION et al., 1966, 1968). In a patient with normal urate clearance, a dose of 300 mg/day of allopurinol gives a plasma level of oxipurinol of about 10 µg/ml.

Since both allopurinol and oxipurinol are dialyzable, patients on hemodialysis who suffer from hyperuricemia require a dose of only about 300 mg of allopurinol after each dialysis to maintain an adequate oxipurinol concentration between dialyses (HAYES et al., 1965; RUNDLES, 1966; ELION, unpublished).

E. Metabolism

The metabolic transformations of allopurinol and oxipurinol are shown in Figure 2. These will be discussed as two categories: 1) plasma and urinary metabolites and 2) tissue metabolites. While all of the plasma metabolites also occur in the tissues, the nucleotides are present only in tissues.

I. Plasma and Urinary Metabolites

The principal metabolic endproduct of allopurinol is oxipurinol. Once the plasma level of oxipurinol has reached a steady state, e.g. after 5–7 days of daily oral doses of allopurinol, the quantity of oxipurinol excreted accounts for 60–70% of the dose

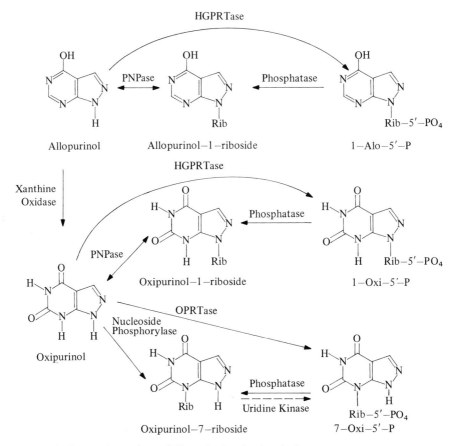

Fig. 2. Metabolic transformations of allopurinol and oxipurinol

(ELION et al., 1966; RODNAN et al., 1975; SIMMONDS, 1969). About 6–12% of allopurinol excreted in the urine is unchanged at the usual therapeutic doses (300–400 mg/day), and an approximately equal amount is excreted as allopurinol-1-ribonucleoside; oxipurinol-7-ribonucleoside accounts for about 3% of the dose (ELION et al., 1966; SIMMONDS, 1969; KRENITSKY et al., 1967).

If animals or human patients are given doses of allopurinol high enough to inhibit allopurinol oxidation (cf. Section IV), the amount of allopurinol in the urine markedly increases. Dogs given 100 mg/kg of allopurinol i.v. excreted 40–50% of the allopurinol unchanged within 24 h (ELION, unpublished). A child orally given 1200 mg of allopurinol excreted approximately 400 mg in the urine as allopurinol (SWEETMAN, 1968).

Patients with xanthinuria have been shown to have little or no xanthine oxidase (ENGELMAN et al., 1964; HOLMES et al., 1974). In such patients one might expect to find no conversion of allopurinol to oxipurinol. This has been the case in two xanthurics studied (ENGELMAN et al., 1964; ELION et al., 1966; SIMMONDS et al., 1974a). However, in two other patients substantial amounts of oxipurinol were

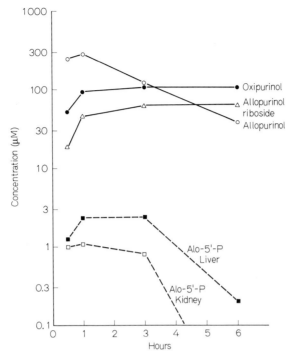

Fig. 3. Plasma and tissue concentrations of allopurinol and its metabolites in the rat at various times following an i.v. injection of 50 mg/kg allopurinol

formed from allopurinol (SIMMONDS, 1969; CHALMERS et al., 1969; AUSCHER et al., 1974). It has been hypothesized (SIMMONDS, 1969) that oxipurinol may be produced via oxipurinol-1-ribonucleotide by the action of inosinate dehydrogenase on allopurinol-1-ribonucleotide. This is unlikely, however, since studies with inosinate dehydrogenase from Sarcoma 180 (MILLER and ADAMCZYK, 1976) have shown that allopurinol-1-ribonucleotide is not a substrate for this enzyme. A more probable explanation is that some xanthuric patients have an active aldehyde oxidase. This is an enzyme which converts allopurinol to oxipurinol, though less efficiently than does xanthine oxidase (KRENITSKY et al., 1972).

Allopurinol ribonucleoside can arise from allopurinol in two different ways: by the action of purine nucleoside phosphorylase (PNPase) on allopurinol and a ribosyl donor (e.g., ribose-1-phosphate, inosine, xanthosine) (KRENITSKY et al., 1967; KRENITSKY, 1967), or by action of phosphatases on allopurinol-1-ribonucleotide (Fig. 2). The nucleoside phosphorylase route appears to be more probable on the basis of drug metabolism and enzyme studies. The pertinent data will be more fully discussed below in connection with tissue metabolites. The data in Figure 3 obtained from studies in the rat following i.v. administration of allopurinol (NELSON et al., 1973) illustrate the close parallel between the plasma levels of allopurinol ribonucleoside and those of oxipurinol, suggesting that both are formed directly from allopurinol. The allopurinol-1-ribonucleotide levels in the livers and kidneys of these animals are lower by 1 or 2 orders of magnitude (Fig. 3).

The small amount of oxipurinol-7-ribonucleoside found in human urine (KRE-
NITSKY et al., 1967; SIMMONDS, 1969) is probably produced by the action of uridine
phosphorylase on oxipurinol (KRENITSKY et al., 1967). Guinea pig intestinal uridine
phosphorylase can also effect this conversion (KRENITSKY et al., 1967). The specificities of the human and guinea pig enzymes are similar, but those of the rat are not
(KRENITSKY et al., 1965). In the rat, no urinary oxipurinol-7-ribonucleoside has been
found in urine after allopurinol administration (NELSON et al., 1973).

No oxipurinol-1-ribonucleoside has been detected in human urine. This may be a
reflection either of its instability (KRENITSKY et al., 1967) or of the fact that, although
oxipurinol binds to purine nucleoside phosphorylase ($K_i = 0.81$ mM) (KRENITSKY et
al., 1968), the velocity of its phosphorylation at 1 mM only 0.15% of that of hypoxanthine (KRENITSKY, 1967).

II. Tissue Metabolites—Nucleotides

Although the conversion of allopurinol to its ribonucleotide had been shown to be
catalyzed by hypoxanthine-guanine phosphoribosyltransferase (HGPRTase) in vitro
(WAY and PARKS, 1958; MCCOLLISTER et al., 1964; KRENITSKY et al., 1969), early
attempts to detect its formation either in vivo or in cell cultures were unsuccessful
(ELION et al., 1966; HITCHINGS, 1969; KELLEY and WYNGAARDEN, 1970). By the use
of [6-^{14}C] allopurinol of high specific activity, the administration of high i.v. doses to
rats, and the extraction of substantial amounts of tissue (5–20 g), it became possible
to isolate, identify, and quantify the amounts of both allopurinol ribonucleotide
(1-alo-5'-P) and two oxipurinol ribonucleotides (1-oxi-5'-P and 7-Oxi-5'-P) formed in
vivo (NELSON et al., 1973). The minimum detectable level of nucleotide metabolites in
these studies was 0.01 nmole/g of tissue. The concentrations of the three mononucleotides were dependent on dose, route of administration, time, and tissue.

The levels of 1-alo-5'-P in the rat following a 50 mg/kg i.v. dose of allopurinol
were highest in the liver and kidneys (Fig. 3); after 6 h, the concentration in the
kidney was undetectable (i.e., <0.01 nmoles/g). At 3 h the level in erythrocytes was
0.27 nmoles/g. The low levels of 1-alo-5'-P attained are not surprising, as the binding
constant of allopurinol to HGPRTase is quite high ($K_i = 0.99$ mM at pH 7.7, 38° C,
for the human erythrocyte enzyme) and its velocity of conversion to ribonucleotide
low (2.7% is the rate of hypoxanthine conversion at 0.125 mM) (KRENITSKY et al.,
1969). The rapid oxidation of allopurinol in vivo results in very low plasma levels
(generally below 10 μM in man after a dose of 300 mg). It is unlikely that allopurinol-
1-ribonucleoside can be phosphorylated to 1-alo-5'-P since there is only marginal
inosine kinase activity in mammalian cells (UTTER, 1960; PAYNE et al., 1970).

The question can now be addressed as to whether the allopurinol-1-ribonucle-
oside found in urine is more likely to arise indirectly via the ribonucleotide or
directly from allopurinol by the action of purine nucleoside phosphorylase. The
quantitative aspects of the metabolic data (cf. Fig. 3) are in favor of the phosphorylase pathway. The apparent binding constant of allopurinol to the nucleoside phosphorylase from human erythrocytes is 0.97 mM (KRENITSKY et al., 1968), similar to
its binding constant to HGPRTase. However, the velocity of conversion of allopurinol to its ribonucleoside is 10% that of hypoxanthine (at 1 mM with ribose-1-
phosphate as ribosyl donor and crystalline calf-spleen nucleoside phosphorylase)

(KRENITSKY, 1967). Moreover, as judged from studies in the monkey, nucleoside phosphorylase activity is manyfold higher than HGPRTase activity in most tissues, particularly in blood cells, liver, kidneys, and lungs (KRENITSKY, 1969).

In children with the Lesch-Nyhan syndrome who lack HGPRTase (SEEGMILLER et al., 1967), very little allopurinol ribonucleoside has been found in the urine following allopurinol administration (SWEETMAN, 1968). This has also been true in one gouty patient lacking HGPRTase (ELION, unpublished). This could be interpreted as indicating that allopurinol-1-ribonucleoside arises from the corresponding ribonucleotide. An alternative explanation is that patients lacking HGPRT have elevated hypoxanthine levels because of their inability to reutilize this purine. Such elevated levels in the serum have indeed been reported (SWEETMAN, 1968). Hypoxanthine is a much better substrate for purine nucleoside phosphorylase than is allopurinol, as its binding constant is 100 times lower than that of allopurinol and its velocity of conversion 10 times greater, and the competition of the two substrates for the enzyme would thus favor the formation of inosine rather than that of allopurinol-1-ribonucleoside. Xanthine is also a competitive substrate with a binding constant 25 times lower and a velocity 5 times greater than allopurinol (KRENITSKY, 1967). While the formation of some allopurinol-1-riboside from the ribonucleotide is not ruled out, the bulk of evidence appears to favor its direct formation from allopurinol.

The concentrations of the oxipurinol ribonucleotides in rats given allopurinol (50 mg/kg i.v.) were lower than those of 1-alo-5'-P and were undetectable in erythrocytes. The highest 7-oxi-5'-P level (2.5 μM) was found in the kidney and the highest 1-oxi-5'-P level (0.73 μM) in the liver, both at 3 h; by 6 h these had declined to 0.39 and 0.09, respectively. Oxipurinol nucleotides were also detected following i.p. administration of ^{14}C-oxipurinol in rats (NELSON et al., 1973).

The formation of 7-oxi-5'-P from oxipurinol and PRPP is catalyzed by orotate phosphoribosyltransferase (OPRTase) from beef erythrocytes (FYFE et al., 1973). This enzyme forms 5'-ribonucleotides from xanthine, uric acid, uracil, and orotic acid (HATFIELD and WYNGAARDEN, 1964, 1964a) with the ribosyl group attached to the N-1 of the 2,4-dioxopyrimidine ring (corresponding to the N-3 of purines and the N-7 in the pyrazolo(3,4-d)-pyrimidine ring system). It is also possible that the oxipurinol-7-ribonucleoside formed by the action of uridine phosphorylase may serve as a substrate for uridine kinase.

The metabolic formation of 1-oxi-5'-P is probably due to the action of HGPRTase on oxipurinol ($K_i > 10$ mM) to this enzyme and the undetectable velocity of conversion in vitro (KRENITSKY et al., 1969) may account for the very low levels of 1-oxi-5'-P found in tissues even at high doses of allopurinol. Attempts to oxidize 1-alo-5'-P to 1-oxi-5'-P with IMP dehydrogenase (derived from Scarcoma 180 ascites cells) in vitro have been unsuccessful, even with a substrate concentration as high as 7.7 mM (MILLER and ADAMCZYK, 1976).

The significance of the quantities of allopurinol and oxipurinol ribonucleoside monophosphates formed in tissues will be discussed below in relation to effects on purine and pyrimidine biosynthesis.

NELSON et al. (1973) found no ribonucleoside di- or triphosphates derived from allopurinol or oxipurinol in the tissues of rats given 50 mg/kg i.v. of a radioactive drug, although the methods used would have detected 10^{-9} M of these compounds. The absence of triphosphates was consistent with the lack of incorporation of allopurinol into nucleic acids both in mouse livers (ELION et al., 1966) and in cultured human fibroblasts (KELLEY and WYNGAARDEN, 1970). Further studies were performed in order to verify the lack of incorporation into nucleic acids under conditions which would present the most severe test, e.g., high dose, high specific activity, rapidly dividing tissue (intestine), and time of maximum mononucleotide formation (NELSON and ELION, 1975). These studies confirmed the previous conclusion that incorporation into nucleic acids does not occur. They also showed no formation of the ribonucleotides of the 4-amino or 6-amino-4-hydroxypyrazolo(3,4-d)pyrimidine (analogs of adenine or guanine) following allopurinol administration. The minute amount of ^{14}C found in the intestinal RNA was solely in the adenine and guanine moieties of the RNA. This is consistent with the ring opening of [6-^{14}C] allopurinol and the loss of a small amount of ^{14}C as radioactive carbon dioxide shown to occur in mice (ELION et al., 1966). It is possible that this carbon is split off as ^{14}C-formate and can then enter the 1-carbon pool to be used in the biosynthesis of purines.

F. Effects on Purine Biosynthesis

The ability of allopurinol to decrease the total purine excretion (hypoxanthine + xanthine + uric acid) in humans and animals who have the enzyme HGPRTase has been mentioned above (cf. Section IIIC). It has been postulated that this is due to reutilization of the oxypurines for nucleic acid synthesis and feedback inhibition of de novo purine biosynthesis by the naturally occurring purine nucleotides and/or allopurinol ribonucleotide. Another possible reason for decreased de novo synthesis is a decrease in phosphoribosylpyrophosphate (PRPP) concentrations, since PRPP is required for the first step of purine biosynthesis, i.e., the reaction with glutamine to form phosphoribosylamine. Either the reutilization of oxypurines or the formation of allopurinol and oxipurinol ribonucleotides would consume PRPP. In addition, the formation of allopurinol ribonucleoside from allopurinol could deplete ribose-1-phosphate, a precursor of PRPP. A decrease in PRPP has been reported in human erythrocytes for a 5 h period following a dose of allopurinol (2–4 mg/kg, p.o.), but not after oxipurinol administration (Fox et al., 1970; Fox and KELLEY, 1971). In human fibroblasts, however, which (unlike erythrocytes) presumably have a functional de novo pathway, there is no significant drop in the PRPP level at an allopurinol concentration of 0.1 mM (10–100 times the plasma level generally found in man) (KELLEY et al., 1971). At the high dose of allopurinol (50 mg/kg i.v.) employed in the rat studies (NELSON et al., 1973; ELION and NELSON, 1974), enough 1-alo-5'-P and 1-oxi-5'-P could have been formed to cause a temporary decrease in PRPP levels in the liver, since the normal PRPP concentration in rat liver is approximately 10 µM (CLIFFORD et al., 1972). However, more needs to be known about the functional capacity of PRPP synthetase and the relative amounts and turnover rates of all the enzymes utilizing PRPP before a conclusion can be reached about the significance of the effect of allopurinol on PRPP levels.

The quantitative determination of 1-alo-5'-P in the tissues of rats at various dose levels of allopurinol helps to elucidate the possible importance of this nucleotide as a pseudofeedback inhibitor. It can be calculated that if 4 µM 1-alo-5'-P is formed in a rat liver when the plasma level (at 1–3 h after an i.v. injection of 50 mg/kg) of allopurinol is between 180–55 µM, then the expected concentration of 1-alo-5'-P in human liver would be $< 0.1\ \mu M$ at plasma levels of $< 10\ \mu M$ allopurinol (following a dose of 300 mg p.o.) (ELION and NELSON, 1974). However, $0.1\ \mu M$ is far below the K_i of $600\ \mu M$ reported for 1-alo-5'-P as an inhibitor of the pigeon liver PRPP amidotransferase (McCOLLISTER et al., 1964). Quantitative considerations, therefore, make it unlikely that this nucleotide is responsible for the feedback inhibition observed in man.

The purine nucleotide pool sizes in rat liver and kidneys at various times after a single i.v. or i.p. dose (20 mg/kg) of allopurinol show only minor transient changes (ELION and NELSON, 1974). In the liver there is a transient decrease in AMP, GMP, GDP, and ATP levels at 1 h with a return to normal or elevated levels at 3 h. In the kidneys, levels of AMP and ATP are slightly elevated at 1 h while GDP levels remained elevated at 24 h. It is apparent that the purine nucleotide pools can fluctuate rapidly and that the fluctuations may be different in different tissues.

In rats fed 0.1% allopurinol of their diet for 1 month, a dose sufficient to reduce allantoin excretion by 50% and to inhibit total purine endproduct excretion (i.e., feedback inhibition), there was no change in mono-, di-, or triphosphates of adenosine or guanosine (ELION and NELSON, 1974). The regulatory mechanisms of purine biosynthesis appear to be very efficient in maintaining normal purine nucleotide levels.

G. Effects on Pyrimidine Biosynthesis

The finding by Fox et al. (1970) and KELLEY and BEARDMORE (1970) that a significant increase in the excretion of orotate and orotidine occurs in both animals and man treated with allopurinol suggests some interference with pyrimidine biosynthesis. Inhibitors of orotidylate decarboxylase are formed when allopurinol or oxipurinol is incubated with red cell lysates and PRPP (Fox et al., 1971; BEARDMORE and KELLEY, 1971) and ^{14}C-orotate metabolism is inhibited in the presence of oxipurinol (KELLEY and BEARDMORE, 1971). This has led both groups of authors to postulate that one or more ribonucleotides of allopurinol or oxipurinol are responsible for this inhibition. Once these nucleotides were isolated and synthesized (FYFE et al., 1973), kinetic studies with orotidylate decarboxylase (ODCase) were possible. The enzyme from yeast and rat liver have exhibited bimodal kinetics (FYFE et al., 1973, 1974), as have the ODCase from human fibroblasts (WORTHY et al., 1974) and human red cell hemolysates (TAX et al., 1976). BROWN et al. (1975) have reported that the partially purified ODCase from human erythrocytes show a triphasic Lineweaver-Burk plot with Km values of 25, 3, and $0.6\ \mu M$ for the monomer, dimer, and tetramer forms of the enzyme, respectively. At levels of OMP above $10\ \mu M$, the K_m $(2\ \mu M)$ and V_{max} are relatively high for the rat liver ODCase and the inhibitors show high K_i values (FYFE et al., 1973). At OMP concentrations below $2\ \mu M$, a lower K_m $(0.5\ \mu M)$ and lower V_{max} and K_i values have been found. These lower K_i values are probably the pertinent ones in vivo (OMP levels in normal rat liver are below $0.1\ \mu M$ and even following high dose allopurinol treatment only reach $5\ \mu M$ (HITCHINGS, 1974)). The low K_i values for 1-alo-5'-P, 1-oxi-5'-P, and 7-oxi-5'-P are: $1 \times 10^{-6}\ M$, $5 \times 10^{-10}\ M$, and $4 \times 10^{-8}\ M$, respectively (FYFE et al., 1973). After high dose of allopurinol i.v. in rats, the maximum levels of the three nucleotides attained in the liver and kidney, particularly the oxipurinol ribonucleotides, exceed these K_i values. If one extrapolates from the plasma levels of oxipurinol in the rat and from comparable levels in man, e.g., 65 µM in man on a 300 mg daily dose, the attainable levels of 1-oxi-5'-P and 7-oxi-5'-P could be as high as 1 µM in tissues such as liver and kidneys (ELION and NELSON, 1974). These levels would be sufficient to produce inhibition of ODCase and the consequent orotic aciduria and orotidinuria which have been observed.

How significant is this inhibition of OMP decarboxylase in relation to the amount of uridine nucleotides available for nucleic acid synthesis in vivo? The experimental evidence indicates that the effects of allopurinol and oxipurinol administration (20 mg/kg, i.v.) on the uridine-containing metabolite pools (UMP, UDP, UTP, and UDP-glucose) are small and transient (NELSON et al., 1973). Even after 7 days of allopurinol treatment at 20 mg/kg/day, the UTP level in rat liver remains unchanged despite a marked elevation of orotidine and orotic acid in the kidneys (possibly in the tubular lumens, since the amount of these compounds in the urine becomes elevated). This apparent contradiction is clarified when the pool sizes of orotic acid and OMP are examined. A remarkable expansion of these pool sizes (to 9 and 73 times control values has been observed in rat livers within one h after allopurinol administration (HITCHINGS, 1974). These would greatly dilute any radioactive precursor used for the measurement of the inhibition of ODCase and make the inhibition appear greater than it actually is. When $NaH^{14}CO_3$ is used as a precursor for uridylate, the rate of incorporation is no lower in the livers of allopurinol-treated rats than in those of normal rats (NELSON, unpublished; cf. HITCHINGS, 1975). It is apparent that the accumulation of OMP, the substrate of the blocked reaction, can partially overcome the inhibition caused by the competitive inhibitors 1-oxi-5'-P and 7-oxi-5'-P. When a steady state is reached, e.g., after 1 week of treatment, a normal turnover of pyrimidines is further aided by an increase in the activity of ODCase. This increased activity may be due to stabilization or activation of the enzyme in vivo (FOX et al., 1971; BEARDMORE et al., 1972; TAX et al., 1976) or to the formation of polymeric forms of the enzyme with lower than normal K_m values (BROWN et al., 1972, 1975; GROBNER and KELLEY, 1975). It has also been suggested that the increased activity may be an artifact of the extraction procedure (BECKER et al., 1974; GROBNER and KELLEY, 1975). In any event, the urinary leakage of orotate and orotidine, which amounts to about 10% of the estimated normal 600 mg/day turnover of pyrimidines in man, appears to be compensated for, as normal pools of uridine nucleotides are maintained.

H. Other Pharmacological Effects

I. Iron Metabolism

Because xanthine oxidase has been thought to have an important physiological role in the transport of iron from liver stores through intestinal mucosa to plasma (MAZUR et al., 1958; MAZUR and CARLETON, 1965), the effect of allopurinol on iron metabolism has been investigated. Rats fed a diet supplemented with 5% ferric ammonium citrate and 0.01% allopurinol have been reported to show a greater increase in hepatic iron content than rats given the iron supplement alone (POWELL, 1966; POWELL and EMMERSON, 1966). However, other investigators using larger numbers of rats and higher doses of allopurinol have found no evidence for excessive iron deposition in allopurinol-treated animals given iron-supplemented diets (UDALL, 1966; GEVIRTZ, 1967; KOZMA et al., 1967; GRACE et al., 1970). Allopurinol administration for 4 months to mice on a normal diet also caused no iron deposition in the liver (KOZMA et al., 1968).

The effect of varying dosage schedules of allopurinol on iron absorption from the gastrointestinal tract of man has been measured using ^{59}Fe. No significant difference has been found between controls and drug-treated groups in the amount of iron absorbed (DAVIS and DELLER, 1966; BOYETT et al., 1968; GREEN et al., 1968). Serum iron levels in patients on allopurinol therapy for months or even years have generally remained within normal limits (EMMERSON, 1966; GREEN et al., 1968; RUNDLES et al., 1966; SCOTT et al., 1966a). However, there is a report of one patient showing a rise in serum iron from 70 to 130 µg/ml during allopurinol therapy (HOENIG et al., 1967). A liver biopsy on a patient who had been treated with allopurinol for 18 months and had received iron therapy periodically during this time showed no abnormal iron deposits (SJOBERG, 1966).

There is still considerable debate as to whether or not xanthine oxidase is required for iron transport or mobilization from ferritin (AYVAZIAN, 1964; SEEGMILLER et al., 1964; ENGELMAN et al., 1964). A patient with xanthinuria who suffered from a gross deficiency of xanthine oxidase in both the intestinal epithelium and the liver was found to be able to absorb orally-administered iron in a normal fashion, and this led ENGELMAN et al. (1964) to conclude that "normal levels of intestinal xanthine oxidase activity are not needed for iron absorption." In any event, it appears that the inhibition of xanthine oxidation achieved clinically with allopurinol, generally under 50%, does not significantly alter iron metabolism.

II. Protection from Ischemia

The damage produced in tissues by ischemia is due mainly to hypoxia. Levels of ATP fall due to dephosphorylation to ADP, AMP, and adenosine; deamination produces inosinate and inosine, and the hypoxanthine resulting therefrom is converted to uric acid and then excreted (IMAI et al., 1964; JONES et al., 1968). The possibility that ATP could be restored to ischemic tissue if the irreversible loss of hypoxanthine by oxidation were prevented has led to an examination of the effects of allopurinol on ischemia and hemorrhagic shock. The resulting reports are somewhat conflicting.

CROWELL et al. (1969) reported that allopurinol pretreatment increases the survival rate in dogs subjected to hemorrhagic shock, but that multiple treatment with allopurinol, hypoxanthine, atropine, heparin, and ouabain is superior to allopurinol alone (CROWELL, 1970). BAKER (1972) found that allopurinol pretreatment alone is not sufficient to protect dogs from irreversible hemhorragic shock but that when allopurinol is combined with hypoxanthine, adenine, inosine, α-ketoglutarate, and oxalacetate, a marked increase in survival rate occurs. LEFER et al. (1969) reported that allopurinol produces a decrease in serum uric acid but has no effect on myocardial ATP and does not lead to increased survival in cats and dogs subjected to hemorrhagic shock. However, HOPKINS et al. (1975) did find an increase in hepatic adenosine nucleotides when oligemic dogs were treated with allopurinol 1 h after reinfusion of blood. LAZARUS et al. (1974) found that allopurinol protects hepatic nuclear RNA synthesis during hemorrhagic shock in dogs.

In dogs and sheep with myocardial ischemia produced by coronary artery ligation, allopurinol has some protective effect (DE WALL et al., 1971). Allopurinol also increases the survival rate in dogs undergoing cardiac arrest induced by electric shock (PARKER and SMITH, 1972) and prevents the rise in serum uric acid usually observed under these conditions. An improved survival rate has also been reported in rats subjected to experimental myocardial infarction and treated pre- and postoperatively with allopurinol (WENZELIDES and MEYER, 1975; WENZELIDES et al., 1975). On the other hand, SHATNEY et al. (1976) found no benefit from postoperative allopurinol treatment in dogs subjected to myocardial infarction.

Of possible relevance to the effects of allopurinol on experimental myocardial ischemia is the increased coronary and aortic flow observed in open-chested dogs treated with relatively high (above 50 mg/kg) i.v. doses of sodium allopurinol (ELLIS et al., 1973; STANLEY, 1971). Moreover, MANZKE and DORNER (1975) found an increase of both ATP and 2,3-diphosphoglycerate levels in erythrocytes of allopurinol-treated patients (7–10 mg/kg p.o. daily) as well as a shifting of the oxygen dissociation curve to the right with an increase in the oxygen desaturation of about 5% at a mean central venous oxygen pressure of 40 mmHg.

During the transplant of organs, the period of warm ischemia often determines the success or failure of the functioning graft. Allopurinol has been reported to reduce damage due to kidney ischemia (VASKO et al., 1972), and pretreatment of canine donor kidneys with allopurinol has been shown to increase the survival time of such allografts (TOLEDO-PEREYRA and NAJARIAN, 1973, 1975; OWENS et al., 1974; CHATTERJEE and BERNE, 1976). Significantly higher levels of ATP, ADP, and AMP were found in the kidneys of allopurinol-treated rats during ischemic and postischemic recovery than in control animals (CUNNINGHAM et al., 1974). TOLEDO-PEREYRA et al. (1975) have found that pretreatment of donor dogs with a combination of allopurinol, isoproterenol, and heparin can prevent the irreversible damage caused by 30 min of liver ischemia prior to the transplant. In a canine model for small bowel preservation and transplant, the addition of allopurinol to the 24 h perfusate has resulted in a significant improvement in the survival of the transplant (TOLEDO-PEREYRA et al., 1975); a similar effect has been noted with pancreatico-duodenal allografts (TERSIGNI et al., 1975). However, in a randomized double-blind clinical study in which allopurinol was either added or withheld from the perfusate used to preserve cadaver kidneys, allopurinol did not show a consistent beneficial effect (TOLEDO-PEREYRA et al., 1977).

Based on the high levels of xanthine oxidase and low levels of plasmalogens found in atherosclerotic plaques, OSTER (1968, 1971) has theorized that xanthine oxidase is responsible for "plasmalogen disease," and that this was a forerunner of atherosclerosis, angina pectoris, and myocardial infarction. OSTER (1968) treated nine angina patients with 600 mg allopurinol/day in an attempt to increase the concentration of plasmalogens in the blood and heart. He reported that this reduced both the number and severity of angina attacks and permitted a reduction in the dose of nitroglycerine. No controlled studies have been reported.

III. Tryptophan Pyrrolase Inhibition

Allopurinol noncompetitively inhibits the activity of rat liver tryptophan pyrrolase in vitro with a $K_i = 8 \times 10^{-7}$ M (BECKING and JOHNSON, 1967); it also inhibits the activity of cortisol-induced or tryptophan-induced enzyme, both in vivo and in vitro (CHYTIL, 1968; GREEN and CURZON, 1968; MOON, 1971; BADAWY and EVANS, 1973; HILLIER et al., 1975; GREEN et al., 1976). HILLIER et al. (1975) reported a reduction in serum tryptophan levels in rats injected intraperitoneally with allopurinol; BECKING and JOHNSON (1967) found no such alteration in plasma tryptophan levels but did report that the rats excreted less kynurenine than normal. It has been suggested that xanthine oxidase participates in the activation of tryptophan pyrrolase (JULIAN and CHYTIL, 1970; CHYTIL, 1968) and that allopurinol exerts its effect via xanthine oxidase inhibition. However, BADAWY and EVANS (1973) have presented evidence to support the idea that the inhibition of rat liver tryptophan pyrrolase by allopurinol is due to prevention of the conjugation of the apoenzyme with its haem activator and not to a regulatory effect of xanthine oxidase on tryptophan pyrrolase activity. A lack of effect of oxipurinol (alloxanthine) on pyrrolase activity in vitro or in vivo has been reported by BADAWY and EVANS (1973). BECKING and JOHNSON (1969), however, have found oxipurinol to be an active inhibitor in vitro.

Since allopurinol prevents the decrease in brain 5-hydroxytryptamine (5-HT) provoked by hydrocortisone (GREEN and CURZON, 1968), it has been suggested (GREEN and CURZON, 1968; HASKOVEC et al., 1972; BADAWY and EVANS, 1974) that allopurinol might have some application in the treatment of depression, particularly if given in conjunction with tryptophan. In a 3 week trial in which allopurinol alone was given to seven depressed patients, no improvement in their condition was noted (HASKOVEC et al., 1972).

IV. Drug Interactions

Since hyperuricemia occurs in a variety of disease states, allopurinol is often given in conjunction with other drugs. Some drug interactions are predictable from the inhibitory effects of allopurinol on xanthine oxidase. The inhibition of the oxidation of 6-MP to thiouric acid (cf. Section III.A.) by allopurinol is evidenced by an increased urinary excretion of 6-MP, an increase in the thiopurine ribonucleotides formed in tissues (ELION, 1975), an increased antitumor activity (ELION et al., 1963; RUNDLES et al., 1963; VOGLER et al., 1966), and an increased toxicity of 6-MP in man and in animals (ELION et al., 1963; LEVINE et al., 1969; RAGAB et al., 1974). One species which does not show this potentiation of toxicity is the rabbit (WALKER et al., 1973), even though the rabbit does show an increased excretion of free 6-MP when given allopurinol at a dose of 50 mg/kg. In humans given high i.v. doses of 6-MP, allopurinol shows no effect on the plasma halflife of 6-MP (COFFEY et al., 1972) although the production of TU is almost completely inhibited. Since the cytotoxicity of 6-MP is due not to the compound itself but to the nucleotides formed from it (HITCHINGS and ELION, 1972), the plasma halflife of 6-MP cannot be correlated with its biological activity. If the capacity of the enzyme systems for the conversion of 6-MP to its nucleotides is insufficient, excess 6-MP will be excreted. The potentiation of the antileukemic activity and toxicity of 6-MP in man (vide supra) have been demonstrated after oral administration of both 6-MP and allopurinol. A similar potentiation occurs with azathioprine, the immunosuppressive agent which is rapidly converted to 6-MP in vivo (ELION and HITCHINGS, 1975).

Several nitrofurans, e.g., nitrofurazone and 2-(2-furyl)-3-(5-nitro-2-furyl) acrylamide, act as electron acceptors for xanthine oxidase, and their metabolism is therefore blocked by allopurinol (TATSUMI et al., 1973). The reduction of the nitrothiazole niridazole by rat liver xanthine oxidase is also inhibited by allopurinol (MORITA et al., 1971). The inhibition of hepatic cytosol nitroreductase activity may be related in rats to the enhancing effect of allopurinol on the bladder carcinogenicity of N-[4-nitro-(5-nitro-2-furyl)-2-thiazolyl] formamide (FANFT) (WANG et al., 1976); allopurinol does not alter the abnormal excretion of tryptophan metabolites related to FANFT administration. Allopurinol has delayed or prevented bladder carcinogenesis in rats fed 2-acetaminofluorene with or without tryptophan (ROMAS et al., 1973).

The oxidation of tolbutamide to carboxytolbutamide, an inactive metabolite, is catalyzed by rat liver xanthine oxidase and aldehyde oxidase (McDANIEL et al., 1969). GLOGNER (1970) has reported the excretion of smaller amounts of carboxytolbutamide in patients given allopurinol 1 h previously.

Allopurinol decreases the therapeutic efficacy of methotrexate against leukemia L 1210 in mice, presumably because of the decreased catabolism of systemic purines; this effect has not been observed in P 288 leukemia (GRINDEY and MORAN, 1975). Coadministration of allopurinol does not alter the toxicity of methotrexate in normal mice.

Because oxipurinol is extensively reabsorbed in the kidney, several interactions occur among drugs which affect renal tubular reabsorption. Uricosuric drugs, e.g. probenecid, increase the excretion of oxipurinol (cf. Section IV). A high dose of aspirin (2.4–3.6 g/day) also increases oxipurinol excretion slightly (RUNDLES and ELION, unpublished), probably because of its uricosuric effect (YÜ and GUTMAN, 1959). Thiazide diuretics, which also inhibit the reabsorption of uric acid and oxipurinol, produce an increased effect of oxipurinol upon pyrimidine metabolism, as shown both by increased orotic acid and orotidine excretion and by increased levels of orotate phosphoribosyltransferase and orotidylate decarboxylase in erythrocytes (WOOD et al., 1972, 1974). The increased excretion of pyrimidine metabolites produced by combined therapy with chlorthiazide and allopurinol amounts to approximately 15% of the total normal production compared to 10% or less with allopurinol alone. However, WOOD et al. (1974) state: "It is doubtful if this interaction presents a sufficient challenge to the patient to contraindicate the use of the combination."

Allopurinol administration has some effect on the metabolism of drugs by liver microsomal enzymes. VESELL et al. (1970) report an increased plasma halflife of dicoumarol and antipyrine in man during allopurinol treatment, with large individual variations in the extent of this prolongation. In dogs given dicoumarol (2 mg/kg every other day) and allopurinol (50 mg/kg/day for 20 days) there has been no significant change in either the plasma level of dicoumarol or the prothrombin clotting times (WELCH, 1973), although the plasma halflife of antipyrine in dogs has been prolonged by allopurinol treatment in a dose-related fashion. RAWLINS and SMITH (1973) have found allopurinol to have no significant effect on steady-state plasma concentrations in patients given warfarin or phenylbutazone. If allopurinol affects the metabolism of dicoumarol in man, the extent of the interaction appears to be below the level of clinical significance.

Because allopurinol and probenecid are often given together in the treatment of tophaceous gout, the effect of allopurinol on the plasma halflife of probenecid has been of interest (TJANDRAMAGA et al., 1972). In 8 out of 14 subjects, a prolongation of the $t_{1/2}$ of probenecid was found during concurrent allopurinol and probenecid treatment; however, there was very considerable individual variation. The increased excretion of oxipurinol caused by the uricosuric action of probenecid makes this drug interaction rather complex.

Cyclophosphamide is both activated and inactivated by liver microsomal enzymes. Although allopurinol prolongs the plasma halflife of cyclophosphamide itself, the plasma alkylating activity and the excretion of cyclophosphamide and its urinary metabolites remain unchanged (BAGLEY et al., 1973). BAGLEY et al. have concluded that alterations in the rate of cyclophosphamide metabolism by drugs in the absence of renal failure do not change toxicity or therapeutic effect. The Boston Collaborative Drug Surveillance Program (1974) reported from a retrospective study greater bone marrow depression in cancer patients given cyclophosphamide and allopurinol than in those given cyclophosphanide alone. LYON (1974) has questioned the interpretation of these data. In an animal study, ALBERTS and VAN DALLEN WETTERS (1975) found that allopurinol potentiated the antileukemic activity of cyclophosphamide while lowering its toxicity to normal marrow.

An increased incidence of ampicillin rashes has been reported in a retrospective study in hospitalized patients receiving allopurinol and ampicillin concomitantly (Boston Collaborative Drug Surveillance Program, 1972). As data on uric acid levels were not available, the authors felt that it was not clear whether the potentiation was due to allopurinol or to hyperuricemia.

V. Reduction of Urinary Calculi

The effectiveness of allopurinol in reducing uric acid urinary calculi (DE VRIES and FRANK, 1967; DE VRIES and SPERLING, 1974) is to be expected from its inhibitory effect on uric acid synthesis. The frequent occurrence of uric acid abnormalities in patients with calcium oxalate nephrolithiasis (COE and KAVALACH, 1974) and the fact that calcium oxalate stones are unusually common in patients with gout (PRIEN and PRIEN, 1968; GUTMAN and YÜ, 1968) suggest that hyperuricosuria and calcium oxalate stone formation might be related (SMITH and BOYCE, 1969; COE and RAISER, 1973). The success of allopurinol treatment in reducing the number of calcium oxalate stones in chronic stone formers has been encouraging (SMITH and BOYCE, 1969; COE and RAISER, 1973; SMITH, 1977; cf. Chapter by F.L. COE). The fact that sodium urate accelerates the precipitation of calcium oxalate in vitro (PAK and ARNOLD, 1975; COE et al., 1975) provides an explanation for the effect of allopurinol, as the reduction of urinary urate concentration would make the heterogeneous nucleation of calcium oxalate stones less likely.

A patient with adenine phosphoribosyltransferase deficiency was found to produce urinary stones of 2,8-dihydroxyadenine (SIMMONDS et al., 1976); allopurinol treatment effectively eliminated these stones. Since 2,8-dihydroxyadenine is the product of adenine oxidation via xanthine oxidase, this effect was anticipated.

J. Toxicology

The acute toxicity of allopurinol in rodents is very low, with an oral $LD_{50} = 700$–2000 mg/kg in mice and an $LD_{50} = > 6000$ mg/kg in rats (Burroughs Wellcome Co., unpublished reports). Female mice and rats tolerate higher doses than do males (IWATA et al., 1969, 1974). Chronic animal studies show that deaths are not due to the drug per se but are rather caused by concretions of xanthine in the kidneys (cf. Section III.C.). The smaller the animal, the higher the ratio of its purine endproduct to the water flux and the greater the danger of xanthine deposits (HITCHINGS, 1966). Dogs have tolerated oral doses of 30 mg/kg daily for a year without toxicity, but have also shown some kidney damage after a year on 90 mg/kg/day (Burroughs Wellcome Co., unpublished reports). Monkeys given very high i.v. doses of allopurinol (1300 mg/M^2/day) for 14 days have shown some anemia and marrow hypocellularity as well as an interstitial nephritis produced by crystalline deposits of oxipurinol in the kidneys (KANN et al., 1968). Oxipurinol urinary stones have also been reported in a child given daily doses of 15 mg/kg oxipurinol together with, 37.5 mg/kg allopurinol (LANDGREBE et al., 1975).

Allopurinol is well tolerated by most patients and serious complications in therapy are rare. The most common side-effect is a maculopapular skin rash which occurs in approximately 3% of all patients and which disappears upon discontinuation of the drug (SCOTT, 1966). A few extreme hypersensitivity reactions of the Stevens-Johnson type have been reported. Gastric irritation and malaise have been noted occasionally but usually do not require that the drug be dropped. Transient leukopenia, thrombocytopenia, leucocytosis, or eosinophilia occurs rarely. A few cases of hepatomegaly and elevated serum glutamic oxalacetic transaminase have been reported; these appear to be related to hypersensitivity to the drug. Patients with poor renal function have more side-effects than do others, possibly as a result of the poor clearance of oxipurinol.

K. Other Xanthine Oxidase Inhibitors

I. Thiopurinol

Another xanthine oxidase inhibitor currently in use for the reduction of hyperuricemia in man is thiopurinol (4-mercaptopyrazolo(3,4-d)pyrimidine), the 4-thio analog of allopurinol (DELBARRE et al., 1968; SERRE et al., 1970; GRAHAME et al., 1974). Thiopurinol is a somewhat weaker competitive inhibitor of xanthine oxidase in vitro than is allopurinol (ELION et al., 1968; DELBARRE et al., 1968; CARTIER and HAMET, 1973) and shows a similar progressive inhibition of the enzyme due to the formation of the tighter binding inhibitor, 6-hydroxy-4-mercaptopyrazolo(3,4-d)pyrimidine (MASSEY et al., 1970). As judged by the urinary excretion of metabolites in man (AUSCHER et al., 1974) and by studies with radioactive compounds in the pig (SIMMONDS et al., 1974), thiopurinol is not as well absorbed from the gastrointestinal tract as is allopurinol. No significant amount of thiopurinol is excreted unchanged; it is rapidly converted in vivo to its 6-hydroxy derivative (AUSCHER et al., 1974; GRAHAME et al., 1974; SIMMONDS et al., 1974). An indication that very little removal of the sulfur occurs in vivo is the virtual absence of oxipurinol in the urine after thiopurinol administration (ELION et al., 1968; GRAHAME et al., 1974; SIMMONDS et al., 1974). Unlike allopurinol and oxipurinol, thiopurinol is bound to plasma and cellular proteins, and approximately 30% of the initially bound material is nondialyzable (DEAN et al., 1974).

It has been generally found that the urinary excretion of oxypurines (xanthine and hypoxanthine) does not rise as much after therapy with thiopurinol as with allopurinol (DELBARRE et al., 1968; SERRE et al., 1970; SIMMONDS et al., 1974; GRAHAME et al., 1974). This has been interpreted in the mouse as being due to the lower degree of xanthine oxidase inhibition achieved with thiopurinol. To achieve similar amounts of oxypurine excretion in the mouse, it has been necessary to give a higher dose of thiopurinol (28 mg/kg) than of oxipurinol (12.5 mg/kg) or allopurinol (3.1 mg/kg) (ELION et al., 1968). When equal doses of allopurinol and thiopurinol are administered to man, allopurinol is approximately twice as effective as thiopurinol in reducing serum urate. A dose of 200–300 mg/day of allopurinol produced reductions in serum urate of 35%, 37%, and 34%, while this dose of thiopurinol reduced serum urate an average of 22%, 26%, 13%, respectively, in three separate studies (DELBARRE et al., 1968, 1968a; RYCKEWAERT, 1970). Since oxypurine excretion is related to the degree of xanthine oxidase inhibition (up to the point where reutilization of oxypurines occurs) (HITCHINGS, 1966), a lower degree of inhibition would be expected to produce lower oxypurine excretion.

It has been suggested (DELBARRE et al., 1968) that, in man, thiopurinol may be a better pseudofeedback inhibitor of purine biosynthesis de novo than is allopurinol. The kinetics of the interactions of both thiopurinol and allopurinol with the HGPRTase from human erythrocytes are comparable (KRENITSKY et al., 1969; CARTIER and HAMET, 1973; AUSCHER et al., 1974a), and there is no indication that the amounts of ribonucleotide formed from the two compounds are appreciably different. Both reduce PRPP levels in erythrocytes (CARTIER and HAMET, 1973). As the amount of allopurinol ribonucleotide formed in vivo is alone not high enough to inhibit PRPP amidotransferase (cf. Section VI), one might assume that thiopurinol ribonucleotide is a more potent inhibitor of the amidotransferase. No evidence for this is available. Patients deficient in HGPRTase show a decrease in uric acid excretion after allopurinol but not after thiopurinol treatment (DELBARRE et al., 1970; GRAHAME et al., 1974; AUSCHER et al., 1974a). This is consistent with the poor in vivo xanthine oxidase inhibition by thiopurinol. Neither allopurinol nor thiopurinol had any effect on oxypurine excretion in a xanthinuric man who was apparently deficient in xanthine oxidase (AUSCHER et al., 1974).

Thiopurinol administration to rats has resulted in an increased urinary excretion of orotic acid and orotidine similar to that seen with allopurinol administration (NELSON, unpublished). SIMMONDS et al. (1974) found no such increase in a study of pigs given 20 mg/kg thiopurinol twice daily; however, this dose also had no effect on the purine metabolism of the pigs. At higher doses (e.g. 300 mg/kg/day), thiopurinol did show a marked effect on allantoin excretion in the pig, but pyrimidine excretion has not been reported (GRAHAME et al., 1976).

II. Other

There is a recent report of a new class of xanthine oxidase inhibitors, 3,5-disubstituted-1,2,4-triazoles (DUGGAN et al., 1975). Several of these compounds have been found to depress urate synthesis in dogs and spider monkeys. No information about their activity in man is available.

References

Ablin, A., Stephens, B. G., Hirata, T., Wilson, K., Williams, H. E.: Nephropathy, xanthinuria, and orotic aciduria complicating Burkitt's lymphoma treated with chemotherapy and allopurinol. Metabolism **21**, 771—778 (1972)

Alberts, D. S., Van Dallen Wetters, T.: Allopurinol potentiates cyclophosphamide antileukemic activity. Proc. Amer. Ass. Cancer Res. **16**, 84 (1975)

Alexander, J. A., Wheeler, G. P., Hill, D. D., Morris, H. P.: Effects of 4-hydroxypyrazolo(3,4-d)pyrimidine upon the catabolism of purines by various tissues of the rat and upon the rate of growth of Morris 5123-C hepatoma. Biochem. Pharmacol. **15**, 881—889 (1966)

Alken, C. E., May, P., Braun, J. S.: Analysis of treatment results in uric acid lithiasis with and without hyperuricemia. Advanc. exp. Med. Biol. **41 B**, 535—540 (1974)

Auscher, C., Mercier, N., Pasquier, C.: Allopurinol and thiopurinol: effect in vivo on urinary oxypurine excretion and rate of synthesis of their ribonucleotides in different enzymatic deficiencies. Advanc. exp. Med. Biol. **41 B**, 657—662 (1974 a)

Auscher, C., Pasquier, C., Mercier, N., Delbarre, F.: Urinary excretion of 6-hydroxylated metabolite and oxypurines in a xanthinuric man given allopurinol or thiopurinol. Advanc. exp. Med. Biol. **41 B**, 663—667 (1974)

Ayvazian, J. H.: Xanthinuria and hemochromatosis. New Engl. J. Med. **270**, 18—22 (1964)

Badawy, A. A.-B., Evans, M.: The mechanism of rat liver tryptophan pyrrolase activity by 4-hydroxypyrazolo[3,4-d]pyrimidine (allopurinol). Biochem. J. **133**, 585—591 (1973)

Badawy, A. A., Evans, M.: Tryptophan plus a pyrrolase inhibitor for depression? Lancet **1974 II**, 1209—1210

Bagley, C. M., Jr., Bostick, F. W., De Vita, V. T., Jr.: Clinical pharmacology of cyclophosphamide. Cancer Res. **33**, 226—233 (1973)

Baker, C. H.: Protection against irreversible haemorrhagic shock by allopurinol. Proc. Soc. exp. Biol. (N.Y.) **141**, 694—698 (1972)

Balis, M. E., Krakoff, I. H., Berman, P. H., Dancis, J.: Urinary metabolites in congenital hyperuricosuria. Science **156**, 1122—1123 (1967)

Band, P. R., Silverberg, D. S., Henderson, J. F., Ulan, R. A., Wensel, R. H., Bannerjee, T. K., Little, A. S.: Xanthine nephropathy in a patient with lymphosarcoma treated with allopurinol. New Engl. J. Med. **283**, 354—357 (1970)

Beardmore, T. D., Cashman, J. S., Kelley, W. N.: Mechanism of allopurinol-mediated increase in cultured human fibroblasts. J. clin. Invest. **51**, 1823—1832 (1972)

Beardmore, T. D., Kelley, W. N.: Mechanism of allopurinol-mediated inhibition of pyrimidine biosynthesis. J. Lab. clin. Med. **78**, 696—704 (1971)

Becker, M. A., Argubright, K. F., Fox, R. M., Seegmiller, J. E.: Oxipurinol-associated inhibition of pyrimidine synthesis in human lymphoblasts. Molec. Pharmacol. **10**, 657—668 (1974)

Becking, G. C., Johnson, W. J.: The inhibition of tryptophan pyrrolase by allopurinol, an inhibitor of xanthine oxidase. Canad. J. Biochem. **45**, 1667—1672 (1967)

Becking, G. C., Johnson, W. J.: Pyrazolo- and triazolopyrimidines as inhibitors of tryptophan pyrrolase. Life Sci. **8 II**, 843—851 (1969)

Boston Collaborative Drug Surveillance Program: Excess of ampicillin rashes associated with allopurinol or hyperuricemia. New Engl. J. Med. **286**, 505—507 (1972)

Boston Collaborative Drug Surveillance Program: Allopurinol and cytotoxic drugs. Interaction in relation to bone marrow depression. J. Amer. med. Ass. **227**, 1036—1040 (1974)

Boyett, J. D., Vogler, W. R., Furtado, V. de P., Schmidt, F. H.: Allopurinol and iron metabolism in man. Blood **32**, 460—468 (1968)

Brown, G. K., Fox, R. M., O'Sullivan, W. J.: Alteration of quarternary structural behavior of an hepatic orotate phosphoribosyltransferase-orotidine-5′-phosphate decarboxylase complex in rats following allopurinol therapy. Biochem. Pharmacol. **21**, 2469—2477 (1972)

Brown, G. K., Fox, R. M., O'Sullivan, W. J.: Interconversion of different molecular weight forms of human erythrocyte orotidylate decarboxylase. J. biol. Chem. **250**, 7352—7358 (1975)

Buchanan, J. M., Flaks, J. G., Hartman, S. C., Levenberg, B., Lukens, L. N., Warren, L.: The enzymatic synthesis of inosinic acid de novo. In: Wolstenholme, G. E. W., O'Connor, C. M. (Eds.): Chemistry and Biology of Purines, Ciba Foundation Symposium, May 1956, pp. 233—252. Boston: Little Brown 1957

Burroughs Wellcome Co.: Unpublished reports

Byers, S. O.: Xanthine oxidase studies. J. Amer. pharm. Ass. sci. Ed. **41**, 611—613 (1952)

Cartier, P. H., Hamet, M.: Mechanism of antiuric action of 4-oxy- and 4-thiopyrazolopyrimidines. Biochem. Pharmacol. **22**, 3061—3075 (1973)

Chalmers, R. A., Kromer, H., Scott, J. T., Watts, R. W. E.: A comparative study of the xanthine oxidase inhibitors allopurinol and oxipurinol in man. Clin. Sci. **35**, 353—362 (1968)

Chalmers, R. A., Parker, R., Simmonds, H. A., Snedden, W., Watts, R. W. E.: The conversion of 4-hydroxypyrazolo[3,4-d]pyrimidine (allopurinol) into 4,6-dihydroxypyrazolo[3,4-d]pyrimidine (oxipurinol) in vivo in the absence of xanthine-oxygen oxido reductase. Biochem. J. **112**, 527—532 (1969)

Chatterjee, S. N., Berne, T. V.: Protective effect of allopurinol in renal ischemia. Amer. J. Surg. **131**, 658—659 (1976)

Chytil, F.: Activation of liver tryptophan oxygenase by adenosine 3′,5′-phosphate and by other purine derivatives. J. biol. Chem. **243**, 893—899 (1968)

Clifford, A., Riumallo, J. A., Baliga, B. S., Munro, H. N., Brown, P. R.: Liver nucleotide metabolism in relation to amino acid supply. Biochim. biophys. (Amst.) Acta **277**, 443—458 (1972)

Coe, F. L., Kavalach, A. G.: Hypercalciuria and hyperuricosuria in patients with calcium nephrolithiasis. New Engl. J. Med. **291**, 1344—1350 (1974)

Coe, F. L., Lawton, R. L., Goldstein, R. B., Tembe, V.: Sodium urate accelerates precipitation of calcium oxalate in vitro. Proc. Soc. exp. Biol. (N.Y.) **149**, 926—929 (1975)

Coe, F. L., Raiser, L.: Allopurinol treatment of uric acid disorders in calcium stone formers. Lancet **1973 I**, 129—131

Coffey, J. J., White, C. A., Lesk, A. B., Rogers, W. I., Serpick, A. A.: Effect of allopurinol on the pharmacokinetics of 6-MP in cancer patients. Cancer Res. **32**, 1283—1289 (1972)

Crowell, J. W.: Oxygen transport in the hypotensive state. Fed. Proc. **29**, 1848—1853 (1970)

Crowell, J. W., Jones, C. E., Smith, E. E.: Effect of allopurinol on hemorrhagic shock. Amer. J. Physiol. **216**, 744—748 (1969)

Cunningham, S. K., Keaveny, T. V., Fitzgerald, P.: Effect of allopurinol on tissue ATP, ADP, and AMP concentrations in renal ischaemia. Brit. J. Surg. **61**, 562—565 (1974)

Davis, P. S., Deller, D. J.: Effect of a xanthine oxidase inhibitor (allopurinol) on radio-iron absorption in man. Lancet **1966 II**, 470—472

Dean, B. M., Perrett, D., Simmonds, H. A., Grahame, R.: Thiopurinol: comparative enzyme inhibition and protein binding studies with allopurinol, oxipurinol and 6-mercaptopurine. Brit. J. clin. Pharmacol. **1**, 119—127 (1974)

Delbarre, F., Auscher, C., De Gery, A., Brouilhet, H., Olivier, J.-L.: Le traitement de la dyspurinurie goutteuse par la mercapto-pyrazolopyrimidine (M.P.P.: thiopurinol). Presse méd. **76**, 2329—2332 (1968)

Delbarre, F., Auscher, C., Thang, K. V., Brouilhet, H., De Gery, A.: Effet de retro-action de certaines pyrazolopyrimidines sur le métabolisme de l'acide urique. C.R. Acad. Sci. (Paris) **267**, 2231—2234 (1968 a)

Delbarre, F., Cartier, P., Auscher, C., De Gery, A., Hamet, M.: Dyspurinies par déficit en hypoxanthine-guanine-phosphoribosyl-transferase. Fréquence et caractères cliniques de l'anenzymose. Presse méd. **78**, 729—734 (1970)

De Vries, A., Frank, M.: Prophylaxis of idiopathic and gouty uric acid lithiasis by allopurinol. Urol. int. **22**, 505—516 (1967)

De Vries, A., Frank, M., Libermon, U. A., Sperling, O.: Allopurinol in the prophylaxis of uric acid stones. Ann. rheum. Dis. **25**, 691—693 (1966)

De Vries, A., Sperling, O.: Recent data on uric acid lithiasis. Adv. Nephrol. **3**, 89—116 (1974)

De Wall, R. A., Vasko, K. A., Stanley, E. L., Kezdi, P.: The responses of the ischemic myocardium to allopurinol. Amer. Heart J. **82**, 362—370 (1971)

Duggan, D. E., Noll, R. M., Baer, J. E., Novello, F. C., Baldwin, J. J.: 3,5-Disubstituted-1,2,4-triazoles, a new class of xanthine oxidase inhibitor. J. med. Chem. **18**, 900—905 (1975)

Edmondson, D., Massey, V., Palmer, G., Beacham, L. M., III, Elion, G. B.: The resolution of active and inactive xanthine oxidase by affinity chromatography. J. biol. Chem. **247**, 1597—1604 (1972)

Elion, G. B.: Unpublished

Elion, G. B.: Enzymatic and metabolic studies with allopurinol. Ann. rheum. Dis. **25**, 608—614 (1966)

Elion, G. B.: Interaction of anticancer drugs with enzymes. In: Pharmacological Basis of Cancer Chemotherapy, pp. 547—564. Baltimore Maryland: Williams and Wilkins Co. 1975

Elion, G. B., Benezra, F. M., Canellas, I., Carrington, L. O., Hitchings, G. H.: Effects of xanthine oxidase inhibitors on purine catabolism. Israel J. Chem. **6**, 787—796 (1968)

Elion, G. B., Bieber, S., Hitchings, G. H.: The fate of 6-mercaptopurine in mice. Ann. N.Y. Acad. Sci. **60**, 297—303 (1954)

Elion, G. B., Callahan, S. W., Hitchings, G. H., Rundles, R. W., Laszlo, J.: Experimental, clinical, and metabolic studies of thiopurines. Cancer Chemother. Rep. **16**, 197—202 (1962)

Elion, G. B., Callahan, S., Nathan, H., Bieber, S., Rundles, R. W., Hitchings, G. H.: Potentiation by inhibition of drug degradation: 6-substituted purines and xanthine oxidase. Biochem. Pharmacol. **12**, 85—93 (1963)

Elion, G. B., Callahan, S., Rundles, R. W., Hitchings, G. H.: Relationship between metabolic fates and antitumor activities of thiopurines. Cancer Res. **23**, 1207—1217 (1963a)

Elion, G. B., Hitchings, G. H.: Azathioprine. In: Sartorelli, A. C., Johns, D. G. (Eds.): Handbook of experimental pharmacology, New Series, Vol. 38, Pt. 2, pp. 404—425. Berlin-Heidelberg-New York: Springer 1975

Elion, G. B., Kovensky, A., Hitchings, G. H., Metz, E., Rundles, R. W.: Metabolic studies of allopurinol, an inhibitor of xanthine oxidase. Biochem. Pharmacol. **15**, 863—880 (1966)

Elion, G. B., Mueller, S., Hitchings, G. H.: Studies on condensed pyrimidine systems XXI. The isolation of synthesis of 6-mercapto-2,8-purinediol (6-thiouric acid). J. Amer. chem. Soc. **81**, 3042—3045 (1959)

Elion, G. B., Nelson, D. J.: Ribonucleotides of allopurinol and oxipurinol in rat tissues and their significance in purine metabolism. Advanc. exp. Med. Biol. **41 B**, 639—652 (1974)

Elion, G. B., Yu, T.-F., Gutman, A. B., Hitchings, G. H.: Renal clearance of oxipurinol, the chief metabolite of allopurinol. Amer. J. Med. **45**, 69—77 (1968)

Ellis, C. H., Touw, K. B., Dickerson, S. W.: Some acute hemodynamic effects of large doses of sodium allopurinol in open-chested dogs. Arch. int. Pharmacodyn. Therap. **205**, 355—367 (1973)

Emmerson, B. T.: Effect of allopurinol on iron metabolism in man. Ann. rheum. Dis. **25**, 700—703 (1966)

Engelman, K., Watts, R. W. E., Klineberg, J. R., Sjoerdsma, A., Seegmiller, J. E.: Clinical, physiological and biochemical studies of a patient with xanthinuria and pheochromocytoma. Amer. J. Med. **37**, 839—861 (1964)

Fox, I. H., Kelley, W. N.: Phosphoribosylpyrophosphate in man: biochemical and clinical significance. Ann. intern. Med. **74**, 424—433 (1971)

Fox, I. H., Wyngaarden, J. B., Kelley, W. N.: Depletion of erythrocyte phosphoribosylpyrophosphate in man—a newly observed effect of allopurinol. New Engl. J. Med. **283**, 117—1182 (1970)

Fox, R. M., Royse-Smith, D., O'Sullivan, W. J.: Orotidinuria induced by allopurinol. Science **168**, 861—862 (1970)

Fox, R. M., Wood, M. H., O'Sullivan, W. J.: Studies on the coordinate activity and lability of orotidylate phosphoribosyl transferase and decarboxylase in human erythrocytes, and the effects of allopurinol administration. J. clin. Invest. **50**, 1050—1060 (1971)

Fyfe, J. A., Miller, R. L., Krenitsky, T. A.: Kinetic properties and inhibition of orotidine 5′-phosphate decarboxylase. J. biol. Chem. **248**, 3801—3809 (1973)

Fyfe, J. A., Nelson, D. J., Hitchings, G. H.: The molecular basis of the effects of allopurinol on pyrimidine metabolism. Adv. exp. Med. Biol. **41 B**, 621—628 (1974)

Gevirtz, N. R.: Allopurinol and iron metabolism. Lancet **1967 II**, 715

Glogner, P.: Metabolism of tolbutamide and cyclamate. Hum. Genet. **9**, 230—232 (1970)

Goldfinger, S., Klinenberg, J. R., Seegmiller, J. E.: The renal excretion of oxypurines. J. clin. Invest. **44**, 623—628 (1965)

Grace, N. D., Greenwald, M. A., Greenberg, M. S.: Effect of allopurinol on iron mobilization. Gastroenterology **59**, 103—108 (1970)

Grahame, R., Simmonds, H. A., Cadenhead, A., Dean, B. M.: Metabolic studies of thiopurinol in man and pig. Advanc. exp. Biol. Med. **41 B**, 597—605 (1974)

Grahame,R., Simmonds,H.A., Cameron,J.S., Cadenhead,A.: Thiopurinol: dose related effect on urinary oxypurine excretion. J. clin. Chem. clin. Biochem. **14**, 291 (1976)

Grayzel,A., Seegmiller,J.E., Lane,E.: Suppression of uric acid synthesis in the gouty human by the use of 6-diazo-5-oxo-L-norleucine. J. clin. Invest. **39**, 447—454 (1960)

Green,A.R., Curzon,G.: Decrease of 5-hydroxytryptamine in the brain provoked by hydrocortisone and its prevention by allopurinol. Nature (Lond.) **220**, 1095—1097 (1968)

Green,R., Levin,N.W., Samassa,D., Charlton,R.W., Bothwell,T.H.: The effect of allopurinol on iron metabolism. S. Afr. med. J. **42**, 776—779 (1968)

Green,A.R., Woods,H.F., Joseph,M.H.: Tryptophan metabolism in the isolated perfused liver of the rat: effects of tryptophan concentration, hydrocortisone and allopurinol on tryptophan concentration, hydrocortisone and allopurinol on tryptophan pyrrolase activity and kynurenine formation. Brit. J. Pharmacol. **57**, 103—114 (1976)

Greenberg,R.: Discussion. In: Wolstenholme,G.E.W., O'Conner,C.M. (Eds.): Chemistry and Biology of Purines, Ciba Foundation Symposium, May 1956, p. 267. Boston: Little Brown 1957

Greene,M.L., Fujimoto,W.Y., Seegmiller,J.E.: Urinary xanthine stones—a rare complication of allopurinol therapy. New Engl. J. Med. **280**, 426—427 (1969)

Grindey,G.B., Moran,R.G.: Effects of allopurinol on the therapeutic efficacy of methotrexate. Cancer Res. **35**, 1702—1705 (1975)

Grobner,W., Kelley,W.N.: Effect on allopurinol and its metabolic derivatives on the configuration of human orotate phosphoribosyltransferase and orotidine 5'-phosphate decarboxylase. Biochem. Pharmacol. **24**, 379—384 (1975)

Gutman,A.B., Yü,T.-F.: Uric acid nephrolithiasis. Amer. J. Med. **45**, 756—779 (1968)

Hamilton,L., Elion,G.B.: The fate of 6-mercaptopurine in man. Ann. N.Y. Acad. Sci. **60**, 304—314 (1954)

Haskovec,L., Dostal,T., Jirak,R.: The action of allopurinol as an inhibitor of liver tryptophan pyrrolase in depressions. Activ. nerv. sup. (Praha) **14**, 131—132 (1972)

Hatfield,D., Wyngaarden,J.B.: 3-ribosylpurines. I. Synthesis (3-ribosyluric acid)5'-phosphate and (3-ribosylxanthine)5'-phosphate by a pyrimidine ribonucleotide pyrophosphorylase of beef erythrocytes. J. biol. Chem. **239**, 2580—2586 (1964)

Hatfield,D., Wyngaarden,J.B.: II. Studies on (3-ribosylxanthine)-5'-phosphate and on ribonucleotide derivatives of certain uracil analogues. J. biol. Chem. **239**, 2587—2592 (1964a)

Hayes,C.P., Jr., Metz,E.N., Robinson,R.R., Rundles,R.W.: The use of allopurinol (HPP) to control hyperuricemia in patients on chronic intermittent hemodialysis. Trans. Amer. Soc. artif. internal Org. **11**, 247—251 (1965)

Hillier,J., Hillier,J.G., Redfern,P.H.: Liver tryptophan pyrrolase activity and metabolism of brain 5-HT in rat. Nature (Lond.) **253**, 566—567 (1975)

Hitchings,G.H.: Effects of allopurinol in relation to purine biosynthesis. Ann. rheum. Dis. **25**, 601—607 (1966)

Hitchings,G.H.: Allopurinol, an inhibitor of xanthine oxidase; physiological and biochemical studies. In: Shugar,D. (Ed.): FEBS Symposium, Biochemical Aspects of Antimetabolites and of Drug Hydroxylation, Vol. 16, pp. 11—22. London-New York: Academic Press 1969

Hitchings,G.H.: Crystals in skeletal muscle. Brit. med. J. **1971 IV**, 555 (1971)

Hitchings,G.H.: Indications for control mechanisms in purine and pyrimidine biosynthesis as revealed by studies with inhibitors. In: Advances in enzyme regulation, Vol. 12, pp. 121—129. Oxford: Pergamon 1974

Hitchings,G.H.: Pharmacology of allopurinol. Arthr. and Rheum. **18**, 863—870 (1975)

Hitchings,G.H., Elion,G.B.: Mechanisms of action of purine and pyrimidine analogues. In: Brodsky,I., Kahn,S.B., Moyer,J.H. (Eds.): Cancer Chemotherapy II, 22nd Hahnemann Symposium, pp. 23—32. New York: Grune and Stratton 1972

Hoenig,V., Brodanonva,M., Strejcek,J., Kordac,V.: Allopurinol and iron metabolism. Lancet **1967 I**, 387

Holmes,E.W., Mason,D.H., Goldstein,L.I., Blount,R.E., Kelley,W.N.: Xanthine oxidase deficiency: studies of a previously unreported case. Clin. Chem. **20**, 1076—1079 (1974)

Hopkins,R.W., Abraham,J., Simeone,F.A., Damewood,C.A.: Effect of allopurinol on hepatic adenosine nucleotides in hemhorrhagic shock. J. Surg. Res. **19**, 381—390 (1975)

Imai,S., Riley,A.L., Berne,R.M.: Effect of ischemia on adenine nucleotides in cardiac and skeletal muscle. Circulat. Res. **15**, 443—450 (1964)

Iwata,H., Yamamoto,I., Huh,K.: Sex differences in allopurinol oxidizing enzyme activity in mouse liver supernatant fraction. Biochem. Pharmacol. **23**, 1144—1146 (1974)

Iwata,H., Yamamoto,I., Muraki,K., Goda,E.: Sex differences of acute toxicity in rats and mice. In: 1st Symp. on Drug Metabolism and Action, Chiba, Japan, Nov. 1969, pp. 124—129

Jones,C.E., Crowell,J.W., Smith,E.E.: Significance of increased blood uric acid following extensive hemhorrage. Amer. J. Physiol. **214**, 1374—1377 (1968)

Julian,J., Chytil,E.: Participation of xanthine oxidase in the activation of liver tryptophan pyrrolase. J. biol. Chem. **245**, 1161—1168 (1970)

Kann,H.E., Jr., Wells,J.H., Galleli,J.F., Schein,P.S., Cooney,D.A., Smith,E.R., Seegmiller,J.E., Carbone,P.P.: The development and use of an intravenous preparation of allopurinol. Amer. J. med. Sci. **256**, 53—63 (1968)

Kelley,W.N., Beardmore,T.D.: Allopurinol: Alteration in pyrimidine metabolism in man. Both allopurinol and oxypurinol inhibit de novo pyrimidine biosynthesis. Science **169**, 388—390 (1970)

Kelley,W.N., Beardmore,T.D., Fox,I.H., Meade,J.C.: Effects of allopurinol and oxipurinol on pyrimidine synthesis in cultured human fibroblasts. Biochem. Pharmacol. **20**, 1471—1478 (1971)

Kelley,W.M., Wyngaarden,J.B.: Effects of allopurinol and oxipurinol on purine synthesis in cultured human cells. J. clin. Invest. **49**, 602—609 (1970)

Klinenberg,J.R., Goldfinger,S.E., Seegmiller,J.E.: Effectiveness of the xanthine oxidase inhibitor allopurinol in the treatment of gout. Ann. intern. Med. **62**, 639—647 (1965)

Kozma,C., Salvador,R.A., Elion,G.B.: Allopurinol and iron storage. Lancet **1967 II**, 1040—1041

Kozma,C., Salvador,R.A., Elion,G.B.: Chronic allopurinol administration and iron storage in mice. Life Sci. **7**, 341—348 (1968)

Krakoff,I.H., Meyer,R.L.: Prevention of hyperuricemia in leukemia and lymphoma. Use of allopurinol, a xanthine oxidase inhibitor. J. Amer. med. Ass. **193**, 89—94 (1965)

Krakoff,I.H., Murphy,M.L.: Hyperuricemia in neoplastic disease in children: prevention with allopurinol, a xanthine oxidase inhibitor. Pediatrics **41**, 52—56 (1968)

Krenitsky,T.A.: Purine nucleoside phosphorylase: kinetics, mechanism, and specificity. Molec. Pharmacol. **3**, 526—536 (1967)

Krenitsky,T.A.: Tissue distribution of purine ribosyl and phosphoribosyl-transferase in the Rhesus monkey. Biochim. biophys. Acta (Amst.) **179**, 506—509 (1969)

Krenitsky,T.A., Elion,G.B., Henderson,A.M., Hitchings,G.H.: Inhibition of human purine nucleoside phosphorylase. J. biol. Chem. **243**, 2876—2881 (1968)

Krenitsky,T.A., Elion,G.B., Strelitz,R.A., Hitchings,G.H.: Ribonucleosides of allopurinol and oxoallopurinol. J. biol. Chem. **242**, 2675—2682 (1967)

Krenitsky,T.A., Mellors,J.W., Barclay,R.K.: Pyrimidine nucleosidases. Their classification and relationship to uric acid ribonucleoside phosphorylase. J. biol. Chem. **240**, 1281—1286 (1965)

Krenitsky,T.A., Neil,S.M., Elion,G.B., Hitchings,G.H.: A comparison of the specificities of xanthine oxidase and aldehyde oxidase. Arch. Biochem. Biophys. **150**, 585—599 (1972)

Krenitsky,T.A., Papaioannau,R., Elion,G.B.: Human hypoxanthine phosphoribosyltransferase. I. purification, properties, and specificity. J. biol. Chem. **244**, 1263—1270 (1969)

Landgrebe,A.R., Nyhan,W.L., Coleman,M.: Urinary-tract stones resulting from the excretion of oxipurinol. New Engl. J. Med. **292**, 626—627 (1975)

Lazarus,H.M., Owens,M.L., Hopfenbeck,A.: Allopurinol protection of hepatic nuclear function during hemorrhagic shock. Surg. Forum **25**, 10—12 (1974)

Lefer,A.M., Daw,C.F., Berne,Q.M.: Cardiac and skeletal muscle metabolic energy stores in hemorrhagic shock. Amer. J. Physiol. **216**, 483—486 (1969)

Levin,N.W., Abrahams,O.L.: Allopurinol in patients with impaired renal function. Ann. rheum. Dis. **25**, 681—687 (1966)

Levine,A.S., Sharp,H.L., Mitchell,J., Krewit,W., Nesbit,M.E.: Combination therapy with 6-mercaptopurine (NSC-755) and allopurinol (NSC-1390) during induction and maintenance of remission of acute leukemia in children. Cancer Chemother. Rep. **53**, 53—57 (1969)

Lyon,G.M.: Allopurinol and cytotoxic agents. J. Amer. med. Ass. **228**, 1371 (1974)

Manzke,H., Dorner,K.: Effect of allopurinol on erythrocyte ATP and a 2,3-diphosphoglycerate levels and hemoglobin oxygen affinity in man. Arch. clin. Pharmacol. Ther. **3**, 107 (1975)

Massey,V., Komai,H., Palmer,G., Elion,G.B.: On the mechanism of inactivation of xanthine oxidase by allopurinol and other pyrazolo(3,4-d)pyrimidines. J. biol. Chem. **245**, 2837—2844 (1970)

Massey,V., Komai,H., Palmer,G., Elion,G.B.: The existence of nonfunctional active sites in milk xanthine oxidase; reaction with functional active site inhibitors. Vitam. Horm. **28**, 505—531 (1970a)

Mazur,A., Carleton,A.: Hepatic xanthine oxidase and ferritin iron in the developing rat. Blood **26**, 317—322 (1965)

Mazur,A., Green,S., Saha,A., Carleton,A.: Mechanism of release of ferritin in vivo by xanthine oxidase. J. clin. Invest. **37**, 1809—1817 (1958)

McCollister,R.J., Gilbert,W.R., Ashton,D.M., Wyngaarden,J.B.: Pseudofeedback inhibition of purine synthesis by 6-mercaptopurine ribonucleotide and other purine analogues. J. biol. Chem. **239**, 1560—1563 (1964)

McDaniel,H.G., Podgainy,H., Bressler,R.: The metabolism of tolbutamide in rat liver. J. Pharmacol. exp. Ther. **167**, 91—97 (1969)

Miller,R.L., Adamczyk,D.L.: Inosine 5'-monophosphate dehydrogenase from sarcoma 180 cells-substrate and inhibitory specificity. Biochem. Pharmacol. **25**, 883—888 (1976)

Moon,R.J.: Tryptophan oxygenase and tryptophan metabolism in endotoxin-poisoned and allopurinol treated mice. Biochim. biophys. Acta (Amst.) **230**, 342—348 (1971)

Morita,M., Feller,D.R., Gillette,J.R.: Reduction of niridazole by rat liver xanthine oxidase. Biochem. Pharmacol. **20**, 217—226 (1971)

Nelson,D.J.: Unpublished

Nelson,D.J., Bugge,C.J.L., Krasny,H.C., Elion,G.B.: Formation of nucleotides of 6-^{14}C oxipurinol in rat tissues and effects on uridine nucleotide pools. Biochem. Pharmacol. **22**, 2003—2033 (1973)

Nelson,D.J., Elion,G.B.: Metabolism of [6-^{14}C] allopurinol-lack of incorporation of allopurinol into nucleic acids. Biochem. Pharmacol. **24**, 1235—1237 (1975)

Oster,K.A.: Treatment of angina pectoris according to a new theory of its origin. Cardiol. Dig. **3**, 29—34 (1968)

Oster,K.A.: Plasmalogen diseases: a new concept of the etiology of the atherosclerotic process. Am. J. Clin. Res. **2**, 30—35 (1971)

Owens,M.L., Lazarus,H.M., Wolcott,M.W., Maxwell,J.G., Taylor,J.B.: Allopurinol and hypoxanthine pretreatment of canine kidney donors. Transplantation **17**, 224—227 (1974)

Pak,C.Y.C., Arnold,L.H.: Heterogeneous nucleation of calcium oxalate by seeds of monosodium urate. Proc. Soc. exp. Biol. (N.Y.) **149**, 930—932 (1975)

Parker,J.C., Smith,E.E.: Effects of xanthine oxidase inhibition in cardiac arrest. Surgery **71**, 339—344 (1972)

Payne,M.R., Dancis,J., Berman,P.H., Balis,M.E.: Inosine kinase in leucocytes of Lesch-Nyhan patients. Exp. Cell Res. **59**, 489—490 (1970)

Pomales,R., Bieber,S., Friedman,R., Hitchings,G.H.: Augmentation of the incorporation of hypoxanthine into nucleic acids by the administration of an inhibitor of xanthine oxidase. Biochim. biophys. Acta (Amst.) **72**, 119—120 (1963)

Pomales,R., Elion,G.B., Hitchings,G.H.: Xanthine as a precursor of nucleic acid purines in the mouse. Biochim. biophys. Acta (Amst.) **95**, 505—506 (1965)

Powell,L.W.: Effects of allopurinol in iron storage in the rat. Ann. rheum. Dis. **25**, 697—699 (1966)

Powell,L.W., Emmerson,B.T.: Haemosiderosis associated with xanthine oxidase inhibition. Lancet **1966 I**, 239—240

Prien,E.L., Prien,E.L.: Composition and structure of urinary stone. Amer. J. Med. **45**, 654—672 (1968)

Ragab,A.H., Gilkerson,E., Myers,M.: The effect of 6-mercaptopurine and allopurinol on granulopoiesis. Cancer Res. **34**, 2246—2249 (1974)

Rawlins,M.D., Smith,S.E.: Influence of allopurinol on drug metabolism in man. Brit. J. Pharmacol. **48**, 693—698 (1973)

Rodnan, G. P., Robin, J. A., Tolchin, S. F., Elion, G. B.: Allopurinol and gouty hyperuricemia. Efficacy of a single daily dose. J. Amer. med. Ass. **231**, 1143—1147 (1975)

Romas, N., Fingerhut, B., Feigelson, P., Veenema, R.: Apparent inhibition of bladder carcinogenesis in the rat by allopurinol. Proc. Amer. Ass. Cancer Res. **14**, 95 (1973)

Rosenbloom, F. M., Kelley, W. N., Miller, J. M., Seegmiller, J. E.: An enzymatic biochemical basis for variation in response to allopurinol. Arthr. and Rheum. **10**, 307 (1967)

Rundles, R. W.: Allopurinol in gouty nephropathy and renal dialysis. Ann. rheum. Dis. **25**, 694—696 (1966)

Rundles, R. W.: Metabolic effects of allopurinol and alloxanthine. Ann. rheum. Dis. **25**, 615—620 (1966a)

Rundles, R. W., Elion, G. B.: Unpublished

Rundles, R. W., Elion, G. B., Hitchings, G. H.: Allopurinol in the treatment of gout and secondary hyperuricemia. Bull. rheum. Dis. **161**, 400—403 (1966a)

Rundles, R. W., Metz, E., Silberman, H. R.: Allopurinol in the treatment of gout. Ann. intern. Med. **64**, 229—258 (1966)

Rundles, R. W., Wyngaarden, J. B., Hitchings, G. H., Elion, G. B.: Drugs and uric acid. Ann. Rev. Pharmacol. **9**, 345—362 (1969)

Rundles, R. W., Wyngaarden, J. B., Hitchings, G. H., Elion, G. B., Silberman, H. R.: Effects of a xanthine oxidase inhibitor on thiopurine metabolism, hyperuricemia and gout. Trans. Ass. Amer. Phycns **76**, 126—140 (1963)

Ryckewaert, A.: Les indications du traitement de fond de la goutte. Cah. Med. **11**, 669—673 (1970)

Scott, J. T. (Ed.): Symposium on allopurinol. Ann. rheum. Dis. **25**(6), 599—718 (1966)

Scott, J. T., Hall, A. P., Grahame, R.: Allopurinol in the treatment of gout. Brit. med. J. **1966II**, 321—327

Seegmiller, J. E., Engelman, K., Klinenberg, J. R., Watts, R. W. E., Sjoerdsma, A.: Xanthine oxidase and iron. New Engl. J. Med. **270**, 534—535 (1964)

Seegmiller, J. E., Rosenbloom, F. M., Kelley, W. N.: Enzyme defect associated with a sex-linked human neurological disorder and excess purine synthesis. Science **155**, 1682—1684 (1967)

Serre, H., Simon, L., Claustre, J.: Les urico-freinateurs dans le traitement de la goutte: à propos de 126 cas. Sem. Hôp. Paris **46**, 3295—3301 (1970)

Shatney, C. H., MacCarter, D. J., Lillehei, R. C.: Effect of allopurinol, propanolol, and methylprednisolone on infarct size in experimental myocardial infarction. Amer. J. Cardiol. **37**, 572—580 (1976)

Simmonds, H. A.: Urinary excretion of purines, pyrimidines, pyrazolopyrimidines in patients treated with allopurinol or oxipurinol. Clin. chim. Acta **23**(2), 353—364 (1969)

Simmonds, H. A., Cadenhead, A., Cameron, J. S., Rising, T. J., Grahame, R., Dean, B. M.: Thiopurinol and purine metabolism. Metabolic and radioisotope studies. Ann. rheum. Dis. **33**, 548—553 (1974)

Simmonds, H. A., Levin, B., Cameron, J. S.: Variations in allopurinol metabolism by xanthinuric subjects. Clin. Sci. molec. Med. **47**, 173—178 (1974a)

Simmonds, H. A., Van Acker, K. J., Cameron, J. S., McBurney, A., Snedden, W.: Purine excretion in complete adenine phosphoribosyltransferase deficiency: effect of diet and allopurinol therapy. J. clin. Chem. clin. Biochem. **14**, 321 (1976)

Sjoberg, K.-H.: Allopurinol therapy of gout with renal complications. Ann. rheum. Dis. **14**, 688—690 (1966)

Skipper, H. E., Robins, R. K., Thomson, J. R., Cheng, C. C., Brockman, R. W., Schabel, F. M. Jr.: Structure activity relationships observed on screening a series of pyrazalopyrimidines against experimental neoplasms. Cancer Res. **17**, 579—596 (1957)

Smith, M. J. V.: Placebo vs. allopurinol for renal calculi. J. Urol. (in press) (1977)

Smith, M. J. V., Boyce, W. H.: Allopurinol and urolithiasis. J. Urol. **102**, 750—753 (1969)

Sorensen, L.: Seminars on the Lesch-Nyhan syndrome; management and treatment, discussion. Fed. Proc. **27**, 1097 (1968)

Spector, T.: Inhibition of urate production by allopurinol. Biochem. Pharmacol. **26**, 355—358 (1977)

Spector, T., Johns, D. G.: Stoichiometric inhibition of reduced xanthine oxidase by hydroxypyrazolo[3,4-d]pyrimidines. J. biol. Chem. **245**, 5079—5085 (1970)

Spector, T., Johns, D. G.: 4-Hydroxypyrazolo(3,4-d)pyrimidine as a substrate for xanthine oxidase: loss of conventional substrate activity with catalytic cycling of the enzyme. Biochem. Biophys. Res. Commun. **38**, 583—589 (1970a)

Stanley, E. L.: Allopurinol, a generalized coronary vasodilator. Circulation **43—44**, 229 (1971)

Sweetman, L.: Urinary and cerebrospinal fluid oxypurine levels and allopurinol metabolism in the Lesch-Nyhan syndrome. Fed. Proc. **27**, 1055—1058 (1968)

Tatsumi, K., Yamaguchi, T., Yoshimura, H.: Metabolsm of drugs. LXXX. The metabolic fate of nitrofuran derivatives. (3) Studies on enzymes in small intestinal mucosa of rat catalyzing degradation of nitrofuran derivatives. Chem. Pharm. Bull. (Tokyo) **21**, 622—628 (1973)

Tax, W. J. M., Veerkamp, J. H., Trijbels, F. J. M., Schretlen, E. D. A. M.: Mechanism of allopurinol-mediated inhibition and stabilization of human orotate phosphoribosyltransferase and orotidine phosphate decarboxylase. Biochem. Pharmacol. **25**, 2025—2032 (1976)

Tersigni, R., Toledo-Pereyra, L. H., Najarian, J. S.: Effects of methylprednisolone, glucagon, and allopurinol in the protection of pancreaticoduodenal allografts perfused for twenty-four hours. Surgery **78**, 599—607 (1975)

Tjandramaga, T. B., Cucinell, S. A., Iscaili, Z. H., Perel, J. M., Dayton, P. G., Yü, T.-F., Gutman, A. B.: Observations on the disposition of probenecid in patients receiving allopurinol. Pharmacology **8**(4—6), 259—272 (1972)

Toledo-Pereyra, L. H., Najarian, J. S.: Total recovery of ischemic kidneys treated with allopurinol before transplantation. Surg. Forum **24**, 302—304 (1973)

Toledo-Pereyra, L. H., Najarian, J. S.: Allopurinol on renal preservation. Transplantation **20**, 256 (1975)

Toledo-Pereyra, L. H., Simmons, R. L., Najarian, J. S.: Protection of the ischemic liver by donor pretreatment before transplantation. Amer. J. Surg. **129**, 513—517 (1975)

Toledo-Pereyra, L. H., Simmons, R. L., Olson, L. C., Najarian, J. S.: Clinical effect of allopurinol on preserved kidney. A randomized double blind study. Ann. Surg. **185**, 128—131 (1977)

Udall, V.: Hepatic iron storage. Ann. Rheum. Dis. **25**, 704 (1966)

Utter, M. F.: Guanosine and inosine nucleotides. In: Boyer, P. D., Lardy, H., Myrbäck, K. (Eds.): The Enzymes, Vol. 2, pp. 75—88. New York: Academic Press 1960

Vasko, K. A., De Wall, R. A., Riley, A. M.: Effect of allopurinol in renal ischemia. Surgery **71**, 787—790 (1972)

Vesell, E. S., Passanti, G. T., Greene, F. E.: Impairment of drug metabolism in man by allopurinol and nortryptyline. New Engl. J. Med. **283**, 1484—1488 (1970)

Vogler, W. R., Bain, J. A., Huguley, C. M., Palmer, H. G. Jr., Lowrey, M. E.: Metabolic and therapeutic effects of allopurinol in patients with leukemia and gout. Amer. J. Med. **40**, 548—549 (1966)

Walker, R. I., Horvath, W. L., Rule, W. S., Herion, J. C., Palmer, J. G.: The failure of allopurinol to enhance 6-mercaptopurine toxicity in rabbits. Cancer Res. **33**, 755—758 (1973)

Wang, C. Y., Hayashida, S., Pamukcu, A. M., Brian, G. T.: Enhancing effect of allopurinol on the induction of bladder cancer in rats by N-[4-(5-nitro-2-furyl)-2-thiazolyl]formamide. Cancer Res. **36**, 1551—1555 (1976)

Watts, R. W. E., Engelman, K., Klinenberg, J. R., Sjoerdsma, A., Seegmiller, J. E.: Enzyme defect in a case of xanthinuria. Nature (Lond.) **201**, 395—396 (1964)

Watts, R. W. E., Snedden, W., Parker, R. A.: A quantitative study of skeletal-muscle purines and pyrazolo(3,4-d)pyrimidines in gout patients treated with allopurinol. Clin. Sci. **41**, 153—158 (1971)

Watts, R. W. E., Watts, J. E. M., Seegmiller, J. E.: Xanthine oxidase activity in human tissues and its inhibition by allopurinol (4-hydroxypyrazolo-[3,4-d]pyrimidine). J. Lab. clin. Invest. **66**, 688—698 (1965)

Way, J. L., Parks, R. E., Jr.: Enzymatic synthesis of 5′-phosphate nucleotides of purine analogs. J. biol. Chem. **231**, 467—480 (1958)

Welch, R. M.: Drug-protein binding: A method for studying the interaction of drugs with bishydroxycoumarin (dicoumarol) in dogs. Ann. N.Y. Acad. Sci. **226**, 259—266 (1973)

Wenzelides, K., Guski, H., Seidler, E., Meyer, R.: The influence of allopurinol on the alterations in the myocardium and the frequency of myocardial infarction in the hearts of rats under various experimental conditions. Dtsch. Gesundh.-Wes. **30**, 183 (1975)

Wenzelides, K., Meyer, R.: The influence of allopurinol upon the size of the experimental myocardial infarction in the rat. Dtsch. Gesundh.-Wes. **30**, 229 (1975)

Westerfeld, W. W., Richert, D. A., Bloom, R. J.: Inhibition of xanthine and succinic oxidases by carbonyl reagents. J. biol. Chem. **234**, 1889—1896 (1959)

Wood, M. H., O'Sullivan, W. J., Wilson, M., Tiller, D. J.: Potentiation of an effect of allopurinol on pyrimidine metabolism by chlorothiazide in man. Clin. exp. Pharmacol. Physiol. **1**, 53—58 (1974)

Wood, M. H., Sebel, E., O'Sullivan, W. J.: Allopurinol and thiazides. Lancet **1972 I**, 751

Worthy, T. E., Grobner, W., Kelley, W. N.: Hereditary orotic aciduria: evidence for structural gene mutation. Proc. nat. Acad. Sci. (Wash.) **71**, 3031—3035 (1974)

Yü, T.-F., Balis, M. E., Krenitsky, T. A., Dancis, J., Silvers, D. N., Elion, G. B., Gutman, A. B.: Rarity of X-linked partial hypoxanthine-guanine phosphoribosyltransferase deficiency in a large gouty population. Ann. intern. Med. **76**, 255—264 (1972)

Yü, T.-F., Gutman, A. B.: Study of the paradoxical effects of salicylate in low, intermediate, and high dosage on the renal mechanisms for excretion of urate in man. J. clin. Invest. **38**, 1298—1315 (1959)

Yü, T.-F., Gutman, A. B.: Effect of allopurinol (4-hydroxypyrazolo(3,4-d)pyrimidine) on serum and urinary uric acid in primary and secondary gout. Amer. J. Med. **37**, 885—898 (1964)

Zuckerman, R., Drell, W., Levin, M. H.: Urinary purines in gout: effect of azaserine. Arthr. and Rheum. **2**, 46—47 (1959)

CHAPTER 22

Enzymatic Uricolysis and Its Use in Therapy

J. M. Brogard, A. Stahl and J. Stahl

A. Introduction

Uric acid is the end product of purine metabolism in some species including man and not in others. In birds and reptiles for example, it is the final metabolite of protein as well as purine degradation. In those organisms in which uric acid is not the terminal excretory product of purine metabolism, the molecule is oxidized to allantoin by the enzyme, urate: O_2-oxidoreductase, also called urate oxidase or uricase (Fig. 1). This enzyme which opens the six-membered ring in the purine molecule, is found in various microorganisms, plants, and the livers and kidneys of most animals. In mammals allantoin is generally the major end product of purine metabolism, but in nonmammalian species there is further metabolism of allantoin. Amphibia and teleost fishes convert allantoin to allantoic acid through the action of the enzyme, allantoinase. The latter opens the five-membered purine ring. Nonteleost fishes contain the enzyme allantoicase which breaks down allantoic acid into urea and glyoxylic acid. Finally, some invertebrates are known to convert urea to ammonia and carbon dioxide through the action of urease.

Man and the great apes differ from other mammals in that they lack the enzyme, urate oxidase. Consequently, uric acid is excreted as such except for that fraction which is degraded by intestinal organisms (see Chapter 12). In these species the renal clearance of urate is modest and thus the circulating level of the compound is higher than in most mammals. This elevated predisposes to gout.

Urate oxidase of fungal origin has been prepared in large amounts and can be highly purified. This preparation has been used in recent years for therapeutic trials. The rationale for this therapy is that the product of the enzyme's action, allantoin, is much more soluble and more readily excreted than is urate.

The first experimental demonstration of enzymatic uricolysis in vivo was made by Oppenheimer and Kunkel [24, 25] in 1941. They injected a colloidal suspension containing uricase of animal origin into chickens, thereby causing a fall in the concentration of urate in plasma. These results were subsequently verified by Altman et al. [2]. Repeated use of the enzyme caused severe anaphylactic reactions, even when soluble preparations were employed.

A cautious attempt to use a purer preparation of animal uricase in man was made by London and Hudson [20] in 1957. This trial was soon abandoned because the hypouricemic action was too weak and too brief.

Laboureur and Langlois [14] isolated urate oxidase from a selected strain of the fungus, *Aspergillus flavus*. The enzyme from this source can be produced on an industrial scale, can be highly purified, and has potent specific activity in vitro. The

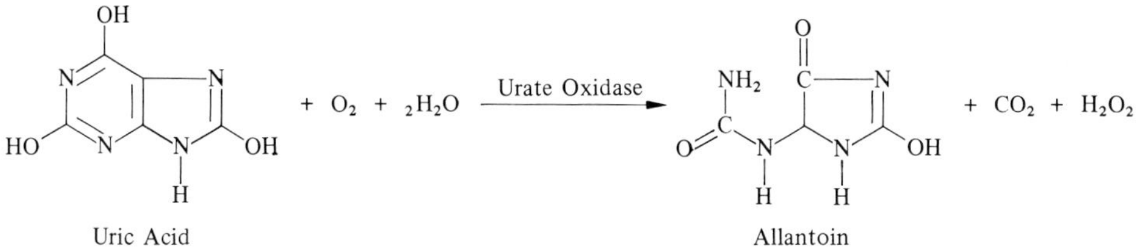

Fig. 1. Enzymatic oxidation of uric acid

powerful uricolytic activity has been demonstrated in chickens and hepatectomized dogs by BRUNAUD et al. [6]. ROYER et al.[26] first demonstrated the uricolytic potency of the preparation in humans. Since then the early observations have been confirmed in physiologic, pharmacologic, and clinical studies.

B. Properties of Urate Oxidase

The enzyme is extracted from large batch cultures of *Aspergillus flavus* Link. After several steps of chromatographic purification, the enzyme solution is lyophilized and sold commercially as a powder with a specific activity of 250 units/mg or in sealed vials containing 1000 units, the usual dosage in man. The powder is easily dissolved in 0.15 M NaCl. Urate oxidase is administered exclusively by the parenteral route, intravenously or intramuscularly. For reasons given below, the enzyme should not be administered in acid solutions.

The enzyme is assayed spectrophotometrically by measuring the decrease of the absorption peak of uric acid at 293 nm; allantoin does not absorb at this wavelength. One unit of urate oxidase is defined as the quantity which oxidizes 0.05 mg of uric acid in ten minutes at pH 8.5 and at $+30°$ C. The optimal pH is 8.5. The stability of the enzyme decreases at pH values below 8.0 and at temperatures above $35°$ C. The deleterious effects of low pH and high temperature are less marked in the presence of serum. The enzyme is poorly soluble in pure water, solubility increasing in the presence of electrolytes and elevation of pH above 7.0. The enzymatic protein emerges as a single, symmetrical peak from a Sephadex G-100 column and migrates as a single band in both paper and polyacrylamide gel electrophoresis. Urate oxidase is a copper-containing enzyme with a molecular weight of 93 000 daltons. The Michaelis constant for uric acid is 6×10^{-5} M. The reaction utilizes oxygen, its velocity being proportional to the partial pressure of O_2. The enzyme is inhibited by ethylenediamine tetraacetic acid, CN^- and Hg^{2+}.

C. Pharmacologic Action of Urate Oxidase

As far as is known urate is the only endogenous, organic substrate for urate oxidase. Uric acid is only slightly soluble in water, 60 mg/liter at $37°$ C. The monosodium salt, the predominant form at pH 7.4, is only slightly more soluble in the presence of normal concentrations of sodium in serum. The solubility of allantoin is much greater, 5.26 g/liter at $37°$ C. Consequently, there is no risk of renal or urinary lithiasis during treatment with urate oxidase. In contrast to agents which inhibit xanthine oxidase, urate oxidase acts at a later stage, i.e., after urate formation (Fig. 1). As a result, no precursors of urate accumulate, such as the relatively insoluble xanthine.

The evidence for the uricolytic action of urate oxidase in vivo is provided by estimation of the levels of urate and allantoin in blood or urine. Urate is estimated either by reduction or by enzymatic methods [11]. Allantoin in urine is determined by the technique of BRUNAUD et al. [6]: allantoin is converted to allantoic acid by alkaline hydrolysis, which in turn is hydrolyzed by hydrochloric acid to glyoxylic acid. The phenylhydrazone of the latter, oxidized by potassium ferricyanide, gives a colored derivative, which is measured at 518 nm.

Allantoin in blood is assayed by the method of STAHL et al. [28], which derives from that of BRUNAUD et al. Interferences due to uric acid, creatinine, glucose, and other aldehydes are eliminated by ion-exchange chromatography and appropriate blank reactions. To avoid further action of urate oxidase in the drawn blood samples, the assay has to be performed either immediately or in the quick-frozen serum (or urine) after storage at $-20°$ C. Addition of $10^{-3} M$ potassium EDTA or cyanide can also inhibit residual urate oxidase activity.

In normal subjects, intravenous administration of a single dose of urate oxidase (1000 units) produces a rapid and marked decline of uricemia, along with a large increase of allantoinemia (Fig. 2). At the same time, one observes a decrease of uricaciduria, associated with a large increase of allantoinuria; the changes in the urinary parameters are very significant in the 3 day period following the injection. During this period, the renal elimination of total purines (uric acid + allantoin, expressed as uric acid) increases. Return to initial values takes place 5 days after the injection. Similar results are observed after administration of a single intramuscular dose of 1000 units of urate oxidase; under these circumstances, however, the changes are less pronounced and occur more slowly (Fig. 3). Repeated intravenous administration of urate oxidase, 800 units/day during 4–5 days (KISSEL et al. [12]), maintains uricemia at levels lower than 20 mg/liter for 1–2 weeks. However, uricemia tends to increase on about the 10th day after the beginning of the treatment (MIZON et al. [22]).

An increase of the renal clearance of urate after urate oxidase treatment was seen in both normal subjects (BROGARD et al. [4]) and hyperuricemic patients (ROYER et al. [27]). This is an important point, since renal excretion of uric acid during gout is lowered, (NUGENT et al., [23]; LATHEM et al. [16]) compared to normal (FONTE-NAILLE et al. [9]). No clear explanation has been furnished as yet for this phenomenon.

The isotopic study of endogenous purine biosynthesis, by measuring the incorporation of ^{14}C-glycine (LEGRAS et al. [17]), demonstrates that hypouricemia, following urate oxidase injection, does not increase purine biosynthesis. The enhanced uric acid excretion would therefore be due to an increased mobilization of uric acid from the tissues.

D. Therapeutic Trials of Enzymatic Uricolysis

I. Urate Oxidase in Primary Hyperuricemia

1. Primary Asymptomatic Hyperuricemia

In these patients, the urate oxidase treatment is followed by a well-defined drop of uricemia. However, this type of hyperuricemia appears to be less sensitive to the action of urate oxidase than the hyperuricemia with gouty manifestations (LOUYOT et al. [21]).

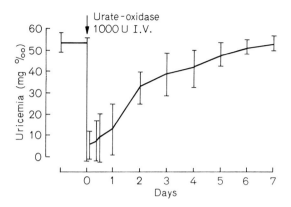

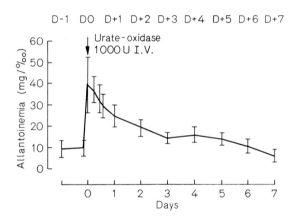

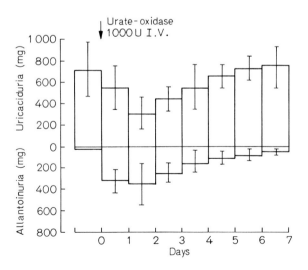

Fig. 2. Uricemia, allantoinemia, and urinary output of uric acid and allantoin, after a single intravenous injection of 1000 urate oxidase units

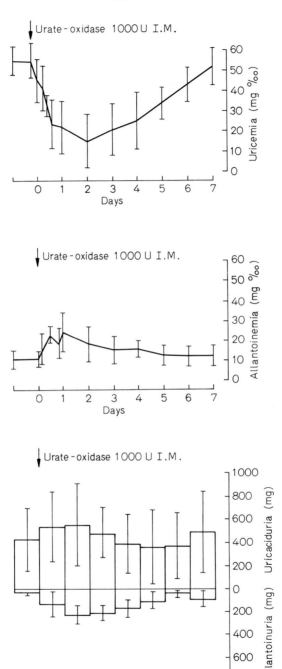

Fig. 3. Uricemia, allantoinemia, and urinary output of uric acid and allantoin, after a single intramuscular injection of 1000 urate oxidase units

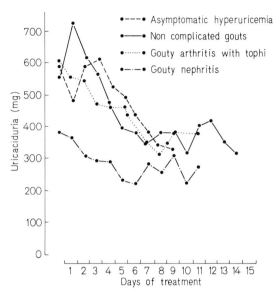

Fig. 4. Evolution of uricaciduria during prolonged treatment with urate oxidase (1000 units/day during 15 consecutive days). Hyperuricemic patients have been divided into four groups (from Louyot et al. [20])

2. Hyperuricemia with Gout

There is general agreement on the efficiency of urate oxidase in the treatment of hyperuricemia with gout. The hypouricemic effect persists 10–15 days after the treatment is completed (Fig. 4). In several cases (Louyot et al. [21]; Hawthorn et al. [10]), softening of tophi has been observed. In long-term therapy, the effect of intravenous or intramuscular administration seems identical. The occurance of acute joint reactions was noticed in some patients and colchicine had to be added. After 2 weeks of uricolytic treatment, the hypouricemic action often abates, but 2–3 months later the initial efficiency returns.

3. Lesch-Nyhan Syndrome

Urate oxidase treatment was unsuccessful in one case of familial hyperuricemic encephalopathy. The allantoinuria increased, but no effect on hyperuricemia was observed; the phenomena remain unexplained (Labrune et al. [15]).

II. Secondary Hyperuricemia

1. In Renal Impairment

In patients with hyperuricemia secondary to renal impairment, the administration of urate oxidase leads also to a decrease of uricemia. The hypouricemic action is equally intense but more prolonged than in normals. The renal failure seems to increase the activity period of urate oxidase, the half-life of which in plasma is lengthened to 6–9 days, as compared with 3–4 days in normal subjects (Devulder et al. [8]).

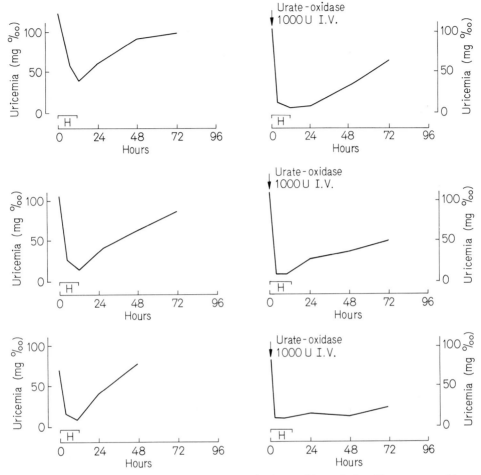

Fig. 5. Evolution of uricemia between two dialysis in three subjects. *Left*: without urate oxidase. *Right*: after intravenous injection of 1000 urate oxidase units at the beginning of the hemo-dialysis (*H*=hemodialysis)

Therapy with urate oxidase has not been associated with any detectable impairment of renal function. The therapy reduces the filtered load of urate, thereby diminishing the probability of crystalluria. The foregoing suggests the potential utility of intermittent treatment of patients with uric acid nephrolithiasis.

Enzymatic uricolysis may also be applied in cases of renal failure treated by long-term hemodialysis, particularly when dialysis does not produce a sufficient decline in plasma urate. The uricolysis induced by the injection of urate oxidase at the beginning of the maintenance dialysis leads to an increased extraction of purine catabolites by the dialyzer; the decrease of uricemia under this condition is more intense than during conventional hemodialysis (Fig. 5). Moreover, the possibility of uricemia arising between two dialyzing procedures is considerably reduced (BROGARD et al. [5]). As the enzyme is not dialyzable, its uricolytic activity persists after completion of the dialyzing procedure (DEVULDER et al. [8]).

2. In Hemopathies

Malignant myeloproliferative syndromes (acute leukemia, myeloid leukemia, lymphosarcoma, myeloma, myelosclerosis) are frequently accompanied by hyperuricemia due to the increased catabolism of the nucleic acids. This hyperuricemia can be enhanced by the cytolysis engendered by therapeutic measures (chemical therapy, radiotherapy, corticoid therapy). The risk of urate precipitation in kidney and urinary tract, already great, is further increased by the acidification of the urine produced by the catabolic waste products. To avoid the occurence of uric acid nephropathy or even anuria, the following measures are usually taken: urinary dilution by forcing of fluids, alkalinization of the urine, and the administration of a xanthine oxidase inhibitor. The same effect can be obtained with uricolytic treatment, which has a hypouricemic action and can thus prevent urate precipitation and the development of renal lithiasis (KISSEL et al. [12], ZITTOUN et al. [29]). The rapidity of the uricolytic effect of urate oxidase avoids postponement of the cytolytic treatment.

3. In Obesity

Weight reduction obtained by caloric restriction or fasting is frequently associated with an increase of uricemia. By combining dietary restriction with administration of urate oxidase, hyperuricemia can be prevented (DEBRY et al. [7]; ASCH [3]). The uricolytic treatment allows to apply fasting diets in hyperuricemic or gouty, obese patients, without risk of renal or gouty complications.

III. Ophthalmology

Senile macular degenerations are relatively often associated with hyperuricemia, and signs of retinal and vitreous uric acid accumulation can be observed. In such patients, improvement of visual acuity may be obtained by uricolytic therapy (ALGAN [1]).

E. Tolerance

I. Clinical Tolerance

More or less painful erythematous reactions can sometimes be seen at the injection points. Signs of general intolerance, such as generalized urticaria, transitory uneasiness, febrile reactions, and shock are rare. The urate oxidase therapy does not seem to lead to hematologic, hepatic, or renal complications. As frequently pointed out, acute attacks of gout may occur during uricolytic treatment.

II. Immunologic Reactions

Immunologic phenomena have been elicited in the sera of patients treated by urate oxidase. The double diffusion method of Ouchterlony or the complement fixation method showed a moderate increase of antienzyme antibodies (ROYER et al. [26]; BROGARD et al. [4]). No clear-cut correlation between immunologic reactivity and the decline of the uricolytic response was noticed (MIZON et al. [22]). Indeed, the enzymatic and antigenic properties of urate oxidase are probably not located at the same sites (ROYER et al. [26]).

The intradermal reaction to urate oxidase can be positive after uricolytic enzyme treatment, which indicates the development of immunity. The reaction, however, tends to diminish with the postponed administration of a new urate oxidase (ROYER et al. [26]).

F. The Use of Uricolytic Therapy: Limits, Indicators, Methods

Theoretically, urate oxidase therapy can reduce all hyperuricemias, except that of the uncommon Lesch-Nyhan syndrome.

The uricolytic treatment meets with two kinds of difficulties: on the one hand, the necessity of parenteral administration of urate oxidase and, on the other hand, the decline of the uricolytic response, which is frequently seen during and after the second week of treatment.

In our view, the administration of urate oxidase is indicated in acute hyperuricemia, whether primary or secondary, when gouty or renal involvements are likely to occur. The following situations are concerned:
— gouty hyperuricemia, mainly the gout with polyarticular tophi
— gout complicated by renal nephropathy
— secondary hyperuricemia, due to renal failure
— hyperuricemia of hemopathies, mainly during the cytolytic treatment of myeloproliferative syndrome
— hypocaloric diets and fasting, essentially when they are applied to gouty and hyperuricemic obese subjects

The uricolytic treatment consisting of intramuscular injections of 1000 units of urate oxidase, repeated daily for 10–15 days, can be resumed at 2 or 3 month intervals if necessary.

After initial treatment of hyperuricemia, the administration of urate oxidase can be replaced by the usual hypouricemic therapy: the previous reduction of the uric acid pool by enzymatic treatment diminishes the risk of uric acid or xanthine precipitation in the urinary tract, which follow the administration of uricosuric substances or of xanthine oxidase inhibitors.

Editor's note: In most countries urate oxidase is not available for use in humans. Clearly, additional studies will be necessary before enzymatic uricolysis can be considered as the treatment of choice in any clinical condition associated with hyperuricemia.

References

1. Algan, B.: Considérations sur l'action de l'urate-oxydase sur des manifestations rétiniennes de l'hyperuricémie. Bull. Soc. belge Ophtal **158**, 332—336 (1971)
2. Altman, K. I., Smull, K., Guzman Barron, E. S. G.: A new method for the preparation of uricase and the effect of uricase on the blood uric acid levels of the chickens. Arch. Biochem. Biophys. **21**, 158—165 (1949)
3. Asch, L.: Expérimentation clinique d'une urate-oxydase. Rev. Rhumatisme **39**, 2, 129—136 (1972)
4. Brogard, J. M., Coumaros, D., Frankhauser, J., Stahl, A., Stahl, J.: Enzymatic uricolysis: a study of the effect of a fungal urate-oxydase. Europ. J. clin. and biol. Res. **17** (9), 890—895 (1972)

5. Brogard, J. M., Frankhauser, J., Stahl, A.: Application de l'uricolyse enzymatique au traitement des hyperuricémies d'origine rénale. Schweiz. med. Wschr. **103**, 404—410 (1973)
6. Brunaud, M., Gros, P., Navarro, J., Raveux, R.: Etude pharmacologique d'une urate-oxydase extraite d'Aspergillus flavus link. Thérapie **24**, 785—795 (1969)
7. Debry, G., David, X., Lorrain, J., Gonand, J. P., Bigard, M. P.: Utilisation de l'urate-oxydase dans les cures de jeûne des obéses. Ann. méd. Nancy **11**, 537—541 (1972)
8. Devulder, B., Plouvier, B., Desprez, Th., Lemaire, P., Tacquet, A.: Influence de l'insuffisance rénale sur la pharmacocinétique et le métabolisme de l'urate-oxydase. Lille Médical **21**, 4, 293—301 (1976)
9. Fontenaille, C., Guiheneuc, P., Prost, A., Heron, B., Royer, R., Boulange, M.: Mode d'élimination rénale de l'acide urique chez les goutteux et les sujets normaux à des taux sanguins comparables. Résultats préliminaires. J. Urol. Néphrol. **78**, 741—743 (1972)
10. Hawthorn, E., Lapousse, J. C., Maestracci, D., D'Omezon, Y.: Traitement de l'uricémie des goutteux par l'urate-oxydase. Lyon-Méditerranée Méd. **8**, 1351—1356 (1972)
11. Kageyama, N.: Enzymatic assay of uric acid. Clin. chim. Acta **31**, 421—426 (1971)
12. Kissel, P., Lamarche, M., Royer, R.: Modification of uricaemia and the excretion of uric acid nitrogen by an enzyme of fungal origin. Nature (Lond.) **217**, 5123, 72—74 (1968)
13. Kissel, P., Schmitt, J., Streiff, F., Makuary, G., Schmidt, C., Toussain, P.: L'urate-oxydase: son intérêt dans la prévention des hyperuricémies thérapeutiques en hématologie. Ann. Méd. Nancy **11**, 519—536 (1972)
14. Laboureur, P., Langlois, C.: Urate-oxydase d'Aspergillus flavus. 1) Obtention, purification, propriétés. 2) Métabolisme, inhibition, spécificité. Bull. Soc. chim. Biol. **50**, 811—841 (1968)
15. Labrune, B., Cartier, P., Bonnenfant, F., Ribierre, M., Mallet, R.: Encéphalopathie familiale avec hyperuricémie. Etude du métabolisme des purines. Essais thérapeutiques. Arch. Franç. Pédiat. **26**, 139—154 (1969)
16. Lathem, W., Rodnan, G. P.: Impairment of uric acid excretion in gout. J. clin. Invest. **41**, 1955—1963 (1962)
17. Legras, B., Royer, R. J., Thomas, J. L.: Effets d'une hypouricémie aigue sur la synthése endogène des purines. Ann. Méd. Nancy **11**, 517—526 (1972)
18. London, M., Finkle, A.: On the potential enzymatic control of uric acid metabolism. J. Urol. **76**, 2, 168—173 (1956)
19. London, M., Hudson, P. B.: Purification and properties of solubilized uricase. Biochem. biophys. Acta **21**, 290—298 (1956)
20. London, M., Hudson, P. B.: Uricolytic activity of purified uricase in two human beings. Science **125**, 937—938 (1957)
21. Louyot, P., Montet, Y., Roland, J., Pourel, J.: L'urate-oxydase dans le traitement de la goutte de l'hyperuricémie. Rev. Rhumatisme Maladies Ostéo-Articulaires **37**, 12, 795—808 (1970)
22. Mizon, J. P., Plaquet, R., Gentit, F., Quiret, J. L.: Orientation nouvelle du traitement de la goutte. Etude clinique et biologique de l'urate-oxydase. Lille Médical **16**, 9, 1332—1345 (1971)
23. Nugent, C. A., Tyler, F. H.: The renal excretion of uric acid in patients with gout and in nongouty subjects. J. clin. Invest. **38**, 1890—1898 (1959)
24. Oppenheimer, E. H.: The lowering of blood uric acid by uricase injections. Bull. Johns Hopkins Hosp. **68**, 190—195 (1941)
25. Oppenheimer, E. H., Kunkel, H. G.: Further observations on the lowering of blood uric acid by uricase injections. Bull. Johns Hopkins Hosp.. **73**, 40—53 (1943)
26. Royer, R., Lamarche, M., Kissel, P.: Etude de l'action d'une urate-oxydase fongique sur l'uricémie et l'excrétion de l'azote urique chez l'homme. Thérapie **22**, 1113—1125 (1967)
27. Royer, R., Vindell, J., Lamarche, M., Kissel, P.: Modalités d'élimination des purines au cours du traitement enzymatique de la goutte et des états hyperuricémiques par une urate-oxydase. Presse méd. **76**, 49, 2325—2328 (1968)
28. Stahl, A., Schang, A. M., Brogard, J. M., Coumaros, D.: Technique de dosage de l'allantoïne sérique et étude de l'action de l'uricase. Ann. biol. Clin. **28**, 377—385 (1970)
29. Zittoun, R., Dauchy, F., Teillaud, C., Barthelemy, M., Bouchard, P.: Le traitement des hyperuricémies en hématologie par l'urate-oxydase et l'allopurinol. Ann. méd. Interne **127**, 6—7, 479—482 (1976)

CHAPTER 23

Pharmacology of Drugs Used in Treatment of Acute Gout

S. L. WALLACE and N. H. ERTEL

A. Introduction

Once the diagnosis of acute gout is made, treatment is generally simple and straightforward. Acute gout is probably the most easily treated of the arthritides, provided that therapy is begun early. Most agents effective in controlling acute gouty inflammation have been in use for years and are well known; several new agents have recently become available (WALLACE, 1975). A number of reports on the treatment of acute gout have been published (GOLDFINGER, 1971; WALLACE, 1972; WYNGAARDEN and KELLEY, 1976). Table 1 lists the major drugs that have been used for this purpose in clinical practice. The pharmacology and mechanisms of action of these drugs are less well appreciated, however, and deserve further emphasis, although a series of reviews of the clinical pharmacology of one of these agents, colchicine, has previously been reported (WALLACE, 1961, 1965; WALLACE and ERTEL, 1969; WALLACE, 1974). Much new recent information has become available.

B. Colchicine

I. Brief History

Colchicine is derived from the seeds and corms of the plant *Colchicum autumnale* (Fig. 1), also known as the meadow saffron or as the autumn crocus. The plant is a member of the lily family, however, and is not a true crocus. Colchicum may have been listed in the Ebers papyrus, an Egyptian document of about 1550 B.C., as a saffron (EIGSTI and DUSTIN, 1955). The first clearly recorded use of extracts of the plant in the treatment of acute gout dates to the sixth century A.D., when Alexander

Table 1. Drugs in the Treatment of Acute Gout

Colchicine orally
Colchicine intravenously
Trimethylcolchicinic acid
Phenylbutazone
Oxyphenbutazone
Indomethacin
Naproxen
Fenoprofen
Adrenocorticotrophic hormone
Adrenocortical steroids orally
Adrenocortical steroids intraarticularly

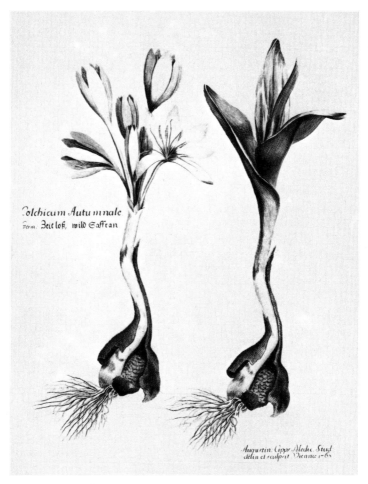

Fig. 1. *Colchicum autumnale*, from STÖRCK *Libellus quo demonstratur Colchici autumnalis radicem* Vienna, Joannis Thomas Trattner, 1763

of Tralles recommended it (HARTUNG, 1954). The drug was reintroduced into therapy by Nicholas Husson, a French Army officer, in Eau Medicinale d'Husson, a patent medicine that he offered as a panacea for innumerable diseases in 1780. The nature of the active ingredient was shown by WANT in 1814 to be colchicum (COPEMAN, 1964; WALLACE, 1973). PELLETIER and CAVENTOU (1820) determined that the active principle of colchicum was the alkaloid colchicine, and they produced a pure preparation. The purified substance has been in constant use in the treatment of acute gout ever since.

II. Structure and Structure/Function Relationships

Colchicine has been synthesized (WOODWARD, 1963), but commercially available preparations are extracted from the plant. Pure colchicine, $C_{22}H_{25}O_6N$, forms fine,

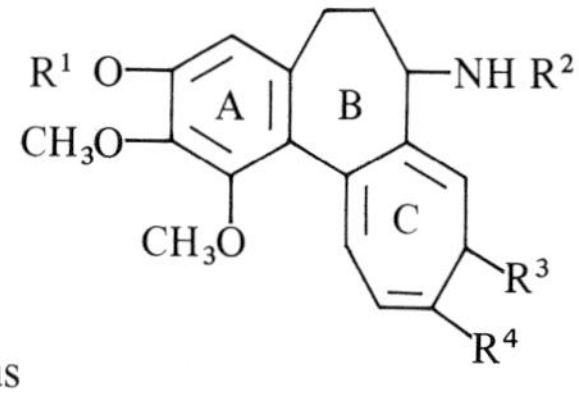

Fig. 2. Central colchicine nucleus

	R_1	R_2	R_3	R_4
Colchicine	CH_3	$COCH_3$	O	OCH_3
Desacetylmethylcolchicine	CH_3	CH_3	O	OCH_3
Desacetylthiocolchicine	CH_3	H	O	SCH_3
Colchicoside	$C_6H_{11}O_5$	$COCH_3$	O	OCH_3
Trimethylcolchicinic acid	CH_3	H	O	OH
Colchiceine	CH_3	$COCH_3$	OH	O

practically colorless needles. It is readily soluble in alcohol, chloroform, or cold water but is less soluble in hot water or cold benzene and is almost insoluble in ether (LOUDON, 1955).

The structure of the molecule was finally determined in 1945, after many years of research by numerous investigators (DEWAR, 1945). The molecule is shown in Figure 2. Its structure contains a number of unusual features, especially the 7 carbon ring B and the tropolonoid configuration of the side chains of the 7 carbon ring C. Three methoxyl groups are attached to the benzenoid first ring. Ring B has an acetylamino side chain, while the tropolonoid features of ring C require a ketone group and another methoxyl group.

Studies have been made of the correlation between the structure of colchicine and some of its analogs (Fig. 2) and the effect of these agents in the treatment of urate crystal-induced inflammation in man (WALLACE, 1959, 1961) and animals (FITZGERALD et al., 1971; ZWEIG et al., 1972; CHANG and MALAWISTA, 1976).

In man, the colchicine analogues tested in the treatment of acute gout were desacetylmethylcolchicine, desacethylthiocolchicine, colchicoside, trimethylcolchicinic acid, and colchiceine. The relationships of each of these compounds to colchicine is shown in Figure 2. These substances were used in the treatment of acute gouty arthritis in man in doses approximately equimolecular to therapeutic amounts of colchicine. Desacetylmethylcolchicine, desacetylthiocolchicine, and trimethylcolchicinic acid were effective; colchicoside was less potent, although it retained some antigout activity, and colchiceine was completely ineffective, both orally and intravenously (WALLACE, 1961). The third ring of colchicine has the configuration of tropolone methyl ether (Fig. 3) (COOK and LOUDON, 1951), and it was concluded that this tropolonoid configuration was necessary for the effectiveness of colchicine in gout (WALLACE, 1959). Tropolone methyl ether has not itself been tested in human gout. A study of the ability of colchicine analogues to suppress human polymorphonuclear leukocyte motility, however, showed that the analogues had about the same order of effectiveness as their clinical potency in treating gout (PHELPS and McCARTY, 1969).

Animal experimentation has yielded somewhat divergent results. FITZGERALD et al. (1971) found colchiceine, trimethylcolchicinic acid, and tropolone all ineffective in

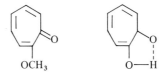

Fig. 3. Tropolone methyl ether and tropolone

suppressing mouse paw swelling induced by urate crystals. They found that both the nitrogen-containing side chain of the second ring and the methoxytropolone structure of the third ring were necessary for suppression of urate-induced inflammation. Conversely, FITZGERALD (1976) found that allocolchicine, in which the third ring of colchicine is benzenoid, without a tropolone formulation, continued to be effective as an antimitotic agent. BENITEZ et al. (1953, 1954), interestingly enough have shown that though tropolone itself did not act on cell mitosis, its presence completely abolished the antimitotic effects of colchicine on rat fibroblast tissue cultures.

ZWEIG and co-workers (1972) found colchiceine to have antiinflammatory potency in urate-induced inflammation in rats, in contrast to both the human (WALLACE, 1959) and mouse studies (FITZGERALD et al., 1971) described above, but found trimethylcolchicinic acid ineffective. The variations among species in drug studies is well known, and extrapolation of animal data to human is risky. CHANG and MALAWISTA (1976) have recently shown that in dogs colchicine suppressed the development of urate crystal-induced inflammation only at a dose that produced drastic drops in peripheral leukocyte counts; doses that did not affect white cell counts did not affect this animal model of gouty inflammation. In ZWEIG et al.'s (1972) studies, colchicine doses necessary to produce 70% suppression of inflammation killed three-quarters of the animals studied. The same doses on a milligram per kilogram basis in humans would be uniformly fatal. It seems clear that animal results, at least in regard to colchicine structure-function relationships, bear no necessary relationship to colchicine pharmacology in humans.

Colchicine is highly light sensitive. Sunlight exposure of colchicine for prolonged periods or to ultraviolet light for shorter periods of time leads to the formation of three photoisomeric products, α, β, and γ-lumicolchicine (Fig. 4) (GREWE and WOLFE, 1951; WILSON and FRIEDKIN, 1966). β and γ-lumicolchicine are stereoisomers (FORBES, 1955), and α-lumicolchicine is a dimer of β-lumicolchicine (WILDMAN and PURSEY, 1968). As can be seen in Figure 4, the tropolonoid structure of colchicine is lost in these photoisomers.

The lumicolchicines did not react with microtubular protein (WILSON and FRIEDKIN, 1967). They were ineffective in arresting mitosis in metaphase in human lymphocyte tissue culture (SAGORIN et al., 1972), in plant secondary root hairs (LINSKENS and WULF, 1953), and in intact grasshopper embryos (WILSON and FRIEDKIN, 1967). The lumicolchicines did not affect plasma protein release from rat hepatocytes as colchicine did (REDMAN et al., 1975). The lumicolchicines were also not antiinflammatory, at least as defined by an inability to inhibit the reverse passive Arthus phenomenon in the rat (MALAWISTA et al., 1972). As far as is known, lumicolchicines have not been purposefully tested in the treatment of acute gout, although large concentrations of lumicolchicines have been found in some batches of colchicine for i.v. injection,

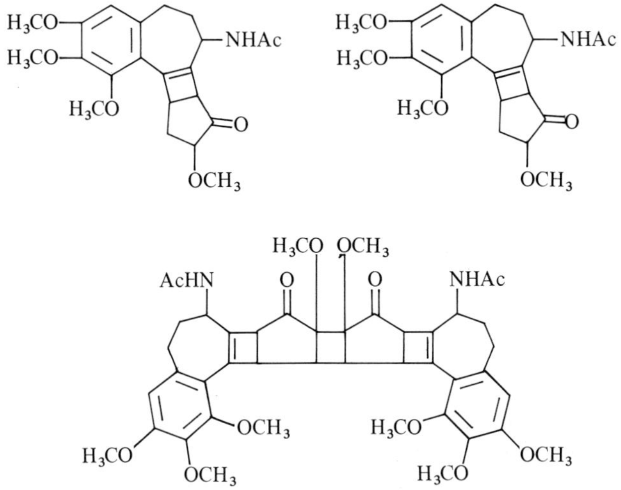

Fig. 4. β, γ, and α lumicolchicine

packaged in clear glass ampules (SAGORIN et al., 1972). If the tropolonoid side chains of the third ring of the colchicine molecule are indeed necessary for its effect on urate crystal-induced inflammation (WALLACE, 1959; FITZGERALD et al., 1971), then the lumicolchicines might be expected in theory not to be effective in the treatment of acute gout.

However, colchicine and the lumicolchicines have been shown to produce similar or identical effects in other cell systems. Both colchicine and the lumicolchicines, but not trimethylcolchicinic acid, inhibited the uptake of adenosine, guanosine, thymidine, and uridine in HeLa cells in a concentration-dependent manner (MIZEL and WILSON, 1972). Similarly, both colchicine and lumicolchicine interfered with nucleoside transport across alveolar macrophage membranes (BERLIN, 1973). Both lumicolchicine and colchicine aggregated plasma membrane intramembranous particles in fibroblasts (FURCHT and SCOTT, 1975). Rat and mouse liver microsomes and nuclear membranes bound about equal amounts of colchicine and lumicolchicine (STADLER and FRANKE, 1974). Finally, both colchicine and lumicolchicine have been shown to inhibit pigment granule aggregation in fiddler crab melanophores (LAMBERT and FINGERMAN, 1976).

III. Metabolism

BOYLAND and MAWSON (1938) first reported a chemical method for measuring colchicine. The alkaloid was converted by hydrolysis in dilute acid solution to colchiceine. The latter was shown to have a green color with ferric chloride in chloroform, which could be measured colorimetrically. This method is quite specific but relatively insensitive. BRUES (1942, 1951) gave colchicine intravenously to mice and measured tissue and body fluid levels by the method of BOYLAND and MAWSON (1938). Following i.v. injection, colchicine rapidly disappeared from the blood stream and extended beyond the extracellular water in a minute or two. The apparent volume of distribution exceeded that of the body water within 0.5 h. Excretion of 10%–20% of the administered dose occurred in the urine during the period of highest blood level. Colchicine was also excreted into the intestine, both by way of bile (shown by biliary fistula) and to a lesser extent directly. Over a several-hour period, one-half to two-thirds of the injected dose appeared within the intestinal tract. Colchicine appeared in the bile almost immediately after injection.

Using a similar colorimetric method, FLEISCHMAN et al. (1965, 1967, 1968), after the administration of very large doses of colchicine to golden hamsters and to gerbils, demonstrated that the drug was excreted in urine, the gastrointestinal tract, and bile.

Other methods have been used for measuring colchicine. LETTRE (1944, 1952) devised a biologic method, extracting blood and tissues containing colchicine and noting the effects of the extracts upon chicken heart fibroblast tissue cultures. Colchicine administered intraperitoneally into the guinea pig was excreted by the liver via bile into the intestine. No urinary excretion was found. PADAWER (1968) also used a morphologic approach to colchicine quantification. He noted the changes in rat peritoneal mast cells associated with various concentrations of the drug. The method was not used, however, in actual studies of colchicine metabolism.

WALASZEK et al. (1952) prepared radioactive, ^{14}C labeled colchicine by growing the plant in a radioactive CO_2 atmosphere and then extracting the colchicine. The labeling was presumably random; the ^{14}C was not located precisely within the colchicine molecule. Studies of these workers were the first approaches to the use of labeled colchicine in studying the metabolism of the drug.

Four hours after the administration of this colchicine preparation to mice, no labeled colchicine was found in the blood, brain, muscle, or heart, but large amounts were present in the intestines, kidney, spleen, and liver (BACK et al., 1951; BACK and WALASZEK, 1953). From 3% to 9% of the administered dose was excreted in the urine as labeled colchicine in the mouse, rat, guinea-pig, and hamster (WALASZEK and KOCSIS, 1956). Exhaled CO_2 containing the label, represented 5%–32% of the administered dose in these animals in 24 h (WALASZEK and KOCSIS, 1956).

Labeled colchicine was given to men (3 mg i.v.), some with gout, others with cancer, and to a third "normal" group without either of these disorders (WALASZEK et al., 1954; WALASZEK et al., 1960). Urinary excretion was much greater in the "normals" than in the gouty or cancer groups. No details of renal function were given. Blood measurements were made in only two men, one with carcinoma of the prostate and one with gout. Peak levels occurred at 0.5 h after i.v. administration and averaged 1 $\mu g/100$ ml. Respiratory excretion was again confirmed (WALASZEK et al., 1960).

As noted above, colchicine is highly light sensitive and under the influence of sunlight or ultraviolet light is altered in part or totally to the lumicolchicines (GREWE and WOLFE, 1951; FORBES, 1955; WILSON and FRIEDKIN, 1966; SAGORIN et al., 1972). WALASZEK and co-workers in the above studies may have underestimated true colchicine levels by the amount converted to lumicolchicine during the studies.

Further and more precise studies of colchicine metabolism, using radioisotopic techniques, required the investigation and solution of two major methodologic problems: 1) the finding of chromatographic systems capable of purifying colchicine with specificity from biologic extracts, and 2) the assessment of the rate of formation of photoisomers of colchicine, when exposed to light and other handling, under various experimental conditions (ERTEL and WALLACE, 1970). Four paper and four thin-layer chromatographic systems were studied for their ability to separate colchicine from its photoisomers and various available colchicine analogues. Two of the paper and two of the thin-layer systems were found to be superior to the others; a thin-layer system, originally devised by WALDI et al. (1961) for the separation of alkaloids was found to be most useful. This system was thin-layer chromatography on silica gel GF_{251} developed for 30 min in chloroform: acetone: diethylamine (50:40:10) (ERTEL and WALLACE, 1970; WALLACE et al., 1970).

Colchicine, labeled with ^{14}C on the methoxyl group of ring C, was used (see Fig. 2) in the study of colchicine metabolism (WALLACE et al., 1970). The prior evidence that the tropolone configuration of the colchicine molecule was necessary for its antigout effect (WALLACE, 1959) suggested the location of the label. Labeled colchicine was mixed with 2 mg cold colchicine and administered intravenously to four groups of patients, one with gout, one with severe renal disease but normal liver function, one with severe liver disease but normal kidney function, and a final group hospitalized with miscellaneous disorders but without gout, renal, or hepatic disease. Blood was obtained at frequent intervals for 2 h.

No colchicine metabolites containing the ^{14}C label were recovered from plasma during the period of study. The apparent volume of distribution for colchicine was much larger than the extracellular fluid volume. The mean apparent volume of distribution for the "normal" individuals (without gout, kidney, or liver disease) was 2.19 ± 0.80 liter/kg body wt. This data confirmed BRUES' (1942, 1951) conclusion that colchicine rapidly goes beyond the extracellular space, inferentially entering cells. For the same group of patients, the plasma half-time for colchicine was only 19.3 ± 7.5 min, again in humans paralleling BRUES' data in mice. The mean calculated zero time colchicine concentration for this group was 1.8 ± 0.7 µg/dl.

Patients with severe hepatocellular disease had higher initial colchicine concentrations, more rapid disappearance, smaller apparent volumes of distribution, shorter colchicine half-times, and greater urinary excretion than did the control "normal" group. Others have shown in animals (LETTRE, 1944; BACK and WALASZEK, 1953) that large amounts of administered colchicine enter the liver. In our studies (WALLACE et al., 1970) the partial exclusion of damaged liver cells from colchicine would logically lead to initially higher plasma colchicine concentrations. With normal renal function, excretion would be more rapid.

Hepatic transport of colchicine in humans has been suggested by clinical evidence (BORUCHOW, 1966). A patient with jaundice due to extrahepatic biliary obstruction demonstrated marked colchicine toxicity on administration of large, but generally nontoxic doses. Biliary excretion of colchicine in rats, hamsters, dogs, and rabbits has been demonstrated after i.v. administration (HUNTER and KLAASEN, 1975). The excretion involved active transport against a concentration gradient. Bile/plasma, liver/plasma, and bile/liver concentrations were consistently greater than 1 and increased with time.

A new radioimmunoassay method for measuring colchicine in plasma and urine has been reported (MITTLER et al., 1975; ERTEL et al., 1976). A different radioimmunoassay method for colchicine, based on antibodies to a conjugate of N-deacetylthiocolchicine and protein, was also described (BOUDENE et al., 1975) at the same time; this assay was 100 times less sensitive than the preceeding one, however, and would not be clinically or pharmacologically useful.

In the Ertel-Mittler assay, colchicine was conjugated to bovine serum albumin through the ketone group on ring C and injected with Freund's adjuvant into New Zealand white rabbits. Antibodies to the colchicine-bovine serum albumin conjugate were produced in one of the rabbits. Colchicine (2 mg i.v.) was given to seven adult males and blood drawn serially for 2 h thereafter. Urine collections were made for up to 10 days after the single colchicine administration.

The calculated zero time plasma colchicine concentration using this method was 2.9 ± 1.5 μg/dl, and the mean half-time was 58 ± 10 min (ERTEL et al., 1976). With the ^{14}C label method (WALLACE et al., 1970), the comparable figures were 1.8 ± 0.7 μg/dl for calculated zero time plasma colchicine concentration and 19.3 ± 7.5 min for plasma half-time. The higher figures with the new method presumably reflect greater sensitivity. Maximal urinary excretion occurred within 2 h after administration of colchicine. Significant amounts of colchicine were still found in the urine up to 10 days after the single dose, an observation also made with the ^{14}C label technique (ERTEL and WALLACE, 1971).

Colchicine's rapid disappearance from the plasma, and equally rapid spread beyond the extracellular fluid, strongly suggests that it enters cells. Colchicine is a lipid-soluble drug and as such crosses lipid cell membrane barriers quickly. Circulating leukocytes represent an excellent tissue for the study of colchicine's entry into cells. They are easily accessible and are thus available for measuring concentrations. Secondly, there is evidence to show that polymorphonuclear leukocytes are necessary for urate crystal-induced inflammation (PHELPS and McCARTY, 1966; CHANG and GRALLA, 1968). A study of leukocyte concentrations of colchicine after i.v. administration using the ^{14}C label method, demonstrated that the peak concentration occurred at 10 min and that stable concentrations, roughly 10 times the maximal plasma concentrations, were maintained for 24 h (ERTEL and WALLACE, 1971). The fall off was slow, and significant concentrations of colchicine were measurable in leukocytes as late as 10 days after a single i.v. dose. These results were based on a method requiring persistence of a ring C methoxyl group containing the ^{14}C tag. Therefore, white cell colchicine concentrations were measured by radioimmunoassay (ERTEL, unpublished data). Preliminary data in two patients showed that in the first 2 h after an i.v. bolus of 3 mg colchicine, the white cell concentration was less than that found in plasma. At 24 h the concentrations were similar. However, 48–96 h after injection, the plasma colchicine concentration declined to low or undetectable levels, while the white cell concentration remained elevated. At 96 h there was a mean white cell colchicine concentration of 1.4 ng/ml. The persistence within the cell undoubtedly is a function of binding to microtubular protein and to other sites (see below). Release of colchicine from cells has been shown to be very slow (reviewed by WALLACE, 1974).

All of the above studies of colchicine metabolism were done after parenteral administration. Plasma levels of colchicine have been measured by the ^{14}C label method after a single oral dose of 1.0 mg (WALLACE and ERTEL, 1973). Peak plasma colchicine concentrations were reached from 0.5 h to 2 h after oral administration. The mean maximal levels were around 0.2 μg/dl, approximately one-tenth the calculated zero time concentrations achieved after the i.v. administration of twice the dose (and using the same method for measurement) (WALLACE et al., 1970).

The location of the colchicine absorption site or sites is not certain. However, the administration of relatively large doses of colchicine has been shown to produce jejunal (RACE et al., 1970) and ileal (WEBB et al., 1968) dysfunction. Presumably, most colchicine absorption occurs in the jejunum and ileum.

Study of colchicine metabolism in man, using either method of measurement, has failed to show evidence of the appearance of metabolites in plasma, urine, or cells (WALLACE et al., 1970; ERTEL and WALLACE, 1971; WALLACE and ERTEL, 1973; ERTEL et al., 1976). SCHOENHARTING et al. (1973) used the Udenfriend system to study colchicine metabolism in vitro. The Udenfriend system is an artificial one that simulates oxidative reactions of liver microsomes in drug metabolism. Colchicine was converted to four metabolic products in this system; three involved mono-demethylation at C 2, C 3, and C 10 (colchiceine), and the fourth was a rearrangement at the tropolone ring C into a benzenoid structure (compare with Fig. 2). Metabolism of colchicine by mammalian liver microsomes in vitro has also been shown (SCHOEN-HARTING et al., 1974). Oxidative monodemethylation has been confirmed in this system as well. It is not clear why metabolites, if they occur in vivo, could not be identified in our studies.

IV. Mechanism of Action

BORISY and TAYLOR (1967) first showed that colchicine binds to microtubular sub-unit protein and interferes with its aggregation into microtubules. This is undoubt-edly the mechanism whereby colchicine leads to the arrest of mitosis at metaphase. Colchicine's action on microtubular function has been studied extensively and has recently been reviewed (MARGOLIS, 1973).

MALAWISTA (1968, 1975) has presented strong arguments to suggest that colchi-cine's mechanism of action in the treatment of acute gout is essentially the same as that in mitosis arrest—an action on microtubule precursors. He demonstrated the presence of microtubules in polymorphonuclear leukocytes and that these microtu-bules were sensitive to colchicine (MALAWISTA and BENSCH, 1967). MALAWISTA (1975) has described the sensitivity of many polymorphonuclear functions to colchi-cine in vitro, although generally at concentrations much higher than those achieva-ble in vivo during therapy (WALLACE et al., 1970; ERTEL et al., 1976).

The only functions of the polymorphonuclear leukocyte consistently interfered with by colchicine in concentrations achievable in vivo, were those concerned with generation of, or response to, a chemotactic stimulus (CANER, 1965; PHELPS, 1970a, b; SPILBERG et al., 1974).

Since the polymorphonuclear leukocyte is necessary for acute urate crystal-in-duced inflammation (PHELPS and MCCARTY, 1966; CHANG and GRALLA, 1968), it has generally been assumed that colchicine acts on this cell. ORTEL and NEWCOMBE (1974) recently described the response of proved acute gouty arthritis to colchicine in a renal transplant patient with virtual absence of polymorphonuclear leukocytes from synovial fluid. The alternative cell suggested to be acted on by colchicine was the phagocytic synoviocyte (ORTEL and NEWCOMBE, 1974; AGUDELO and SCHU-MACHER, 1973).

There are, however, a number of contrary arguments to the Malawista hypothe-sis—whether the pertinent cell is the polymorphonuclear leukocyte or the synovio-cyte or both. One of these is the demonstration that trimethylcolchicinic acid, a colchicine analogue (see Fig. 2) effective in the treatment of acute gout (WALLACE, 1959, 1961; SMYTH and FRANK, 1962) had *no* effect on microtubular precursor protein, not even in concentrations 1000 times higher than effective concentrations of colchicine (MIZEL and WILSON, 1972). As one would expect, if trimethylcolchicinic acid does not act on microtubular precursor protein, it is not antimitotic. There is a plentitude of confirmatory evidence, summarized by WALLACE (1975).

MALAWISTA (1975) has suggested that because of the similarity between the colchicine and trimethylcolchicinic acid molecules, in vivo metabolic changes in the latter might change it to the former, or some other colchicine analogue with antimicrotubule effect. There are very good arguments against this hypothesis. SCHOENHARTING et al. (1973, 1974) have shown in vitro that colchicine metabolism (if it occurs in vivo) is primarily one of demethylation by liver microsomes, plus a change of the tropolonoid structure of ring C to a benzene ring configuration. Similar changes to the trimethylcolchicinic acid molecule would not produce a substance with antimitotic effect. As noted above (WALLACE, 1959; FITZGERALD et al., 1971), the tropolone configuration of the third ring of colchicine is *necessary* for its antigout effect although not for its antimitotic effect (FITZGERALD, 1976); this configuration is lost in colchicine (and presumably would be in trimethylcolchicinic acid) during the in vitro metabolic studies of SCHOENHARTING et al. (1973, 1974).

PHELPS and MCCARTY (1969) have shown, in an in vitro system where drug metabolism is essentially precluded, that trimethylcolchicinic acid is nearly as effective as colchicine in interfering with human polymorphonuclear leukocyte motility. There is one further piece of evidence demonstrating that trimethylcolchicinic acid is not likely to be converted to colchicine in vivo. Trimethylcolchicinic acid has been given in doses as high as 16–25 mg over a 2-day period to men with gout; no colchicine-like (or other) side effects ensued (WALLACE, 1959; SMYTH and FRANK, 1962).

One can only conclude that if trimethylcolchicinic acid is effective in gout, has no effect on microtubules, and is chemically so similar to colchicine, then colchicine's effect in gout is most likely mediated by some other mechanism.

Another colchicine analog, desacetamidocolchicine, with greater antimitotic potency than colchicine, had very little antiinflammatory effect against urate crystal-induced inflammation in animals (FITZGERALD et al., 1971).

WILSON and BRYAN (1974) have noted that "a potential hazard associated with the use of the colchicine-binding reaction to measure tubulin quantitatively is the assumption that all macromolecularly bound colchicine in a particular cell extract is bound solely to tubulin." There is now a multiplicity of evidence that cellular substances other than microtubular protein bind colchicine. A study of the autoradiographic localization of colchicine binding sites demonstrated that colchicine was bound largely to nuclear material rather than to microtubules (FRANKE et al., 1972). In rat liver homogenate, colchicine binding proteins were found by chemical means in crude nuclei, in mitochondrial and ergastoplasmic fractions, and in microsomal fractions. Only 22% of the colchicine was found in the microtubular fraction (STADLER and FRANKE, 1972). Colchicine has been shown to bind to membranes; the binding capability is very high in nuclear membranes from mammalian liver. This liver membrane binding of colchicine differs in a series of ways from colchicine binding to microtubular protein. Differences include heat stability, dependence on drug concentration, and evidence that liver microsomes and nuclear membranes bind equal amounts of colchicine and lumicolchicine (STADLER and FRANKE, 1974).

In the section of this chapter on colchicine's structure/function relationships, a number of other ways in which colchicine and lumicolchicine behave similarly were cited. Both substances inhibited nucleoside transport across membranes (MIZEL and WILSON, 1972; BERLIN, 1973). Both aggregated plasma membrane particles in fibroblasts (FURCHT and SCOTT, 1975). Both functioned similarly in other ways. And yet lumicolchicines *do not* react with microtubular protein (WILSON and FRIEDKIN, 1967).

Colchicine, it is clear, has cellular functions other than microtubular ones. A possible additional site where colchicine may exert its effect is the plasma or other cell membrane. According to the fluid mosaic model of cell surfaces, proteins are free to diffuse in cell membranes and thus should assume a random or homogeneous distribution. Colchicine-sensitive proteins have been shown to modify the movement of lectin-binding sites in cell membranes (OLIVER et al., 1974). These authors demonstrated a specific effect of colchicine on concavalin-binding sites on polymorphonuclear leukocyte cell membranes. Isolated polymorphonuclear leukocyte membranes, exposed to colchicine, showed decreased concavalin-binding sites compared to control membranes (OLIVER et al., 1974). This effect could not have been exerted by way of the microtubules.

Colchicine's inhibition of nucleoside transport across the HeLa cell membrane (MIZEL and WILSON, 1972) was independent of temperature, in contrast to a microtubular protein effect, as well as being sensitive to lumicolchicine. This action on cell membrane transport was specific for nucleosides and did not affect the transport of a nonmetabolizable sugar or a nonmetabolizable amino acid. BERLIN (1973) showed that colchicine interfered with nucleoside transport across alveolar macrophage membranes. This effect was also accomplished by lumicolchicine but not by vinblastine at a concentration that disrupted microtubules.

Plasma proteins produced by the liver are synthesized on polysomes attached to the membrane of endoplasmic reticulum and are then transported stepwise from the lumen of rough endoplasmic reticulum to the smooth and thus to the Golgi complex. Finally, Golgi-derived vesicles containing the secretory proteins migrate to the sinusoidal cell surface, fuse with the plasma membrane and empty their contents. Colchicine inhibited the late events, after filling of the Golgi-derived vesicles but before fusion of the vesicles to the plasma membrane (REDMAN et al., 1975). At the time this colchicine effect was maximal, neither the concentration nor the arrangement of microtubules was altered by the colchicine. In fact, microtubules were still detected in the Golgi regions, along bile capillaries, and along the sinusoidal front of the hepatocyte, hours after this maximal effect. The authors concluded that the inhibitory effect of colchicine on plasma protein secretion could not be ascribed to microtubule failure of assembly.

LAMBERT and FINGERMAN (1976) concluded that colchicine's activity in inhibiting pigment granule aggregation in melanophores in the fiddler crab was not due to microtubular action, but that the effect was at the cell membrane. WUNDERLICH et al. (1973) noted a direct action of colchicine on the membranes of the ciliate protozoan, *Tetrahymene pyriformis*, impairing the temperature-induced motility of particles of the alveolar membrane. In the concentration used peripheral microtubules were not disaggregated.

In general, colchicine is known to alter the function (MIZEL and WILSON, 1972; PESANTI and AXLINE, 1975), and topographic distribution (UKENA and BERLIN, 1972) of plasma membrane transport sites, to inhibit pinocytic activity (PESANTI and AXLINE, 1975) and to prevent induction of lysosomal acid hydrolases by endocytosis in macrophages (PESANTI and AXLINE, 1975). Abnormal function of the Golgi apparatus (REDMAN et al., 1975; EHRLICH et al., 1974) and stimulation of cellular autophagy (HIRSIMAKI et al., 1975), have been reported for other cells. Not all of these activities have been clearly shown to be unrelated to action on tubulin, but some membranes certainly are affected separately by colchicine.

V. Clinical Use

Colchicine is valuable in gout in three ways: it is an effective treatment for the acute attack (WALLACE et al., 1967); it is a potent prophylactic agent (YÜ and GUTMAN, 1961; PAULUS et al., 1974); and the response to colchicine therapy has diagnostic value (WALLACE et al., 1967).

In the treatment of acute gout, colchicine may be given by two routes, orally or intravenously. The drug is usually taken by mouth, in multiple, fairly frequent, small doses. This method of therapy is designed to minimize the ultimate severity of toxic gastrointestinal effects (see below), rather than in relation to controlling the attack. When first given, 0.5 or 0.6 mg colchicine is given hourly (or twice as much every 2 h) until the first of three possible end results occurs: 1) improvement in the attack of gout; 2) the earliest evidence of gastrointestinal side effects; or 3) if neither of the above occur first, the completion of a maximum dose preselected according to body weight. The range of maximal total doses given by mouth for a single attack is usually 8–16 mg colchicine. Doses of this size cause side effects in many patients. When the effective, or toxic, or maximal dose is established for the patient during his first attack treated with colchicine, in general the same benefit and/or side effects will be obtained with the same dose in subsequent attacks. To speed the response to therapy, half the total dose can be given at once, and the remainder on an hourly or two-hourly basis, with the same three end points.

Generally gastrointestinal toxicity appears before therapeutic benefit, the side effects within 8–12 h and the benefit from 12–48 h after initiating therapy by mouth. About 75% of unselected patients with acute gout will respond rapidly and objectively to colchicine therapy (WALLACE et al., 1967). Delay in beginning treatment is the reason for at least part of the failures with colchicine.

Colchicine is as effective given intravenously as it is by mouth. The major advantage of the i.v. route is that it avoids almost completely the gastrointestinal side effects associated with oral administration of colchicine. Benefit also occurs more rapidly, within 6–24 h, sometimes sooner. In the postoperative patient with acute gout, usually colchicine given intravenously is the treatment of choice. The most significant risk with i.v. colchicine is that of extravasation. The colchicine solution is remarkably irritating, and local sloughs may occur. Care must be taken to ensure that the administering needle is well within the vein, and the colchicine dose should be given slowly. Some recommend diluting the colchicine with 20 ml normal saline prior to administration, to minimize venous inflammation (WYNGAARDEN and KELLEY, 1976), which otherwise would occur with some frequency. The local phlebitis from i.v. colchicine usually has little clinical import, however.

Since i.v. administration of colchicine is rarely if ever associated with significant gastrointestinal side effects, one need not give multiple, fractional doses by this route. We have found a single dose of 3 mg as effective as divided doses in treatment of acute gout (WALLACE, 1974) without the added risk of extravasation or local venous irritation associated with each additional dose. Other investigators (GOLDFINGER, 1971) suggest an initial dose of 2–3 mg. If prompt relief is not obtained, additional doses of 1 mg are given every 6 h. It must be remembered that response to i.v. colchicine may take longer than 6 h.

The recurrence of acute gout can be totally prevented or minimized by the daily administration of small doses of colchicine. Doses ranging from one tablet (0.5–0.6 mg) every other day to four tablets daily (the preponderant dose being 1.0–1.2 mg/day) have been shown to eradicate attacks completely or reduce their frequency significantly in 93% of a large series of patients with gout (YÜ and GUTMAN, 1961).

The value of colchicine as an aid in the diagnosis of gout has diminished with the increasing dependence upon demonstration of the urate crystal as an absolute criterion for the diagnosis. When crystals are not searched for (or rarely, when searched for and not found), the response of the patient to a full course of colchicine may have some diagnostic usefulness. Three studies attest to this. LOCKIE (1939) was the first modern investigator to compare the effects of colchicine upon acute gout with its results in other disorders. All of 75 patients with acute gout responded with marked relief of symptoms, while none of 50 patients with other rheumatic diseases had significant benefit. KANTOR and BROWN (1966) treated 51 patients, 20 with gout and the remainder with other rheumatic disorders, with i.v. colchicine. They concluded that colchicine was highly specific in the treatment of acute gout.

WALLACE et al. (1967) devised rather rigid criteria for the therapeutic response to colchicine to maximize its diagnostic value. A response was defined as a greater than 50% reduction in the inflammatory manifestations of the acute attack within 24–48 h and no recurrence of another episode within 7 days of treatment. Only 75% of the patients with acute gout responded dramatically, while 3 patients of 62 with other rheumatic disorders also met the criteria.

Responses to colchicine in other disorders have been reviewed in WALLACE (1974). Occasional patients with sarcoid arthritis (KAPLAN, 1960, 1963), hydroxyapatite inflammation (THOMPSON et al., 1968), and calcium pyrophosphate crystal-induced arthritis (McCARTY, 1976) may also respond dramatically to colchicine. Patients with sarcoid arthritis may usually be distinguished from those with acute gout by the presence of physical features of sarcoidosis. Calcium pyrophosphate inflammation can best be differentially diagnosed by a search for the appropriate crystal, while hydroxyapatite disease is best recognized radiologically.

VI. Toxicology

The toxic gastrointestinal effects associated with colchicine administration by mouth have been recognized as long as the drug has been in use. Historically, Sydenham may have been responsible in part for the disappearance of colchicum from gout therapy by his strong opposition to purgation in treatment (HARTUNG, 1957). Hyperperistalsis, abdominal cramping pain, a watery diarrhea, nausea and/or vomiting occur in about 80% of patients who take a full therapeutic dose of the drug for the attack; similar symptoms occasionally occur after a period of weeks in patients who take the larger prophylactic doses.

Intravenous administration does not cause the same side effects. The logical assumption must be that the process of gastrointestinal absorption of the drug, presumably in the jejunum and ileum, leads to intestinal cell changes that in themselves produce these symptoms (WALLACE, 1974).

A group of human volunteers were studied, receiving doses of 1.9–3.6 mg colchicine per day for periods up to 3 weeks, but mostly for 4–8 days (FALOON et al., 1966; WEBB et al., 1968; RACE et al., 1970; FALOON, 1970; RUBULIS et al., 1970). All patients developed diarrhea; steatorrhea occurred with the larger dosages. A fall in serum cholesterol associated with enhanced excretion of bile acids and sterol compounds in stool occurred (FALOON et al., 1966; FALOON, 1970; RUBULIS et al., 1970). This increased excretion was presumably due to impaired reabsorption of acidic and neutral sterols in the distal ileum, thus interfering with the enterohepatic cycle of steroids and bile acids. Parenteral colchicine was without effect on serum cholesterol levels or fecal fat excretion (RUBULIS et al., 1970).

Serum carotene levels also fell. d-Xylose absorption was decreased to below normal in all individuals studied during colchicine administration (RACE et al., 1970). There were consistent and marked increases in fecal sodium and potassium and somewhat lesser increases in fecal nitrogen. These changes were dose related. There was a definite decrease in absorption of B_{12} during oral colchicine administration (WEBB et al., 1968). These results were not simply due to diarrhea, because they were not reproduced by cascara.

Histologic studies on jejunal mucosa during colchicine therapy revealed edema and round-cell infiltration in three of five patients. Mucosal lactase and sucrase activities were reduced (RACE et al., 1970). Gastric mucosa was normal on biopsy (WEBB et al., 1968). FALOON (1970) concluded that colchicine affected both the jejunum and the ileum. Decreased absorption of d-xylose and of carotene and reduced enzyme activity in jejunal mucosa were jejunal effects of colchicine. Ileal activity of the drug was manifested by decreased B_{12} absorption and increased excretion of bile acids and sterols in the feces, associated with a fall in serum cholesterol.

There have been a number of animal studies of the effect of colchicine on intestinal mucosa. HERBST et al. (1970) noted, on giving colchicine to rats, a mild diarrhea but general good health. Intestinal lactase activity was most severely depressed, invertase less markedly, and maltase not at all. Alkaline phosphatase, another brush border enzyme, was also depressed. Histologically, there was only a mild increase in inflammatory and goblet cells. In the guinea-pig, colchicine reduced sucrase and maltase levels but not gamma glutamyl transpeptidase (COHEN and McNAMARA, 1970). Colchicine caused reduced dehydrogenase activity in intestinal mucosa in mice (MYREN et al., 1966) and depressed xylose absorption in dogs (LUKETIC and SHAPIRO, 1964). The drug, given orally to dogs 4 mg/day for 14 days, produced severe malabsorption, as demonstrated by increased fecal fat, lowered xylose absorption, decreased serum cholesterol levels, and depressed disaccharidase activity (HILL, 1972).

Intraperitoneal colchicine administered to rats resulted in a delay and a decrease in lymphatic absorption of oleic acid administered per duodenum (GLICKMAN et al., 1976). Colchicine had no effect on protein synthesis nor on glucose transport in the intestinal cells. Lipoprotein release, however, occurs at the same location in the cell plasma membrane as glucose transport, and yet the effects were disparate. The authors could not be certain whether the mechanism was related to a direct effect on the plasma membrane, interfering with exocytosis, or to an effect on microtubule assembly. ARREAZE-PLAZA et al. (1976) also showed that colchicine in rats interfered with the intracellular phase of fat absorption, with a rise in intestinal fat content and inhibition of release of absorbed fat to the chyle.

In the human, colchicine overdoses, whether therapeutic (STENNERMAN and HAY-ASHI, 1971) or suicidal (GAULTIER et al., 1969) have been associated with more severe and more general toxic manifestations. The gastrointestinal side effects described above may lead to a classical cholera-like syndrome, with profound dehydration, hypokalemia, hyponatremia, metabolic acidosis, renal shutdown, and death. Shock may occur, secondary to the profound dehydration or to septicemia associated with severe intestinal wall damage. Death can occur with any overdose but is invariable after the ingestion of more than 40 mg (GAULTIER et al., 1969). The smallest dose recorded as fatal was 7 mg given over a 4-day period (McLEOD and PHILLIPS, 1947). Another patient, with inoperable cancer, died after 12 mg in 4 days (BROWN and SEED, 1945). The risk of colchicine toxicity is greater in patients with chronic renal or chronic hepatic disease (WALLACE et al., 1970).

Earliest hematologic manifestation of colchicine toxicity is disseminated intra-vascular coagulation; maximal abnormalities occurred about 25 h after suicidal ingestion of a large, single dose (CRABIE et al., 1970). A rise in leukocyte count was often seen early. Marrow failure, characterized usually by leukopenia and by throm-bocytopenia and bleeding, occurred later, reaching its peak at about the fifth day (GAULTIER et al., 1969).

A new hematologic manifestation has recently been reported; large, dark staining (on Wright-Giemsa stain) single inclusions in 7–15% of the neutrophils in an 18-year old poisoned with colchicine. There was vacuolization in the cytoplasm and nuclei of the cells (POWELL and WOLF, 1976).

Other toxic manifestations of colchicine overdose include hepatocellular failure (BRUNS, 1968; GAULTIER et al., 1969), late central nervous system dysfunction, in-cluding convulsive seizures and loss of deep tendon reflexes (CARR, 1965; BRUNS, 1968; GAULTIER et al., 1969), myopathy (KONTOS, 1962), hypocalcemia (ELLWOOD and ROBB, 1971; HEATH et al., 1972; POWELL and WOLF, 1976), alopecia and stomati-tis (BRUNS, 1968; POWELL and WOLF, 1976), and porphyria cutanea tarda (KUOKKA-NEN, 1971).

Prophylactic therapy with colchicine has been associated with rare gonadal side effects. One man developed azospermia while receiving 0.6 mg twice daily; his sperm count was normal on 0.6 mg once a day (MERLIN, 1972). Colchicine was given to men in doses of 1.8–2.4 mg/day for up to 6 months without producing any effects on sperm count, luteinizing hormone, follicle-stimulating hormone, or testosterone lev-els (BREMNER and PAULSEN, 1976). Ovulation was not affected in women receiving 1.2 mg colchicine daily (BOARD, 1964).

YÜ and GUTMAN (1961) studied 34 male patients in whom colchicine prophylaxis began before age 40. All the children born to these fathers both before and after taking colchicine were normal and healthy. However, two reports (CESTARI et al., 1965; FERREIRA and BUONICONTI, 1968) described the birth of children with Down's syndrome, whose fathers had been receiving colchicine prophylaxis at the time of conception. Others, summarized in WALLACE and ERTEL (1969), suggested that the

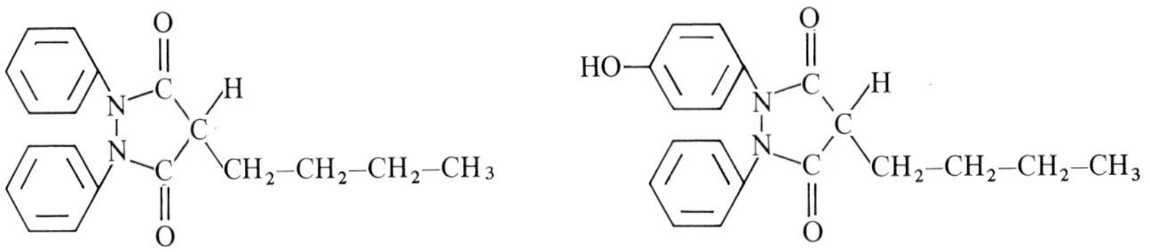

Fig. 5. Phenylbutazone and oxyphenbutazone

greater age of the gouty patients and their wives, and perhaps the genetic makeup of the gouty individual, was more likely than the drug to explain the seeming relationship.

Treatment of colchicine toxicity is symptomatic. If the patient is seen soon enough after ingestion, gastric lavage might be of value. Otherwise, treatment is directed at correcting the dehydration, electrolyte imbalance, metabolic acidosis and shock, and supporting the patient during intravascular coagulation and marrow hypofunction. Attempts at hemodialysis and exchange transfusion have failed (ELLWOOD and ROBB, 1971), which is not surprising, since so little of the toxic material remains in the blood (WALLACE et al., 1970; ERTEL et al., 1976).

C. Phenylbutazone and Oxyphenbutazone

I. Structure and Function

Phenylbutazone is a pyrazolone derivative, 3–5-dioxy-1,2-diphenyl-4-n-butylpyrazolidine (Fig. 5) and has antiinflammatory and uricosuric activity. Two metabolites were found in the urine, oxyphenbutazone (Fig. 5), where one of the benzene rings is hydroxylated in the para position, and a second metabolite, in which a hydroxyl group has been introduced in the 3 position of the butyl side chain (BURNS et al., 1955). The two metabolites have split the two major effects of the parent compound; oxyphenbutazone is antiinflammatory but not uricosuric, while the second metabolite is uricosuric but not significantly antiinflammatory (YÜ et al., 1958).

II. Metabolism

The initial studies on phenylbutazone metabolism (BURNS et al., 1953) demonstrated that peak plasma phenylbutazone levels after single oral doses of 800 mg were reached within 2 h. Phenylbutazone was 98% bound to albumin in the serum at therapeutic concentrations; only the free drug was available for metabolic transformation and for therapeutic or toxic effects. Disappearance from plasma was slow, averaging 21%/day. Almost no phenylbutazone appeared in the urine and less than 5% of the drug appeared in the feces.

Increases in doses over 800 mg did not lead to further rises in plasma levels; daily doses of 400–600 mg produced plasma levels only slightly lower than at 800 mg (BURNS et al., 1953). Plasma levels of 20–40 µg/ml were found as long as 7 days after therapy was discontinued (SOLBERG, 1975). Maximal plasma concentrations ranged around 100 µg/ml (BRODIE, 1965). The mean half-life of phenylbutazone was 3.16 ± 0.19 days (ALVARES et al., 1975).

More recent studies of phenylbutazone metabolism have been performed with the drug labeled with ^{14}C (DIETERLE et al., 1976). After a single oral dose, absorption from the gastrointestinal tract was rapid and complete. Excretion was slow; 21 days after the single dose, only 88% had been recovered, 61% from urine and 27% from feces. The fecal elimination probably represented intestinal secretion, because excretion by this route was slow. Peak plasma concentration occurred at 3 h, with slow decay of the curve between 7 and 336 h and a half-life of 88 h (3.66 days, not remarkably different from the results cited above).

Phenylbutazone is metabolized by hepatic microsomal hydroxylase enzymes. The drug acts as an enzyme inducer, accelerating its own metabolism. The limiting plasma level is about 100 µg/ml (BRODIE, 1965). With higher plasma levels, less phenylbutazone is protein bound, more is free, and more is metabolized in the liver.

Large individual differences in plasma half-lives of phenylbutazone and oxyphenbutazone have been shown (DAVIES and THORGEIRSSON, 1971), due at least in part to differences in liver enzyme activity on the drugs. These differences among individuals are genetically controlled; monozygotic twins had very similar phenylbutazone half-lives, while significantly greater differences occurred in dizygotic twins (VESELL and PAGE, 1968).

DIETERLE et al. (1976) noted three different pathways of formation of phenylbutazone metabolites—oxidation to oxyphenbutazone, γ hydroxyphenylbutazone, and ϱ, γ dihydroxyphenylbutazone; O glucuronidation of these three primary metabolites; and C^1 glucuronidation of phenylbutazone itself. C^1 glucuronidation is a novel form of drug metabolism (RICHTER et al., 1975). Phenylbutazone glucuronides were conjugates in which $C(1^1)$ of the glucuronic acid ligand was directly attached to $C(4)$ of the pyrazolidine ring (RICHTER et al., 1975). One percent of an administered dose was excreted as unchanged drug; more than 50% of the dose excreted in the urine was as C glucuronide (DIETERLE et al., 1976).

VAN PETTEN et al. (1971) compared different brands of phenylbutazone after oral administration and noted wide variability in absorption. Peak blood levels after a 200 mg dose varied between 12 and 50 µg/ml, and times necessary to reach mean peak blood levels ranged from 2.4 to 8.4 h.

Phenylbutazone metabolism has been studied in patients with chronic liver disease, with differing results. Earlier studies (BURNS et al., 1953; WEINER et al., 1954) found that disappearance curves and half-lives were not altered by liver disease. More recent investigators disagreed. LEVI et al. (1968) found that the half-life of phenylbutazone was prolonged in patients with chronic liver disease, while HVIDBERG et al. (1974) found that the plasma phenylbutazone half-life in cirrhotics correlated with the galactose elimination capacity, a liver-function test.

Phenylbutazone metabolism in the rat with adjuvant-induced arthritis was studied (PERREY et al., 1976). During the acute phase of the arthritis, there was a marked reduction in the elimination rate of phenylbutazone and a significant increase in the volume of distribution. The former was due to reduced hepatic biotransformation; the latter was attributed to the decrease in serum albumin and consequent reduced plasma binding capacity. With the chronic phase of arthritis, metabolism became normal. A study of phenylbutazone metabolism in the patient with acute gout might be of interest.

Phenylbutazone and oxyphenbutazone are prime examples of the problems physicians face in considering pharmacokinetic drug interactions. Drug absorption of phenylbutazone, at least in the rat, can be reduced by the tricyclic antidepressants imipramine and desimipramine, presumably because the latter drugs have atropine-like activity, slowing gastric emptying, and leading to delayed small intestinal absorption (PRESCOTT, 1969). It is possible that any drug capable of delaying gastric emptying would produce similar results.

Of greater clinical significance, a number of acidic drugs compete for the same albumin binding sites with phenylbutazone and oxyphenbutazone (SOLOMON et al., 1968). One acidic drug may be displaced from albumin by another, increasing, at least temporarily, the concentration of the free first drug. Such highly bound drugs include phenylbutazone, oxyphenbutazone, warfarin, bishydroxycoumarin, ethylbis-coumacetate, tolbutamide, and other sulfonureas, and the sulfonamides. Phenylbutazone and oxyphenbutazone can potentiate the effects of these drugs. The margin between the therapeutic and the toxic potentials of unbound drug in the tissues may be very small.

Albumin binding competition between phenylbutazone and other drugs has been studied most intensively with warfarin (SOLOMON and SCHROGIE, 1967; SOLOMON et al., 1968; SCHARY et al., 1975). Warfarin is 97% bound to albumin; bishydroxycoumarin is 99% bound. Warfarin and phenylbutazone share a common albumin receptor site. A 10-fold increase in free warfarin resulted after phenylbutazone in an in vitro study simulating in vivo situations (SOLOMON and SCHROGIE, 1967). Long-term, multiple-dose phenylbutazone caused a rise in unbound warfarin, leading to a significantly increased effect (SCHARY et al., 1975). Warfarin has been shown to exist as a racemic mixture of equal parts of two isomeric forms, R- and S-warfarin (LEWIS et al., 1974). The S form was five times more potent as an anticoagulant than the R form; phenylbutazone interfered with S-isomer metabolism. The effect on albumin binding was minor; the most significant effect in this study was on hepatic microsomal metabolism of S-warfarin.

More than 200 drugs, insecticides, herbicides, polycyclic hydrocarbons, dye stuffs, and naturally occurring compounds are known to influence the activity of drug metabolizing enzymes in liver microsomes (CONNEY, 1967; PRESCOTT, 1969). The drugs include, in addition to phenylbutazone and oxyphenbutazone, the barbiturates; the sedatives gluthemide, methylprylone and chloral hydrate; the tranquilizers meprobamate, chlordiazepoxide, and chlorpromazine; the anticonvulsants diphenylhydantoin, methylphenylhydantoin and paramethadione; and tolbutamide (CONNEY, 1967). Phenobarbital has been shown to shorten phenylbutazone half-life by inducing metabolizing enzymes (LEVI et al., 1968). The interrelationships between phenylbutazone and oxyphenbutazone and the large number of other drugs and chemicals that affect hepatic microsomal enzyme activity have not been studied. However, patients with gout are frequently on other medications; the physician treating such patients must be aware of the possible interrelationships among these drugs and must protect the patient against the effects of inadvertent excessive or inadequate drug blood levels.

Drug interference involving phenylbutazone and oxyphenbutazone is possible even at the renal level. Only small amounts of unchanged drug are excreted in the urine (DIETERLE et al., 1976). However, phenylbutazone and oxyphenbutazone are actively secreted in the tubule (GUTMAN et al., 1960). The hypoglycemic effect of

acetohexamide was enhanced by the simultaneous administration of phenylbutazone, apparently due to the inhibition by phenylbutazone of the renal excretion of
hydrohexamide, an active metabolite of acetohexamide. Oxyphenbutazone slowed
the renal excretion of penicillin in man (PRESCOTT, 1969).

III. Clinical Use

Phenylbutazone and oxyphenbutazone are very effective drugs in the treatment of
acute gout—even more effective than colchicine. A response to phenylbutazone or its
analogue has no diagnostic specificity; these agents are equally effective in the treatment of acute pseudogout and are of benefit in many other forms of inflammatory
arthritis. Once the diagnosis of gout is made, especially if i.v. forms of colchicine are
not available, phenylbutazone or oxyphenbutazone is the drug of choice in treating
acute gout in suitable patients.
The optimal dose of either of these two drugs in the treatment of acute gout is about
600 mg/day. Larger doses do not produce very much greater blood levels (BURNS et
al., 1953; BRODIE, 1965). There is no particular advantage in giving large loading
doses; 200 mg three times daily is as effective as other regimens. To combat the acute
attack of gout and to minimize the likelihood of the recurrence of further inflammation on cessation of therapy, 3–5 days of therapy are generally necessary.

MAUER (1955) has summarized the toxic effects of phenylbutazone, reviewing
nearly 4000 patients. The most frequent side effects were upper gastrointestinal
symptoms, such as nausea, vomiting, and epigastric pain, seen in more than 10% of
patients; edema and cardiac decompensation in 9%; and rashes in 5%. It must be
remembered that his survey was largely of long-term administration of the drug in
rheumatoid arthritis. The serious and/or fatal reactions were agranulocytosis, occurring from day 7 to day 60 of therapy; severe gastrointestinal side effects, with onset
between day 7 and day 34 of therapy; and toxic hepatitis, very infrequent, but
appearing as early as day 3 and with a total dose as low as 1.5 g phenylbutazone.

In the treatment of acute gout, phenylbutazone is customarily given for no longer
than 5 days. The most likely side effect to occur in this brief period is worsening of an
already-present peptic ulcer; gastric or duodenal ulceration is for this reason an
absolute contraindication to phenylbutazone/oxyphenbutazone therapy. Edema and
cardiac decompensation may occur; the risk of giving these drugs to a patient
already in congestive heart failure must be considered. Marrow depression and skin
rashes are very unlikely during short-term treatment. Toxic hepatitis is an idiosyn-
cratic reaction, fortunately very rare.

The problems associated with drug interference between phenylbutazone or oxyphenbutazone and other agents have been discussed above. Close attention must be
paid to this possibility whenever phenylbutazone or oxyphenbutazone are used.

D. Indomethacin

I. Structure

Indomethacin (Fig. 6) is 1-(p-chlorobenzoyl)-5-methoxy-2-methylindol-3-acetic acid.
It is a weak organic acid that was discovered in a search for serotonin-like compounds with antiinflammatory activity (WYNGAARDEN and KELLEY, 1976).

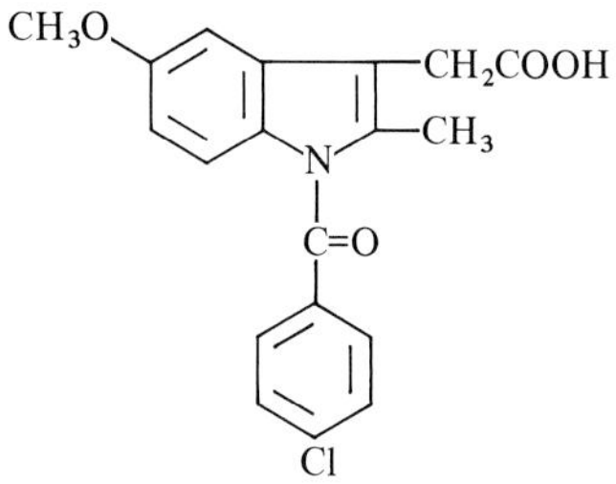

Fig. 6. Indomethacin

II. Metabolism

Initial studies of indomethacin metabolism in man (HUCKER et al., 1966) described rapid absorption, with peak plasma levels at 1 h. In 24 h, 42% of the administered dose was excreted in the urine, with an additional 8% in the next 24 h. In 24 h, 20% of the dose was excreted by way of the feces. In that same period of time, 15% of the administered dose was excreted in the bile, chiefly as the glucuronide (MILLBURN, 1970). Plasma half-life in man was about 2 h.

More recent metabolic studies have adduced new information. Indomethacin undergoes extensive O-demethylation and N-deacylation in man (DUGGAN et al., 1972). Demethylation followed by deacylation constituted the major pathway for catabolism; direct deacylation was a minor pathway. The hepatic microsomal enzymes were involved in demethylation but not in deacylation. There was minimal or no enterohepatic recycling of indomethacin in man. Fecal excretion ranged from 21% to 42% of the administered dose, predominantly of the two demethylated metabolites.

After oral administration of ^{14}C labeled indomethacin (DUGGAN et al., 1972), plasma levels of total radioactivity increased at variable rates to peak between 40 and 180 min. Nearly all the radioactivity represented indomethacin itself at that time. In the first 4 h, indomethacin and its glucuronide were the chief excretory products in urine. After that the demethylated and demethylated deacylated compounds and their glucuronides predominated. The metabolites were all devoid of antiinflammatory effect.

Pharmacokinetics of indomethacin in man is best interpreted according to a two-compartment open model (PALMER et al., 1974; ALVAN et al., 1975). The mean half-life of the initial phase was 0.77 h with a range 0.3–1.2 h. The mean half-life of the terminal phase was 7.2 h, with a range 4.0–11.2 h. This prolonged plasma life fits more closely with indomethacin's known prolonged clinical effect and suggests that a steady state can be achieved on three times daily dosing in many patients. EMORI et al. (1973) also found a prolonged indomethacin half-life both in serum and in synovial fluid. There was no evidence with indomethacin of dose-dependent metabolism, in contrast to phenylbutazone (ALVAN et al., 1975).

Indomethacin is transported in blood 90% bound to plasma proteins, predominantly albumin, over a wide range of concentrations (MASON and McQUEEN, 1974). The binding is primarily to a single site on the albumin molecule, with a strong affinity constant. It has been suggested that indomethacin binding to albumin is most likely through its indole-ring system, since tryptophane and other indole compounds are bound as well (SJÖHALIN and SJÖDIN, 1972). Indomethacin displaces phenylbutazone competitively from binding to albumin, while salicylate, in turn, interferes with indomethacin binding in clinically available concentrations (MASON and MCQUEEN, 1974). In contrast, indomethacin and warfarin failed to interact in any way (VESELL et al., 1975), and other investigators failed to demonstrate any influence of indomethacin or salicylate on each other's metabolism (CHAMPION et al., 1972; LINDQUIST et al., 1974).

Indomethacin is excreted by the kidney by means of tubular secretion. This process may be inhibited by probenecid (SKEITH et al., 1968).

III. Mechanism of Action

There is now a profusion of evidence that indomethacin can inhibit prostaglandin synthetase activity (FERREIRA et al., 1971; VANE, 1971; HAMBERG, 1972; FLOWER, 1974). HAMBERG (1972) used the concentration of the major metabolite of prosta-glandin E_1 and E_2 in the urine of man as an index of whole-body prostaglandin synthesis. Indomethacin in a dose of 50 mg four times daily produced 77–98% inhibition. Return of the metabolite concentration to normal took 24–48 h after stopping the drug.

Inflammatory joint fluids have much higher prostaglandin concentrations than do noninflammatory fluids (ROBINSON and LEVINE, 1974). Treatment of the patient with indomethacin reduced the elevated synovial fluid prostaglandin level to normal.

Many antiinflammatory drugs have been shown to interfere with prostaglandin synthetase activity in vitro (FLOWER, 1974). In order of decreasing potency, such drugs are meclofenamic acid > niflumic acid or indomethacin > mefenemic acid > flu-fenemic acid > naproxen > phenylbutazone > aspirin or ibuprofen. It is clear that in vitro effectiveness in suppressing prostaglandin synthesis bears no direct relationship to the activity of these same drugs in the treatment of acute gout.

Indomethacin has been shown to have other effects that might influence its antiinflammatory function. It inhibited prostaglandin catabolism (PACE-ASCIAK and COLE, 1975) as well as synthesis. It reduced plasma kininogen levels in patients with classical rheumatoid arthritis within 15 min of drug administration (SHARMA et al., 1975). It inhibited leukocyte motility at concentrations as low as 0.01 μM (PHELPS, 1969).

IV. Clinical Use and Toxicity

Indomethacin in large dosage (200 mg or more per day in divided doses for 5–6 days) was as effective in the treatment of acute gout as phenylbutazone (EMMERSON, 1967; SMYTH, 1970). These large doses, however, are likely to produce frequent gastrointes-tinal or central nervous system side effects. Of EMMERSON's 22 patients (1967), 10 had such ill effects. In another study (BOARDMAN and HART, 1967), more than 60% of patients on relatively high doses of indomethacin (a mean of 2.9 mg/kg/day) had side effects, mostly within 48 h of initiating therapy. O'BRIEN (1968) surveyed clinical trials with indomethacin and found that at doses of 150–200 mg/day, 60–70% of patients developed toxic effects.

New and potentially serious side effects of indomethacin have recently been described. Its salt-retaining, edema-producing effect has long been known (O'BRIEN, 1968). A study has shown that patients with normal blood pressure and others with essential hypertension, when treated with indomethacin in doses of 200 mg/day, had a significant increase in mean blood pressure in both groups (PATAK et al., 1975). This was not related to sodium retention, weight gain, or presumably to volume expansion. Indomethacin interfered with the usual side effects of furosemide therapy as well and suppressed renin and aldosterone excretion. Others have shown that indomethacin caused a significant reduction in plasma renin activity within 1 h, even after a single dose of 50 mg (RUMPF et al., 1975; DONKER et al., 1976). This action was not related to natriuresis. The effect was attributed to inhibition of synthesis of renal prostaglandins, causing potentiation of endogenous angiotensin II (DONKER et al., 1976). In the anesthetized dog (FEIGEN et al., 1976), indomethacin decreased renal blood flow, increased aortic pressure and increased calculated renal vascular resistance. Further studies of the effect of indomethacin on the kidney and on blood pressure under clinical circumstances are necessary, especially since hypertension and renal disease are so frequent in gout (WALLACE, 1975 b).

E. Naproxen

I. Chemical Structure

Naproxen is related to the arylacetic acid class of drugs and has the formula d-2-(6^1-methoxy-2^1-naphthyl) propionic acid. The d isomer possess the antiinflammatory properties of the drug, while the l isomer is inactive. Only the d form of naproxen is included in the final therapeutic formulation (HARRISON et al., 1970).

II. Metabolism

Naproxen was rapidly and completely absorbed from the gastrointestinal tract in man. Peak plasma levels were reached 2 h after a single dose (DESAGER et al., 1976); a steady state was achieved after four or five doses (RUNKEL et al., 1973; SEGRE, 1975). The drug is acidic and highly bound (99%) to albumin. With doses over 500 mg twice daily, albumin transport capacity was exceeded, and there followed a transiently higher plasma level and increased metabolism and renal clearance. This accelerated renal clearance limited naproxen levels in man (RUNKEL et al., 1973; SEGRE, 1975).

Naproxen had a small volume of distribution, approximately twice plasma volume. It also had a relatively long half-life in man, with a mean of 13 h (SEGRE, 1975). Naproxen was present in the blood only as the unchanged drug. Excretion was almost totally in the urine, as the glucuronide, as the demethylated (at the 6 methyl position) drug and as the glucuronide of the latter. Less than 10% of the administered dose appeared in the urine as unchanged naproxen (RUNKEL et al., 1973). None of the metabolites have therapeutic activity.

Bicarbonate increased the rapidity of naproxen absorption, while antacids, such as aluminum hydroxide and magnesium oxide, inhibited absorption (SEGRE, 1975). When naproxen and aspirin were given together, the peak concentration of naproxen was decreased and the time of reaching the peak delayed. There was no reciprocal effect on salicylate concentrations (SEGRE et al., 1974). The presumed mechanism was by competition for albumin binding. There are no reports as yet of drug interactions with warfarin or the sulfonureas.

III. Mechanism of Action

Naproxen is one of the many nonsteroidal antiinflammatory drugs that interfere with the synthesis of prostaglandins (TOMLINSON et al., 1972; FLOWER, 1974). Whether this is its only mechanism is uncertain. It was antiinflammatory in the cotton pellet-induced granuloma system in adrenalectomized rats; it did not have thymolytic activity (ROZKOWSKI et al., 1971).

IV. Clinical Use

The treatment with naproxen of 40 patients with acute gout has been reported (CUQ, 1973; WILLKENS and CASE, 1973; WILLKENS et al., 1976). The doses used were larger in general than those shown to lead to maximal plasma levels (see above); totals ranged from 350 to 1750 mg on day 1. Smaller doses were used in succeeding days.

CUQ (1973) had a 75% success rate in his 20 patients with acute gout; four patients had mild side effects—headache, nausea, abdominal pain. WILLKENS et al. (1976) reported that 15 of his 20 patients showed significant clearing of objective inflammatory changes within 24–48 h of therapy. One patient with cardiovascular disease and borderline cardiac decompensation gained 4 kg during therapy. Another developed bladder atony. One patient had a rebound flare of gouty arthritis.

F. Fenoprofen

I. Chemical Structure

Fenoprofen is another propionic acid analogue, the calcium salt of 2-(3-phenoxy-phenyl) propionic acid.

II. Metabolism

The calcium salt of fenoprofen, given by mouth, was about 80% absorbed. However, there was a lag time of 10–15 min before absorption began, or at least before minimal measurable quantities could be shown in plasma (RUBIN et al., 1974; GRUBER, 1976). The absorption occurred both in the stomach and in the small intestine (RUBIN et al., 1972), and was interfered with by food. Peak plasma levels occurred at 2 h after oral administration. The half-life for disappearance from plasma was about 3 h.

When fenoprofen was administered repeatedly, an equilibrium was rapidly achieved. Accumulation was minimal (GRUBER, 1976). Fenoprofen did not influence its own rate of metabolism, even on repeated administration (RUBIN et al., 1974).

Fenoprofen in plasma was 99% albumin bound. Metabolism was in the liver. 90% of the drug was excreted in the urine, nearly half as hydroxyfenoprofen glucuronide and an equivalent amount as fenoprofen glucuronide. Only 3% of the administered dose was excreted as unchanged fenoprofen (GRUBER, 1976). Renal clearance of the unchanged fenoprofen was about 40 ml/min, suggesting that the drug underwent tubular reabsorption (RUBIN et al., 1972). The metabolites were cleared rapidly without reabsorption.

Salicylate reduced fenoprofen blood levels and led to increased excretion of the hydroxylated form but not to increased total excretion. The precise mechanism of this drug interference was unclear; it apparently did not involve albumin binding (GRUBER, 1976). Phenobarbital also lowered fenoprofen concentrations. Warfarin, indomethacin, phenylbutazone, as well as aspirin did not alter fenoprofen binding to albumin in clinical concentrations (RUBIN et al., 1974).

III. Mechanism of Action

Fenoprofen also has been shown to inhibit prostaglandin synthesis (Ho and EASTER-MAN, 1974). In a group of aspirin-sensitive asthmatics, both fenoprofen and ibuprofen also induced bronchoconstriction, suggesting that this effect is mediated by reduction of prostaglandin levels (SCZEKLIK et al., 1976).

IV. Clinical Use

WALLACE (1975a) administered fenoprofen in doses of 800 mg every 6 h for periods ranging from 3 to 8 days to 10 patients with acute gout. Initial improvement was apparent within 6 h in all patients. Five of the 10 patients had dramatic objective improvement within 48 h, while another two had a good response but less than the above.

In a second report, WANASUKAPUNT et al. (1976) treated 27 patients with acute gout, with a total of 36 joints involved. At 48 h, 14 of the 36 joints had an excellent response, and another 14 had had a good response. Fenoprofen is clearly a moderately effective drug in the treatment of acute gouty arthritis.

References

Agudelo, C. A., Schumacher, H. R.: The synovitis of acute gouty arthritis: a light and electron microscopic study. Hum. Pathol. **4**, 265—279 (1973)

Alvan, G., Orme, M., Bertelsson, L., Ekstrand, R., Palmer, L.: Pharmacokinetics of indomethacin. Clin. Pharmacol. Ther. **18**, 364—373 (1975)

Alvares, A. P., Kapelner, S., Sassa, S., Kappas, A.: Drug metabolism in normal children, lead poisoned children, and normal adults. Clin. Pharmacol. Ther. **17**, 179—186 (1975)

Arreaza-Plaza, C. A., Bosch, V., Otayek, M. A.: Lipid transport across the intestinal epithelial cell: effect of colchicine. Biochim. Biophys. Acta (Amst.) **431**, 297—302 (1976)

Back, A., Walaszek, E. J.: Studies with radioactive colchicine. I. The influence of tumors on the tissue distribution of radioactive colchicine in mice. Cancer Res. **13**, 552—555 (1953)

Back, A., Walaszek, E. J., Uyeki, E.: Distribution of radioactive colchicine in some organs of normal and tumor-bearing mice. Proc. Soc. exp. Biol. (N.Y.) **77**, 667—669 (1951)

Benitez, H. H., Murray, M. R., Chargaff, E.: Antagonism between colchicine and tropolone in rat fibroblast cultures. Experientia (Basel) **9**, 426—427 (1953)

Benitez, H. H., Murray, M. R., Chargaff, E.: Studies of the inhibition of the colchicine effect on mitosis. Ann. N.Y. Acad. Sci. **58**, 1288—1302 (1954)

Berlin, R. D.: Temperature dependence of nucleoside membrane transport in rabbit alveolar macrophages and polymorphonuclear leukocytes. J. biol. Chem. **248**, 4724—4730 (1973)

Board, J. A.: Effects of colchicine on human ovulation. Amer. J. Obstet. Gynec. **89**, 830—831 (1964)

Boardman, P. L., Hart, F. D.: Side effects of indomethacin. Ann. Rheum. Dis. **26**, 127—132 (1967)

Borisy, G. G., Taylor, E. W.: The mechanism of action of colchicine. Binding of colchicine-H^3 to cellular protein. J. Cell Biol. **34**, 525—533 (1967)

Boruchow, I. B.: Bone marrow depression associated with acute colchicine toxicity in the presence of hepatic dysfunction. Cancer **19**, 541—543 (1966)

Boudene, C., Duprey, F., Buohon, C.: Radioimmunoassay of colchicine. Biochem. J. **151**, 413—415 (1975)

Boyland, E., Mawson, E. H.: The conversion of colchicine into colchiceine. Biochem. J. **32**, 1204—1206 (1938)

Bremner, W. J., Paulsen, C. A.: Colchicine and testicular function in man. New Engl. J. Med. **294**, 1384—1385 (1976)

Brodie, B. B.: Displacement of one drug by another from carrier or receptor sites. Proc. roy. Soc. Med. **58**, 946—955 (1965)

Brown, W. O., Seed, L.: Effect of colchicine on human tissues. Amer. J. Clin. Pathol. **15**, 189—195 (1945)

Brues, A. M.: The fate of colchicine in the body. J. clin. Invest. **21**, 646 (1942)

Brues, A. M.: Discussion of a paper by M. Levine. Ann. N. Y. Acad. Sci. **51**, 1406—1408 (1951)

Bruns, B. J.: Colchicine toxicity. Aust. Ann. Med. **17**, 341—344 (1968)

Burns, J. J., Rose, R. K., Chenkin, T., Goldman, A., Schulert, A., Brodie, B. B.: The physiologic disposition of phenylbutazone in man, and a method for its estimation in biologic material. J. Pharmacol. exp. Ther. **109**, 346—357 (1953)

Burns, J. J., Rose, R. K., Goodwin, S., Reichenthal, J., Horning, E. C., Brodie, B. B.: The metabolic fate of phenylbutazone in man. J. Pharmacol. exp. Ther. **113**, 481—489 (1955)

Caner, J. E. Z.: Colchicine inhibition of chemotaxis. Arthr. and Rheum. **8**, 757—761 (1965)

Carr, A. A.: Colchicine toxicity. Arch. intern. Med. **115**, 29—33 (1965)

Cestari, A. N., Botelho Viera Filho, J. P., Yonenaga, Y., Magnelli, N., Imada, J.: A case of human reproductive abnormalities induced by colchicine treatment. Rev. Bras. Biol. **25**, 253—256 (1965)

Champion, G. D., Paulus, H. E., Mongan, E.: The effect of aspirin on serum indomethacin. Clin. Pharmacol. Ther. **13**, 239—244 (1972)

Chang, Y.-H., Gralla, E. J.: Suppression of urate crystal-induced canine joint inflammation by heterologous anti-polymorphonuclear leukocyte serum. Arthr. and Rheum. **11**, 145—150 (1968)

Chang, Y.-H., Malawista, S. E.: Mechanism of action of colchicine IV. Failure of non-leukopenic doses of colchicine to suppress urate crystal-induced canine joint inflammation. Inflammation **1**, 143—150 (1976)

Cohen, M., McNamara, H.: The effect of colchicine on guinea pig intestinal enzyme activity. Amer. J. dig. Dis. **15**, 247—250 (1970)

Conney, A. H.: Pharmacological implications of microsomal enzyme induction. Pharmacol. Rev. **19**, 317—366 (1967)

Cook, J. W., Loudon, J. D.: The tropolones. Quart. Rev. **5**, 99—130 (1951)

Copeman, W. S. C.: A Short History of the Gout and the Rheumatic Diseases. Berkeley-Los Angeles: University of California Press 1964

Crabie, P., Pollet, J., Pebay-Peyroula, F.: Etude de l'hemostase au cours des intoxications aigues par la colchicine. Europ. J. Toxicol. Environ. Hyg. **3**, 373—385 (1970)

Cuq, P.: Experience française du traitement de la crise de goutte aigue par le Naproxen. Scand. J. Rheumatol. Suppl. **2**, 64—68 (1973)

Davies, D. S., Thorgeirsson, S. S.: Individual differences in plasma half-lives of lipid-soluble drugs in man. Acta Pharmacol. Toxicol. (Kbh.) **29**, 181—190 (1971)

Desager, J. P., Vanderbist, M., Harvengt, C.: Naproxen plasma levels in volunteers after single dose administration by oral and rectal routes. J. clin. Pharmacol. **16**, 189—193 (1976)

Dewar, M. J. S.: Structure of colchicine. Nature (Lond.) **155**, 141—142 (1945)

Dieterle, W., Faigle, J. W., Früh, F., Mory, H., Theobald, W., Alt, K. O., Richter, W. J.: Metabolism of phenylbutazone in man. Arzneimittel-Forsch. **26**, 572—577 (1976)

Donker, A. J. M., Arisz, L., Brentjens, J. R. H., Van den Hern, G. K., Hollemans, H. J. G.: Effect of indomethacin on kidney function and plasma renin activity in man. Nephron **17**, 288—290 (1976)

Duggan, D. E., Hogans, A. F., Kwan, K. C., McMahon, F. G.: The metabolism of indomethacin in man. J. Pharmacol. exp. Ther. **181**, 563—575 (1972)

Ehrlich, H. P., Ross, R., Bornstein, P.: Effect of microtubular agents and secretion of collagen, a biochemical and morphological study. J. Cell Biol. **62**, 390—405 (1974)

Eigsti, O. J., Dustin, P., Jr.: Colchicine in Agriculture, Medicine, Biology, and Chemistry. Ames, Iowa: Iowa State College Press 1955

Ellwood, M. G., Robb, G. H.: Self-poisoning with colchicine. Postgrad. med. J. **47**, 129—131 (1971)

Emmerson, B. T.: Regimen of indocin therapy in acute gouty arthritis. Br. Med. J. **1967** II, 272—274

Emori, W., Paulus, H. E., Bluestone, R., Pearson, C. M.: The pharmacokinetics of indomethacin in serum. Clin. Pharmacol. Ther. **14**, 134 (1973)

Ertel, N. H., Mittler, J. C., Akgun, S., Wallace, S. L.: A radioimmunoassay for colchicine in plasma and urine. Science **193**, 233—235 (1976)

Ertel, N. H., Wallace, S. L.: Purification of colchicine, its photoisomers and some congeners by paper and thin-layer chromatography. Biochem. Med. **4**, 181—192 (1970)

Ertel, N. H., Wallace, S. L.: Measurement of colchicine in urine and peripheral leukocytes. Clin. Res. **19**, 348 (1971)

Faloon, W. W.: Drug production of intestinal malabsorption. N.Y. State J. Med. **70**, 2189—2192 (1970)

Faloon, W. W., Webb, D. I., Race, T. F.: Cholesterol lowering effect of colchicine. Ann. intern. Med. **66**, 1058 (1966)

Feigen, L. P., Klainen, E., Chapnick, B. M., Kadowitz, P. J.: The effect of indomethacin on renal function in pentobarbital anesthetized dogs. J. Pharmacol. exp. Ther. **198**, 457—463 (1976)

Ferreira, N. R., Buoniconti, A.: Trisomy after colchicine therapy. Lancet **1968** II, 1304

Ferreira, S. H., Moncada, S., Vane, J. R.: Indomethacin and aspirin abolish prostaglandin release from spleen. Nature (Lond.) [New Biol.] **231**, 237—239 (1971)

Fitzgerald, T. J.: Molecular features of colchicine associated with antimitotic activity and inhibition of tubulin polymerization. Biochem. Pharmacol. **25**, 1383—1387 (1976)

Fitzgerald, T. J., Williams, B., Uyeki, E.: Colchicine on sodium urate-induced paw swelling in mice: structure-activity relationships of colchicine derivatives. Proc. Soc. exp. Biol. (N.Y.) **136**, 115—120 (1971)

Fleischman, W., Price, H. G., Fleischman, S. K.: Fate of intraperitoneally administered colchicine in the golden hamster. Med. Pharmacol. Exp. **12**, 172—176 (1965)

Fleischman, W., Price, H. G., Fleischman, S. K.: Fate of intraperitoneally administered colchicine in the Mongolian gerbil. Med. Pharmacol. Exp. **17**, 323—326 (1967)

Fleischman, W., Price, H. G., Fleischman, S. K.: Pathways of excretion of colchicine in the golden hamster. Pharmacology **1**, 48—52 (1968)

Flower, R. J.: Drugs which inhibit prostaglandin synthesis. Pharmacol. Rev. **26**, 33—67 (1974)

Forbes, E. J.: Colchicine and related compounds part 14. Structure of B- and γ-lumicolchicine. J. chem. Soc. 3864—3870 (1955)

Franke, W. W., Stadler, J., Krein, S.: Autoradiographic localization of colchicine-binding sites. Beitr. Pathol. **146**, 289—291 (1972)

Furcht, L. T., Scott, R. E.: Effect of vinblastine sulfate, colchicine and lumicolchicine on membranous organization of normal and transformed cells. Exp. Cell Res. **96**, 271—282 (1975)

Gaultier, M., Kaufer, A., Bismuth, C., Crabie, P., Fréjaville, J.-P.: Données actuelles sur l'intoxication aigue par la colchicine. Ann. Med. Interne **12** 605—618 (1969)

Glickman, R. M., Perretto, J. L., Kirsch, K.: Intestinal lipoprotein formation: effect of colchicine. Gastroenterology **70**, 347—352 (1976)

Goldfinger, S. E.: Treatment of gout. New Engl. J. Med. **285**, 1303—1306 (1971)

Grewe, R., Wolfe, W.: Umwandlung des Colchizins durch Sonnenlicht. Chem. Ber. **84**, 621—625 (1951)

Gruber, C. M.: Clinical pharmacology of fenoprofen, a review. J. Rheumatol. Suppl. **2**, 8—17 (1976)

Gutman, A. B., Dayton, P. G., Yü, T.-F., Berger, L., Chen, W., Sican, L. E., Burns, J. J.: A study of the inverse relationships between pKa and rate of renal excretion of phenylbutazone analogues in man and dog. Amer. J. Med. **29**, 1017—1033 (1960)

Hamberg, M.: Inhibition of prostaglandin synthesis in man. Biophys. Res. Commun. **49**, 720—726 (1972)

Harrison, I. T., Lewis, B., Nelson, P., Rooks, W., Roszkowski, A., Tomolonis, A., Fried, J. H.: Non-steroidal anti-inflammatory agents. I. 6-substituted 2 naphylacetic acids. J. med. Chem. **13**, 203—205 (1970)

Hartung, E. F.: History of the use of colchicum and related medicaments in gout. Ann. rheum. Dis. **13**, 190—200 (1954)

Hartung, E. F.: Historical considerations. Metabolism **6**, 196—208 (1957)

Heath, D. A., Palmer, J. S., Aurbach, G. D.: The hypocalcemic action of colchicine. Endocrinology **50**, 1589—1593 (1972)

Herbst, J. J., Hurwitz, R., Sunshine, P., Kretschmer, N.: The effect of colchicine on intestinal disaccharides: correlation with biochemical aspects of cellular renewal. J. clin. Invest. **49**, 530—536 (1970)

Hill, F. W. G.: Malabsorption in dogs induced with oral colchicine. Brit. Vet. J. **128**, 372—378 (1972)

Hirsimaki, G., Arstelo, A., Trump, B. F.: Autophagocytosis: in vitro induction by microtubule poisons. Exp. Cell Res. **92**, 11—14 (1975)

Ho, P. P. K., Easterman, M. A.: Fenoprofen inhibition of prostaglandin synthesis. Prostaglandins **6**, 107—113 (1974)

Hucker, H. B., Zacchei, A. G., Cox, S. V., Brodie, D. A., Cantwell, N. H. R.: Studies on the absorption, distribution and excretion of indomethacin in various species. J. Pharmacol. exp. Ther. **153**, 237—249 (1966)

Hunter, A. L., Klaasen, C. D.: Biliary excretion of colchicine. J. Pharmacol. exp. Ther. **192**, 605—617 (1975)

Hvidberg, E. F., Andreasen, P. B., Ranek, L.: Plasma half-life of phenylbutazone in patients with impaired liver function. Clin. Pharmacol. Ther. **15**, 171—177 (1974)

Kantor, T. G., Brown, R.: Test of non-specific anti-inflammatory activity of colchicine. Arthr. and Rheum. **9**, 862 (1966)

Kaplan, H.: Sarcoid arthritis with a response to colchicine. New Engl. J. Med. **263**, 778—781 (1960)

Kaplan, H.: Further experiences with colchicine in the treatment of sarcoid arthritis. New Engl. J. Med. **268**, 761—764 (1963)

Kontos, H. A.: Myopathy associated with chronic colchicine toxicity. New Engl. J. Med. **266**, 38—39 (1962)

Kuokkanen, K.: Porphyria cutanea tarda due to colchicine in a patient with gout. Acta Derm. Venereol. **51**, 318—320 (1971)

Lambert, D. T., Fingerman, M.: Evidence for a non-microtubular effect in pigment granule aggregation in melanophores of the fiddler crab, *Uca pugilator*. Comp. Biochem. Physiol. [C] **53**, 25—28 (1976)

Lettre, H.: Some investigations on cell behavior under various conditions. Cancer Res. **12**, 847—860 (1952)

Lettre, H., Lutze, M.: Beitrag zur Verteilung und Wirkung der Colchizine in Tierkörper. Z. physiol. Chem. **281**, 58—64 (1944)

Levi, A. J., Sherlock, S., Walker, D.: Phenylbutazone metabolism in patients with liver disease in relation to previous drug therapy. Lancet **1968 I**, 1275—1279

Lewis, R. J., Trager, W. F., Chan, K. K., Breckenridge, A., Orme, M., Roland, M., Schary, W.: Warfarin: stereochemical aspects of its metabolism and the interaction with phenylbutazone. J. clin. Invest. **53**, 1607—1617 (1974)

Lindquist, B., Jensen, K. M., Johansson, H., Hansen, T.: Effect of administration of aspirin and indomethacin on serum concentration. Clin. Pharmacol. Ther. **15**, 247—252 (1974)

Linskens, H. F., Wulf, W.: Über die Trennung und Mitosewirkung der Lumicolchicine. Naturwissenschaften **40**, 487—488 (1953)

Lockie, L. M.: A discussion of a therapeutic test and a provocative test in gouty arthritis. Ann. intern. Med. **13**, 755—760 (1939)

Loudon, J. D.: Chemistry of colchicine. In: Colchicine in Agriculture, Medicine, Biology, and Chemistry. Ames, Iowa: Iowa State College Press 1955

Luketic, G. C., Shapiro, M.: Effect of colchicine on xylose absorption in dogs. Clin. Res. **11**, 31 (1964)

McCarty, D. J.: Calcium pyrophosphate crystal deposition disease-1975. Arthr. and Rheum. **19**, 275—285 (1976)

McLeod, J. G., Phillips, L.: Hypersensitivity to colchicine. Ann. rheum. Dis. **6**, 224—229 (1947)

Malawista, S. E.: Colchicine: a common mechanism for its anti-inflammatory and antimitotic effects. Arthr. and Rheum. **11**, 191—197 (1968)

Malawista, S. E.: The action of colchicine in acute gouty arthritis. Arthr. and Rheum. **18**, 835—846 (1975)

Malawista, S. E., Bensch, K. G.: Human polymorphonuclear leukocytes: demonstration of microtubules and effect of colchicine. Science **156**, 521—522 (1967)

Malawista, S. E., Chang, Y.-H., Wilson, L.: Lumicolchicine: lack of anti-inflammatory effect. Arthr. and Rheum. **15**, 641—643 (1972)

Margolis, L.: Colchicine-sensitive microtubules. Int. Rev. Cytol. **34**, 333—361 (1973)

Mason, R. W., McQueen, E. G.: Protein binding of indomethacin: binding of indomethacin to human plasma albumin and its displacement from binding by ibuprofen, phenylbutazone and salicylate in vitro. Pharmacology **12**, 12—19 (1974)

Mauer, E. F.: The toxic effects of phenylbutazone. New Engl. J. Med. **253**, 404—410 (1955)

Merlin, H. E.: Azospermia caused by colchicine. Fertil. Steril. **23**, 180—181 (1972)

Millburn, P.: Factors in the biliary excretion of organic compounds. In: Metabolic Conjugation and Metabolic Hydrolysis, Vol. 2. New York: Academic Press 1970

Mittler, J. C., Ertel, N. H., Akgun, S., Wallace, S. L.: A radioimmunoassay for colchicine in plasma and urine. Clin. Res. **23**, 222 (1975)

Mizel, S. B., Wilson, L.: Nucleoside transport in mammalian cells: inhibition by colchicine. Biochemistry **11**, 2573—2578 (1972)

Myren, J., Luketic, G. C., Ceballos, R., Sachs, G., Hirschowitz, B. I.: Effects of colchicine on intestinal mucosal disaccharidases. Amer. J. Dig. Dis. **11**, 394—403 (1966)

O'Brien, W. M.: Indomethacin: a survey of clinical trials. Clin. Pharmacol. Ther. **9**, 94—107 (1968)

Oliver, J. M., Ukena, T. E., Berlin, R. D.: Effects of phagocytosis and colchicine on the lectin-binding sites on cell surfaces. Proc. nat. Acad. Sci. (Wash.) **71**, 394—398 (1974)

Ortel, R. W., Newcombe, D. S.: Acute gouty arthritis and response to colchicine in the virtual absence of synovial fluid leukocytes. New Engl. J. Med. **290**, 1363—1364 (1974)

Pace-Asciak, C., Cole, S.: Inhibitors of prostaglandin catabolism. Experientia (Basel) **31**, 143—145 (1975)

Padawer, J.: Paramitotic effects of colchicine: further studies of the mast cell assay. Proc. Soc. exp. Biol. (N.Y.) **127**, 194—199 (1968)

Palmer, L., Bertilsson, L., Alvan, G., Orme, M., Sjögvist, F., Holmstedt, B.: Indomethacin: quantative determination in plasma by mass fragmentography, including pilot pharmaco-kinetics in man. In: Prostaglandin Synthetase Inhibitors. New York: Raven Press 1974

Patak, R. V., Mookerjee, B. K., Bentzel, C. J., Hysert, P. E., Babej, M., Lee, J. B.: Antagonism of the effects of furosemide by indomethacin in normal and hypertensive man. Prostaglandins **10**, 649—659 (1975)

Paulus, H. E., Schlosstein, L. H., Godfrey, R. G., Klinenberg, J. R., Bluestone, R.: Prophylactic colchicine therapy of intercritical gout. Arthr. and Rheum. **17**, 609—614 (1974)

Pelletier, P. J., Caventou, J.-B.: Examen chimique de plusiers vegetaux de la famille des colchicées et du principe actif qu'ils renferment. Ann. Chim. Phys. **14**, 69—83 (1820)

Perry, K., Jonen, H. G., Kahl, G. F., Jähnshen, E.: Elimination and distribution of phenylbutazone in rats during the course of adjuvant-induced arthritis. J. Pharmacol. exp. Ther. **197**, 470—477 (1976)

Pesanti, E. L., Axline, S. G.: Colchicine effects on lysosomal enzyme induction and intracellular degradation in the cultivated macrophage. J. exp. Med. **141**, 1030—1046 (1975)

Phelps, P.: Polymorphonuclear leukocyte motility in vitro. II. Stimulatory effect of monosodium urate crystals and urate in solution. Arthr. and Rheum. **12**, 189—196 (1969)

Phelps, P.: Appearance of chemotactic activity following intraarticular injection of monosodium urate crystals: effect of colchicine. J. Lab. clin. Med. **76**, 622—631 (1970a)

Phelps, P.: Polymorphonuclear leukocyte activity in vitro IV. Arthr. and Rheum. **13**, 1—9 (1970b)

Phelps, P., McCarty, D. J.: Crystal-induced inflammation in canine joints. II. Importance of polymorphonuclear leukocytes. J. exp. Med. **124**, 115—126 (1966)

Phelps, P., McCarty, D. J.: Crystal induced arthritis. Postgrad. med. **45**, 87—93 (1969)

Powell, H. C., Wolf, P. L.: Neutrophilic leukocyte inclusions in colchicine intoxication. Arch. Path. Lab. Med. **100**, 136—138 (1976)

Prescott, L. F.: Pharmocokinetic drug interactions. Lancet **1969 II**, 1239—1243

Race, T. F., Paes, I. C., Faloon, W. W.: Intestinal malabsorption induced by oral colchicine. Amer. J. Med. Sci. **259**, 32—41 (1970)

Redman, C. M., Benerjee, D., Howell, K., Palade, G. E.: Colchicine inhibition of plasma protein release from rat hepatocytes. J. Cell Biol. **66**, 42—59 (1975)

Richter, W. J., Alt, K. O., Dieterle, W., Faigle, J. W., Kriemler, H.-P., Mory, H., Winkler, T.: C-glucuronides, a novel type of drug metabolite. Helv. chim. Acta **58**, 2512—2517 (1975)

Robinson, D. R., Levine, L.: Prostaglandin concentrations in synovial fluid in rheumatic diseases: action of indomethacin and aspirin. In: Prostaglandin Synthetase Inhibitors. New York: Raven Press 1974

Roszkowski, A. P., Rooks, W. H., Tomolonis, A. J., Miller, L. M.: Anti-inflammatory and analgetic properties of d-2-(6¹-methoxy-2¹-naphthyl)-propionic acid (naproxen). J. Pharmacol. exp. Ther. **179**, 114—123 (1971)

Rubin, A., Chernish, S. M., Crabtree, R., Gruber, C. M., Helleberg, L., Rodda, B. E., Warrick, P., Wolen, R. L., Ridolfo, A. S.: A profile of the physiologic disposition and gastrointestinal effects of fenoprofen in man. Curr. Med. Res. Opin. **2**, 529—544 (1974)

Rubin, A., Rodda, B. E., Warrick, P., Ridolfo, A. S., Gruber, C. M.: Physiologic disposition of fenoprofen in man. II. Plasma and urine pharmacokinetics after oral and intravenous administration. J. Pharm. Sci. **61**, 739—745 (1972)

Rubulis, A., Rubert, M., Faloon, W. W.: Cholesterol lowering, fecal bile acid and sterol changes during neomycin and colchicine. J. clin. Nutr. **23**, 1251—1259 (1970)

Rumpf, K. W., Frenzel, S., Lowitz, H. D., Scheler, F.: The effect of indomethacin on plasma renin activity in man under normal conditions and after stimulation of the renin-angiotensin system. Prostaglandins **10**, 641—648 (1975)

Runkel, R., Forchielli, E., Boost, G., Chaplin, M., Hill, R., Sevelius, H., Thompson, G., Segre, E.: Naproxen metabolism, excretion and comparative pharmacokinetics. Scand. J. Rheumatol. Suppl. **2**, 29—36 (1973)

Sagorin, C., Ertel, N. H., Wallace, S. L.: Photoisomerization of colchicine. Loss of significant antimitotic activity in tissue culture. Arthr. and Rheum. **15**, 213—217 (1972)

Schary, W. L., Lewis, R. J., Rowland, M.: Warfarin-phenylbutazone interaction in man: a long-term multiple dose study. Res. Commun. Chem. Pathol. Pharmacol. **10**, 663—672 (1975)

Schoenharting, M., Mende, G., Siebert, G.: The metabolic transformation of colchicine. II. The metabolism of colchicine by mammalian liver microsomes. Hoppe-Seylers Z. physiol. Chem. **355**, 1391—1399 (1974)

Schoenharting, M., Pfaender, P., Ricker, A., Siebert, G.: The metabolic transformation of colchicine. I. The oxidative formation of products from colchicine in the Udenfriend system. Hoppe-Seylers Z. physiol. Chem. **354**, 421—436 (1973)

Segre, E. J.: Naproxen metabolism in man. J. Clin. Pharmacol. **15**, 316—323 (1975)

Segre, E. J., Runkel, R., Chaplin, M., Sevelius, H., Forchielli, E.: Naproxen-aspirin interactions in man. Clin. Pharmacol. Ther. **15**, 374—379 (1974)

Sharma, J. N., Zeitlin, I. J., Brooks, P. M., Dick, W. C.: Raised plasma kininogen levels in rheumatoid arthritis. Response to indomethacin and relationship to clinical indices. Ann. rheum. Dis. **34**, 464 (1975)

Sjöhalin, I. S., Sjödin, T.: Binding of drugs to human serum albumin. Biochem. Pharmacol. **21**, 3041—3052 (1972)

Skeith, M. D., Simkin, P. A., Healey, L. A.: The renal excretion of indomethacin and its inhibition by probenecid. Clin. Pharmacol. Ther. **9**, 89—93 (1968)

Smyth, C. J.: Indomethacin—its rightful place in treatment. Ann. intern. Med. **72**, 430—432 (1970)

Smyth, C. J., Frank, L. S.: Treatment of acute gouty arthritis. Rheumatism. **18**, 2—8 (1962)

Solberg, C. O.: Influence of therapeutic concentrations of phenylbutazone on granulocyte function. Acta path. microbiol. scand. **B 83**, 100—104 (1975)

Solomon, H. M., Schrogie, J. J.: The effect of various drugs on the binding of warfarin-C[14] to human albumin. Biochem. Pharmacol. **16**, 1219—1226 (1967)

Solomon, H. M., Schrogie, J. J., Williams, D.: The displacement of phenybutazone-^{14}C and warfarin-^{14}C from human albumin by various drugs and fatty acids. Biochem. Pharmacol. **17**, 143—151 (1968)

Spilberg, I., Mandell, B., Wochner, R. D.: Studies in crystal induced chemotactic factor. J. Lab. clin. Med. **83**, 56—63 (1974)

Stadler, J., Franke, W. W.: Colchicine-binding proteins in chromatin and membranes. Nature (Lond.) New Biol. **237**, 237—238 (1972)

Stadler, J., Franke, W. W.: Characterization of the colchicine binding of membrane fractions from rat and mouse liver. J. Cell Biol. **60**, 297—303 (1974)

Stennerman, G. N., Hayashi, T.: Colchicine intoxication: a reappraisal of its pathology based on a study of three fatal cases. Hum. Pathol. **2**, 321—332 (1971)

Sczeklik, A., Gryglewski, R. J., Czerndawski-Mysik, G., Zmuda, A.: Aspirin-induced asthma. Hypersensitivity to fenoprofen and ibuprofen in relation to their inhibitory action on prostaglandin generation. J. Allergy Clin. Immunol. **58**, 10—18 (1976)

Thompson, G. R., Ting, Y. M., Riggs, G. A.: Calcific tendonitis and soft tissue calcification resembling gout. J. Amer. med. Ass. **203**, 464—472 (1968)

Tomlinson, R. V., Ringold, H., Quereshi, M. C., Forchielli, E.: Relationship between inhibition of prostaglandin synthesis and drug efficacy. Biochim. Biophys. Res. Commun. **45**, 552—559 (1972)

Ukena, T. D., Berlin, R. D.: Effect of colchicine and vinblastine on the topographical separation of membrane functions. J. exp. Med. **136**, 1—7 (1972)

Vane, J. R.: Inhibition of prostaglandin synthesis as a mechanism of action for aspirin-like drugs. Nature (Lond.) New Biol. **231**, 232—235 (1971)

Van Petten, A. R., Feng, H., Withey, R. J., Littau, H. F.: The physiologic availability of solid dosage forms of phenylbutazone. J. Clin. Pharmacol. **11**, 177—186 (1971)

Vesell, E. S., Page, J. G.: Genetic control of drug levels in man: phenylbutazone. Science **159**, 1479—1480 (1968)

Vesell, E. S., Passananti, G. T., Johnson, A. O.: Failure of indomethacin and warfarin to interact in normal human volunteers. J. Clin. Pharmacol. **15**, 486—495 (1975)

Walaszek, E. J., Kelsey, F. E., Geiling, E. M. K.: Biosynthesis and isolation of radioactive colchicine. Science **116**, 225—227 (1952)

Walaszek, E. J., Kocsis, J. J.: Excretion of ^{14}C labelled colchicine. Fed. Proc. **15**, 495 (1956)

Walaszek, E. J., Kocsis, J. J., Le Roy, G. V., Geiling, E. M. K.: Studies on the excretion of radioactive colchicine. Arch. int. Pharmacodyn. Ther. **125**, 371—382 (1960)

Walaszek, E. J., Le Roy, G. V., Geiling, E. M. K.: Renal excretion of radioactive colchicine in patients with and without neoplastic disease. Fed. Proc. **13**, 413 (1954)

Waldi, D., Schnackerz, K., Munter, F.: Eine systematische Analyse von Alkaloiden auf Dünnschichtplatten. J. Chromatog. **6**, 61—73 (1961)

Wallace, S. L.: Colchicine analogues in the treatment of acute gout. Arthr. and Rheum. **2**, 389—395 (1959)

Wallace, S. L.: Colchicine: clinical pharmacology in acute gouty arthritis. Amer. J. Med. **30**, 439—448 (1961)

Wallace, S. L.: Mechanism of action of colchicine. Arthr. and Rheum. **8**, 744—748 (1965)

Wallace, S. L.: The treatment of gout. Arthr. and Rheum. **15**, 317—323 (1972)

Wallace, S. L.: Colchicum. The panacea. Bull. N.Y. Acad. Med. **40**, 130—135 (1973)

Wallace, S. L.: Colchicine. Semin. Arthr. and Rheum. **3**, 369—381 (1974)

Wallace, S. L.: Colchicine and new anti-inflammatory drugs in the treatment of acute gout. Arthr. and Rheum. **18**, 847—850 (1975a)

Wallace, S. L.: Gout and hypertension. Arthr. and Rheum. **18**, 721—725 (1975b)

Wallace, S. L., Bernstein, D., Diamond, H.: Diagnostic value of the colchicine therapeutic trial. J. Amer. med. Ass. **199**, 525—528 (1967)

Wallace, S. L., Ertel, N. H.: Colchicine: current problems. Bull. rheum. Dis. **20**, 582—587 (1969)

Wallace, S. L., Ertel, N. H.: Plasma levels of colchicine after oral administration of a single dose. Metabolism **22**, 749—753 (1973)

Wallace, S. L., Omokoku, B., Ertel, N. H.: Colchicine plasma levels. Implications as to pharmacology and mechanism of action. Amer. J. Med. **48**, 443—448 (1970)

Wanasukapunt, S., Lertratanakul, Y., Rubenstein, H. M.: Effect of fenoprofen calcium on acute gouty arthritis. Arthr. and Rheum. **19**, 933—935 (1976)

Webb, D. I., Chodos, R. B., Maher, C. Q., Faloon, W. W.: Mechanism of vitamin B 12 malabsorption in patients receiving colchicine. New Engl. J. Med. **279**, 845—850 (1968)

Weiner, M., Chenkin, T., Burns, J. J.: Observations on the metabolic transformation and effects of phenylbutazone in subjects with hepatic disease. Amer. J. Med. Sci. **228**, 36—39 (1954)

Wildman, W. C., Pursey, B. A.: Colchicine and related compounds. In: The Alkaloids, Vol. II. New York: Academic Press 1968

Willkens, R. F., Case, J. B.: Treatment of acute gout with naproxen. Scand. J. Rheumatol. Suppl. **2**, 69—71 (1973)

Willkens, R. F., Case, J. B., Huix, F. J.: The treatment of acute gout with naproxen. J. clin. Pharmacol. **15**, 363—366 (1976)

Wilson, J., Bryan, J.: Biochemical and pharmacologic properties of microtubules. In: Advances in Cell and Molecular Biology. New York: Academic Press 1974

Wilson, L., Friedkin, M.: The biochemical events of mitosis. I. Synthesis and properties of colchicine labelled with tritium in its acetyl moiety. Biochemistry **5**, 2463—2468 (1966)

Wilson, L., Friedkin, M.: The biochemical events of mitosis. II. The in vivo and in vitro binding of colchicine in grasshopper embryos and its possible relation to the inhibition of mitosis. Biochemistry **6**, 3126—3135 (1967)

Woodward, R. B.: A total synthesis of colchicine. In: The Harvey Lectures, Series 59. New York-London: Academic Press 1967

Wunderlich, F., Müller, R., Speth, V.: Direct evidence for a colchicine-induced impairment in the mobility of membrane components. Science **182**, 1136—1138 (1973)

Wyngaarden, J. B., Kelley, W. N.: Gout and Hyperuricemia. New York: Grune and Stratton 1976

Yü, T.-F., Burns, J. J., Paton, B. C., Gutman, A. B., Brodie, B. B.: Phenylbutazone metabolites; antirheumatic, sodium-retaining, and uricosuric effects in man. J. Pharmacol. exp. Ther. **123**, 63—69 (1958)

Yü, T.-F., Gutman, A. B.: Efficacy of colchicine prophylaxis. Ann. intern. Med. **55**, 179—192 (1961)

Zweig, M. H., Maling, H. M., Webster, M. E.: Inhibition of sodium urate rat hind paw edema by colchicine derivatives. Correlation with antimitotic activity. J. Pharmacol. exp. Ther. **182**, 344—350 (1972)

Author Index

Page numbers in *italics* indicate References

Subject Index

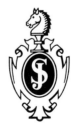

Springer-Verlag
Berlin
Heidelberg
New York

Handbook of Experimental Pharmacology

Continuation of "Handbuch der experimentellen Pharmakologie"

Heffter-Heubner, New Series

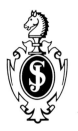

Springer-Verlag
Berlin
Heidelberg
New York